Surgical Critical Care and Emergency Surgery:
Clinical Questions and Answers

# Surgical Critical Care and Emergency Surgery

Clinical Questions and Answers

Second Edition

*Edited by*

**Forrest "Dell" Moore, MD, FACS**
*Vice Chief of Surgery*
*Associate Trauma Medical Director*
*John Peter Smith Health Network/Acclaim Physician Group*
*Fort Worth, TX, USA*

**Peter Rhee, MD, MPH, FACS, FCCM, DMCC**
*Professor of Surgery at USUHS, Emory, and Morehouse*
*Chief of Surgery and Senior Vice President of Grady*
*Atlanta, GA, USA*

**Gerard J. Fulda, MD, FACS, FCCM**
*Associate Professor, Department of Surgery*
*Jefferson Medical College, Philadelphia, PA*
*Chairman Department of Surgery*
*Physician Leader Surgical Service Line*
*Christiana Care Health Systems, Newark, DE, USA*

**WILEY** Blackwell

This second edition first published 2018
© 2018 by John Wiley & Sons Ltd

*Edition History*
John Wiley & Sons Ltd (1e, 2012)

*Registered Office(s)*
John Wiley & Sons, Inc., 111 River Street, Hoboken, NJ 07030, USA
John Wiley & Sons Ltd, The Atrium, Southern Gate, Chichester, West Sussex, PO19 8SQ, UK

*Editorial Office*
9600 Garsington Road, Oxford, OX4 2DQ, UK

For details of our global editorial offices, customer services, and more information about Wiley products visit us at www.wiley.com.

Wiley also publishes its books in a variety of electronic formats and by print-on-demand. Some content that appears in standard print versions of this book may not be available in other formats.

*Library of Congress Cataloging-in-Publication Data*

Names: Moore, Forrest "Dell", editor. | Rhee, Peter, 1961– editor. | Fulda, Gerard J., editor.
Title: Surgical critical care and emergency surgery : clinical questions and answers / edited by
    Forrest "Dell" Moore, Peter Rhee, Gerard J. Fulda.
Description: 2e. | Hoboken, NJ : Wiley, 2017. | Includes bibliographical references and index. |
Identifiers: LCCN 2017054466 (print) | LCCN 2017054742 (ebook) | ISBN 9781119317982 (pdf) | ISBN 9781119317951 (epub) |
    ISBN 9781119317920 (pbk.)
Subjects: | MESH: Critical Care–methods | Surgical Procedures, Operative–methods | Wounds and Injuries–surgery |
    Emergencies | Critical Illness–therapy | Emergency Treatment–methods | Examination Questions
Classification: LCC RD93 (ebook) | LCC RD93 (print) | NLM WO 18.2 | DDC 617/.026–dc23
LC record available at https://lccn.loc.gov/2017054466

Cover Design: Wiley
Cover Images: (Background) © Paulo Gomez/Hemera/Gettyimages;
(Inset image) © jacoblund/Gettyimages

Set in 10/12pt Warnock by SPi Global, Pondicherry, India

Printed and bound by CPI Group (UK) Ltd, Croydon, CR0 4YY

10  9  8  7  6  5  4  3  2  1

**Part One**

**Surgical Critical Care**

# 1

# Respiratory and Cardiovascular Physiology

*Marcin Jankowski, DO and Frederick Giberson, MD*

1 *All of the following are mechanisms by which vasodilators improve cardiac function in acute decompensated left heart failure except:*
   A *Increase stroke volume*
   B *Decrease ventricular filling pressure*
   C *Increase ventricular preload*
   D *Decrease end-diastolic volume*
   E *Decrease ventricular afterload*

Most patients with acute heart failure present with increased left-ventricular filling pressure, high systemic vascular resistance, high or normal blood pressure, and low cardiac output. These physiologic changes increase myocardial oxygen demand and decrease the pressure gradient for myocardial perfusion resulting in ischemia. Therapy with vasodilators in the acute setting can often improve hemodynamics and symptoms.

Nitroglycerine is a powerful venodilator with mild vasodilatory effects. It relieves pulmonary congestion through direct venodilation, reducing left and right ventricular filling pressures, systemic vascular resistance, wall stress, and myocardial oxygen consumption. Cardiac output usually increases due to decreased LV wall stress, decreased afterload, and improvement in myocardial ischemia. The development of "tachyphylaxis" or tolerance within 16–24 hours of starting the infusion is a potential drawback of nitroglycerine.

Nitroprusside is an equal arteriolar and venous tone reducer, lowering both systemic and vascular resistance and left and right filling pressures. Its effects on reducing afterload increase stroke volume in heart failure. Potential complications of nitroprusside include cyanide toxicity and the risk of "coronary steal syndrome."

In patients with acute heart failure, therapeutic reduction of left-ventricular filling pressure with any of the above agents correlates with improved outcome.

Increased ventricular preload would increase the filling pressure, causing further increases in wall stress and myocardial oxygen consumption, leading to ischemia.

**Answer: C**

Marino, P. (2014) *The ICU Book*, 4th edn, Lippincott Williams & Wilkins, Philadelphia, PA, chapter 13.
Mehra, M.R. (2015) Heart failure: management, in *Harrison's Principles of Internal Medicine*, 19th edn (eds D. Kasper, A. Fauci, S. Hauser, *et al.*), McGraw-Hill, New York.

2 *Which factor is most influential in optimizing the rate of volume resuscitation through venous access catheters?*
   A *Laminar flow*
   B *Length*
   C *Viscosity*
   D *Radius*
   E *Pressure gradient*

The forces that determine flow are derived from observations on ideal hydraulic circuits that are rigid and the flow is steady and laminar. The Hagen-Poiseuille equation states that flow is determined by the fourth power of the inner radius of the tube ($Q = \Delta p \pi r^4 / 8\mu L$), where P is pressure, $\mu$ is viscosity, L is length, and r is radius. This means that a two-fold increase in the radius of a catheter will result in a sixteen-fold increase in flow. As the equation states, the remaining components of resistance, such as pressure difference along the length of the tube and fluid viscosity, are inversely related and exert a much smaller influence on flow. Therefore, cannulation of large central veins with long catheters are much less effective than cannulation of peripheral veins with a short catheter. This illustrates that it is the size of the catheter and not the vein that determines the rate of volume infusion (see Figure 1.1).

**Answer: D**

Marino, P. (2014) *The ICU Book*, 4th edn, Lippincott Williams & Wilkins, Philadelphia, PA, chapter 12.

*Surgical Critical Care and Emergency Surgery: Clinical Questions and Answers*, Second Edition.
Edited by Forrest "Dell" Moore, Peter Rhee, and Gerard J. Fulda.
© 2018 John Wiley & Sons Ltd. Published 2018 by John Wiley & Sons Ltd.
Companion website: www.wiley.com/go/moore/surgical_criticalcare_and_emergency_surgery

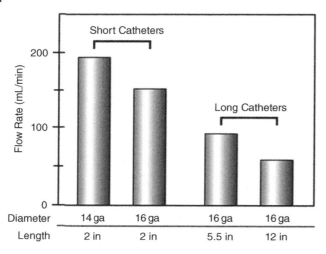

**Figure 1.1** The influence of catheter dimensions on the gravity-driven infusion of water.

**3** *Choose the correct physiologic process represented by each of the cardiac pressure-volume loops in Figure 1.2.*
   **A** 1) *Increased preload, increased stroke volume,*
      2) *Increased afterload, decreased stroke volume*
   **B** 1) *Decreased preload, increased stroke volume,*
      2) *Decreased afterload, increased stroke volume*
   **C** 1) *Increased preload, decreased stroke volume,*
      2) *Decreased afterload, increased stroke volume*
   **D** 1) *Decreased preload, decreased stroke volume,*
      2) *Increased afterload, decreased stroke volume*
   **E** 1) *Decreased preload, increased stroke volume,*
      2) *Increased afterload, decreased stroke volume*

One of the most important factors in determining stroke volume is the extent of cardiac filling during diastole or the end-diastolic volume. This concept is known as the Frank–Starling law of the heart. This law states that, with all other factors equal, the stroke volume will increase as the end-diastolic volume increases. In Figure 1.2A, the ventricular preload or end-diastolic volume (LV volume) is increased, which ultimately increases stroke volume defined by the area under the curve. Notice the LV pressure is not affected. Increased afterload, at constant preload, will have a negative impact on stroke volume. In Figure 1.2B, the ventricular afterload (LV pressure) is increased, which results in a decreased stroke volume, again defined by the area under the curve.

**Answer: A**

Mohrman, D. and Heller, L. (2014) *Cardiovascular Physiology*, 8th edn, McGraw-Hill, New York, chapter 3.

**4** *A 68-year-old patient is admitted to the SICU following a prolonged exploratory laparotomy and extensive lysis of adhesions for a small bowel obstruction. The patient is currently tachycardic and hypotensive. Identify the most effective way of promoting end-organ perfusion in this patient.*
   **A** *Increase arterial pressure (total peripheral resistance) with vasoactive agents*
   **B** *Decrease sympathetic drive with heavy sedation*
   **C** *Increase end-diastolic volume with controlled volume resuscitation*
   **D** *Increase contractility with a positive inotropic agent*
   **E** *Increase end-systolic volume*

This patient is presumed to be in hypovolemic shock as a result of a prolonged operative procedure with inadequate perioperative fluid resuscitation. The insensible losses of an open abdomen for several hours in addition to significant fluid shifts due to the small bowel obstruction can significantly lower intravascular volume. The low urine output is another clue that this patient would benefit from controlled volume resuscitation.

(A)

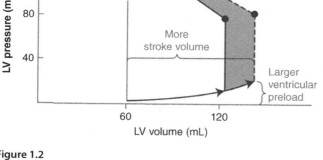

(B)

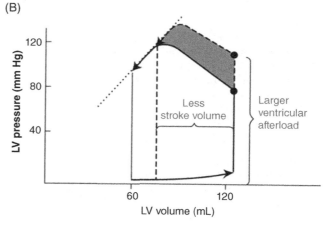

**Figure 1.2**

Starting a vasopressor such as norepinephrine would increase the blood pressure but the effects of increased afterload on the heart and the peripheral vasoconstriction leading to ischemia would be detrimental in this patient. Lowering the sympathetic drive with increased sedation will lead to severe hypotension and worsening shock. Increasing contractility with an inotrope in a hypovolemic patient would add great stress to the heart and still provide inadequate perfusion as a result of low preload. An increase in end-systolic volume would indicate a decreased stroke volume and lower cardiac output and would not promote end-organ perfusion.

$$CO = HR \times SV$$
$$SV = EDV - ESV$$

According to the principle of continuity, the stroke output of the heart is the main determinant of circulatory blood flow. The forces that directly affect the flow are preload, afterload and contractility. According to the Frank–Starling principle, in the normal heart diastolic volume is the principal force that governs the strength of ventricular contraction. This promotes adequate cardiac output and good end-organ perfusion.

**Answer: C**

Levick, J.R. (2013) *An Introduction to Cardiovascular Physiology*, Butterworth and Co. London.

5 *Which physiologic process is least likely to increase myocardial oxygen consumption?*
 A *Increasing inotropic support*
 B *A 100% increase in heart rate*
 C *Increasing afterload*
 D *100% increase in end-diastolic volume*
 E *Increasing blood pressure*

Myocardial oxygen consumption ($MVO_2$) is primarily determined by myocyte contraction. Therefore, factors that increase tension generated by the myocytes, the rate of tension development and the number of cycles per unit time will ultimately increase myocardial oxygen consumption. According to the Law of LaPlace, cardiac wall tension is proportional to the product of intraventricular pressure and the ventricular radius.

Since the $MVO_2$ is closely related to wall tension, any changes that generate greater intraventricular pressure from increased afterload or inotropic stimulation will result in increased oxygen consumption. Increasing inotropy will result in increased $MVO_2$ due to the increased rate of tension and the increased magnitude of the tension. Doubling the heart rate will approximately double the $MVO_2$ due to twice the number of tension cycles per minute. Increased afterload will increase

$MVO_2$ due to increased wall tension. Increased preload or end-diastolic volume does not affect $MVO_2$ to the same extent. This is because preload is often expressed as ventricular end-diastolic volume and is not directly based on the radius. If we assume the ventricle is a sphere, then:

$$V = \frac{4}{3}\pi \cdot r^3$$

Therefore

$$r \propto \sqrt[3]{V}$$

Substituting this relationship into the Law of LaPlace

$$T \propto P \cdot \sqrt[3]{V}$$

This relationship illustrates that a 100% increase in ventricular volume will result in only a 26% increase in wall tension. In contrast, a 100% increase in ventricular pressure will result in a 100% increase in wall tension. For this reason, wall tension, and therefore $MVO_2$, is far less sensitive to changes in ventricular volume than pressure.

**Answer: D**

Klabunde, R.E. (2011) *Cardiovascular Physiology Concepts*, 2nd edn. Lippincott, Williams & Wilkins, Philadelphia, PA.
Rhoades, R. and Bell, D.R. (2012) *Medical Physiology: Principles for Clinical Medicine*, 4th edn, Lippincott, Williams & Wilkins, Philadelphia, PA.

6 *A 73-year-old obese man with a past medical history significant for diabetes, hypertension, and peripheral vascular disease undergoes an elective right hemicolectomy. While in the PACU, the patient becomes acutely hypotensive and lethargic requiring immediate intubation. What effects do you expect positive pressure ventilation to have on your patient's cardiac function?*
 A *Increased pleural pressure, increased transmural pressure, increased ventricular afterload*
 B *Decreased pleural pressure, increased transmural pressure, increased ventricular afterload*
 C *Decreased pleural pressure, decreased transmural pressure, decreased ventricular afterload*
 D *Increased pleural pressure, decreased transmural pressure, decreased ventricular afterload*
 E *Increased pleural pressure, increased transmural pressure, decreased ventricular afterload*

This patient has a significant medical history that puts him at high risk of an acute coronary event. Hypotension and decreased mental status clearly indicate the need for immediate intubation. The effects of positive pressure ventilation will have direct effects on this patient's cardiovascular function. Ventricular afterload is a transmural force so it is directly affected by the pleural pressure on the outer surface of the heart. Positive pleural pressures will enhance ventricular emptying by promoting the inward movement of the ventricular wall during systole. In addition, the increased pleural pressure will decrease transmural pressure and decrease ventricular afterload. In this case, the positive pressure ventilation provides cardiac support by "unloading" the left ventricle resulting in increased stroke volume, cardiac output and ultimately better end-organ perfusion.

**Answer: D**

Cairo, J.M. (2016) Extrapulmonary effects of mechanical ventilation, in *Pilbeam's Mechanical Ventilation. Physiological and Clinical Applications*, 6th edn, Elsevier, St. Louis, MO, pp. 304–314

7  Following surgical debridement for lower extremity necrotizing fasciitis, a 47-year-old man is admitted to the ICU. A Swan-Ganz catheter was inserted for refractory hypotension. The initial values are CVP = 5 mm Hg, MAP = 50 mm Hg, PCWP = 8 mm Hg, $PaO_2$ = 60 mm Hg, CO = 4.5 L/min, SVR = 450 dynes · sec/cm$^5$, and $O_2$ saturation of 93%. The hemoglobin is 8 g/dL. The most effective intervention to maximize perfusion pressure and oxygen delivery would be which of the following?
  A  Titrate the $FiO_2$ to a $SaO_2$ > 98%
  B  Transfuse with two units of packed red blood cells
  C  Fluid bolus with 1 L normal saline
  D  Titrate the $FiO_2$ to a $PaO_2$ > 80
  E  Start a vasopressor

To maximize the oxygen delivery ($DO_2$) and perfusion pressure to the vital organs, it is important to determine the factors that directly affect it. According to the formula below, oxygen delivery ($DO_2$) is dependent on cardiac output (Q), the hemoglobin level (Hb), and the $O_2$ saturation ($SaO_2$):

$$DO_2 = Q \times (1.34 \times Hb \times SaO_2 \times 10) + (0.003 \times PaO_2)$$

This patient is likely septic from his infectious process. In addition, the long operation likely included a significant blood loss and fluid shifts so hypovolemic/hemorrhagic shock is likely contributing to this patient's hypotension. The low CVP, low wedge pressure indicates a need for volume replacement. The fact that this patient is anemic as a result of significant blood loss means that transfusing this patient would likely benefit his oxygen-carrying capacity as well as provide volume replacement. Fluid bolus is not inappropriate; however, two units of

packed red blood cells would be more appropriate. Titrating the $PaO_2$ would not add any benefit because, according to the above equation, it contributes very little to the overall oxygen delivery. Starting a vasopressor in a hypovolemic patient is inappropriate at this time and should be reserved for continued hypotension after adequate fluid resuscitation. Titrating the $FiO_2$ to a saturation of greater than 98% would not be clinically relevant. Although the patient requires better oxygen-carrying capacity, this would be better solved with red blood cell replacement.

**Answer: B**

Marino, P. (2014) *The ICU Book*, 4th edn, Lippincott Williams & Wilkins, Philadelphia, PA, chapter 2.

8  To promote adequate alveolar ventilation, decrease shunting, and ultimately improve oxygenation, the addition of positive end-expiratory pressure (PEEP) in a severely hypoxic patient with ARDS will:
  A  Limit the increase in residual volume (RV)
  B  Limit the decrease in expiratory reserve volume (ERV)
  C  Limit the increase in inspiratory reserve volume (IRV)
  D  Limit the decrease in tidal volume (TV)
  E  Increase $pCO_2$

Patients with ARDS have a significantly decreased lung compliance, which leads to significant alveolar collapse. This results in decreased surface area for adequate gas exchange and an increased alveolar shunt fraction resulting in hypoventilation and refractory hypoxemia. The minimum volume and pressure of gas necessary to prevent small airway collapse is the critical closing volume (CCV). When CCV exceeds functional residual capacity (FRC), alveolar collapse occurs. The two components of FRC are residual volume (RV) and expiratory reserve volume (ERV).

The role of extrinsic positive end-expiratory pressure (PEEP) in ARDS is to prevent alveolar collapse, promote further alveolar recruitment, and improve oxygenation by limiting the decrease in FRC and maintaining it above the critical closing volume. Therefore, limiting the decrease in ERV will limit the decrease in FRC and keep it above the CCV thus preventing alveolar collapse.

Limiting an increase in the residual volume would keep the FRC below the CCV and promote alveolar collapse. Positive-end expiratory pressure has no effect on inspiratory reserve volume (IRV) or tidal volume (TV) and does not increase $pCO_2$.

**Answer: B**

Rimensberger, P.C. and Bryan, A.C. (1999) Measurement of functional residual capacity in the critically ill. Relevance for the assessment of respiratory mechanics during mechanical ventilation. *Intensive Care Medicine,* **25** (5), 540–542.

Sidebotham, D., McKee, A., Gillham, M., and Levy, J. (2007) *Cardiothoracic Critical Care,* Butterworth-Heinemann, Philadelphia, PA.

**9** *Which of the five mechanical events of the cardiac cycle is described by an initial contraction, increasing ventricular pressure and closing of the AV valves?*
 A *Ventricular diastole*
 B *Atrial systole*
 C *Isovolumic ventricular contraction*
 D *Ventricular ejection (systole)*
 E *Isovolumic relaxation*

The repetitive cellular electrical events resulting in mechanical motions of the heart occur with each beat and make up the cardiac cycle. The mechanical events of the cardiac cycle correlate with ECG waves and occur in five phases described in Figure 1.3.

1) Ventricular diastole (mid-diastole): Throughout most of ventricular diastole, the atria and ventricles are relaxed. The AV valves are open, and the ventricles fill passively.
2) Atrial systole: During atrial systole a small amount of additional blood is pumped into the ventricles.
3) Isovolumic ventricular contraction: Initial contraction increases ventricular pressure, closing the AV valves. Blood is pressurized during isovolumic ventricular contraction.
4) Ventricular ejection (systole): The semilunar valves open when ventricular pressures exceed pressures in the aorta and pulmonary artery. Ventricular ejection (systole) of blood follows.
5) Isovolumic relaxation: The semilunar valves close when the ventricles relax and pressure in the ventricles decreases. The AV valves open when pressure in the ventricles decreases below atrial pressure.

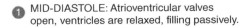
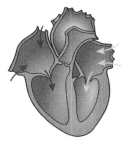
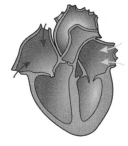
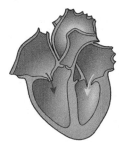
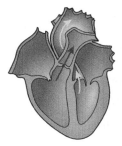
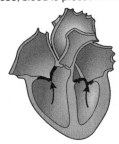

**Figure 1.3** The cardiac cycle illustrated.

Atria fill with blood throughout ventricular systole, allowing rapid ventricular filling at the start of the next diastolic period.

**Answer: C**

Kibble, J.D. and Halsey, C.R. (2015) Cardiovascular physiology, in *Medical Physiology: The Big Picture*, McGraw-Hill, New York, pp. 131–174.

Barrett, K.E., Barman, S.M., Boitano, S., and Brooks, H.L. (2016) The heart as a pump, in *Ganong's Review of Medical Physiology* (K. E. Barrett, S.M. Barman, S, Boitano, and H.L. Brooks, eds), 25th edn, McGraw-Hill, New York, pp. 537–553.

10  *A recent post-op 78-year-old man is admitted to the STICU with an acute myocardial infarction and resulting severe hypotension. A STAT ECHO shows decompensating right-sided heart failure. CVP = 23 cm H$_2$0. What is the most appropriate therapeutic intervention at this time?*
   A *Volume*
   B *Vasodilator therapy*
   C *Furosemide*
   D *Inodilator therapy*
   E *Mechanical cardiac support*

The mainstay therapy of right-sided heart failure associated with severe hypotension as a result of an acute myocardial infarction is volume infusion. However, it is important to carefully monitor the CVP or PAWP in order to avoid worsening right heart failure resulting in left-sided heart failure as a result of interventricular interdependence. A mechanism where right-sided volume overload leads to septal deviation and compromised left ventricular filling. An elevated CVP or PAWP of > 15 should be utilized as an endpoint of volume infusion in right heart failure. At this point, inodilator therapy with dobutamine or levosimendan should be initiated. Additional volume infusion would only lead to further hemodynamic instability and potential collapse. Vasodilator therapy should only be used in normotensive heart failure due to its risk for hypotension. Diuretics should only be used in normo- or hypertensive heart failure patients. Mechanical cardiac support should only be initiated in patients who are in cardiogenic shock due to left-sided heart failure.

Acute decompensated heart failure (ADHF) can present in many different ways and require different therapeutic strategies. This patient represents the "low output" phenotype that is often associated with hypoperfusion and end-organ dysfunction. See Figure 1.4.

**Answer: D**

Mehra, M.R. (2015) Heart failure: management, in *Harrison's Principles of Internal Medicine*, 19th edn (D. Kasper, A. Fauci, S. Hauser, *et al.*, eds), McGraw-Hill, New York, chapter 280.

11  *The right atrial tracing in Figure 1.5 is consistent with:*
   A *Tricuspid stenosis*
   B *Normal right atrial waveform tracing*
   C *Tricuspid regurgitation*
   D *Constrictive pericarditis*
   E *Mitral stenosis*

The normal jugular venous pulse contains three positive waves (Figure 1.6). These positive deflections, labeled "a," "c," and "v" occur, respectively, before the carotid upstroke and just after the P wave of the ECG (a wave); simultaneous with the upstroke of the carotid pulse (c wave); and during ventricular systole until the tricuspid valve opens (v wave). The "a" wave is generated by atrial contraction, which actively fills the right ventricle in end-diastole. The "c" wave is caused either by transmission of the carotid arterial impulse through the external and internal jugular veins or by the bulging of the tricuspid valve into the right atrium in early systole. The "v" wave reflects the passive increase in pressure and volume of the right atrium as it fills in late systole and early diastole.

Normally the crests of the "a" and "v" waves are approximately equal in amplitude. The descents or troughs of the jugular venous pulse occur between the "a" and "c" wave ("x" descent), between the "c" and "v" wave ("x" descent), and between the "v" and "a" wave ("y" descent). The x and x' descents reflect movement of the lower portion of the right atrium toward the right ventricle during the final phases of ventricular systole. The y descent represents the abrupt termination of the downstroke of the v wave during early diastole after the tricuspid valve opens and the right ventricle begins to fill passively. Normally the y descent is neither as brisk nor as deep as the x descent.

**Answer: C**

Hall, J.B., Schmidt, G.A., and Wood, L.D.H. (eds) (2005) *Principles of Critical Care*, 3rd edn, McGraw-Hill, New York.

McGee, S. (2007) *Evidence-based Physical Diagnosis*, 2nd edn, W. B. Saunders & Co., Philadelphia, PA.

Pinsky, L.E. and Wipf, J.E. (n.d.) University of Washington Department of Medicine. *Advanced Physical Diagnosis. Learning and Teaching at the Bedside.* Edition 1, http://depts.washington.edu/physdx/neck/index.html (accessed November 6, 2011).

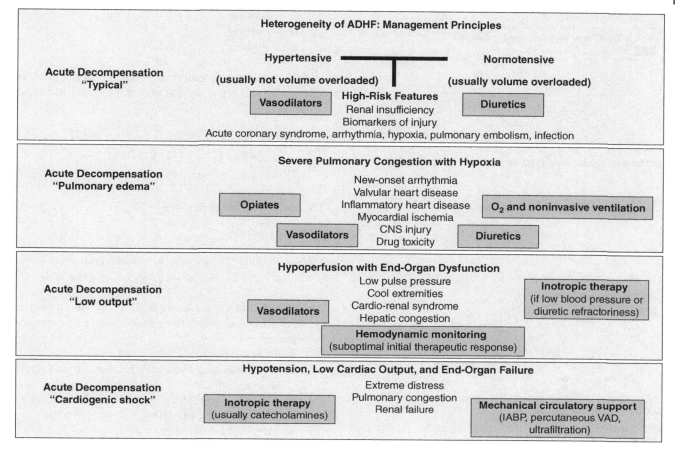

**Figure 1.4**

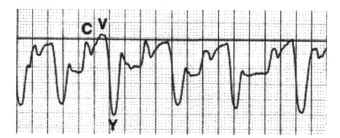

**Figure 1.5**

**12** *The addition of PEEP in optimizing ventilatory support in patients with ARDS does all of the following except:*
  **A** *Increases functional residual capacity (FRC) above the alveolar closing pressure*
  **B** *Maximizes inspiratory alveolar recruitment*
  **C** *Limits ventilation below the lower inflection point to minimize shear-force injury*
  **D** *Improves V/Q mismatch*
  **E** *Increases the mean airway pressure*

The addition of positive-end expiratory pressure (PEEP) in patients who have ARDS has been shown to be beneficial.

By maintaining a small positive pressure at the end of expiration, considerable improvement in the arterial $PaO_2$ can be obtained. The addition of PEEP maintains the functional residual capacity (FRC) above the critical closing volume (CCV) of the alveoli, thus preventing alveolar collapse. It also limits ventilation below the lower inflection point minimizing shear force injury to the alveoli. The prevention of alveolar collapse results in improved V/Q mismatch, decreased shunting, and improved gas exchange. The addition of PEEP in ARDS also allows for lower $FiO_2$ to be used in maintaining adequate oxygenation.

PEEP maximizes the expiratory alveolar recruitment; it has no effect on the inspiratory portion of ventilatory support.

**Answer: B**

Gattinoni, L,, Cairon, M., Cressoni, M., *et al.* (2006) Lung recruitement in patients with acute respiratory distress syndrome. *New England Journal of Medicine* **354**, 1775–1786.

West, B. (2008) *Pulmonary Pathophysiology – The Essentials*, 8th edn, Lippincott, Williams & Wilkins, Philadelphia, PA.

(A) Tricuspid stenosis.

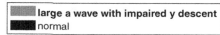

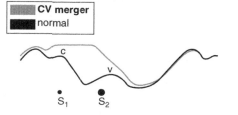

(B) Normal jugular venous tracing.

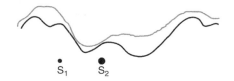

(C) Tricuspid regurgitation.

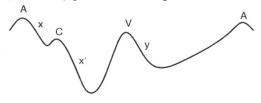

(D) Constrictive pericarditis

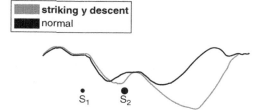

**Figure 1.6**

**13** *A 70-year-old man with a history of diabetes, hypertension, coronary artery disease, asthma and long-standing cigarette smoking undergoes an emergency laparotomy and Graham patch for a perforated duodenal ulcer. Following the procedure, he develops acute respiratory distress and oxygen saturation of 88%. Blood gas analysis reveals the following:*
*pH = 7.43*
*paO$_2$ = 55 mm Hg*
*HCO$_3$ = 23 mmol/L*
*pCO$_2$ = 35 mm Hg*

*Based on the above results, you would calculate his A-a gradient to be (assuming atmospheric pressure at sea level, water vapor pressure = 47 mm Hg):*
**A** *8 mm Hg*
**B** *15 mm Hg*

**C** *30 mm Hg*
**D** *51 mm Hg*
**E** *61 mm Hg*

The A-a gradient is equal to PAO$_2$ – PaO$_2$ (55 from ABG). The PAO$_2$ can be calculated using the following equation:

$$PaO_2 = FiO_2 (P_B - P_{H2O}) - (PaCO_2 / RQ)$$
$$= 0.21(760 - 47) - (35 / 0.8)$$
$$PaO_2 = 106 \, mm \, Hg$$

Therefore, A-a gradient (PaO$_2$ – PAO$_2$) = 51 mm Hg.

**Answer: D**

Marino, P. (2007) *The ICU Book*, 3rd edn, Lippincott Williams & Wilkins, Philadelphia, PA, chapter 19.

**14** *What is the most likely etiology of the patient in question 13's respiratory failure and the appropriate intervention?*
**A** *Pulmonary edema, cardiac workup*
**B** *Neuromuscular weakness, intubation, and reversal of anesthetic*
**C** *Pulmonary embolism, systemic anticoagulation*
**D** *Acute asthma exacerbation, bronchodilators*
**E** *Hypoventilation, pain control*

Disorders that cause hypoxemia can be categorized into four groups: hypoventilation, low inspired oxygen, shunting, and V/Q mismatch. Although all of these can potentially present with hypoxemia, calculating the alveolar-arterial (A-a) gradient and determining whether administering 100% oxygen is of benefit, can often determine the specific type of hypoxemia and lead to quick and effective treatment.

Acute hypoventilation often presents with an elevated PaCO$_2$ and a normal A-a gradient. This is usually seen in patients with altered mental status due to excessive sedation, narcotic use, or residual anesthesia. Since this patient's PaCO$_2$ is low (35 mm Hg), it is not the cause of this patient's hypoxemia.

Low inspired oxygen presents with a low PO$_2$ and a normal A-a gradient. Since this patient's A-a gradient is elevated, this is unlikely the cause of the hypoxemia.

A V/Q mismatch (pulmonary embolism or acute asthma exacerbation) presents with a normal PaCO$_2$ and an elevated A-a gradient that does correct with administration of 100% oxygen. Since this patient's hypoxemia does not improve after being placed on the nonrebreather mask, it is unlikely that this is the cause.

Shunting (pulmonary edema) presents with a normal PaCO$_2$ and an elevated A-a gradient that does *not* correct with the administration of 100% oxygen. This patient has a normal $PaCO_2$, an elevated A-a gradient and hypoxemia that does not correct with the administration of 100% oxygen. This patient has a pulmonary shunt.

Although an A-a gradient can vary with age and the concentration of inspired oxygen, an A-a gradient of 51 is clearly elevated. This patient has a normal $PaCO_2$ and an elevated A-a gradient that did not improve with 100% oxygen administration therefore a shunt is clearly present. Common causes of shunting include pulmonary edema and pneumonia.

Reviewing this patient's many risk factors for a postoperative myocardial infarction and a decreased left ventricular function makes pulmonary edema the most likely explanation.

**Answer: A**

Weinberger, S.E., Cockrill, B.A., and Mande, J. (2008) *Principles of Pulmonary Medicine*, 5th edn. W.B. Saunders, Philadelphia, PA.

15  *You are taking care of a morbidly obese patient on a ventilator who is hypotensive and hypoxic. His peak airway pressures and plateau pressures have been slowly rising over the last few days. You decide to place an esophageal balloon catheter. The values are obtained:*

$$Pplat = 45 cm H_2O$$
$$\Delta tP = 15 cm H_2O$$
$$\Delta Pes = 5 cm H_2O$$

*What is the likely cause of the increased peak airway pressures and what is your next intervention?*
 A *Decreased lung compliance, increase PEEP to 25 cm $H_2O$*
 B *Decreased lung compliance, high frequency oscillator ventilation*
 C *Decreased chest wall compliance, increase PEEP to 25 cm $H_2O$*
 D *Decreased chest wall compliance, high-frequency oscillator ventilation*
 E *Decreased lung compliance, bronchodilators*

The high plateau pressures in this patient are concerning for worsening lung function or poor chest-wall mechanics due to obesity that don't allow for proper gas exchange. One way to differentiate the major cause of these elevated plateau pressures is to place an esophageal balloon. After placement, measuring the proper pressures on inspiration and expiration reveals that the largest contributing factor to these high pressures is the weight of the chest wall causing poor chest-wall compliance. The small change in esophageal pressures, as compared with the larger change in transpulmonary pressures, indicates poor chest-wall compliance and good lung compliance. It is why the major factor in this patient's high inspiratory pressures is poor chest-wall compliance. The patient is hypotensive, so increasing the PEEP would likely result in further drop in blood pressure. This is why high-frequency oscillator ventilation would likely improve this patient's hypoxemia without affecting the blood pressure.

**Answer: D**

Talmor, D., Sarge, T., O'Donnell, C., and Ritz, R. (2006) Esophageal and transpulmonary pressures in acute respiratory failure. *Critical Care Medicine*, **34** (5), 1389–1394.

Valenza, F., Chevallard, G., Porro, G.A., and Gattinoni, L. (2007) Static and dynamic components of esophageal and central venous pressure during intra-abdominal hypertension. *Critical Care Medicine*, **35** (6), 1575–1581.

16  *All of the following cardiovascular changes occur in pregnancy except:*
 A *Increased cardiac output*
 B *Decreased plasma volume*
 C *Increased heart rate*
 D *Decreased systemic vascular resistance*
 E *Increased red blood cell mass – "relative anemia"*

The following cardiovascular changes occur during pregnancy:

- Decreased systemic vascular resistance
- Increased plasma volume
- Increased red blood cell volume
- Increased heart rate
- Increased ventricular distention
- Increased blood pressure
- Increased cardiac output
- Decreased peripheral vascular resistance

**Answer: B**

DeCherney, A.H. and Nathan, L. (2007) *Current Diagnosis and Treatment: Obstetrics and Gynecology*, 10th edn, McGraw-Hill, New York, chapter 7.

Yeomans, E.R. and Gilstrap, L.C., III. (2005) Physiologic changes in pregnancy and their impact on critical care. *Critical Care Medicine*, **33**, 256–258.

17  *Choose the incorrect statement regarding the physiology of the intra-aortic balloon pump:*

A *Shortened intraventricular contraction phase leads to increased oxygen demand*

B *The tip of catheter should be between the second and third rib on a chest x-ray*

C *Early inflation leads to increased afterload and decreased cardiac output*

D *Early or late deflation leads to a smaller afterload reduction*

E *Aortic valve insufficiency is a definite contraindication*

Patients who suffer hemodynamic compromise despite medical therapies may benefit from mechanical cardiac support of an intra-aortic balloon pump (IABP). One of the benefits of this device is the decreased oxygen demand of the myocardium as a result of the shortened intraventricular contraction phase. It is of great importance to confirm the proper placement of the balloon catheter with a chest x-ray that shows the tip of the balloon catheter to be 1 to 2 cm below the aortic knob or between the second and third rib. If the balloon is placed too proximal in the aorta, occlusion of the brachiocephalic, left carotid, or left subclavian arteries may occur. If the balloon is too distal, obstruction of the celiac, superior mesenteric, and inferior mesenteric arteries may lead to mesenteric ischemia. The renal arteries may also be occluded, resulting in renal failure.

Additional complications of intra-aortic balloon-pump placement include limb ischemia, aortic dissection, neurologic complications, thrombocytopenia, bleeding, and infection.

The inflation of the balloon catheter should occur at the onset of diastole. This results in increased diastolic pressures that promote perfusion of the myocardium as well as distal organs. If inflation occurs too early it will lead to increased afterload and decreased cardiac output. Deflation should occur at the onset of systole. Early or late deflation will diminish the effects of afterload reduction. One of the definite contraindications to placement of an IABP is the presence of a hemodynamically significant aortic valve insufficiency. This would exacerbate the magnitude of the aortic regurgitation.

**Answer: A**

Ferguson, J.J., Cohen, M., Freedman, R.J., *et al.* (2001) The current practice of intra-aortic balloon counterpulsation: results from the Benchmark Registry. *Journal of American Cardiology*, **38**, 1456–1462.

Hurwitz, L.M. and Goodman, P.C. (2005) Intraaortic balloon pump location and aortic dissection. *American Journal of Roentgenology*, **184**, 1245–1246.

Sidebotham, D., McKee, A., Gillham, M., and Levy, J. (2007) *Cardiothoracic Critical Care*, Butterworth-Heinemann, Philadelphia, PA.

18 *Choose the **incorrect** statement regarding the West lung zones:*

A *Zone 1 does not exist under normal physiologic conditions*

B *In hypovolemic states, zone 1 is converted to zone 2 and zone 3*

C *V/Q ratio is higher in zone 1 than in zone 3*

D *Artificial ventilation with excessive PEEP can increase dead space ventilation*

E *Perfusion and ventilation are better in the bases than the apices of the lungs*

The three West zones of the lung divide the lung into three regions based on the relationship between alveolar pressure (PA), pulmonary arterial pressure (Pa) and pulmonary venous pressure (Pv).

Zone 1 represents alveolar dead space and is due to arterial collapse secondary to increased alveolar pressures (PA > Pa > Pv).

Zone 2 is approximately 3 cm above the heart and represents and represents a zone of pulsatile perfusion (Pa > PA > Pv).

Zone 3 represents the majority of healthy lungs where no external resistance to blood flow exists promoting continuous perfusion of ventilated lungs (Pa > Pv > PA).

Zone 1 does not exist under normal physiologic conditions because pulmonary arterial pressure is higher than alveolar pressure in all parts of the lung. However, when a patient is placed on mechanical ventilation (positive pressure ventilation with PEEP) the alveolar pressure (PA) becomes greater than the pulmonary arterial pressure (Pa) and pulmonary venous pressure (Pv). This represents a conversion of zone 3 to zone 1 and 2 and marks an increase in alveolar dead space. In a hypovolemic state, the pulmonary arterial and venous pressures fall below the alveolar pressures representing a similar conversion of zone 3 to zone 1 and 2. Both perfusion and ventilation are better at the bases than the apices. However, perfusion is better at the bases and ventilation is better at the apices due to gravitational forces.

**Answer: B**

Lumb, A. (2000) *Nunn's Applied Respiratory Physiology*, 5 edn, Butterworth-Heinemann, Oxford.

West, J., Dollery, C., and Naimark, A. (1964) Distribution of blood flow in isolated lung; relation to vascular and alveolar pressures. *Journal of Applied Physiology*, **19**, 713–724.

19 *Choose the correct statement regarding clinical implications of cardiopulmonary interactions during mechanical ventilation:*

**A** *The decreased trans-pulmonary pressure and decreased systemic filling pressure is responsible for decreased venous return*

**B** *Right ventricular end-diastolic volume is increased due to increased airway pressure and decreased venous return*

**C** *The difference between trans-pulmonary and systemic filling pressures is the gradient for venous return*

**D** *Patients with severe left ventricular dysfunction may have decreased transmural aortic pressure resulting in decreased cardiac output*

**E** *Patients with decreased PCWP usually improve with additional PEEP*

The *increased* trans-pulmonary pressure and decreased systemic filling pressure is responsible for decreased venous return to the heart resulting in hypotension. This phenomenon is more pronounced in hypovolemic patients and may worsen hypotension in patients with low PCWP.

Right ventricular end-diastolic volume is *decreased* due to the increased transpulmonary pressure and decreased venous return.

Patients with severe left ventricular dysfunction may have decreased transmural aortic pressure resulting in *increased* cardiac output.

**Answer: C**

Hurford, W.E. (1999) Cardiopulmonary interactions during mechanical ventilation. *International Anesthesiology Clinics*, 37 (3), 35–46.

Marino, P. (2007) *The ICU Book*, 3rd edn, Lippincott Williams & Wilkins, Philadelphia, PA.

**20** *The location of optimal PEEP on a volume-pressure curve is:*

**A** *Slightly below the lower inflection point*

**B** *Slightly above the lower inflection point*

**C** *Slightly below the upper inflection point*

**D** *Slightly above the upper inflection point*

**E** *Cannot be determined on the volume-pressure curve*

In ARDS, patients often have lower compliant lungs that require more pressure to achieve the same volume of ventilation. On a pressure-volume curve, the lower inflection point represents increased pressure necessary to initiate the opening of alveoli and initiate a breath. The upper inflection point represents increased pressures with limited gains in volume. Conventional ventilation often reaches pressures that are above the upper inflection point and below the lower inflection point. Any ventilation above the upper inflection point results in some degree of over-distention and leads to volutrauma. Ventilating below the lower inflection point results in under-recruitment and shear force injury. The ideal mode of ventilation works between the two inflection points eliminating over distention and volutrauma and under-recruitment and shear force injury. Use tidal volumes that are below the upper inflection point and PEEP that is above the lower inflection point.

**Answer: B**

Lubin, M.F., Smith, R.B., Dobson, T.F., *et al.* (2010) *Medical Management of the Surgical Patient: A Textbook of Perioperative Medicine*, 4th edn, Cambridge University Press, Cambridge.

Ward, N.S., Lin, D.Y., Nelson, D.L., *et al.* (2002) Successful determination of lower inflection point and maximal compliance in a population of patients with acute respiratory distress syndrome. *Critical Care Medicine*, 30 (5), 963–968.

**21** *Identify the correct statement regarding the relationship between oxygen delivery and oxygen uptake during a shock state:*

**A** *Oxygen uptake is always constant at tissue level due to increased oxygen extraction*

**B** *Oxygen uptake at tissue level is always oxygen supply dependent*

**C** *Critical oxygen delivery is constant and clinically predictable*

**D** *Critical oxygen delivery is the lowest level required to support aerobic metabolism*

**E** *Oxygen uptake increases with oxygen delivery in a linear relationship*

As changes in oxygen supply ($DO_2$) vary, the body's oxygen transport system attempts to maintain a constant delivery of oxygen ($VO_2$) to the tissues. This is possible due to the body's ability to adjust its level of oxygen extraction. As delivery of oxygen decreases, the extraction ratio will initially increase in a reciprocal manner. This allows for a constant oxygen supply to the tissues. Unfortunately, once the extraction ratio reaches its limit, any additional decrease in oxygen supply will result in an equal decrease of oxygen delivery. At this point, critical oxygen delivery is reached representing the lowest level of oxygen to support aerobic metabolism. After this point, oxygen delivery becomes supply dependent and the rate of aerobic metabolism is directly limited by the oxygen supply. Therefore, oxygen uptake is only constant until it reaches maximal oxygen extraction and becomes oxygen-supply dependent.

Oxygen uptake at the tissue level is only oxygen-supply dependent only after the critical oxygen delivery is reached and dysoxia occurs. Unfortunately, identifying the critical oxygen delivery in ICU patients is not possible and is clinically irrelevant.

**Answer: D**

Marino, P. (2007) *The ICU Book*, 3rd edn, Lippincott Williams & Wilkins, Philadelphia, PA, chapter 1.

Schumacker, P.T. and Cain, S.M. (1987) The concept of a critical oxygen delivery. *Intensive Care Medicine*, **13**(4), 223–229.

**22** *You are caring for a patient in ARDS who exhibits severe bilateral pulmonary infiltrates. The cause for his hypoxia is related to trans-vascular fluid shifts resulting in interstitial edema. Identify the primary reason for this pathologic process.*

   **A** *Increased capillary and interstitial hydrostatic pressure gradient*

   **B** *Increased oncotic reflection coefficient*

   **C** *Increased capillary and interstitial oncotic pressure gradient*

   **D** *Increased capillary membrane permeability coefficient*

   **E** *Increased oncotic pressure differences*

This question refers to the Starling equation which describes the forces that influence the movement of fluid across capillary membranes.

$$J_v = K_f\left([P_c - P_i]\right) - \sigma\left[\pi_c - \pi_i\right]$$

$P_c$ = Capillary hydrostatic pressure

$P_i$ = Interstitial hydrostatic pressure

$\pi_c$ = Capillary oncotic pressure

$\pi i$ = Interstitial oncotic pressure

$K_f$ = Permeability coefficient

$\sigma$ = Reflection coefficient

In ALI/ARDS, the oncotic pressure difference between the capillary and the interstitium is essentially zero due to the membrane damage caused by mediators, which allows for large protein leaks into the interstitium, causing equilibrium. The oncotic pressure difference is zero, so the product with the reflection coefficient is essentially zero. According to this equation only two forces determine the extent of transmembrane fluid flux: the permeability coefficient and the hydrostatic pressure. In this case, the increased permeability coefficient is the major determinant of overwhelming interstitial edema since high hydrostatic pressures are often seen in congestive heart failure and not in ALI/ARDS.

**Answer: D**

Hamid, Q., Shannon, J., and Martin, J. (2005) *Physiologic Basis of Respiratory Disease*, B.C. Decker, Hamilton, ON, Canada.

Lewis C.A. and Martin, G.S. (2004) Understanding and managing fluid balance in patients with acute lung injury. *Current Opinion in Critical Care*, **10** (1), 13–17.

## 2

## Cardiopulmonary Resuscitation, Oxygen Delivery, and Shock

*Filip Moshkovsky, DO, Luis Cardenas, DO and Mark Cipolle, MD*

**1** *A patient is in ventricular fibrillation with cardiac arrest. Administration of what treatment option is no longer recommended in the updated 2015 American Heart Association guidelines for CPR:*
  **A** *Magnesium sulfate*
  **B** *Monophasic shock with 360 J*
  **C** *Epinephrine HCl*
  **D** *Lidocaine*
  **E** *Vasopressin*

The updated guidelines from the American Heart Association in 2015 no longer recommend administration of vasopressin in any of the ACLS algorithms. There has been no advantage in substituting epinephrine with vasopressin and therefore has been completely removed as a recommended chemical agent for cardiac arrest. Magnesium sulfate is recommended in cardiac arrest if torsades de pointes is identified. Monophasic shock with 360 J is recommended. Alternatively, biphasic shock can be administered set to the highest manufacturer recommended setting. Lidocaine can be administered if first- line recommended antiarrhythmic, amiodarone, is not available.

**Answer: E**

American Heart Association (2015) Part 7: adult advanced cardiovascular life support: 2015 American Heart Association guidelines update for CPR and emergency cardiovascular care. *Circulation*, **132** (suppl 2), S444–S464.

**2** *All of the following are positive predictors of survival after sudden cardiac arrest except:*
  **A** *Witnessed cardiac arrest*
  **B** *Initiation of CPR by bystander*
  **C** *Initial rhythm of ventricular tachycardia (VT) or ventricular fibrillation (VF)*
  **D** *Chronic diabetes mellitus*
  **E** *Early access to external defibrillation*

Significant underlying comorbidities such as prior myocardial ischemia and diabetes have no role in influencing survival rates from sudden cardiac arrest. Survival rates are extremely variable and range from 0 to 18%. There are several factors that influence these survival rates. Community education plays a large role in the survival of patients who have undergone a significant cardiac event. Cardiopulmonary resuscitation certification, as well as apid notification of emergency medical services (EMS), and rapid initiation of CPR and defibrillation all contribute to improving survival. Other factors include witnessed versus non-witnessed cardiac arrest, race, age, sex, and initial VT or VF rhythm. The problem is that only about 20 to 30% of patients have CPR performed during a cardiac arrest. As the length of time increases, the chance of survival significantly falls. Patients who are initially in VT or VF have a two to three times greater chance of survival than patients who initially present in pulseless electrical activity (PEA) arrest.

**Answer: D**

Cummins, R.O., Ornato, J.P., Thies, W.H., and Pepe, P.E. (1991) Improving survival from sudden cardiac arrest: the "chain of survival" concept. A statement for health professionals from the Advanced Cardiac Life Support Subcommittee and the Emergency Cardiac Care Committee, American Heart Association. *Circulation*, **83**, 1832–1847.

Deutschman, C. and Neligan, P. (2010) *Evidence-Based Practice of Critical Care*, W. B. Saunders & Co., Philadelphia, PA.

Zipes, D. and Hein, W. (1998) Sudden cardiac death. *Circulation*, **98**, 2334–2351.

**3** *For prehospital VF arrest, compared to lidocaine, amiodarone administration in the field:*
  **A** *Improves survival to hospital admission*
  **B** *Decreases the rate of vasopressor use for hypotension*

*Surgical Critical Care and Emergency Surgery: Clinical Questions and Answers*, Second Edition.
Edited by Forrest "Dell" Moore, Peter Rhee, and Gerard J. Fulda.
© 2018 John Wiley & Sons Ltd. Published 2018 by John Wiley & Sons Ltd.
Companion website: www.wiley.com/go/moore/surgical_criticalcare_and_emergency_surgery

C *Decreases use of atropine for treatment of bradycardia*

D *Improves survival to hospital discharge*

E *Results in a decrease in ICU days*

Dorian evaluated this question and found more patients receiving amiodarone in the field had a better chance of survival to hospital admission than patients in the lidocaine group (22.8% versus 12.0%, P = 0.009). Results showed that there was no significant difference between the two groups with regard to vasopressor usage for hypotension, or atropine usage for bradycardia. Results also revealed that there was no difference in the rates of hospital discharge between the two groups (5.0% versus 3.0%). The ALIVE trial results did support the 2005 American Heart Association (AHA) recommendation to use amiodarone as the first-line antiarrhythmic agent in cardiac arrest. The updated 2015 guidelines from AHA continue to recommend amiodarone as the first line anti-arrhythmic agent. The guidelines state that amiodarone should be given as a 300 mg intravenous bolus, followed by one dose of 150 mg intravenously for ventricular fibrillation, paroxysmal ventricular tachycardia, unresponsive to CPR, shock, or vasopressors.

**Answer: A**

American Heart Association (2015) Part 7: Adult advanced cardiovascular life support: 2015 American Heart Association guidelines update for CPR and emergency cardiovascular care. *Circulation*, **132** (suppl 2), S444–S464.

Deutschman, C. and Neligan, P. (2010) *Evidence-Based Practice of Critical Care*, W.B. Saunders & Co., Philadelphia, PA.

Dorian, P., Cass, D., Schwartz, B., *et al.* (2002) Amiodarone as compared with lidocaine for shock-resistant ventricular fibrillation. *New England Journal of Medicine*, **346**, 884–890.

4 *All of the following are underlying causes of PEA arrest except:*

A *Tension pneumothorax*

B *Hyperkalemia*

C *Hypomagnesemia*

D *Hypothermia*

E *Cardiac tamponade*

Hypomagnesemia is not commonly associated with PEA arrest. PEA is defined as cardiac electrical activity on the monitor with the absence of a pulse or blood pressure. Recent studies using ultrasound showed evidence of mechanical activity of the heart, however, there was not enough antegrade force to produce a palpable pulse or a blood pressure. Medications to treat PEA arrest include epinephrine, and in some cases, atropine. Definitive treatment of PEA involves finding and treating the underlying cause. The causes are commonly referred to as the six "Hs" and the five "Ts". The six "H's" include hypovolemia, hypoxia, hydrogen ion (acidosis), hypo/hyperkalemia, hypoglycemia, and hypothermia. The five "Ts" include toxins, tamponade (cardiac), tension pneumothorax, thrombosis (cardiac or pulmonary), and trauma. Hypomagnesemia manifests as weakness, muscle cramps, increased CNS irritability with tremors, athetosis, nystagmus, and an extensor plantar reflex. Most frequently, hypomagnesemia is associated with torsades de pointes, not PEA.

**Answer: C**

American Heart Association (2015) Part 7: adult advanced cardiovascular life support: 2015 American Heart Association guidelines update for CPR and emergency cardiovascular care. *Circulation*, **132** (suppl 2), S444–S464.

American Heart Association (2016) Part 5: cardiac arrest: pulseless electrical activity. *Advanced Cardiovascular Life Support – Provider manual.*

5 *CPR provides approximately what percentage of myocardial blood flow and what percentage of cerebral blood flow?*

A *10–30% of myocardial blood flow and 30–40% cerebral blood flow*

B *30–40% of myocardial blood flow and 10–30% of cerebral blood flow*

C *50–60% of myocardial blood flow and cerebral blood flow*

D *70–80% of myocardial blood flow and cerebral blood flow*

E *With proper chest compressions, approximately 90% of normal myocardial blood flow and cerebral blood flow*

Despite proper CPR technique, standard closed-chest compressions provide only 10–30% of myocardial blood flow and 30–40% of cerebral blood flow. Most studies have shown that regional organ perfusion, which is achieved during CPR, is considerably less than that achieved during normal sinus rhythm. Previous research in this area has stated that a minimum aortic diastolic pressure of approximately 40 mm Hg is needed to have a return of spontaneous circulation. Patients who do survive cardiac arrest typically have a coronary perfusion pressure of greater than 15 mm Hg.

**Answer: A**

Del Guercio, L.R.M., Feins, N.R., Cohn, J., *et al.* (1965) Comparison of blood flow during external and internal cardiac massage in man. *Circulation*, **31/32** (suppl. 1), 171.

Kern, K. (1997) Cardiopulmonary resuscitation physiology. *ACC Current Journal Review*, **6**, 11–13.

**6** *All of the following are recommended in the 2005 AHA guidelines and the 2015 AHA update regarding CPR and sudden cardiac arrest, except:*
  **A** *Use a compression to ventilation ratio (C/V ratio) of 30:2*
  **B** *Initiate chest compressions prior to defibrillation for ventricular fibrillation in sudden cardiac arrest*
  **C** *Deliver only one shock when attempting defibrillation*
  **D** *Use high-dose epinephrine after two rounds of unsuccessful defibrillation*
  **E** *Moderately induced hypothermia in survivors of in-hospital or out-of-hospital cardiac arrest*

The use of high-dose epinephrine has not been shown to improve survival after sudden cardiac arrest. Epinephrine at a dose of 1 mg is still the current recommendation for patients with any non-perfusing rhythm. The recommendation of C/V ratio 30:2 in patients of all ages except newborns is unchanged in the 2015 AHA updated guideline. This ratio is based on several studies showing that over time, blood-flow increases with more chest compressions. Performing 15 compressions then two rescue breaths causes the mechanism to be interrupted and decreases blood flow to the tissues. The 30:2 ratio is thought to reduce hyperventilation of the patient, decrease interruptions of compressions and make it easier for healthcare workers to understand. Compression first, versus shock first, for ventricular fibrillation in sudden cardiac arrest, is based on studies that looked at the interval between the call to the emergency medical services and delivery of the initial shock if the interval was 4–5 minutes or longer. A period of CPR before attempted shock improved survival in these patients. One shock versus the three-shock sequence for attempted defibrillation is the latest recommendation from 2005 guidelines and has not changed in the updated 2015 guidelines. The guidelines state that only one shock of 150 J or 200 J using a biphasic defibrillator or 360 J of a monophasic defibrillator should be used in these patients. In an effort to decrease transthoracic impedence, a three-shock sequence was used in rapid succession. Because the new biphasic defibrillators have an excellent first shock efficacy, the one-shock method for attempted defibrillation continues to be part of the guidelines.

**Answer: D**

American Heart Association (2015) Part 7: adult advanced cardiovascular life support: 2015 American Heart Association guidelines update for CPR and emergency cardiovascular care. *Circulation*, **132** (suppl 2), S444–S464.

Deutschman, C. and Neligan, P. (2010) *Evidence-Based Practice of Critical Care*, W.B. Saunders & Co., Philadelphia, PA.

Zaritsky, A. and Morley, P. (2005) American Heart Association guidelines for cardiopulmonary resuscitation and emergency cardiovascular care. Editorial: the evidence evaluation process for the 2005 International Consensus on Cardiopulmonary Resuscitation and Emergency Cardiovascular Care Science with Treatment Recommendations. *Circulation*, **112**, 128–130.

**7** *A 67-year-old man was discharged 3 days ago after elective colostomy reversal. He has chest pain and a witnessed cardiac arrest. ACLS was provided and ROSC was obtained after 5 minutes of CPR. The patient was intubated secondary to his comatose state with concern for inability to protect his airway. The following will increase his likelihood of a meaningful recovery:*
  **A** *Early tracheostomy placement*
  **B** *Continue with 80% $FiO_2$ for 8 hours after obtaining ROSC*
  **C** *Initiate targeted temperature management immediately, maintaining temperature at 30 °C*
  **D** *Avoid use of pressors given the recent colostomy reversal*
  **E** *If there is concern for a cardiac cause of cardiac arrest, obtain coronary intervention even if patient is unstable on pressors*

The new updated 2015 guidelines for cardiac arrest recommend initiating coronary intervention in suspected cardiac etiology for out-of-hospital cardiac arrest. This should not be delayed even if the patient is requiring pressor support and is unstable. Also recommended in the 2005 guidelines and the 2015 update is the use of hypothermia after cardiac arrest. This should not delay coronary intervention but should be started as soon as possible. The new updates also change the range of hypothermia to include 32–36 °C. Brain neurons are extremely sensitive to a reduction in cerebral blood flow which can cause permanent brain damage in minutes. Two recent trials demonstrated improved survival rates in patients that underwent mild hypothermia as compared to patients who received standard therapy. Both studies also showed an improvement in neurologic function after hypothermia treatment. In several small studies, high-dose epinephrine failed to show any survival benefit in patients that have suffered cardiac arrest.

**Answer: E**

American Heart Association (2015) Part 8: post cardiac arrest care: 2015 American Heart Association guidelines update for CPR and emergency cardiovascular care. *Circulation*, **132** (suppl 2), S465–S482.

Parrillo, E.J. and Dellinger, R.P. (2014) *Critical Care Medicine: Principles of Diagnosis and Management in the Adult*, 4th edn. W.B. Saunders & Co., Philadelphia, PA

**8** *What is the oxygen content ($CaO_2$) in an ICU patient who has a hemoglobin of 11.0 gm/dL, an oxygen saturation ($SaO_2$) of 96%, and an arterial oxygen partial pressure of ($PaO_2$) of 90 mm Hg.*
   **A** *10 mL/dL*
   **B** *11 mL/dL*
   **C** *12 mL/dL*
   **D** *13 mL/dL*
   **E** *14 mL/dL*

The oxygen content of the blood can be calculated from knowing the patient's hemoglobin, oxygen saturation, and partial pressure of arterial oxygen and the following formula.

$$CaO_2 = (1.3 \times Hb \times SaO_2) + (0.003 \times PaO_2)$$
$$CaO_2 = (1.3 \times 11 \times 0.96) + (0.003 \times 90)$$
$$CaO_2 = (13.72) + (0.27)$$
$$= 13.99 \text{ or } 14 \text{ mL/dL}$$

The equation can be simplified by ignoring the second half of the equation due to the very small amount of dissolved oxygen in blood. In this case, only 0.27 mL/dL of oxygen is dissolved and this is less then 2% of the total oxygen found in the blood. In order to simplify the equation, the accuracy of the oxygen content will be slightly off but still reflect greater than 98% of the true oxygen in the blood.

The simplified equation is:

$$CaO_2 = 1.34 \times Hb \times SaO_2$$

**Answer: E**

Marino, P. (2014) *The ICU Book*, 4th edn, Lippincott Williams & Wilkins, Philadelphia, PA.

**9** *What is the oxygen delivery ($DO_2$) of an ICU patient with hemoglobin of 10.0 gm/dL; an oxygen saturation of 98% on room air, $PaO_2$ of 92 mm Hg, and a cardiac output of 4 L/min?*
   **A** *410 mL/min*
   **B** *510 mL/min*
   **C** *521 mL/min*
   **D** *700 mL/min*
   **E** *610 mL/min*

Oxygen delivery can be calculated knowing the patient's hemoglobin, oxygen saturation, partial pressure of arterial oxygen, and cardiac output using the following formula.

$$DO_2 = Q \times CaO_2 \text{ or } DO_2 = Q((1.3 \times Hb \times SaO_2)$$
$$+ (0.003 \times PaO_2)) \times 10$$

$Q$ = cardiac output, $CaCo_2$ = oxygen content of the blood

$$DO_2 = 4 \times ((1.3 \times 10 \times 0.98) + (0.003 \times 92)) \times 10$$
$$DO_2 = 520.6 \text{ or } 521 \text{ mL/min}$$

The equation is multiplied by 10 to convert volumes percent to mL/min. This equation can be simplified as well with ignoring the dissolved oxygen in the blood. Multiplying $(0.003 \times 92) = 0.27$ which is a small fraction of the total number. The simplified equation can be used as follows:

$$DO_2 = CO \times CaO_2 \times 10$$

A $DO_2$ index can be calculated by substituting the cardiac index for the cardiac output, which is the cardiac output divided by the body surface area (BSA).

**Answer: C**

Marino, P. (2014) *The ICU Book*, 4th edn, Lippincott Williams & Wilkins, Philadelphia, PA.

**10** *Calculate the oxygen consumption ($\dot{V}O_2$) in a ventilated patient in your ICU with a cardiac output of 5 L/min, a Hb of 12.0 gm/dL, $PaO_2$ 90 mm Hg, an $SaO_2$ of 95%, and an $SvO_2$ of 60%.*
   **A** *178 mL/min*
   **B** *281 mL/min*
   **C** *378 mL/min*
   **D** *478 mL/min*
   **E** *578 mL/min*

Oxygen uptake/consumption ($\dot{V}O_2$), can be calculated using the patients hemoglobin, arterial oxygen saturation and venous oxygen saturation. The constant of 1.34 is the maximum saturation of hemoglobin with oxygen. Given that dissolved oxygen in the blood is an extremely small amount, this may be omitted from the equation.

$$\dot{V}O_2 = CO \times (1.34 \times Hb) \times (SaO_2 - SvO_2) \times 10.$$
$$\dot{V}O_2 = 5 \text{ L/min} \times (1.34 \times 12 \text{ gm/dL}) \times (0.95 - 0.60) \times 10$$

**Answer: B**

Marino, P. (2014) *The ICU Book*, 4th edn, Lippincott Williams & Wilkins, Philadelphia, PA.

**11** *A 47-year-old man presents with pancreatitis. He has not been able to eat or drink for 2 days and states he last urinated over 24 hours ago. He is admitted to the ICU and the following data was obtained: $SvO_2$ of 40%, Cardiac Index of 1.6 L/min/$m^2$, Hb of 16 gm/dL and $SaO_2$ of 100%. An expected oxygen extraction would be?*

**A** *10%*
**B** *30%*
**C** *40%*
**D** *60%*
**E** *70%*

Hypovolemic shock will lead to decreased mixed venous oxygen saturation and decreased cardiac index. Because of the decreased oxygen delivery secondary to decreased cardiac output the body can compensate delivery of oxygen to the tissues by increasing the oxygen extraction ($O_2ER$). $O_2ER$ is the ratio of oxygen uptake ($\dot{V}O_2$) of the tissue to the oxygen delivery ($DO_2$). Oxygen that is not extracted returns to the mixed venous circulation and the normal mixed venous saturation ($SvO_2$) from the pulmonary artery is approximately 75%. The equation for oxygen extraction is: $O_2ER = VO_2/DO_2$ This ratio is written out as follows:

$$O_2ER = \left[ CO \times (1.34 \times Hb) v (SaO_2 - SvO_2) \times 10 \right] / \left[ CO \times (1.34 \times Hb) \times SaO_2 \right]$$

A significant portion of the equation cancels out and is simplified as:

$$O_2ER = (SaO_2 - SvO_2) / SaO_2$$

From the question above the equation is calculated as follows:

$$O_2ER = (1 - 0.4) / 1$$

0.6 converts to 60% extraction.

This equation implies that the mixed venous blood is extracted from the pulmonary artery since blood from the vena cava may not be a reliable representation of true whole body mixed venous blood saturation. The heart has the highest oxygen extraction and in the ICU patient, may significantly alter this equation if blood from the vena cava, and not the pulmonary artery, is used. Different tissues/organs have different maximal extraction rates with the heart being able to extract the most, nearing 100%, while kidneys may be able to extract 50%. If the supply of the oxygen to the tissues is less than tissue demand, or because of limited extraction of any tissue causes dysoxia, this will lead to cell dysfunction and decreased ATP production with ensuing tissue/organ dysfunction such as seen in shock.

**Answer: D**

Fink, M.P., Abraham, E., Vincent, J.L., and Kochanek, P.M. (2005) *Text Book of Critical Care*, 5th edn, W.B. Saunders & Co., Philadelphia, PA.

Marino, P. (2014) *The ICU Book*, 4th edn, Lippincott Williams & Wilkins, Philadelphia, PA.

Parrillo, E.J. and Dellinger, R.P. (2014) *Critical Care Medicine: Principles of Diagnosis and Management in the Adult*, 4th edn, W.B. Saunders & Co., Philadelphia, PA.

**12** *All of the following shift the oxygen-dissociation curve to the left except:*
**A** *Fetal Hb*
**B** *Carboxyhemoglobin*
**C** *Respiratory alkalosis*
**D** *Hypercapnia*
**E** *Hypothermia*

The oxygen-dissociation curve is a great tool to help understand how hemoglobin carries and releases oxygen. This curve explains how and why oxygen is released at the peripheral capillaries but has increased uptake in the pulmonary capillaries. The sinusoidal curve plots the proportion of saturated hemoglobin on the vertical axis presented as a percentage against partial pressure of oxygen on the horizontal axis. There are multiple factors that will shift the curve either to the right or to the left. A rightward shift indicates that the hemoglobin has a decreased affinity for oxygen and will therefore release oxygen from the hemoglobin into the capillary bed. In other words, it is more difficult for hemoglobin to bind to oxygen but easier for the hemoglobin to release oxygen bound to it. The added effect of this rightward shift increases the partial pressure of oxygen in the tissues where it is mostly needed, such as during strenuous exercise, or various shock states. In contrast, a leftward shift indicates that the hemoglobin has an increased affinity for oxygen, so that the hemoglobin binds oxygen more easily but unloads it more judiciously. The following are common causes for a left shift: alkalemia, hypothermia, decreased $CO_2$, decreased 2,3 DPG and carboxyhemoglobin. The opposite will shift the curve to the right: acidemia, hyperthermia, increased $CO_2$, and increased 2,3 DPG.

**Answer: D**

Marini, J.J. and Wheeler, A.P. (2006) *Critical Care Medicine, The Essentials*, Lippincott Williams & Wilkins, Philadelphia, PA.

Marino, P. (2014) *The ICU Book*, 4th edn, Lippincott Williams & Wilkins, Philadelphia, PA.

**13** *The diagnosis of SIRS may include all of the following except:*
   **A** *A blood pressure of 86/40 mm Hg*
   **B** *Temperature of 35.6 °C*
   **C** *Heart rate of 103 beats/min*
   **D** *$PaCO_2$ of 27 mm Hg*
   **E** *WBC of $15.5 \times 10^3$/microL*

Hypotension is not included in the criteria for the diagnosis of systemic inflammatory response syndrome (SIRS). This is a syndrome characterized by abnormal regulation of various cytokines leading to generalized inflammation, organ dysfunction, and eventual organ failure. The definition of SIRS was formalized in 1992 following a consensus statement between the American College of Chest Physicians and the Society of Critical Care Medicine. SIRS is defined as being present when two or more of the following criteria are met:

Temperature : > 38°C or < 36°C

Heart rate : > 90 beats/min

Respiratory rate > 20 breaths/min or $PaCO_2$ < 32 mm Hg

WBC > 12 000/microL or < 4000/microL

The causes of SIRS can be broken down into infectious causes, which include sepsis, or noninfectious causes, which include trauma, burns, pancreatitis, hemorrhage, and ischemia. Treatment should be directed at treating the underlying etiology.

**Answer: A**

Marini, J.J. and Wheeler, A.P. (2006) *Critical Care Medicine, The Essentials*, Lippincott Williams & Wilkins, Philadelphia, PA.
Marino, P. (2014) *The ICU Book*, 4th edn, Lippincott Williams & Wilkins, Philadelphia, PA.

**14** *All of the following are consistent with cardiogenic shock except:*
   **A** *PAWP > 18 mm Hg*
   **B** *C.I. < 2.2 L/min/m²*
   **C** *$SaO_2$ of 86%*
   **D** *Pulmonary edema*
   **E** *$S_V O_2$ of 90%*

An $S_V O_2$ of 90% is increased from the normal range of 70–75%, which would be consistent with septic shock, not cardiogenic shock. The $S_V O_2$ is decreased in cardiogenic shock. Cardiogenic shock results from either a direct or indirect insult to the heart, leading to decreased cardiac output, despite normal ventricular filling pressures. Cardiogenic shock is diagnosed when the cardiac index is less than 2.2 L/min/m², and the pulmonary

wedge pressure is greater than 18 mm Hg. The decreased contractility of the left ventricle is the etiology of cardiogenic shock. Because the ejection fraction is reduced, the ventricle tries to compensate by becoming more compliant in an effort to increase stroke volume. After a certain point, the ventricle can no longer work at this level and begins to fail. This failure leads to a significant decrease in cardiac output, which then leads to pulmonary edema, an increase in myocardial oxygen consumption, and an increased intrapulmonary shunt, resulting in decreasing $SaO_2$.

**Answer: E**

Marini, J.J. and Wheeler, A.P. (2006) *Critical Care Medicine, The Essentials*, Lippincott Williams & Wilkins, Philadelphia, PA.
Marino, P. (2014) *The ICU Book*, 4th edn, Lippincott Williams & Wilkins, Philadelphia, PA.
Parrillo, E.J. and Dellinger, R.P. (2014) *Critical Care Medicine: Principles of Diagnosis and Management in the Adult*, 4th edn, W.B. Saunders & Co, Philadelphia, PA

**15** *All of the following statements regarding* pulsus paradoxus *are true except:*
   **A** *It is considered a normal variant during the inspiratory phase of respiration*
   **B** *It has been shown to be a positive predictor of the severity of pericardial tamponade*
   **C** *A slight increase in blood pressure occurs with inspiration, while a drop in blood pressure is seen during exhalation*
   **D** *Heart sounds can be auscultated when a radial pulse is not felt during exhalation*
   **E** *Cardiac cause may include constrictive pericarditis*

*Pulsus paradoxus* is defined as a decrease in systolic blood pressure greater than 10 mm Hg during the inspiratory phase of the respiratory cycle, and may be considered a normal variant. Under normal conditions, there are several changes in intrathoracic pressure that are transmitted to the heart and great vessels. During inspiration, there is distention of the right ventricle due to increased venous return. This causes the interventricular septum to bulge into the left ventricle, which then causes increased pooling of blood in the expanded lungs, further decreasing return to the left ventricle and decreasing stroke volume of the left ventricle. This fall in stroke volume of the left ventricle is reflected as a fall in systolic pressure. On clinical examination, you are able to auscultate the heart during inspiration but do lose a signal at the radial artery. *Pulsus paradoxus* has been shown to be a positive predictor of the severity of pericardial tamponade as demonstrated by Curtiss *et al.* *Pulsus paradoxus* has been linked to several disease processes that can be separated into cardiac, pulmonary, and noncardiac/nonpulmonary causes. Cardiac causes are tamponade, constrictive pericarditis, pericardial effusion, and cardiogenic shock. Pulmonary causes include pulmonary embolism, tension pneumothorax, asthma, and COPD. Noncardiac/nonpulmonary causes include anaphylactic reactions and shock, and obstruction of the superior vena cava.

**Answer: C**

Curtiss, E.I., Reddy, P.S., Uretsky, B.F., and Cecchetti, A.A. (1988) Pulsus paradoxus: definition and relation to the severity of cardiac tamponade. *American Heart Journal*, **115** (2), 391–398.

Guyton, A.G. (1963) *Circulatory Physiology: Cardiac Output and Its Regulation*, W. B. Saunders & Co., Philadelphia, PA.

**16** *Compared to neurogenic shock, spinal shock involves:*
   **A** *Loss of sensation followed by motor paralysis and gradual recovery of some reflexes*
   **B** *A distributive type of shock resulting in hypotension and bradycardia that is from disruption of the autonomic pathways within the spinal cord*
   **C** *A sudden loss of sympathetic stimulation to the blood vessels*
   **D** *The loss of neurologic function of the spinal cord following a prolonged period of hypotension*
   **E** *Loss of motor paralysis, severe neuropathic pain, and intact sensation*

Spinal shock refers to a loss of sensation followed by motor paralysis and eventual recovery of some reflexes. Spinal shock results in an acute flaccidity and loss of reflexes following spinal cord injury and is not due to systemic hypotension. Spinal shock initially presents as a complete loss of cord function. As the shock state improves some primitive reflexes such as the bulbocavernosus will return. Spinal shock can occur at any cord level. Neuropathic pain is not a usual symptom.

Neurogenic shock involves hemodynamic compromise associated with bradycardia and decreased systemic vascular resistance that typically occurs with injuries above the level of T6. Neurogenic shock is a form of distributive shock which is due to disruption of the sympathetic autonomic pathways within the spinal cord, resulting in hypotension and bradycardia. Treatment consists of volume resuscitation and vasopressors (pure alpha-agonist) for blood pressure control.

**Answer: A**

Marini, J.J. and Wheeler, A.P. (2006) *Critical Care Medicine, The Essentials*, Lippincott Williams & Wilkins, Philadelphia, PA.

Mattox, L.K., Moore, E.E., and Faliciano, V.D. (2013) *Trauma*, 7th edn, McGraw-Hill. New York, NY.

Piepmeyer, J.M., Lehmann, K.B. and Lane, J.G. (1985) Cardiovascular instability following acute cervical spine trauma. *Central Nervous System Trauma*, **2**, 153–159.

**17** *A patient sustains significant thoracoabdominal injuries from a 20-foot fall. His hemodynamic profile is as follows: decreased cardiac output, increased systemic vascular resistance, decreased pulmonary wedge pressure, decreased CVP and decreased mixed venous oxygen. All of the following may be appropriate to administer except:*
   **A** *Steroids*
   **B** *Blood products*
   **C** *Colloids*
   **D** *Isotonic solution*
   **E** *Hypertonic solution*

The importance of recognizing hypovolemic/hemorrhagic shock is paramount to timely and accurate treatment. It is fundamental to understand that in hypovolemic shock, the treatment is to stop the loss of volume and or hemorrhage and to restore volume. Isotonic and hypertonic solution may be used for the purpose of restoring intravascular volume. In the case of hemorrhagic shock, it is even more important to restore the oxygen-carrying capabilities while restoring volume with blood products capable of transporting oxygen from the lungs to the organs and tissues. Steroids have no role in hypovolemic/hemorrhagic shock.

**Answer: A**

Mattox, L.K., Moore, E.E., and Faliciano, V.D. (2013) *Trauma*, 7th edn. McGraw-Hill. New York, NY

Parrillo, E.J. and Dellinger, R.P. (2014) *Critical Care Medicine: Principles of Diagnosis and Management in the Adult*, 4th edn, W.B. Saunders & Co., Philadelphia, PA

# 3

# ECMO

*Andy Michaels, MD*

1 *Which of the following is not a relative contraindication for ECMO in adults with ARDS?*
   A *Mechanical ventilation for more than 7 days with "high" ventilator settings (i.e., $FiO_2 > 0.9$, Pplat > 30 cm $H_2O$)*
   B *Major immunosuppression (absolute neutrophil count < 400/$mm^3$)*
   C *Recent trauma*
   D *Non-recoverable comorbidity such as major CNS damage or terminal malignancy*
   E *Age greater than 65 years*

The indications for ECMO are fairly clear. For respiratory failure with severe hypoxia (PF ratio < 100 on a $FiO_2 > 0.9$) or hypercarbia (pH < 7.2 despite maximal safe ventilation), veno-venous (VV) ECMO is indicated. Other respiratory indications include massive air leak and bridge to pulmonary transplant. For cardiac indications, typically, veno-arterial (VA) ECMO is used. The indications include refractory cardiogenic shock, massive pulmonary embolus, cardiac arrest or failure to wean from bypass after cardiac surgery.

Contraindications for ECMO are less well defined and, as the extent of international experience has illuminated the discussion, some experts suggest that there are no absolute contraindications to the use of ECMO. Most practitioners however would recognize the list above as "relative" contraindications except for patients with non-recoverable comorbidity such as major CNS damage or terminal malignancy. The term "relative contraindication" has historical interest only as many patients with recent trauma, immunosuppression, lung injurious pre-ECMO ventilation and advanced age have been successfully treated with ECMO in recent years.

**Answer D**

Bartlett, R.H. (2016) Extracorporeal membrane oxygenation (ECMO) in adults, *Up To Date*, September.
ELSO Adult Respiratory Failure Supplement to the ELSO General Guidelines, December 2013.

2 *A 30-year-old woman with group A beta-hemolytic streptococcal sepsis is placed on veno-arterial ECMO by a percutaneous femoro-femoral route. She was cannulated with a 19 French arterial and a 25 French venous cannula. She was on both dobutamine and epinephrine drips at the initiation of ECMO and her $PaO_2$:$FiO_2$ ratio was 80 on a $FiO_2$ of 100% with APRV of 35 mm Hg over 15 mm Hg. She has a creatinine of 3.5 and is oliguric. After being placed on ECMO, her $PaO_2$ rises to 200 in the right radial arterial line with an $O_2$ saturation of 97%. An ECHO shows severe left ventricular hypokinesis. After 6 hours on ECMO her pressors have been weaned off and her mean arterial pressure is 65 mm Hg and pulsatile, however her $O_2$ saturation measured by a pulse oximeter on the right hand falls to 67%. The ECMO circuit appears to be functioning well, flow is unchanged at 5Lpm and her ECMO circuit arterial saturation has remained 100%.*
   *The appropriate maneuver is to:*
   A *Place another venous cannula to improve flow rates*
   B *Place a distal perfusion cannula in her femoral artery and perform a 4-compartment fasciotomy*
   C *Place a dialysis circuit into the ECMO circuit and begin CVVH*
   D *Perform a cutdown on her axillary artery with an end to side graft, cannulate her right jugular vein and reinstitute VA ECMO by a proximal route*
   E *Place a right jugular venous infusion catheter, initiate veno-venous ECMO and remove her femoral arterial cannula.*

This patient has developed what is known as the "Harlequin Syndrome" where her native cardiac output has improved and she has competing flow in the descending aorta between her recovering native cardiac output and her retrograde ECMO inflow. The result is a well-oxygenated lower body, a relatively hypoxic upper body and left ventricular strain.

*Surgical Critical Care and Emergency Surgery: Clinical Questions and Answers,* Second Edition.
Edited by Forrest "Dell" Moore, Peter Rhee, and Gerard J. Fulda.
© 2018 John Wiley & Sons Ltd. Published 2018 by John Wiley & Sons Ltd.
Companion website: www.wiley.com/go/moore/surgical_criticalcare_and_emergency_surgery

Generally, despite the need for pressor and evidence of renal injury, veno-venous (VV) ECMO is a better choice for a patient like the one described. It is unlikely that her lungs have recovered and the scenario described is typical for a patient who is placed on veno-arterial (VA) ECMO through the groin when VV would have been more appropriate.

She will still need ECMO for hypoxia for several days and so VV ECMO should be initiated to support her now. The best option is to place a right IJ infusion cannula, remove the femoral cannula and repair the femoral artery. The VA configuration, while initially tolerable, is now inappropriate and is causing harm. The pressor requirements and cardiac failure in acute sepsis often recover rapidly with the delivery of oxygen and frequently a similar progression of cardiac recovery is seen when VV is used in a patient like the one described. Occasionally poor flow can be improved by the placement of a second venous cannula but that is not the problem described and that is why A is not the answer. Answer B is not correct as the problem is not due to lack of flow in the leg. If a femoral arterial cannula is placed, especially in a patient with small vessels, distal ischemia may result. If this is discovered after the fact, a distal perfusion catheter +/- fasciotomies is indicated, but it is better to place a perfusion catheter at the time of cannulation. Option C is not the answer because the presence of renal insufficiency and need for renal replacement therapy has nothing to do with and will not correct the described physiology. Option D is not the answer as the current circuit is flowing well and has not changed.

**Answer E**

Madershahian, N., Nagib, R., Wippermann, J., *et al.* (2006) A simple technique of distal limb perfusion during prolonged femoro-femoral cannulation. *Journal of Cardiac Surgery*, **21** (2), 168–169.

Rupprecht, L., Lunz, D., Philipp, A., *et al.* (2015) Pitfalls in percutaneous ECMO cannulation. *Heart Lung and Vessels*, **7** (4), 320–326.

**3** *A 5 foot 8 inch, 250 pound man (BMI 38) is placed on VV ECMO for H1N1 pneumonia. His pre-ECMO PF ratio is 70 and his $O_2$ saturation is 78% on PRVC with PEEP of 15 and $FiO_2$ of 100%. He is cannulated with a 31 French dual lumen cannula in the right internal jugular vein and after ECMO is initiated he is placed on SIMV 40%, rate of 12, PEEP of 5 mm Hg and TV of 500 cc. His ECMO circuit has an arterial saturation of 100% and a venous saturation of 60% with flow of 5 Lpm. His $SaO_2$ in the radial arterial line is 80%. His hemoglobin is 10 g/dL, his creatinine is 1.3, he is not on any pressors agents and his pH is 7.34.*

*The next appropriate maneuver is to:*

**A** *Transfuse him to a hemoglobin of > 12 g/dL*
**B** *Convert his right internal jugular dual lumen veno-venous (RIJ DLVV) cannula to a drainage cannula, place a femoral arterial cannula and convert him to VA ECMO*
**C** *Increase the ECMO flow rate to 7 Lpm*
**D** *Increase the ECMO sweep to clear $CO_2$*
**E** *Do nothing, he has adequate support*

A thorough understanding of oxygen delivery and consumption is essential to manage many adult ECMO patients because their oxygen saturations may seem low while their $O_2$ delivery, and more importantly, their delivery:consumption ratio ($DO_2$:$VO_2$) is adequate. This patient is in no distress, has adequate support and requires no intervention. His $SaO_2$ is 80% and his $SvO_2$ (as measured in the ECMO venous line) is 60%. Even though his arterial saturation is only 80% on ECMO his "mixed venous" saturation is 60% and this represents $DO_2$:$VO_2$ of 4:1 [80%/(80%−60%)] which is sufficient to maintain aerobic metabolism with reserve. Answer A is not correct because even though transfusions in ECMO is controversial and the current ELSO guidelines suggest that adults on ECMO for ARDS should be transfused to a hemoglobin of 12–14 g/dL, many centers follow general ICU guidelines for transfusion and the current hemoglobin of 10 g/dL is adequate. Answer C is not correct because increased ECMO flow (and 7 Lpm as listed is a very high rate of flow) is unnecessary as the patient does not have any indication that the delivery of oxygen is inadequate. B and D are not the answer as the patient does not have high $CO_2$ and there is no indication to convert to VA as the patient currently has adequate support.

**Answer E**

ELSO Guidelines for Cardiopulmonary Extracorporeal Life Support Extracorporeal Life Support Organization, Version 1.3 November 2013 Ann Arbor, MI, www.elsonet.org (accessed November 2013).

Montisci, A., Maj, G., Zangrillo, A., *et al.* (2015) Management of refractory hypoxemia during venovenous extracorporeal membrane oxygenation for ARDS. *ASAIO (American Society for Artificial Internal Organs) Journal*, **61**, 227–236.

**4** *Which of the following adult ECMO patients is most likely to be discharged alive from the hospital after treatment for refractory hypoxemic respiratory failure?*
**A** *62-year-old man with bacterial pneumonia who has been on the ventilator for 4 days and has had neuromuscular blockade. The patient's $PaO_2$:$FiO_2$ ratio is 80*

B *25-year-old woman who has bacterial pneumonia and bacterial endometritis following childbirth. She has been on the ventilator for 36 hours and has been treated with nitric oxide. The patient's PaO$_2$:FiO$_2$ ratio is 100*

C *32-year-old male trauma patient who has been on the ventilator for 5 days and has been treated with neuromuscular blockade. The patient's PaO$_2$:FiO$_2$ ratio is 56*

D *18-year-old woman with viral pneumonia who has been ventilated for 3 days and has had peak airway pressures > 42 cm H$_2$O and pCO$_2$ > 75 mm Hg. The patient's PaO$_2$:FiO$_2$ ratio is 96*

E *52-year-old man who aspirated and suffered a cardiac arrest with return of spontaneous circulation. He has been ventilated for three days and has a PaO$_2$:FiO$_2$ ratio of 88*

Patient selection is an essential skill for physicians treating adult respiratory failure with ECMO. There are many factors to consider and one tool that synthesizes many of the variables is the RESP score. Developed in a cohort of 2355 patients and based in a multivariate logistic regression the scale utilizes a number of variables that are available for assessment prior to the initiation of ECMO. Based on the values of these variables, candidates for ECMO support may be stratified based upon expected survival. There are five categories and expected survival ranges from 18% to 92% based on which category a patient is placed within.

In general, the age of an adult patient is not a factor until they are older than 50 years. Beyond that, there is no upper age limit for the use of ECMO but expected survival decreases with increasing age. The time a patient has been treated with mechanical ventilation negatively impacts survival, particularly if there is evidence of ventilator induced lung injury (VILI). Evidence of VILI includes, but is not limited to, elevated peak airway pressures. The maneuvers performed prior to initiation also affect outcome. Patients treated with neuromuscular blockade were more likely to survive while those treated with nitric oxide did less well.

Evidence of secondary problems is associated with poor outcome. Additional non-pulmonary sources of infection, CNS dysfunction, immunocompromised status or poor perfusion (bicarbonate drip or cardiac arrest) all were associated with a reduced expected survival. Finally, the primary respiratory diagnosis had much effect on outcome with asthma being the most favorable followed by aspiration and the bacterial, viral or ARDS related to trauma and burns. Non-respiratory and chronic respiratory indications have the poorest prognosis.

Table 3.1 and the website www.respscore.com may be helpful to understand the variables that comprise the

**Table 3.1** The RESP score at ECMO initiation.

| Parameter | Score |
|---|---|
| Age, yr | |
| 18 – 49 | 0 |
| 50 – 59 | −2 |
| ≥60 | −3 |
| Immunocompromised status* | −2 |
| Mechanical ventilation prior to initiation of ECMO | |
| <48 h | 3 |
| 48 h – 7 d | 1 |
| >7 d | 0 |
| Acute respiratory diagnosis group (select only one) | |
| Viral pneumonia | 3 |
| Bacterial pneumonia | 3 |
| Asthma | 11 |
| Trauma and burn | 3 |
| Aspiration pneumonitis | 5 |
| Other acute respiratory diagnoses | 1 |
| Nonrespiratory and chronic respiratory diagnoses | 0 |
| Central nervous system dysfunction[†] | −7 |
| Acute associated (nonpulmonary) infection[‡] | −3 |
| Neuromuscular blockade agents before ECMO | 1 |
| Nitric oxide use before ECMO | −1 |
| Bicarbonate infusion before ECMO | −2 |
| Cardiac arrest before ECMO | −2 |
| PaCO$_2$, mm Hg | |
| <75 | 0 |
| ≥75 | −1 |
| Peak inspiratory pressure, cm H$_2$O | |
| <42 | 0 |
| ≥42 | −1 |
| Total score | −22 to 15 |

**Hospital Survival by Risk Class**

| Total RESP Score | Risk Class | Survival |
|---|---|---|
| ≥6 | I | 92% |
| 3 to 5 | II | 76% |
| −1 to 2 | III | 57% |
| −5 to −2 | IV | 33% |
| ≤−6 | V | 18% |

*Definition of abbreviations*: ECMO = extracorporeal membrane oxygenation; RESP = Respiratory ECMO Survival Prediction.
An online calculator is available at www.respscore.com.
* "Immunocompromised" is defined as hematological malignancies, solid tumor, solid organ transplantation, human immunodeficiency virus, and cirrhosis.
† "Central nervous system dysfunction" diagnosis combined neurotrauma, stroke, encephalopathy, cerebral embolism, and seizure and epileptic syndrome.
‡ "Acute associated (nonpulmonary) infection" is defined as another bacterial, viral, parasitic, or fungal infection that did not involve the lung.

RESP score and their relationship to survival to discharge. Based on the data used to derive the RESP score, the patient with the highest RESP score and the best chance of survival to discharge is the trauma patient in option C.

**Answer C**

Schmidt, M., Bailey, M., Sheldrake, J., *et al.* (2014) Predicting survival after ECMO for severe acute respiratory failure: the respiratory ECMO survival prediction (RESP)-score. *American Journal of Respiratory and Critical Care Medicine*, **189** (11), 1374–1382.

5 *In adults who have suffered traumatic injury, the use of ECMO to treat acute hypoxic respiratory failure is:*
   A *Contra-indicated because of the required anti-coagulation for ECMO*
   B *Shown to have no benefit in addition to the use of the APRV (airway pressure release ventilation) mode of ventilation*
   C *Only indicated after 72 hours has elapsed from the most recent operation or injury*
   D *Associated with a higher rate of survival to discharge in patients with refractory hypoxemic ARDS compared with those treated by conventional means*
   E *A new application of the technology emerging in practice many years after the use of ECMO for other causes of lung failure*

ECMO has been used for the injured since the beginning of its clinical use and thus answer E is not correct. In 1972, the first adult treated with ECMO for lung failure was a trauma patient. With improvements in ECMO technology and anti-coagulation practices, ECMO has been used increasingly in the injured with excellent results. ECMO may be used for cardiopulmonary support in refractory shock with a VA approach, but the more frequent (and described above) scenario is ECMO VV support for acute refractory hypoxemic ARDS. The early application of ECMO for patients with $PaO_2:FiO_2$ ratio $< 80$ on a $FiO_2 > 0.9$ compared with a matched cohort treated with current standard ventilation protocols using APRV and/or HFV showed that 65% of the patients treated with ECMO survived to hospital discharge vs 24% of the patients treated by conventional means. ECMO can be used for acute ARDS or cardiovascular support even during the initial resuscitative operations and modern circuits are able to function for many days with no heparin at all and thus answer A is not correct. The early institution of ECMO for patients with refractory ARDS prevents further consequences of

hypoxia and, if properly utilized with "lung rest" ventilator settings on ECMO, prevents ventilator induced lung injury. This lung injury is found with all forms of mechanical ventilation.

**Answer D**

Guirand, D.M., Okoye, O.T., Schmid, B.St., *et al.* (2014) Venovenous extracorporeal life support improves survival adult trauma patients with acute hypoxemic respiratory failure: a multicenter retrospective cohort study. *The Journal of Trauma and Acute Care Surgery*, **76**, 1275–1281.
Hill, J.D., O'Brien, T.G., Murray, J.J., *et al.* (1972) Prolonged extra-corporeal oxygenation for acute post-traumatic respiratory failure (shock-lung syndrome). Use of the Bramson membrane lung. *New England Journal of Medicine*, **286**, 629–634.

6 *Which of the following is NOT a component of coagulopathy associated with ECMO?*
   A *Thrombocytopenia*
   B *Pharmacologic anticoagulation*
   C *Acquired von Willebrand syndrome*
   D *Platelet dysfunction*
   E *Antithrombin III deficiency*

All of the defects in the clotting cascade listed above are found in patients placed on ECMO, but antithrombin III (ATIII) deficiency is not characterized by coagulopathy. This situation is noted when the amount of heparin necessary to anticoagulate a patient to a desired level increases without explanation. This is because ATIII is essential to heparin's mode of activity which enhances the thrombin:antithrombin complex formation. In the situation of increasing heparin dose required to maintain a stable level of anticoagulation it is appropriate to check the antithrombin III level and replace it if it is below 80% with either a concentrate or fresh frozen plasma.

The other defects in the clotting cascade listed above are common factors in any ECMO case, particularly if there is bleeding involved. ECMO is associated with thrombocytopenia, platelet dysfunction, pharmacologic anticoagulation (utilizing heparin or other anticoagulants), and acquired von Willebrand syndrome.

**Answer E**

Murphy, D.A., Hockings, L.E., Andrews, R.K., *et al.* (2015) Extracorporeal membrane oxygenation–hemostatic complications. *Transfusion Medicine Reviews*, **29**, 90–101.

7 *A 56-year-old female is on VV ECMO for acute hypoxemic ARDS due to H1N1 pneumonia. It is ECMO day three. Her $PaCO_2$ is 52 and her pH is 7.34 and her serum lactate is 1.3 mmol/dL.*

*To correct her acid:base abnormality, she should be treated by:*

A *Increasing her minute ventilation on the ventilator*

B *Adding a second venous line to the ECMO circuit*

C *Increasing the rate of sweep gas in the ECMO circuit*

D *Increasing the flow of the ECMO circuit*

E *Starting a bicarbonate drip*

This appears to be an acute, uncompensated respiratory acidosis. The scenario does not discuss her degree of oxygenation nor does it describe any evidence of metabolic acidosis. The only thing necessary to correct the $pCO_2$ and the pH is to increase the rate of sweep gas in the ECMO circuit thus answer C is correct. It would be an error try to utilize the ventilator and try to increase the minute ventilation of the injured lungs during the acute hypoxic phase for either oxygenation or ventilation and thus answer A is not correct. There are many strategies for "lung rest" on ECMO but only high airway pressures after ECMO has been initiated are associated with poor outcomes. Adding a second venous drainage cannula is only useful in some cases if the flow is limited by venous return to the circuit and thus answer B is not correct. Increasing the rate of flow of the ECMO circuit will increase oxygen delivery but not ventilation and thus answer D is also incorrect. Likewise, adding additional drainage may improve flow and oxygen delivery but will not affect the $pCO_2$. Although occasionally a bicarbonate drip is used in a patient is weaning from ECMO who is not able to fully normalize $pCO_2$ even though their ability to oxygenate has recovered it is not indicated when the circuit is still available and necessary for the support of oxygenation.

**Answer C**

Neto, A.S., Schnidt, M., Azevedo, L.C., *et al.* (2016) Associations between ventilator settings during extracorporeal membrane oxygenation for refractory hypoxemia and outcome in patients with acute respiratory distress syndrome: a pooled individual patient data analysis. *Intensive Care Medicine*, **42**, 1672–1684.

8 *An adult with ARDS from bacterial pneumonia has been on ECMO for 4 days because of severe hypoxia. ECMO flow is at 5 Lpm and the arterial saturation is 88%. The ventilator is set to PCV 20/10, FiO₂ of 30% with RR of 10.*

   *The best indicator that it is time to trial off ECMO is:*

A *The $pCO_2$ decreases when the ventilator is set to PCV 35/12, FiO₂ 0.80*

B *When the ventilator is set to FiO₂ of 100% the patient arterial saturation increases to 100%*

C *The ECMO sweep gas has been reduced by half to maintain the same $pCO_2$*

D *The patient is weaned from inotropic medications and able to be diuresed*

E *The patient is interactive with minimal sedation and their chest x-ray is beginning to clear*

There are a number of ways to evaluate a patient on ECMO, but the most important consideration is the original indication for ECMO and the resolution of that problem. The patient presented above is in a simple situation of hypoxia from pneumonia. When the native lung achieves significant function, recruitment and weaning should be initiated. The maneuver described in choice B is called the Cilley test and is simply setting the FiO₂ to 100% on the ventilator with no other changes. A positive test is a rapid increase of $SaO_2$ to 100%. When this condition is met, the native lung is contributing significant oxygenation and efforts to recruit the pulmonary reserve should begin. In contrast to the relative harmlessness of changing the FiO₂ on the ventilator for a patient on ECMO, adjusting the pressures to try to "open" the lung and test ventilation is ill advised and could be harmful. Thus answer A is not correct. The decrease in sweep gas on the ECMO circuit is a good indicator of improving native ventilation but is not an indicator of improved oxygenation and thus answer C is not correct. Patient's cardiovascular and neurologic states should be managed to achieve normal physiology as soon as possible and throughout their care but does not indicate whether the lungs have improved enough to be wean off ECMO. Thus answer D and E are not correct.

**Answer B**

ELSO Adult Respiratory Failure Supplement to the ELSO General Guidelines, December 2013.

Van Meurs, K., Zwischenberger and the Extracorporeal Life Support Organization (2005) *ECMO Extracorporeal Cardiopulmonary Support in Critical Care*, 3rd edn, Extracorporeal Life Support Organization, Ann Arbor, Michigan

9 *In a patient who is on ECMO for severe ARDS and begins to bleed several hundred cc/shift from a previously placed chest tube that had not been draining blood before the best option listed is to:*

A *Transfuse platelets to above 150 000 /uL*

B *Adjust the heparin infusion for an anti-Xa level of 0.70*

C *Adjust the heparin infusion for an ACT 180–220*

D *Begin aminocaproic acid for fibrinolysis*

E *Place another chest tube to prevent retained hemothorax*

The central principle in the management of bleeding on ECMO is to prevent it. All maneuvers must be conducted with great care, modified techniques and thoughtful timing to prevent and reduce the negative impact of one of the most frequent and damaging complications on ECMO. There are several factors involved in the complex scenario of bleeding on ECMO. Systemic anticoagulation predisposes the patient to hemorrhage, both intervention stimulated and spontaneous. There have been no noted differences in bleeding incidence between anticoagulation agents and most programs utilize adjusted dose heparin with a target activated clotting time (ACT) of >1.5 times the measured normal value for that device. This generally is an ACT of 140–160. Both the anti-Xa level of 0.70 and the ACT of 180–220 listed above reflect more significant anticoagulation.

The general principles for bleeding depend on two major variables – where is the patient bleeding and what is the status of the patient's coagulation system. The most common site for bleeding is the cannulation site and meticulous technique, careful securing of the lines to include a purse-string stitch and aggressive management of oozing generally will suffice. Additionally, significant bleeding may occur, either spontaneously of after instrumentation from mucous membranes, the GI or GU tract or spontaneously into the injured lung, airway or pleural space. Spontaneous bleeding into the head is a generally lethal complication and not rare.

Manipulation of the clotting system is generally necessary for bleeding that requires transfusion, especially from operative sites. The first step is to reduce (or eliminate) the systemic anticoagulation. Second is to assure that the platelet count is > 100 000, the INR is < 1.5 and that there is no hypofibrinogenemia or significant fibrinolysis taking place. Blood and products should be used appropriately to restore normal levels of factors, platelets, and fibrinogen. Various means for determining clotting status exist and there is growing enthusiasm for bedside thromboelastography (TEG or ROTEM). If fibrinolysis is demonstrated or suspected, antifibrinolytics should be used. It has long been common practice to use ε-aminocaproic acid in conjunction with operative interventions.

Finally, surgical interventions to correct hemorrhage must be carefully chosen, timed, and conducted. Often, collaboration with interventional radiology may provide a less damaging approach to vascular, soft tissue, and even chest wall bleeding. All procedures should be conducted with absolute attention to hemostasis and the liberal use of electrocautery, topical hemostatic agents and, if necessary, packing and repeated operations. Placing chest tubes can be cause significant complications in this scenario of spontaneous bleeding from coagulopathy. Chest tubes may also bleed several days after placement

and this is generally from the chest wall at the insertion site. A basic principle is to limit instrumentation and to place chest tubes only if the drainage will prevent a major complication or hasten recovery.

One useful caveat is that for patients on VV ECMO, all bleeding from the chest will be bright red even though it may be venous.

**Answer D**

Mazzeffi, M., Greenwood, J., Tanaka, K., *et al.* (2016) Bleeding, transfusion, and mortality on extracorporeal life support: ECLS working group on thrombosis and hemostasis. *The Annals of Thoracic Surgery*, **101** (2), 682–689.

Murphy, D.A., Hockings, L.E., Andrews, R.K., *et al.* (2015): Extracorporeal membrane oxygenation-hemostatic complications. *Transfusion Medicine Reviews*, **29** (2), 90–101.

Paden, M.L., Conrad, S.A., Rycus, P.T., *et al.* (2013) Extracorporeal Life Support Organization Registry report 2012. *ASAIO Journal*, **59**, pp. 202–210.

**10**  *The following are all complications of a right internal jugular dual lumen veno-venous ECMO cannula placement except:*
   **A**  *Cardiac Tamponade*
   **B**  *Hepatic vein cannulation*
   **C**  *Pneumothorax*
   **D**  *Recirculation*
   **E**  *Harlequin Syndrome*

The use of the Avalon Elite BiCaval Dual Lumen catheter (Avalon Laboratories, LLC, CA) has become increasingly popular in the treatment of adults with ARDS for several reasons. First, it involves a single site of cannulation and reduces all the risks of vascular access (infection, injury, thrombosis, catheter dislodgement, nursing care, etc.) by half. Second, with the groin free, patients may be managed with less sedation and they can participate in their care more actively. There is also less recirculation and flows of 6 Lpm may be achieved with the 31 French model.

There are many known complications of this procedure and they fall into three general categories, each with an imaging adjuvant that reduces these risks. First, there are all the issues of vascular access in the right neck. Recommendations include using real-time ultrasound guidance and a more posterior-superior approach to allow the catheter a more gradual path into the vein. Local bleeding at the cannulation site is the most common problem and a well-placed purse-string stitch and several fixation stitches reduce this. Second, there are problems with the placement of the wire by Seldinger technique and subsequent vascular injuries by serial dilation or ultimate malposition. The best way to avoid these problems is to use real-time fluoroscopy to visualize the wire position and observe the passages of the dilators. Common malposition errors include coiling within the right atrium leading to malposition or perforation of the heart with tamponade or placement of the distal drainage ports in the hepatic veins. Some practitioners utilize a more stiff wire (Amplatz) for the final steps to better support the cannula during placement.

Finally, there can be significant flow and/or recirculation issues if the infusion port is not within the right atrium and oriented towards the tricuspid valve. Transesophageal echocardiography (TEE) is instrumental to assuring that the inflow jet is properly positioned.

The Harlequin Syndrome is a complication of femoral arterial cannulation for VA ECMO and does not occur with either dual lumen or dual cannula VV ECMO.

**Answer E**

Javidfar, J., Wang, D., Zwischenberger, J.B., *et al.* (2011) Insertion of Bicaval Dual Lumen extracorporeal membrane oxygenation catheter with image guidance. *ASAIO Journal,* **57**, 203–205.

Reeb, J., Olland, A., Renaud, S., *et al.* (2016) Vascular access for extracorporeal life support: tips and tricks. *Journal of Thoracic Disease,* **8** (Suppl 4), S353–S363.

**The next five questions are variations of the following scenario (references are combined).**

*You have been consulted to consider a 32-year-old woman with viral pneumonia for ECMO. She has been on a ventilator for 36 hours with ARDSnet protective settings and a PEEP of 16 cm H$_2$O. The FiO$_2$ on the ventilator is 80% and her arterial blood gas measurements (from a right radial arterial line) are 7.25 / 62 / 75 / 26 (90%). Her only interventions have been bronchoscopy, inhaled nitric oxide and neuromuscular blockade. A transthoracic cardiac ECHO shows moderate right ventricular dilation and mild tricuspid regurgitation. A PA catheter shows PA pressures of 42/12 mm Hg with a PA wedge of 20 mm Hg and SvO$_2$ of 50. She is not on pressors and is making urine.*

11  *The best choice for her at this point would be to:*
   A *Not escalate care*
   B *Be placed on a bicarbonate drip to correct her respiratory acidosis from permissive hypercapnia*
   C *Be placed on VA ECMO because she is showing evidence of acute cor pulmonale*
   D *Be placed on VV ECMO for profound hypoxemic ARDS*
   E *Be placed in a prone position*

The patient described has severe ARDS by the Berlin criteria (PaO$_2$:FiO$_2$ ratio < 100) and is facing a predicted mortality of 45%. She is being ventilated with accepted standards and is suffering from acute hypoxemic ARDS. A pH of 7.25 due to mild hypercapnia does not need to be addressed by either increasing her minute ventilation or by adding a solution of bicarbonate. In fact, mild to moderate hypercapnia is the direct result of limiting the amount of ventilation and hence ventilator induced lung injury. Given her degree of hypoxia ECMO is a consideration at this point, but she has not had a trial of prone positioning. Many patients respond to positional therapy with intermittent prone positioning with much improved respiratory dynamics and performance and require no further interventions. It is always challenging to apply positional therapy to a patient this compromised so this should only be done in an ICU with experience in this type of care.

The classic criteria for ECMO for respiratory failure are similar in most programs and involve either severe hypercapnia or hypoxemia *DESPITE and AFTER* optimal care. This level of care currently includes protective ventilation and advanced ventilatory modes, neuromuscular blockade, inhaled nitric oxide or prostacyclin and positional therapy. The degree of impairment varies from program to program but ECMO is typically considered if PF ratio is < 80 on a FiO$_2$ of > 0.80 or if pH is < 7.2 on maximal safe ventilator settings.

If proning is not an option, she has a PF ratio of 94 and is on 80% FiO$_2$ and is clearly nearing the threshold for ECMO. VA ECMO would be inappropriate. Her right heart strain is very mild and typical for a patient with ARDS. This will resolve with the provision of oxygenated blood to the currently hypoxic and vaso-constricting pulmonary vasculature. If she is to be placed on ECMO, VV, preferably with a dual lumen catheter would be the choice.

**Answer E**

*She responds well to prone positioning and is started on the ICU proning protocol with several positional changes each day. Initially her PF ratio improves to 160, her pCO$_2$ declines to 45 and she is able to be weaned to an FiO$_2$ of 0.6.*

12  *The best choice for her at this point would be to:*
   A *Not escalate care*
   B *Be placed on a bicarbonate drip to correct her respiratory acidosis from permissive hypercapnia*
   C *Be placed on VA ECMO because she is showing evidence of acute cor pulmonale*
   D *Be placed on VV ECMO for profound hypoxemic ARDS*
   E *Be placed in a prone position*

She has improved as the prone position helped with the hypoxia through recruitment and with the hypercarbia which is now down to 45 mm Hg. She thus does not need a bicarbonate drip, nor ECMO at this time.

**Answer A**

*Two days later you are called to the bedside by the nurse who reports a new fever, progressive oliguria and decreasing $O_2$ saturation and blood pressure. The patient is now on 10 mcg of dopamine and milrinone has just been started. Her current ventilator settings are APRV 32/15, 100% and her PF ratio is 75. Her PA saturation is 47% and the PA pressures are 48/12 mm Hg. Her systemic pressures are 110/70 mm Hg and her heart rate is 96 beats/min.*

13  The best choice for her at this point would be to:
   A  Undergo bronchoscopy and washing sent for bacteriology and started on empiric antibiotics for hospital-acquired pneumonia
   B  Initiate acute renal replacement therapy due to volume overload
   C  Be placed on VA ECMO because now she is showing evidence of shock in addition to acute cor pulmonale
   D  Be placed on VV ECMO for profound hypoxemic ARDS
   E  Be sent to the CT scanner to identify the source of her new infection

She has had some sort of second insult and hospital acquired pneumonia is the likely cause, but this is incidental to the observation that she has changed from a patient with adequate support to one who is decompensating. She will surely require antibiotics and may need renal replacement therapy but the most threatening aspect of her situation is profound hypoxemia and the exhaustion of all available measures short of VV ECMO. Depending on the set up of the facility, it may be possible to place a DLVV cannula (if fluoroscopy is available in the ICU to supplement U/S and TEE), but more likely, due to the risk of intra-hospital transfer to the angiography suite, she will need to have a two-cannula system placed in the ICU.

Again, the modest hemodynamic instability, renal injury, and elevated PA pressures and RV strain are typical of ARDS with sepsis and will resolve on VV ECMO. It is important to manage patients with ARDS in a euvolemic state. Often crystalloids are limited to prevent the accumulation of extravascular lung water but this is erroneous thinking because the edema of ARDS is not hydrostatic and is non-cardiogenic. On the other hand, exuberant use of high levels of PEEP may decrease venous return and lead to increasing IV replacement to increase the CVP and restore cardiac output.

VA ECMO is indicated for pulmonary hypertension but typically in patients with end stage lung disease and PA pressures > 50% of systemic. Even if she should become more compromised including the need for renal replacement therapy and vasopressor support, the correct choice is VV ECMO.

**Answer D**

*After an uncomplicated placement of a 27 French venous cannula in the right femoral vein and a 21 French arterial cannula in the right internal jugular vein ECMO flow is initiated. She has oximeters on her left index finger, the tip of her PA catheter and the venous line of her ECMO circuit. For the next questions, assume that the oxygen provided to the ECMO circuit is adequate and stable, pump flow is 5 Lpm and circuit pressures are acceptable and unchanged.*

14  Her PA saturation is now 65% and her $SaO_2$ is 82% and her ECCV (ECMO venous saturation) is 77%. The next maneuver should be to:
   A  Transfuse her because she needs more oxygen carrying capacity
   B  Add CVVH to her ECMO circuit to accelerate the mobilization of extravascular lung water
   C  Switch to VA ECMO because she is not receiving adequate support
   D  Increase her ECMO flow rate
   E  Withdraw the groin cannula several centimeters

The physiology demonstrated is recirculation. More oxygenated blood from the IJ cannula is going through the venous line (sat 75%) than through her pulmonary artery (sat 65%). There are a number of causes for recirculation but the most frequent is that the drainage cannula is too close to the infusion cannula and "steals" flow away from the tricuspid valve. The ideal place for a venous cannula is just below the right atrium in the retro-hepatic portion of the inferior vena cava.

When oxygen delivery is insufficient, both increasing the hemoglobin and increasing the ECMO flow will increase delivery, but first it is essential to assure the circuit is configured and functioning properly. The fact that there is more oxygen in the venous drainage cannula than the pulmonary artery indicates that the circuit is not ideal and that there is recirculation. Likewise, achieving euvolemia and eliminating the effects of fluid overload is a necessary step during recovery but will not address the problem described.

Recirculation is always present to some degree with VV ECMO but is decreased with greater distance between cannulas, lower flow rates and reduced pulmonary artery pressures.

**Answer E**

*After adjustment of the cannula she demonstrates systemic SaO$_2$ of 94%, PA saturations of 94% and ECCV (ECMO circuit venous) saturations of 65%. Her ventilator is placed to "rest settings" (IMV 6, TV 400 cc, FiO$_2$ 30% and PEEP 5) and she continues to have SaO$_2$ in the low/mid 90%s and gradually weans off of her pressors.*

*You receive a call several hours later that she now has SaO$_2$ of 84%, SvO$_2$ of 82% and an ECCV of 55%.*

**15** *This acute change most likely represents:*
   **A** *Oxygenator failure*
   **B** *Increased oxygen consumption*
   **C** *Respiratory decompensation from too rapid of ventilator weaning*
   **D** *Native cardiac output has increased and her ECMO support is relatively less*
   **E** *A blood clot in the venous line*

The most likely acute change is the development of a hyper-dynamic state in the patient. As native cardiac output increases, the relative contribution of the 5 Lpm from the ECMO circuit is decreased and oxygen saturation would fall in all distributions. In this case there is little to do unless there is evidence of evolving cellular ischemia such as an increasing lactate, base deficit or other inflammatory markers. If the determination is that she requires a greater delivery to consumption ratio to meet her demands there are several options to do so. The circuit flow rate could be increased to match her increased CO, she could be transfused to increase the oxygen carrying capacity of her blood or she could benefit from prone positioning which might improve the native lung function and often decreases the intrapulmonary shunt. Finally, her consumption could be decreased with sedation, neuromuscular blockade and mild hypothermia. This scenario is typical of a patient still in the acute inflammatory phase of care or one developing a new infectious source. Modern oxygenators rarely fail early or quickly so this would be low on the differential. If increased consumption was involved the ECMO circuit arterial saturation (ECCA) and arterial saturation would be maintained while the ECCV (ECMO drainage) saturation would fall. A thrombosis of the venous line would manifest with flow and pressure changes, not oxygenation issues. There is almost no situation in which the ventilator should be increased above rest settings during ECMO for ARDS.

**Answer D**

ELSO Adult Respiratory Failure Supplement to the ELSO General Guidelines, December 2013.

Guerin,, C., Reignier, J., Richard, J., et al. (2013) Prone positioning in severe acute respiratory distress syndrome. *New England Journal of Medicine*, **368**, 2159–2168.

Lazzeri, C., Cianchi, G., Bonizzoli, M., et al. (2016) Right ventricle dilation as a prognostic factor in refractory acute respiratory distress syndrome requiring venovenous extracorporeal membrane oxygenation. *Minerva Anestesiol.* **82** (10), 1043–1049.

Montisci, A., Maj, G., Zangrillo, A., et al. (2015) Management of refractory hypoxemia during venovenous extracorporeal membrane oxygenation for ARDS. *ASAIO Journal*, **61**, 227–236.

# 4

# Arrhythmias, Acute Coronary Syndromes, and Hypertensive Emergencies

*Rondi Gelbard, MD and Omar K. Danner, MD*

1 *A 66-year-old man with diabetes, hypertension, and atrial fibrillation on warfarin is scheduled to undergo a symptomatic ventral hernia repair. He has a remote history of a TIA, and had an MI two years ago. His blood pressure is currently well controlled on a beta-blocker. Which of the following is the next best step in management prior to proceeding with surgery?*

A *Continue warfarin*

B *Discontinue warfarin and start clopidogrel*

C *Bridge with IV unfractionated heparin prior to surgery*

D *Discontinue warfarin 5 days prior to scheduled surgery*

E *Switch to dabigatran*

The management of anticoagulation for atrial fibrillation in the perioperative period depends on a patient's risk of having a thromboembolic event, which is determined by their CHADS$_2$ or more recent CHA$_2$DS$_2$-VASc (which includes additional stroke risk factors – see Table 4.1) score. This patient's CHADS$_2$ score is 3 (and CHA$_2$DS$_2$-VASc score is 5) putting him at approximately 6% annual stroke risk. Anyone with a score of 2 or greater should undergo long-term anticoagulation. In terms of periprocedural interruption of anticoagulation, patients with low short-term risk (CHADS$_2$ 0–2) and duration of interruption less than 1 week do not require bridging with heparin. For those at moderate risk (CHADS$_2$ 3–4), bridging may be reasonable and for those with high-risk features (CHADS$_2$ 5–6), bridging is recommended. Clopidogrel alone does not confer an advantage over warfarin for preventing stroke. Dabigatran, an alternative to warfarin, is a direct thrombin inhibitor with no available reversal agent; therefore, it should not be initiated prior to surgery.

**Answer: C**

Yarmohammadi, H., Varr, B.C., Puwanant, S., *et al.* (2012) Role of CHADS2 score in evaluation of thromboembolic risk and mortality in patients with atrial fibrillation undergoing direct current cardioversion (from the ACUTE Trial Substudy), *American Journal of Cardiology*, **110** (2), 222–226.

2 *A 52-year-old woman with a history of hypertension and STEMI 6 months ago requiring percutaneous coronary intervention (PCI) with a bare metal stent presents with a symptomatic inguinal hernia. Her symptoms have been increasing in frequency and duration and she wants to undergo a hernia repair. Her current medications include aspirin, clopidogrel, and metoprolol. On exam, her blood pressure is 128/67 mm Hg and her pulse is 68 p/min. Her cardiovascular exam is normal. Which of the following is the next best step in management?*

A *Discontinue aspirin and clopidogrel and proceed with surgery*

B *Discontinue aspirin and clopidogrel and start dipyridamole*

C *Continue aspirin and clopidogrel and proceed to surgery*

D *Delay surgery for an additional six months*

E *Discontinue clopidogrel, continue aspirin and proceed with surgery*

According to recent guidelines, in patients with acute coronary syndrome treated with bare metal or drug eluting stent implantation, dual antiplatelet therapy (DAPT) with aspirin and clopidogrel, prasugrel, or ticagrelor should be continued for at least 12 months. Elective noncardiac surgeries should be delayed in order to complete a full year of DAPT. Discontinuing DAPT increases the risk of stent thrombosis and subsequent myocardial infarction. Dipyridamole is not approved for DAPT.

*Surgical Critical Care and Emergency Surgery: Clinical Questions and Answers*, Second Edition.
Edited by Forrest "Dell" Moore, Peter Rhee, and Gerard J. Fulda.
© 2018 John Wiley & Sons Ltd. Published 2018 by John Wiley & Sons Ltd.
Companion website: www.wiley.com/go/moore/surgical_criticalcare_and_emergency_surgery

**Table 4.1** CHA$_2$DS$_2$-VASc calculation.

| | Condition | Points |
|---|---|---|
| **C** | Congestive heart failure (or Left ventricular systolic dysfunction) | 1 |
| **H** | Hypertension: blood pressure consistently above 140/90 mm Hg (or treated hypertension on medication) | 1 |
| **A$_2$** | Age ≥ 75 years | 2 |
| **D** | Diabetes Mellitus | 1 |
| **S$_2$** | Prior Stroke or TIA or thromboembolism | 2 |
| **V** | Vascular disease (e.g., peripheral artery disease, myocardial infarction, aortic plaque) | 1 |
| **A** | Age 65–74 years | 1 |
| **Sc** | Sex category (i.e., female sex) | 1 |

Proceeding with elective surgery while on DAPT would lead to an increased risk of bleeding. If the surgery is more urgent, aspirin should be continued and clopidogrel discontinued and restarted as soon as possible after surgery. In this case, the inguinal hernia repair is an elective surgery and clopidogrel should not be discontinued.

**Answer: D**

Collet, J.P., Silvain, J., Barthélémy, O., *et al.* (2014) Dual-antiplatelet treatment beyond 1 year after drug-eluting stent implantation (ARCTIC-Interruption): a randomised trial. *Lancet*, **384**,1577–1585.

Levine, G.N., Bates, E.R., Bittl, J.A., *et al* (2016) ACC/AHA guideline focused update on duration of dual antiplatelet therapy in patients with coronary artery disease. *Journal of the American College of Cardiology*, **68** (10), 1082–1115.

**3** *A 21-year-old football player is evaluated for symptomatic tachycardia. He first noticed the symptoms at age 9 while running and has noticed the episodes are becoming more frequent and lasting longer. He describes atypical chest pain, slight dyspnea, and palpitations but has never lost consciousness. His stress echocardiogram was normal and his baseline EKG is shown in Figure 4.1. Based upon your patient's symptoms and the EKG findings, which of the following is the most likely diagnosis?*

**A** *First-degree AV block*
**B** *Atrial fibrillation with slow ventricular response*
**C** *SVT with functional bundle branch block or aberrant conduction*
**D** *Wolff–Parkinson–White syndrome*
**E** *Mobitz Type II AV block*

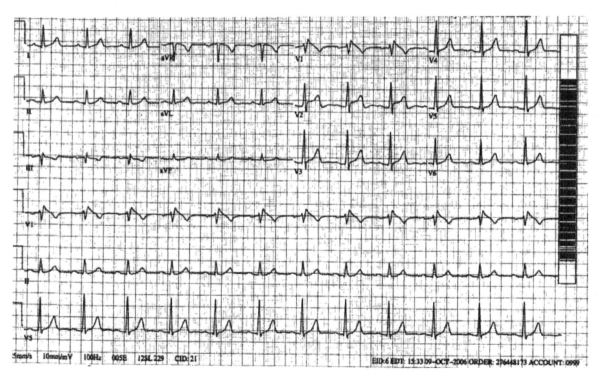

**Figure 4.1**

Wolff–Parkinson–White syndrome is a pre-excitation syndrome associated with an atrioventricular reentrant tachycardia. The tachycardia is due to an accessory pathway within the conduction system of the heart known as the Bundle of Kent. Certain medications, physical activity, and stress can send the electrical impulse into the accessory Bundle of Kent causing the prior unidirectional block to quickly recover its excitability thus sending the impulse back to reenter the circuit. Most patients remain asymptomatic throughout their lives; however, a small percentage of patients become symptomatic and progress to ventricular fibrillation, which then causes sudden death. People who are symptomatic during episodes of tachycardia experience palpitations, dizziness, shortness of breath, and fainting or near-fainting spells. Classic EKG findings include a short P-R interval (<0.12 s), a wide QRS complex (>0.12 s), slurring of the initial upstroke of the QRS complex (delta wave), and abnormal T waves indicating problems with repolarization. A classic delta wave can be seen in the precordial leads. Acute treatment in a hypotensive patient involves cardioversion and amiodarone or procainamide in a more stable patient. Treatment is based on risk stratification of the individual but the definitive treatment for WPW syndrome usually involves radiofrequency ablation of the accessory pathway. First-degree AV block is incorrect because it is characterized by a PR interval > 0.2 s due to a delay in impulse conduction in the AV node and is typically asymptomatic. Atrial fibrillation with slow ventricular response is associated with an absence of clear P waves on EKG. SVT with functional bundle branch block or aberrant conduction may appear as a wide QRS complex on EKG but is not associated with a delta wave. Mobitz Type II AV block would appear as a dropped QRS complex with no change in the preceding PR intervals.

**Answer: D**

Marini, J.J. and Wheeler, A.P. (2006) *Critical Care Medicine, The Essentials*, Lippincott Williams & Wilkins, Philadelphia, PA.

Skanes, A.C., Obeyesekere, M., and Klein, G.J. (2015) Electrophysiology testing and catheter ablation are helpful when evaluating asymptomatic patients with Wolff-Parkinson-White pattern: the con perspective. *Cardiac Electrophysiology Clinics*, 7 (3), 377–383.

**4**  *A 40-year-old Asian man with controlled hypertension suddenly collapses while eating. His son promptly initiates CPR. Upon arrival of the paramedics, he is in ventricular fibrillation and is successfully converted to normal sinus rhythm with external defibrillation. In the emergency room, the EKG shown in Figure 4.2*

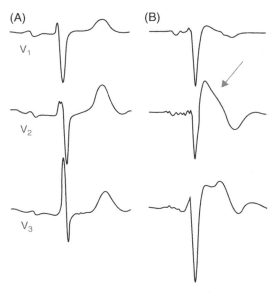

**Figure 4.2** (A) Normal electrocardiogram pattern in the precordial leads V1–3. (B) changes in Brugada syndrome (type B).

*was obtained. He had a second episode of ventricular fibrillation in the ED and was again successfully defibrillated. Definitive treatment for this patient's diagnosis would be:*

**A** *Observation*
**B** *Isoproterenol*
**C** *Propanolol*
**D** *Implantable cardiac defibrillator*
**E** *Surgical revascularization*

The clinical scenario and classic EKG findings suggest Brugada syndrome. Placement of an implantable cardiac defibrillator is the only definitive treatment for this cardiac pathology. Brugada syndrome has an autosomal dominant pattern of transmission and is characterized by cardiac conduction delays, which can lead to ventricular fibrillation and sudden cardiac death. It is more common in men and Asians. EKG findings typically include a right bundle branch block with ST segment elevations in the precordial leads. The pathophysiology is thought be an alteration in the transmembrane ion currents that together constitute the cardiac action potential. In this case, observation would not be correct. Even though the patient remains in normal sinus rhythm, the underlying problem has not been fixed, and he would likely revert to ventricular fibrillation. Isoproterenol is an option to help treat ventricular tachycardia storms by augmenting the cardiac L-type channels; however, it is not a definitive treatment. Propanolol is incorrect. Beta-blockers are drugs of choice for patients with long QT syndrome, which is the most common type of inherited arrhythmia. Surgical revascularization is not an option in these patients. An ICD should be surgically placed, which will then be programmed to fire when it detects an unstable rhythm.

**Answer: D**

Alings, M. and Wilde, A. (1999) "Brugada" syndrome: clinical data and suggested pathophysiological mechanism. *Circulation*, **99** (5), 666–673.

5 *A 57-year-old woman is admitted to the ICU after being intubated for respiratory failure following an asthma attack. Several hours after intubation she remains hypotensive. Her EKG is concerning for ST segment elevations in the precordial leads. Troponin is elevated at 0.56 μg/L. Cardiac catheterization demonstrates that her vessels are completely normal. Bedside echocardiogram is done, which reveals an ejection fraction of approximately 25% and significant hypokinesis of the mid and apical segments of the left ventricle. Which of the following is the most likely diagnosis?*
  A *Broken heart syndrome*
  B *Myocardial infarction*
  C *Acute pericarditis*
  D *Pulmonary embolism*
  E *Hypertrophic cardiomyopathy*

Takotsubo's syndrome or broken heart syndrome is a transient cardiomyopathy that causes significant cardiac depression and closely resembles acute coronary syndromes. Patients typically present with respiratory failure after a significant upper airway problem with EKG changes including ST segment elevation and T wave inversion, and mildly elevated cardiac enzymes. However, there is characteristic ballooning of the left ventricle on echocardiogram and no significant stenotic lesions of the coronary vessels on catheterization. Takotsubo's is thought to be due to stress-induced catecholamine release, with toxicity to and subsequent stunning of the myocardium. Acute coronary syndrome should be the diagnosis until proven otherwise. However, unlike Takotsubo's, myocardial infarction is typically associated with significantly elevated cardiac enzymes and evidence of coronary artery occlusion on cardiac catheterization. Acute pericarditis is incorrect as it is associated with diffuse ST segment elevation on EKG. Pulmonary embolism is characterized by a prominent S wave in lead I, a Q wave and inverted T wave in lead III, sinus tachycardia, and signs of right heart strain on echocardiogram. Hypertrophic cardiomyopathy would appear as increased QRS voltage and upright T waves (in the leads with Q waves), and disproportionate hypertrophy (particularly of the septum), hyperdynamic or preserved ejection fraction, atrial enlargement and diastolic dysfunction on echocardiogram. The prognosis for Takotsubo's is excellent. Most patients experience a complete recovery in about four to eight weeks and recurrence is less than 3%.

**Answer: A**

Dorfman, T.A. and Iskandrian, A.E. (2009) Takotsubo cardiomyopathy: state-of-the-art review. *Journal of Nuclear Cardiology*, **16** (1), 122–134.

Kawai, S., Kitabatake, A., and Tomoike, H. (2007) Guidelines for diagnosis of Takotsubo (ampulla) cardiomyopathy. *Circulation Journal*, **71** (6), 990–992.

6 *A 76-year-old man comes to the emergency room after his wife states that "he has been falling a lot lately." He is immediately placed on the cardiac monitor and a 12-lead EKG is obtained, which is shown in Figure 4.3. Which of the following diagnoses is seen on the EKG?*
  A *Complete heart block*
  B *Second degree heart block (Mobitz type II)*
  C *Second degree heart block (Mobitz type I - Wenckebach)*
  D *Myocardial infarction*
  E *First degree heart block*

This patient has type I second-degree heart block (Mobitz type I, Wenckebach), usually caused by disease within the AV node. Patients often present with a history of falling or syncope. EKG findings for type I second degree heart block include progressive prolongation of the P-R interval on consecutive beats, followed by a dropped QRS complex (due to conduction failure). There is a relatively fixed interval between non-conducted beats. Type II second-degree AV block (Mobitz type II) is almost always a disease of the distal conduction system (Bundle of His). On EKG, Mobitz type II is characterized by a dropped QRS complex with no change in the preceding PR intervals. Mobitz type II AV block can progress to complete heart block leading to sudden cardiac death. First-degree heart block is characterized by a P-R interval greater than 0.2 s, which is not seen in this EKG. The EKG findings of complete heart block, or third-degree heart block, include no concordance between the P waves and the QRS complexes. The most definitive treatment for AV nodal blocks is an implantable pacemaker. Myocardial infarction is not typically associated with prolongation of the PR interval or dropped QRS complex on EKG.

**Answer: C**

Barold, S.S. and Hayes, D.L. (2001) Second-degree atrioventricular block: a reappraisal. *Mayo Clinical Proceedings*, **76** (1), 44–57.

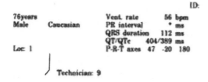

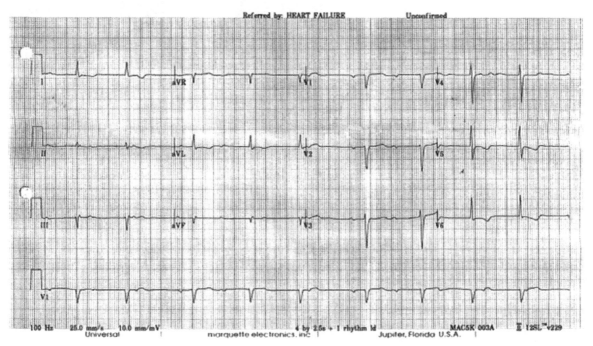

**Figure 4.3**

Heart Block, Second Degree (2009) http://emedicine.medscape.com/article/758383-overview (accessed February 26, 2011).

**7** *A 67-year-old man presents to your office for follow up after a recent acute anterior myocardial infarction. EKG demonstrates abnormal left axis deviation, QRS prolongation > 100 and poor R wave progression in leads V1–V3. Which of the following is the most likely diagnosis?*

**A** *Left ventricular hypertrophy*
**B** *Left bundle branch block*
**C** *Right bundle branch block*
**D** *Left anterior fascicular block*
**E** *Left posterior fascicular block*

Left anterior fascicular block is the most common conduction block in general and the most common conduction delay seen in acute anterior wall myocardial infarction due to occlusion of the left anterior descending artery. LAFB is classically associated with *left axis deviation* in a frontal plane usually –45 to –90 degrees. There is no specific treatment for the different types of

hemiblocks other than diagnosing and treatment the underlying cardiac ischemia. The EKG criteria are as follows:

Left axis deviation (usually –45 to –90 degrees);
rS complexes in leads II, III, aVF;
Small q-waves in leads I and/or aVL;
R-peak time in lead aVL < 0.04 s, often with slurred R wave downstroke;
QRS duration usually > 0.12 s unless there is coexisting RBBB;
Poor R wave progression in leads V1–V3 and deeper S-waves in leads V5 and V6

A left posterior fascicular block (LPFB) is a rare condition where the left posterior fascicle, which travels to the inferior and posterior portion of the left ventricle does not conduct the electrical impulses from the AV node, but rather through the left anterior fascicle and right bundle branch, leading to a right axis deviation seen on the EKG. A left bundle branch block would have a more prolonged QRS complex (>0.12 s). A right bundle branch block would have an extra deflection in the QRS complex (as well as a terminal R wave in V1 and a slurred S wave in leads I and V6) but would not show left axis deviation. A left posterior fascicular block is characterized by right axis deviation on EKG.

**Answer: D**

Da Costa, D., Brady, W.J., and Edhouse, J. (2002). Bradycardias and atrioventricular conduction block. *British Medical Journal*, **324**, 535–538.
Raoof, S., George, L., Saleh, A., and Sung, A. (2009) *ACP Manual of Critical Care*, McGraw-Hill, New York.

**8** *A 34-year-old woman with chronic hypertension is in her first trimester of pregnancy. Prior to becoming pregnant, her blood pressure was well controlled on lisinopril. Which of the following antihypertensive medications would be safe to continue throughout her pregnancy?*
  **A** *Enalapril*
  **B** *Amiodarone*
  **C** *Losartan*
  **D** *Labetalol*
  **E** *Atenolol*

Data are limited on the safety of most cardiovascular medications during pregnancy and should only be used when necessary. Beta-blockers cross the placenta and can cause significant levels in the fetus. While Atenolol can cause premature delivery and low birth weight and should be avoided during pregnancy, labetalol and metoprolol have been found to be safe in pregnancy. ACE inhibitors, angiotensin receptor blockers and aldosterone agonists should all be avoided due to teratogenicity. Amiodarone can cause fetal hypothyroidism and prematurity and should be avoided if possible.

**Answer: D**

Task Force on the Management of Cardiovascular Diseases During Pregnancy of the European Society of Cardiology (2003) Expert consensus document on management of cardiovascular diseases during pregnancy. *European Heart Journal*, **24**, 761–781.

**9** *Two weeks following a myocardial infarction, a 64-year-old man is admitted to the trauma service with multiple rib fractures and a pulmonary contusion after a motor vehicle collision. He has a history of alcohol abuse and has been noncompliant with his cardiac medications. On examination he has a pulse of 100 beats/min, blood pressure 100/70 mm Hg, respirations 20 breaths/min, tenderness and bruising along the right lateral chest wall. A 12-lead ECG confirms a recent inferior myocardial infarction and an echocardiogram is shown in Figure 4.4.*

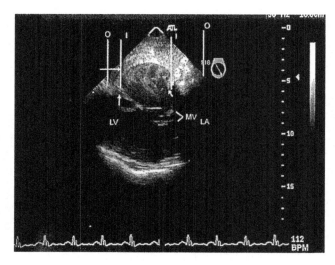

**Figure 4.4**

*In view of this finding, which of the following is the most appropriate management for this patient?*
  **A** *Confirmatory cardiac catheterization*
  **B** *Six months of oral anticoagulation*
  **C** *Pericardiocentesis*
  **D** *NSAIDs for six weeks*
  **E** *Immediate referral to the cardiothoracic surgical service*

The echocardiogram reveals a very large left ventricular pseudoaneurysm. The outer boundary of the pseudoaneurysm is marked by vertical lines O and the communication with the left ventricle by vertical lines l. A pseudoaneurysm (false aneurysm) results from a free wall rupture of the left ventricle, usually as a result of a previous myocardial infarction. The rupture is contained by overlying pericardium and lacks any organized cardiac structures, unlike a true ventricular aneurysm. The occurrence of free-wall rupture is less than 1%; however, the mortality is significant and one-half of the ruptures will result in out-of-hospital sudden deaths. Diagnosis is usually made within six months of infarction. Surgical intervention for a large or expanding pseudoaneurysm is recommended. Answer choice A is incorrect because contrast ventriculography is diagnostic in only half of patients compared to 97% for 2D echocardiography. Pericardiocentesis would not treat the pseudoaneurysm and could lead to free rupture. NSAIDs would not be helpful for managing a pseudoaneurysm. Although Coumadin is of value in circumstances of left-ventricular clot in the setting of a true left-ventricular aneurysm, it is contraindicated in this setting.

**Answer: E**

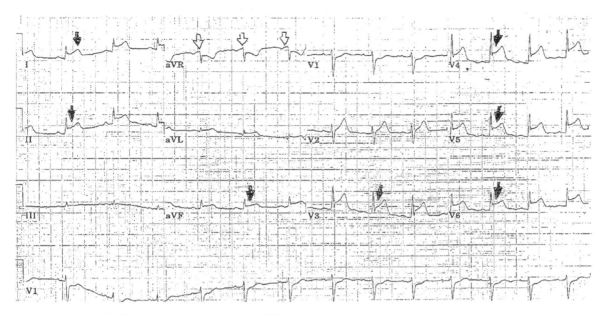

**Figure 4.5** 12-lead ECG with arrows showing pericarditis.

Atik, F.A. and Lytle, B.W. (2007) Surgical treatment of post infarction left ventricular pseudoaneurysm. *The Annals of Thoracic Surgery*, **83**, 526–531.

Califf, R. and Roe, M. (2010) *Acute Coronary Syndrome Essentials*. Jones & Bartlett Learning, Sudbury, MA.

**10** *A 39-year-old obese man presents to the emergency room the evening prior to elective hernia surgery with several hours of sudden onset chest pain and shortness of breath. He admits to being anxious concerning the morning surgery. His medications include albuterol and Lipitor. His pulse is regular and he has a blood pressure of 165/89 mm Hg and a respiratory rate of 22 breaths/min. He is sitting at the edge of the examining table and states he finds it "easier to breath" and feels better in that position. His electrocardiogram is shown in Figure 4.5. Which of the following would be indicated based on his electrocardiogram and clinical findings?*

**A** *Cardiac catheterization*
**B** *Echocardiogram*
**C** *Albuterol*
**D** *Thrombolytics*
**E** *Sublingual nitroglycerin*

Based on the electrocardiogram findings and his history, the most likely diagnosis is acute pericarditis. The EKG reveals ST elevation (Figure 4.6) and diffuse J-point elevation throughout the electrocardiogram (solid arrows) with no localization to coronary artery distribution. There is atrial segment elevation in leads aVR (hollow arrows).

Diffuse ST segment elevation and PR segment elevation in lead aVR strongly support the diagnosis of acute pericarditis, which should be distinguished from acute myocardial injury. Answer choice B would be the most appropriate answer as an echocardiogram, in the absence of a prior myocardial infarction, demonstrates normal LV function without wall motion abnormality. It would also demonstrate the presence or absence of a pericardial effusion which occurs in up to 30% of patients with acute pericarditis. Cardiac catheterization is not indicated for the diagnosis or management of pericarditis. Albuterol, a bronchodilator, would not be helpful for treating pericarditis. Thrombolytics would be inappropriate as they may result in the development of a hemorrhagic pericardial effusion and possible cardiac tamponade. Sublingual nitroglycerin would be appropriate for the treatment of acute coronary syndrome, not pericarditis. Anti-inflammatory medications are the primary treatment modality for acute pericarditis, including high dose aspirin (or NSAIDs in the absence of an MI). Indomethacin and corticosteroids have been relegated to refractory cases due to concerns regarding increased coronary vascular resistance, and increased risk of myocardial rupture in the setting of a healing previously unrecognized myocardial infarction.

**Answer: B**

Califf, R. and Roe, M. (2010) *Acute Coronary Syndrome Essentials*, Jones & Bartlett Learning, Sudbury, MA.

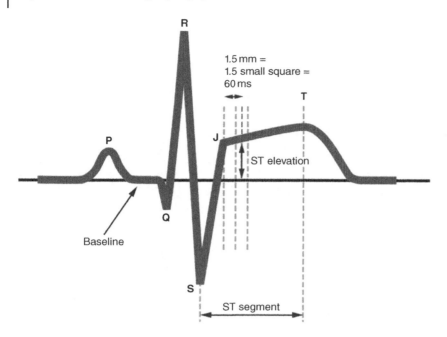

**Figure 4.6** How to measure ST elevation.

Parillo, J.E. and Dellinger, R.D. (2008) *Critical Care Medicine: Principles of Diagnosis and Management in the Adult.* Mosby, Philadelphia, PA.

**11** Ten days after undergoing a laparoscopic right inguinal hernia repair, a 69-year-old man presents to your office complaining of worsening fatigue and shortness of breath. Physical examination reveals a blood pressure of 115/69 mm Hg, pulse 111 beats/min, and respiratory rate 22 breaths/min. He has marked rales at both lung bases, and a 4/6 holosystolic murmur auscultated best at the base of the heart. An electrocardiogram is performed and reveals evidence of a recent inferior myocardial infarction. Chest x-ray reveals bilateral pulmonary edema. His echocardiogram is shown in Figure 4.7.

Which of the following statements is true in regards to the myocardial complication demonstrated?

**A** The anterior lateral papillary muscle is supplied by dual blood supply but is the most likely to rupture

**B** The posteromedial papillary muscle is supplied only by the right coronary artery and is the most common form of papillary muscle rupture after an infarct

**C** The severity of mitral regurgitation following an acute myocardial infarction is not an independent predictor of survival

**D** Intra-aortic balloon pump utilization is of little use in reducing the risk of significant left ventricular overload in this type of case

**E** Papillary muscle rupture rarely occurs in the first two to nine days after a significant myocardial infarction

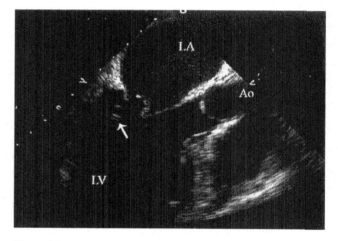

**Figure 4.7**

Rupture of the posteromedial papillary muscle represents the most common form of papillary muscle rupture as it is exclusively supplied by the posterior descending branch of the right coronary artery. Answer choice A is incorrect because the anterolateral papillary muscle is less likely to rupture given its dual blood supply from both the diagonal branches of the left anterior descending and branches off of the circumflex marginal artery. In this clinical scenario, a myocardial infarction was precipitated by the stress of the laparoscopic inguinal hernia repair. When pulmonary edema develops two to nine days after an infarction and coincides with necrosis of the papillary head, papillary muscle rupture should be seriously considered in the differential diagnosis. On physical examination, a new apical systolic murmur, audible at the base of the heart, is often present and ends just prior to the second heart sound, S2. It is uncommon to have a palpable thrill.

Prolapse of the posterior mitral leaflet into the left ventricle (the arrow is pointing to the vague outline of the ruptured head of the papillary muscle) can be seen on echocardiogram. Choice C is incorrect because significant correlation exists between mortality and worsening severity of mitral regurgitation on echocardiography in the setting of acute infarction. Acute mitral regurgitation results in a sudden state of volume overload of the left ventricle. Dilation of the left ventricle does not have time to develop under these circumstances, and there is an abrupt rise in left ventricular end-diastolic and left atrial pressure. This phenomenon may subsequently result in pulmonary hypertension, pulmonary edema, and acute right ventricular dysfunction followed by cardiogenic shock. Consequently, definitive treatment is expedient cardiac surgery. However, stabilization of the cardiovascular system requires administration of vasodilators and intra-aortic balloon counter pulsation therapy to promote forward flow.

**Answer: B**

Gabelli, A., Layon, A.J., and Yu, M. (2012) *Civetta, Taylor & Kirby's Critical Care.* Lippincott Williams and Wilkins: Philadelphia, PA.

Parillo, J.E. and Dellinger, R.D. (2014) *Critical Care Medicine: Principles of Diagnosis and Management in the Adult.* Mosby: Philadelphia, PA.

Thompson, C.R., Buller, C.E., Sleeper, L.A., *et al.* (2000) Cardiogenic shock due to acute severe mitral regurgitation complicating acute myocardial infarction: a report from the SHOCK Trial Registry. Journal of the American College of Cardiology, **36** (3) (Suppl. I), 1104–1109.

**12**  *A 59-year-old woman with a history of depression and alcohol abuse is admitted to the hospital for management of acute diverticulitis. She is started on a course of levofloxacin. On exam her heart rate is 60 beats/min, blood pressure is 110/70 mm Hg, and respiratory rate 17 breaths/min. Her ionized calcium is 2.9 mg/dL and her serum phosphorus is 1.8 mg/dL. Her electrocardiogram is illustrated in Figure 4.8.*

*Two days after admission, the patient becomes profoundly hypertensive, and the rhythm strip shown in Figure 4.9 is obtained:*

*The patient is immediately electrically cardioverted with a return to her baseline sinus rhythm on the monitor and improvement in her blood pressure to 115/80 mm Hg. Following cardioversion, which of the following medications should be given next?*
**A** *IV amiodarone*
**B** *IV lidocaine*

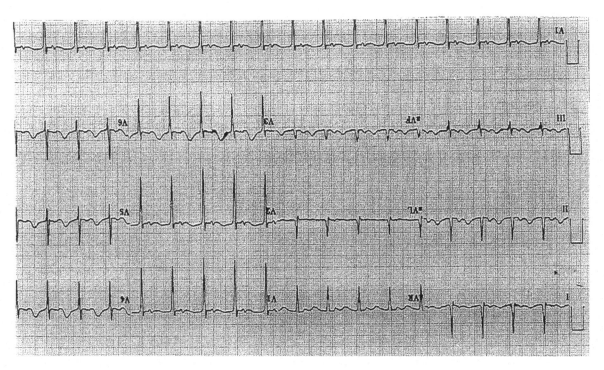

**Figure 4.8**

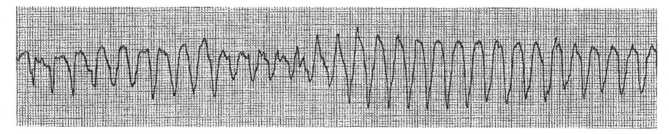

**Figure 4.9**

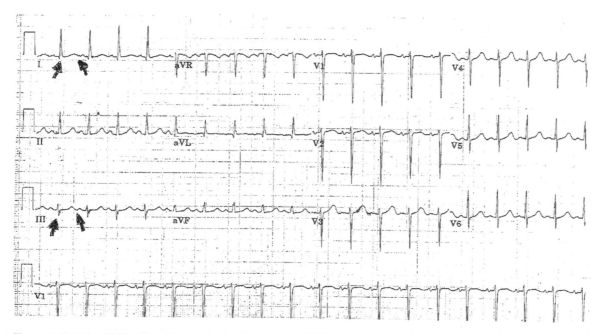

**Figure 4.10** 12 lead ECG with solid arrows showing prolonged QT interval.

**C** *IV magnesium*
**D** *IV sotalol*
**E** *IV ibutilide*

The rhythm strip is consistent with torsades de pointes, a classic form of polymorphic ventricular tachycardia characterized by a gradual change in the amplitude and twisting of the QRS complexes around the isoelectric line. It is associated with a prolonged QT interval (Figure 4.10), which may be congenital or acquired. Risk factors including hypokalemia, hypomagnesemia, bradycardia and certain medications including fluoroquinolones and antiarrhythmic medications.

Polymorphic ventricular tachycardia is poorly tolerated by patients and may degenerate into ventricular fibrillation. Consequently, intravenous magnesium (dose of 1–2 gm) should be given over one to two minutes after the immediate cardioversion. In addition, correction of any underlying electrolyte abnormality should be undertaken. On the contrary, ibutilide, sotalol and amiodarone

are contraindicated as they worsen QT prolongation. Lastly, lidocaine has been proven to be ineffective.

**Answer: C**

Aggerwal, R., Prakash, O., and Medii, B. (2006) Drug induced Torsades de Pointes. *Journal of Medical Education and Research*, **8** (4), 185–189.

Gabelli, A., Layon, A.J., and Yu, M. (2012) *Civetta, Taylor & Kirby's Critical Care*, Lippincott Williams and Wilkins, Philadelphia, PA.

Parillo, J.E. and Dellinger, R.D. (2014) *Critical Care Medicine: Principles of Diagnosis and Management in the Adult*. Mosby, Philadelphia, PA.

**13** *A 67-year-old man presents to your clinic with a 3-day history of fatigue, nausea, vomiting, and obstipation. He is noted to be hypokalemic and mildly hypomagnesemic. He is admitted to the hospital for further workup. His initial electrocardiogram in the*

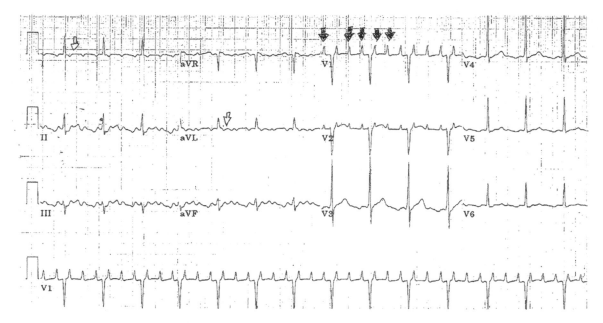

**Figure 4.11**

*emergency room just prior to transfer to the ward is illustrated in Figure 4.11.*

*Four hours later he complains of retrosternal chest pain relieved by sublingual nitroglycerin. His daughter states that her father has been complaining of "fluttering in his chest" for the past several days and has a history of compensated "congestive heart failure." On physical examination, his heart rate is 95 beats/min and irregular, blood pressure is 121/79 mm Hg, respiratory rate is 18 breaths/min, and oxygen saturation of 96% on 40% face mask. Which would be most appropriate next step in management?*

**A** *Synchronized monophasic cardioversion*

**B** *Intravenous amiodarone and anticoagulation*

**C** *Intravenous ibutilide*

**D** *Intravenous beta blocker and diltiazem*

**E** *Carotid massage*

The 12-lead EKG demonstrates atrial flutter with a rapid ventricular response rate in lead V1. The rate of atrial activity is 275 beats/min. The discrete regular atrial waves are consistent with atrial flutter (represented by the solid arrows). Ventricular conduction is occurring at a frequency of 3:1 with stimulation of one QRS complex per three flutter waves. This is an unusual finding as atrial flutter is typically associated with a fixed even conduction ratio of 2:1 or 4:1. When atrial flutter is transmitted through the AV node in a 1:1 ratio, it often conducts aberrantly with a wide QRS complex tachycardia which may be easily mistaken for ventricular tachycardia. Therefore, it is not uncommon that atrial flutter presents with atrial undulations at a rate of 240–340

beats/min. The atrial flutter morphology is classically described as inverted flutter waves that lack an isoelectric base in leads I, II, and aVF. In addition, they are associated with small, positive deflections with a characteristic isoelectric baseline which can be observed in lead V1 as demonstrated in this case. The ECG in Figure 4.11 shows the baseline artifact in the inferior leads. There are also subtle non-specific ST & T wave changes noted (see hollow arrows).

This patient is hemodynamically stable and by history, he has probably been in flutter for at least 96 hours before his admission. Prior to performing cardioversion in a patient with a history of atrial flutter greater than 48 hours, an echocardiogram should be performed to rule out the existence of a left atrial thrombus, which can potentially lead to thromboembolic events. An atrial thrombus may be present in 10 to 34% of patients after being in atrial flutter for > 72 hours. Furthermore, anticoagulation should be initiated for at least three weeks prior to undergoing attempted cardioversion in a relatively stable patient after the echocardiography has been performed. Amiodarone has proven to be effective in the setting of systolic dysfunction and ischemic episodes.

Although ibutilide has been used as an option in the conversion of atrial flutter, it is contraindicated in the setting of acute coronary syndromes and electrolyte disturbances, such as hypokalemia and clinically significant hypomagnesiumia, as seen in the case above. This is due to a higher propensity for the patient to develop Torsades de pointes. Beta-blockers are frequently recommended for rate control in setting of atrial flutter, but when used in conjunction with diltiazem, they can lead to profound bradycardia and heart block. Carotid massage is another technique that can be used to unmask flutter waves, and can help confirm the diagnosis of atrial flutter in the presence of a 2:1 AV block. However, it is ineffective in the conversion of the arrhythmia to normal rate and rhythm; the original ventricular rate predictably resumes upon discontinuation. Therefore, based on the options listed above, the combination of anticoagulation plus amiodarone would be the most suitable choice in this particular scenario.

**Answer: B**

Field, J., Gonzales, L., and Hazinski, M. (2013) *Advanced Cardiac Life Support Manual*. American Heart Association, Dallas, TX.

Parillo, J.E. and Dellinger, R.D. (2014) *Critical Care Medicine: Principles of Diagnosis and Management in the Adult*. Mosby: Philadelphia, PA.

**14** *Which of the following statements regarding the utilization of coronary artery bypass grafting (CABG) for acute coronary syndrome is true?*

  **A** *Diabetics with multivessel disease and prior PTCA have worse outcomes with CABG versus repeat PTCA*

  **B** *Perioperative mortality for elective CABG is increased three to seven days after acute MI and therefore cannot be done safely*

  **C** *Clopidogrel should be held for five to seven days prior to CABG*

  **D** *CABG following fibrinolytic therapy leads to reoperation for bleeding in less than 1%*

  **E** *Mortality rates for emergent CABG following failed fibrinolytic therapy is 50%*

Clopidogrel (Plavix) should be held for five to seven days prior to CABG to minimize the risk of perioperative bleeding. CABG for patients with preserved LV function who require revascularization can be safely performed within a few days of a STEMI. CABG following fibrinolytic therapy leads to a reoperation for bleeding in ~ 4% of patients. Mortality rates for emergent CABG after failed fibrinolytic therapy remains about 15%. Diabetics with multivessel disease and prior PTCA have better outcomes with CABG versus repeat PTCA.

**Answer: C**

Califf, R. and Roe, M. (2010) *Acute Coronary Syndrome Essentials*, Jones and Bartlett Learning, Sudbury, MA.

Parillo, I.E. and Dellinger, R.D. (2014) *Critical Care Medicine: Principles of Diagnosis and Management in the Adult*. Mosby, Philadelphia, PA.

The BARI (Bypass Angioplasty Revasculization Investigation) Investigators (2000) Seven year outcome by treatment. *Journal of the American College of Cardiology*, **35**, 1122–1129.

**15** *A 69-year-old woman undergoes a sigmoid colectomy. She has a history of type II diabetes mellitus and hypercholesterolemia. Forty-eight hours after the procedure, she complains of worsening epigastric discomfort after coming back from physical therapy. A stat electrocardiogram is obtained and is shown in Figure 4.12.*

  *She is initially treated conservatively, but 3 days later she is noted to have a new holo-systolic murmur and a palpable thrill along the left sternal border. An echocardiogram is performed, shown in Figure 4.13.*

  *Which of the following statements concerning rupture of the interventricular septum is correct?*

  **A** *Most commonly occurs with anterior myocardial infarctions*

  **B** *If pulmonary artery catheterization were performed you would expect a prominent v-wave in the pulmonary capillary wedge pressure tracing*

  **C** *This complication is found in 5–6% of acute myocardial infarctions*

  **D** *The expected mortality would be 40–60% with medical therapy, and is equivalent to surgical intervention at one year*

  **E** *Survival is the same with inferior posterior infarctions compared to anterior infarctions*

The patient has a post-myocardial infarction ventriculoseptal defect (VSD), which complicates 0.5–2% of acute myocardial infarctions. VSDs typically occur two to five days following the myocardial event. Patients are usually older and have multi-vessel disease. Rupture of the interventricular septum is more common with anterior myocardial infarctions because the septum is supplied by the septal perforating branches of the left anterior descending artery. Evidence of septal necrosis is heralded by the development of a holo-systolic murmur at the left sternal border, which indicates a significant VSD. Diagnosis is confirmed using two-dimensional echocardiography combined with Doppler flow studies. The echocardiogram illustrated in Figure 4.13 shows an inferior septal defect with thinning of portions of the necrotic septal wall (arrows). Pulmonary artery catheterization with oximetry demonstrates a greater than 5–7% step-up in oxygenation between the right atrium and ventricle. In addition, an absence of V waves is present in the pulmonary artery wedge pressure tracing, which differentiate a ventricular septal defect from a papillary muscle rupture. VSD is the cause of death in 5% of all fatal myocardial infarctions. The SHOCK study revealed

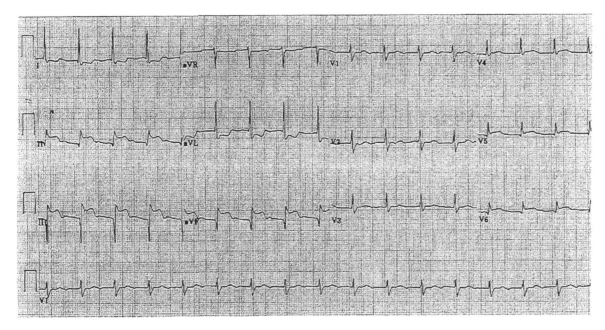

**Figure 4.12**

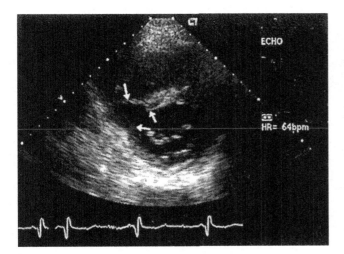

**Figure 4.13**

that 25% of patients die in the first 24 hours and 50% at one week with a 90% in-hospital mortality rate when there is associated cardiogenic shock. The survival for posterior-inferior or right ventricular associated ventricular septal defects is significantly worse than for those with anterior myocardial infarctions.

**Answer: A**

Blanche, C., Khan, S.S., Choux, A., and Metloff, J.M. (1994) Post infarction ventricular septal defect in the elderly: analysis and results. *The Annals of Thoracic Surgery*, **57**, 91–98.

Parillo, J.E. and Dellinger, R.D. (2014) *Critical Care Medicine: Principles of Diagnosis and Management in the Adult*, Mosby, Philadelphia, PA.

Topaz, O. and Taylor, A.L. (1992) Interventricular septal rupture complicating acute myocardial infarction: from pathophysiologic features to the role of invasive and noninvasive diagnostic modalities in current management. *American Journal of Medicine*, **93**, 683–688.

**16** *A 63-year-old man develops angina pectoris on the postoperative day four following emergent right hemicolectomy for an obstructing right colon neoplasm. His postoperative course has been complicated by persistent emesis. The patient subsequently develops progressive hypotension. On physical examination, he is noted to have a positive Kussmaul's sign. An initial electrocardiogram is performed with results as illustrated in Figure 4.14.*

*A Swan–Ganz catheter is inserted and the patient's hemodynamic profile is assessed. His ratio of right atrial pressure to wedge pressure is noted to be less than 0.8. A selective right-sided chest lead ECG is carried out a few hours later with results as shown in Figure 4.15.*

*Which of the following statements regarding this condition is correct?*

**A** *Patients with this type of myocardial infarction complication are older*

**B** *Hospital mortality is 25% with defibrillation*

**C** *More commonly associated with multi-vessel disease*

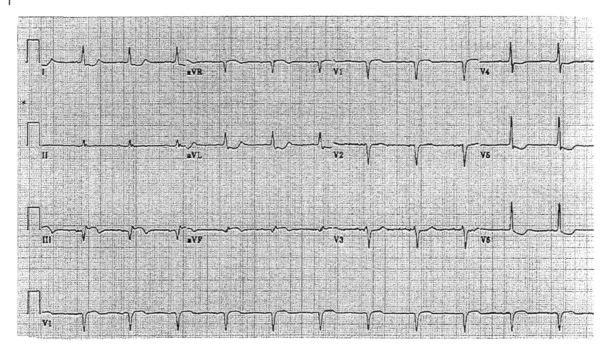

**Figure 4.14**

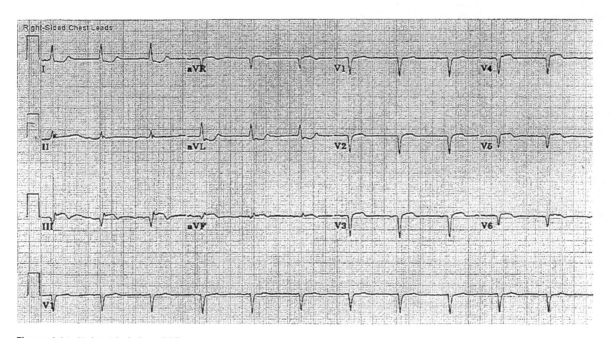

**Figure 4.15** Right-sided chest ECG.

**D** *Bezold-Jarisch reflex is associated with cardioversion*
**E** *The patient should undergo volume expansion to overcome his right ventricular dysfunction*

This patient has a significant right-sided ventricular infarction. Right-ventricular infarctions occur in approximately 30% of inferior infarcts and 10% of anterior infarcts. The initial 12 lead typically exhibits ST segment elevation and T wave inversion in the inferior leads (solid arrows). There is also a 1 mm of ST segment elevation in lead V1 (hollow arrows). Furthermore, lateral ST segment depression is also identifiable. This constellation of findings is consistent with an acute right ventricular

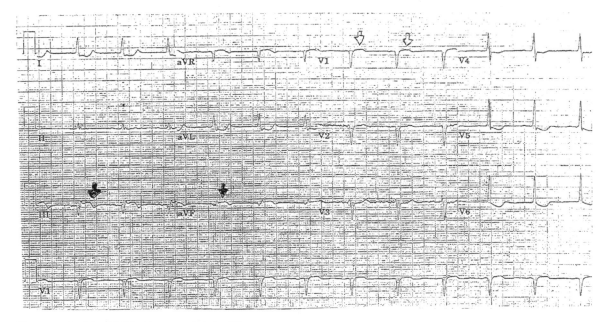

**Figure 4.16** 12 lead ECG with arrows inferior MI.

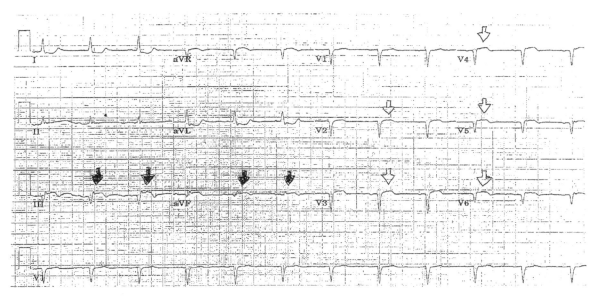

**Figure 4.17** RT sided chest lead ECG.

infarction. Verification should be obtained by performing a right-sided ECG tracing. It is important to assess leads V1-2 for ST segment elevation and prominent R waves, which may be representative of a right-ventricular or posterior myocardial infarction.

The right-sided ECG in Figure 4.16 demonstrates inferior Q wave formation (solid arrows) and ST elevation (hollow arrows). These findings are indicative of an acute inferior myocardial infarction. In addition, ST elevation is present in leads the precordial leads V2–6R, which is

consistent with an acute right-ventricular infarction (Figure 4.17).

The presence of a right ventricular infarction is suggested by identification of Kussmaul's sign (jugular venous distention on inspiration) in the face of hypotension accompanied by inferior myocardial infarctions. Pulmonary artery catheterization reveals the right atrial pressure exceeds 10 mm Hg and the ratio of right atrial pressure to wedge pressure is classically less than 0.8. Treatment requires early reperfusion by mechanical or thrombolytic means. The Bezold–Jarisch reflex is the sudden development of bradycardia associated with hypotension, which can be seen after the reopening of an occluded right coronary artery. This is referred to as a sympathoinhibitory reflex. Maintenance of RV preload is important and should be accomplished by aggressive volume expansion. However, administration of nitrates and diuretics should be avoided.

**Answer: E**

Gabelli, A., Layon, A.J., and Yu, M. (2012) *Civetta, Taylor & Kirby's Critical Care*. Lippincott Williams and Wilkins: Philadelphia, PA.

Jacobs, A., Leopold, J., Bates, E., *et al.* (2003) Cardiogenic shock caused by rt ventricular infarction: a report from the SHOCK registry. *Journal of the American College of Cardiology*, **41**, 1273–1279.

Lim, S.T. and Goldstein, J.A. (2001) RT ventricular infarction. *Current Treatment Options in Cardiovascular Medicine*, **3**, 95–101.

17 *A 60-year-old woman with hypertension and hyperlipidemia presents to the Emergency Department for acute onset of chest pain 90 minutes ago and is found to have ST-segment elevation in leads V2–V4 and ST-segment depression in leads II, III and aVF. She is immediately started on thrombolytic therapy. Which of the following statements regarding thrombolytics in acute coronary syndromes is true?*

A *Thrombolytics obtain acute patency rates of 70–80%*

B *Thrombolytics are indicated in patients with RBBB presenting within 24 hours of symptoms*

C *Thrombolytics have an associated risk of intracranial hemorrhage of 0.5–1.5%*

D *Thrombolytic therapy can be administered within 1 month of an ischemic stroke*

E *Thrombolytics can be administered in select patients with severe but controllable hypertension on presentation (systolic BP > 200 mm Hg or diastolic BP > 120 mm Hg)*

Fibrinolytic therapy is associated with certain limitations. This includes acute patency rates of occluded vessels of approximately 50–60%. The incidence of intracranial hemorrhage occurs at a relatively low rate of 0.5–1.5%. The indications for use of thrombolytics are as follows: acute myocardial infarction associated with ST-segment elevation or left bundle branch block (LBBB) that presents within 12 hours of onset. Absolute contraindications include:

• Any prior intracranial hemorrhage, trauma, lesion, or neoplasm

• Prior ischemic stroke within 3 months
• Active bleeding

Relative contraindication includes:

• Uncontrolled hypertension on presentation (systolic BP > 180 mm Hg or diastolic BP > 110 mm Hg)

**Answer: C**

Antman, E.A., Anbe, T.O., Armstrong, P.W., *et al.* (2013) ACC/AHA guidelines for management of patients with ST elevation myocardial infarctions. *Journal of the American College of Cardiology*, **61**, 485–510.

Califf, R. and Roe, M. (2010) *Acute Coronary Syndrome Essentials*, Jones and Bartlett Learning, Sudbury, MA.

Parillo, J.E. and Dellinger, R.D. (2014) *Critical Care Medicine: Principles of Diagnosis and Management in the Adult*. Mosby, Philadelphia, PA.

18 *Which of the following statements regarding complications after myocardial infarction is true?*

A *Right ventricular infarcts are associated with a decreased right atrial pressure (RAP), a RAP/PCWP ratio > 0.8, and an increased cardiac output (CO)*

B *Cardiogenic shock leads to decreased BP, decreased CO, increased PCWP, and increased systemic vascular resistance (SVR)*

C *Acute mitral regurgitation causes a decrease in PCWP (prominent V-wave may be seen) and decreased CO*

D *Cardiac tamponade is associated with increased BP, pulsus paradoxus, decreased CO as well as absent X descent on central venous pressure (CVP) tracing*

E *Oxygen tension is decreased from RA to RV/PA in patients with acute ventricular septal defects. VSDs increase right-to-left shunting with decreased pulmonary blood flow*

It is important to recognize the hemodynamic variations that exist between the different surgical complications associated with acute myocardial infarctions as their management will differ. Cardiogenic shock (answer B) leads to decreased BP, decreased CO, increased PCWP and increased SVR. Answer A is incorrect because right ventricular infarcts are associated with increased right atrial pressure, a RAP/PCWP ratio > 0.8, and a decreased cardiac output (CO). Acute mitral regurgitation causes an increase in PCWP, prominent V-wave, and decreased CO. Cardiac tamponade is associated with decreased BP and pulsus paradoxus which is a decrease in systolic blood pressure during inspiration. In cardiac tamponade, the RAP approximates PCWP, which is referred to as equalization of pressures. It leads to decreased CO as well as prominent X decent on central venous pressure tracings. In patients with acute ventricular septal defects, oxygen tension is stepped-up from the RA to the RV and PA. VSDs increase left-to-right shunting with increased pulmonary blood flow, which results in a falsely elevated CO.

**Answer: B**

Gabelli, A., Layon, A.J., and Yu, M. (2012) *Civetta, Taylor & Kirby's Critical Care*, Lippincott, Butterworth Heinemann, Philadelphia, PA.

Parrillo, J.E. and Dellinger, R.P. (2014) *Critical Care Medicine: Principles of Diagnosis and Management in the Adult*, Mosby, Philadelphia, PA.

Sidenbotham, D., Mckee, A., Gillham, M., and Levy, J.H. (2007) *Cardio Thoracic Critical Care*, Butterworth Heinemann, Philadelphia, PA.

**19** *A 65-year-old man with a history of peptic ulcer disease (PUD), myocardial infarction 5 years ago, hypertension and tobacco use presents to your office for his annual physical exam. His current medications include a proton pump inhibitor, simvastatin, and metoprolol. He walks 2 miles every other day for exercise. On exam, he is 5 feet 10 inches tall and weighs 200 lb. His blood pressure is 129/78 mm Hg and his pulse is 80 beats/min. Laboratory workup reveals a normal triglyceride level and a hemoglobin A1c level of 5.6%. Which of the following modifications would you recommend to reduce his cardiac risk?*

**A** *Initiation of daily Aspirin 81 mg*
**B** *Increase his dose of metoprolol*
**C** *Stop smoking*
**D** *Start an oral antihyperglycemic agent*
**E** *Start an Ace-inhibitor*

Smoking is a major contributor to the development of CAD, acute myocardial infarction, and heart failure.

Smoking cessation can significantly reduce mortality among patients with CAD, with the greatest benefit seen after three years. Based on ACC/AHA guidelines, target blood pressure among patients with CAD is less than 130/80. This patient meets this criterion so no additional antihypertensive medications are necessary. While daily aspirin is widely accepted for the secondary prevention of cardiovascular events, it should be used with caution in patients with a history of PUD. There is no proven benefit to strict glycemic control on the risk of macrovascular disease. An A1c level of below 5.7% is considered normal and 5.7–6.4% signals pre-diabetes.

**Answer: C**

Smith, S.C., Jr, Allen, J., Blair, S.N., *et al.* (2006) AHA/ACC guidelines for secondary prevention for patients with coronary and other atherosclerotic vascular disease: 2006 update endorsed by the National Heart, Lung, and Blood Institute. *Journal of the American College of Cardiology*, **47**, 2130.

Ittaman, S.V., VanWormer, J.J., and Rezkalla, S.H. (2014) The role of aspirin in the prevention of cardiovascular disease. *Clinical Medicine and Research*, **12**, 147–154.

**20** *A 72-year-old man on postoperative day 5 following a Nissen fundoplication for severe gastroesophageal reflux disease is discovered to have new-onset ST changes on a routine electrocardiogram. The patient has not complained of any chest pain or discomfort. You decide to draw a set of cardiac enzymes. Later that evening, the patient suddenly develops the rhythm shown in Figure 4.18 after being found unresponsive. His blood pressure is 50/20 mm Hg and there is no detectable pulse. Cardioversion is attempted immediately without success and repeated cycles of CPR and epinephrine via ACLS protocol are initiated along with vasopressin followed by repeated cardioversion. The rhythm remains unchanged and the patient remains hypotensive.*

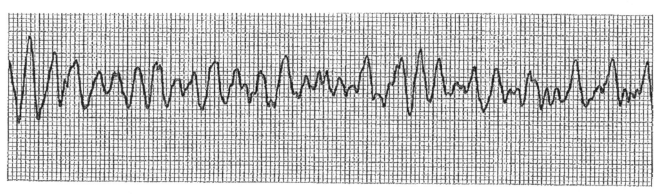

**Figure 4.18**

*What would be the next most appropriate step in the management of the patient in this clinical setting?*

**A** *IV procainamide*

**B** *IV amiodarone*

**C** *IV magnesium*

**D** *IV lidocaine*

**E** *IV bretylium tosylate*

Ventricular fibrillation (VF) occurs within the first four hours following a MI in 4% of patients. VF can usually be cardioverted within the first minute but is less than 25% successful when initiated after 4 minutes. Current ACLS guidelines for witnessed arrest recommend immediate unsynchronized defibrillation at 120–200 J monophasic followed by resumption of CPR for 2 minutes or five cycles. Epinephrine 1 mg IV push every 3–5 minutes or vasopressin 40 U IV once, for persistent VF. After five cycles of CPR, if the patient persists in VF, another shock should be delivered. If VF persists, amiodarone (300 mg IV bolus) should be given (may repeat with 150 mg dose). Alternatively, lidocaine is given in a first dose of 1–1.5 mg/kg IV, followed by 0.5–0.75 mg/kg, for a maximum of 3 doses or 3 mg/kg. Magnesium (1–2 gm IV bolus over 5 min) would be recommended for Torsades de Pointes. Compared to lidocaine, amiodarone has demonstrated increased survival to hospital admission. Procainamide is not recommended acutely due to its long administration time. Bretylium tosylate is no longer recommended for use in cardiac arrest.

**Answer: B**

Gabelli, A., Layon, A.J., Yu, M. (2012) *Civetta, Taylor & Kirby's Critical Care*, Lippincott, Williams and Wilkins, Philadelphia, PA.

Field, J., Gonzales, L., and Hazinski, M. (2015) *Advanced Cardiac Life Support*, American Heart Association.

Sidebotham, D., Mckee, A., Gillham, M., and Levy, J.H. (2007) *Cardio Thoracic Critical Care*, Butterworth Heinemann, Philadelphia, PA.

# 5

## Sepsis and the Inflammatory Response to Injury
*Juan C. Duchesne, MD and Marquinn D. Duke, MD*

**Questions 1 and 2 refer to the following case.**
*A 80-year-old man presents to the emergency department with a 2-day history of fever, chills, cough, and right-sided pleuritic chest pain. On the day of admission, the patient's family noted that he was more lethargic and dizzy and was falling frequently. The patient's vital signs are: temperature 101.5°F; heart rate 120 beats/min; respiratory rate 30 breaths/min; blood pressure 70/35 mm Hg; and oxygen saturation as measured by pulse oximetry, 80% without oxygen supplementation. A chest radiograph shows a right lower lobe infiltrate.*

1  *This patient's condition can best be defined as which of the following?*
  **A** *Multi-organ dysfunction syndrome (MODS)*
  **B** *Sepsis*
  **C** *Septic shock*
  **D** *Severe sepsis*
  **E** *Systemic inflammatory response syndrome (SIRS)*

The patient fulfills criteria for severe sepsis, defined as sepsis with evidence of organ dysfunction, hypoperfusion, or hypotension. SIRS is defined as an inflammatory response to insult manifested by two of the following: temperature greater than 38°C (100.4°F) or less than 36°C (96.8°F), heart rate greater than 90 beats/min, respiratory rate greater than 20 breaths/min, and white blood cell count greater that $12 \times 10/\mu L$, less than $4 \times 10/\mu L$, or 10% bands. A diagnosis of sepsis is given if infection is present in addition to meeting criteria for SIRS. Septic shock includes sepsis-induced hypotension (despite fluid resuscitation) along with evidence of hypoperfusion. MODS is the presence of altered organ function such that hemostasis cannot be maintained without intervention. This patient's lack of fluid resuscitation classifies him as having severe sepsis rather than septic shock.

**Answer: D**

Bone, R.C., Balk, R.A., Cerra, F.B., *et al.* (1992) Definition for sepsis and organ failure and guidelines for the use of innovative therapies in sepsis. The ACCP/SCCM Consensus Conference Committee. American College of Chest Physicians/Society of Critical Care Medicine. *Chest*, **101**, 1644–1555.

Holmes, C.L. and Walley, K.R. (2003) The evaluation and management of shock. *Clinics in Chest Medicine*, **24**, 775–789.

2  *What is the first step in the initial management of this patient?*
  **A** *Antibiotic therapy*
  **B** *β-Blocker therapy to control heart rate*
  **C** *Intravenous (IV) fluid resuscitation*
  **D** *Supplemental oxygen and airway management*
  **E** *Vasopressor therapy with dopamine*

The initial evaluation of any critically ill patient in shock should include assessing and establishing an airway, evaluating breathing (which includes consideration of mechanical ventilator support), and restoring adequate circulation. Adequate oxygenation should be ensured with a goal of achieving an arterial oxygen saturation of 90% or greater.

**Answer: D**

Bone, R.C., Balk, R.A., Cerra, F.B., *et al.* (1992) Definition for sepsis and organ failure and guidelines for the use of innovative therapies in sepsis. *The ACCP/SCCM Consensus Conference Committee. American College of Chest Physicians/Society of Critical Care Medicine. Chest*, **101**, 1644–1555.

Holmes, C.L. and Walley, K.R. (2003) The evaluation and management of shock. *Clinics in Chest Medicine*, **24**, 775–789.

*Surgical Critical Care and Emergency Surgery: Clinical Questions and Answers*, Second Edition.
Edited by Forrest "Dell" Moore, Peter Rhee, and Gerard J. Fulda.
© 2018 John Wiley & Sons Ltd. Published 2018 by John Wiley & Sons Ltd.
Companion website: www.wiley.com/go/moore/surgical_criticalcare_and_emergency_surgery

**3** *Which of the following is an indication for using corticosteroids in septic shock?*
 **A** *Acute respiratory distress syndrome (ARDS)*
 **B** *Necrotizing pneumonia*
 **C** *Peritonitis*
 **D** *Sepsis responding well to fluid resuscitation*
 **E** *Vasopressor-dependent septic shock*

An inappropriate cortisol response is not uncommon in patients with septic shock. Low-dose IV corticosteroids (hydrocortisone 200–300 mg/day) are recommended in patients with vasopressor-dependent septic shock. However, steroids should not be used in the absence of vasopressor requirement. Higher doses of corticosteroids have been shown to be harmful in severe sepsis. The use of adrenal function tests to guide decisions on corticosteroid therapy is no longer recommended prior to initiation of corticosteroids. Historically, an absolute incremental increase of 9 μg/dL at 30 or 60 minutes after administration of 250 μg of corticotropin was found as the best cutoff value to distinguish between adequate adrenal response (responders) and relative adrenal insufficiency (non-responders).

**Answer: E**

Bone, R.C., Fisher, C.J., and Clemmer, T.P. (1987) A controlled clinical trial of high-dose methylprednisolone in the treatment of severe sepsis and septic shock. *New England Journal of Medicine*, **317**, 653–658.

Keh, D. and Sprung, C.L. (2004) Use of corticosteroid therapy in patients with sepsis and septic shock: an evidence-based review. *Critical Care Medicine*, **32** (11 Suppl), S527–S533.

Rivers, E.P., Gaspari, M., Saad, G.A., *et al.* (2001) Adrenal insufficiency in high-risk surgical ICU patients. *Chest*, **119**, 889–896.

**4** *Which one of the following would be most likely to cause early onset (within the first 4 days of hospitalization) ventilator-associated pneumonia (VAP)?*
 **A** Streptococcus pneumonia
 **B** Staphylococcus aureus
 **C** Acinetobacter
 **D** Pseudomonas aeruginosa
 **E** Klebsiella pneumonia

Early-onset VAP occurs within the 1<sup>st</sup> 4 days of hospitalization and most commonly is caused by community acquire pathogens such as *S. pneumonia* and Haemophilus species. In 20–50% of cases, VAP is caused by a polymicrobial infection. The role of anaerobic bacteria and VAP is not clear. In general, it appears that oropharyngeal bacteria, rather than gastric bacteria, are the major sources of VAP. The most common pathogens isolated in VAP are *Staph. aureus*, Pseudomonas, Enterobacter species, and Klebsiella species. It appears that VAP caused by Pseudomonas and Acinetobacter species are factors for higher mortality. Acinetobacter species are not common pathogens in early VAP.

**Answer: A**

Craven, D.E. and Steger, K.A. (1995) Nosocomial pneumonia in mechanically ventilated adult patients: epidemiology and prevention in 1996. *Seminars in Respiratory Infections*, 11, 32–53.

Safdar, N., Dezfulian, C., Collard, H.R., and Saint, S. (2005) Clinical and economic consequences of ventilator-associated pneumonia: A systematic review. *Critical care Medicine*, **33** (10), 2184–2193.

**5** *Which one of the following is supportive of a diagnosis of VAP?*
 **A** *Positive culture (more than $10^3$ colony forming units [CFUs]/ml) from an endobronchial aspirate*
 **B** *Positive culture (more than $10^2$ CFUs/ml) from a protected brush specimen (PBS) performed during bronchoscopy*
 **C** *Positive culture (more than $10^2$ CFUs/ml) from a PBS obtained blindly without bronchoscopy*
 **D** *Positive culture (more than $10^4$ CFUs/ml) from a bronchoalveolar lavage (BAL)*
 **E** *Positive culture (more than $10^2$ CFUs/ml) from a BAL*

The use of quantitative microbiology to make the diagnosis of VAP offers multiple options. Sources of specimens can be from bronchoscopic bronchoalveolar lavage, protected brush specimen, or blind BAL. The following criteria must be met for the following quantitative modalities to confirm the diagnosis of VAP: Endobronchial aspirate, more than $10^6$ CFU/mL; PSB from bronchoscopy, more than $10^3$ CFU/mL; PSB obtained blindly, more than $10^3$ CFU/mL; and BAL with or without protected catheter, more than $10^4$ CFU/mL. Therefore, a BAL culture with more than $10^4$ CFU/mL will meet criteria for the diagnosis of VAP.

**Answer: D**

Ewig, S., Bauer, T., and Torres, A. (2002) The pulmonary physician in critical care • 4: nosocomial pneumonia. *Thorax*, **57** (4), 366–371.

Rea-Neto, A., Youssef, N., Tuche, F., *et al.* (2008) Diagnosis of ventilator-associated pneumonia: a systematic review of the literature. *Critical Care*, **12** (2), R56.

**6** *Which one of the following has the strongest causative association with VAP?*
**A** *Gastric bacteria*
**B** *Nasal bacteria*
**C** *Oropharyngeal bacteria*
**D** *Skin bacteria*
**E** *Small bowel translocation*

Oropharyngeal bacteria are the major source of VAP, not gastric bacteria. It does not appear that nasal bacteria independently play a significant role in the development of VAP. Other sources exist exogenously, such as bacteria transferred from healthcare provider to patient from inadequately washing hands, inadequately disinfected respiratory therapy equipment and contaminated medication biopsies. Aspiration of oropharyngeal bacteria into the lower respiratory tract and reduced host defense mechanisms are risk factors for the development of VAP.

**Answer: C**

Kollef, M.H., Skubas, N.J., and Sundt, T.M. (1999) A randomized clinical trial of continuous aspiration of subglottic secretions in cardiac surgery patients. *Chest*, **116**, 1339–1346.
Pneumatikos, I.A., Dragoumanis, C.K., and Bouros, D.E. (2009) Ventilator-associated pneumonia or endotracheal tube-associated pneumonia?: An approach to the pathogenesis and preventive strategies emphasizing the importance of endotracheal tube. *Anesthesiology*, **110** (3), 673–680.

**7** *Which one of the following antibiotics would be effective in treating an infection caused by an extended-spectrum B-lactamase-producing strain of Enterobacter species?*
**A** *Piperacillin/tazobactam*
**B** *Ampicillin/sulbactam*
**C** *Ceftazidime*
**D** *Cefoxitine*
**E** *Ciprofloxacin*

When an organism is identified as producing an extended-spectrum beta-lactamase, the efficacy of all third-generation cephalosporins, monobactams, extended-spectrum beta-lactams, and beta-lactamase inhibitor combinations are suspect. The cephamycins, which includes cefoxitin and cefotetan, are effective agents. Other effective agents include the carbapenems, fourth-generation cephalosporins, the fluoroquinolones and the aminoglycosides. The presence of broad-spectrum beta-lactamase is most often found on isolates of Enterobacter, Citrobacter, and Serratia organism. Klebsiella pneumonia that produces ESBL has also been encountered.

**Answer: D**

Bassetti, M.I., Righi, E., Fasce, R., *et al.* (2007) Efficacy of ertapenem in the treatment of early ventilator-associated pneumonia caused by extended-spectrum beta-lactamase-producing organisms in an intensive care unit. *Journal of Antimicrobial Chemotherapy*, **60** (2), 433–435.
Grgurich, P.E., Hudcova, J., Lei, Y., *et al.* (2014) Management and prevention of ventilator-associated pneumonia caused by multidrug-resistant pathogens. *Expert Review of Respiratory Medicine*, **6** (5), 533–555.

**8** *Which one of the following organisms may be effectively treated by removal of the catheter alone?*
**A** *Enterococcal species*
**B** Klebsiella pneumonia
**C** Candida albicans
**D** Staphylococcus aureus
**E** *Pseudomonas spp*

There are several important issues to consider when treating catheter-related bloodstream infection. *Staph epidermidis* is often a contaminant, however, when it is responsible for bloodstream infection, it tends to behave in non-virulent manner. Thus, it usually can be treated by removing the catheter with or without the addition of a short course of antibiotics.

**Answer: A**

Pérez Parra, A., Cruz Menárquez, M., Pérez Granda, M.J. (2010) A simple educational intervention to decrease incidence of central line-associated bloodstream infection (CLABSI) in intensive care units with low baseline incidence of CLABSI. *Infection Control and Hospital Epidemiology*, **31** (9), 964–967.
Pronovost, P., Needham, D., Berenholtz, S., *et al.* (2006) An intervention to decrease catheter-related bloodstream infections in the ICU. *New England Journal of Medicine*, **355** (26), 2725–2732. Erratum in: *New England Journal of Medicine* (2007) **356** (25), 2660.

**9** *Which antifungal has excellent CSF penetration for treatment of cryptococcal meningitis?*
**A** *Capsofungin*
**B** *Fluconazole*
**C** *Itraconazole*
**D** *Ketoconazole*
**E** *Clotrimazole*

The azole antifungals work by inhibiting the activity of lanosterol demethylase, blocking the production of fungal cell walls. As opposed to amphotericin B, which is fungicidal, these agents are fungistatic. The most common side effect of azoles is hepatic dysfunction, resulting in elevation of transaminases. Fluconazole, the most widely used of the azoles, has excellent activity against most of the Candida species. Although its widespread use has made resistance among the Candida species common, it remains first-line therapy for invasive candidiasis. It has a great bioavailability and can easily penetrate the CSF. Fluconazole can be used in central nervous system infection including those caused by Cryptococcus species.

**Answer: B**

Menichetti, F., Fiorio, M., Tosti, A., *et al.* (1996) High-dose fluconazole therapy for cryptococcal meningitis in patients with AIDS. *Clinical Infectious Diseases*, **22** (5), 838–840.

Van der Horst, C.M., Saag, M.S., Cloud, G.A., *et al.* (1997) Treatment of cryptococcal meningitis associated with the acquired immunodeficiency syndrome. *New England Journal of Medicine*, **337** (1), 15–21.

10 *A patient with large-cell lung cancer presents to the ED with a fever 102°F and a non-productive cough. The patient is on a chemotherapy regimen and her WBC is 0.4 cells/mm$^3$. Which of the following will be the best treatment regimen?*
   A *Antibiotic double-coverage for gram-negative bacteria*
   B *Empiric antifungal therapy*
   C *Removal of any long-term catheters*
   D *Continuation of antibiotic therapy until resolution of neutropenia*
   E *Empiric antiviral therapy*

Neutropenia represents a common complication of chemotherapeutic agents. An absolute neutrophil count less than 500 /mm$^3$ places patients at greater risk of infection. Anaerobic and gram-negatives bacteria aren't the most common pathogens in the neutropenic population and include *Enterobacter coli*, Klebsiella and Pseudomonas. While empiric combination antibiotic therapy may seem reasonable in this condition, no studies have proven a mortality benefit over monotherapy. In general, if fever persists, then therapies are continued during the course of neutropenia to prevent break-through bacteremia. If the cause is identified, 10–14 days of therapy is usually sufficient. If no source is identified, therapy is stopped once the absolute neutrophil count exceeds 1000 cells/uL or fever resolves. Neutropenic patients who've failed to improve despite empiric antibiotic therapy may require the addition of antifungal therapy within 4–7 days. Catheters do not necessarily need to be removed in febrile neutropenic patients if there is no evidence of infection.

**Answer: D**

Anaissie, E.J., Vartivarian, S., Bodey, G. P., *et al.* (1996) Randomized comparison between antibiotics alone and antibiotics plus granulocyte-macrophage colony-stimulating factor (*Escherichia coli*-derived) in cancer patients with fever and neutropenia. *The American Journal of Medicine*, **100** (1), 17–23.

Paul, M., Yahav, D., Fraser, A., and Leibovici, L. (2006) Empirical antibiotic monotherapy for febrile neutropenia: systematic review and meta-analysis of randomized controlled trials. *Journal of Antimicrobial Chemotherapy*, **57** (2): 176–189.

11 *While working on his farm an 18-year-old man lacerates his forearm on a rusted iron fence. Which one of the following is correct regarding tetanus?*
   A *Tetanus is a disease of the young with most cases occurring in young adults under the age of 20 years*
   B *The severity of illness is greater if the incubation period is short*
   C *The tetanus toxin is carried by anterograde axonal transport where it promotes neuronal transmitter release*
   D *Neuromuscular blockade is first-line therapy to control severe muscle rigidity*
   E *The wound needs to only be irrigated and closed*

Tetanus, a fatal disease, is caused by the exotoxin of *Clostridium tetani*. While common in less developed countries, tetanus vaccine has made the disease extremely rare in the USA, where it has become a disease of adults. Vaccination eliminates the likelihood of disease. The median time to disease onset is approximately 6 days. The exotoxin travels to the peripheral motor neurons by retrograde axonal transport and blocks inhibitory impulses, causing prolonged muscle spasms. This patient should be admitted to the intensive care unit and initial treatment should include human tetanus immunoglobulin and extensive wound debridement. Supportive measures such as mechanical ventilation should be implemented if needed. Following these initial steps, control of muscle hypertonicity with benzodiazepines is preferred.

**Answer: B**

Rhee, P., Nunley, M.K., Demetriades, D., *et al.* (2005) Tetanus and trauma: a review and recommendations. *The Journal of Trauma*, **58** (5), 1082–1088.

Talan, D.A. (2004) Tetanus immunity and physician compliance with tetanus prophylaxis practices among emergency department patients presenting with wounds. *Annals of Emergency Medicine*, **43** (3), 305–314.

**12** *Which of the following is NOT a common causative organism for ventilator-associated pneumonia?*
  **A** *MRSA*
  **B** *Pseudomonas*
  **C** *Enterobacter*
  **D** *Mycoplasma*
  **E** Legionella

Pseudomonas and MRSA are the two most common organisms for ventilator-associated infections (VAP). Hence, in mechanically ventilated patients at risk for VAP, empiric antibiotic coverage should generally cover these organisms (i.e., vancomycin and pipercillin-tazobactam), especially if ventilated greater than 72 hours, until culture results are available. Other gram-negative organisms such as Acinetobacter and Enterobacter are also common. Mycoplasma is not a common VAP organism. *Legionella pneumophila* are nutritionally fastidious, intracellular bacilli, gram-negative organisms. Infection with *Legionella* is associated with exposure to artificial water systems, condensers, and respiratory therapy equipment. Use of PCR as a rapid and specific diagnostic method for *Legionella* infection overcame the long culture time needed for its growth (3–5 days) and the need of media supplemented with iron and cysteine as well as difficult colonial identification in mixed cultures.

**Answer: D**

Grossman, R.F. and Fein, A. (2000) Evidence-based assessment of diagnostic tests for ventilator-associated pneumonia. *Chest*, **117** (4, suppl 2), 177S–181S.
Topley, W. and Wilson, S. (2008) *Topley and Wilson's Microbiology and Microbial Infections*, 10th edn., Hodder and Arnold, London.

**13** *A 26-year-old man presents to the ED with a 3-day history of fever and increasing fatigue and malaise. Vital signs are temperature 101.9°F, heart rate 125 beats/minute, RR 30 breaths/minute and BP 70/30 mm Hg. His exam is notable for lethargy with evidence of cellulitis and blebs on his extremities. His skin is flushed and warm and his pulses are 2+. Lung exam reveals rales bilaterally. He is intubated, receives 1 liter of normal saline and dopamine is started at 8 ug/kg/min. He is then transferred to the ICU. As you evaluate him, his heart rate is 140 beats/minute and his BP is 60/35 mm Hg. You order another liter NS bolus with no effect on heart rate or blood pressure. What is the most appropriate therapy at this time?*
  **A** *Vasopressin*
  **B** *Methylprednisolone*
  **C** *Increase dopamine to 20 mcg/kg/min*
  **D** *Norepinephrine*
  **E** *Hypertonic saline*

This patient has septic shock with evidence of "warm" or vasodilatory shock on physical exam. He has already received 60 cc/kg NS and appears to be fluid refractory at this time. While it would be reasonable to increase the dopamine infusion, the most appropriate choice would be to order a vasoconstrictive agent such as norepineprhine in order to improve blood pressure and perfusion. Dopamine has fallen out of favor due to potential immunomodulatory effects, reliance on endogenous catecholamines, tachyarrhythmias, and so on.

**Answer: D**

Avni, T., Lador, A., Lev, S., *et al.* (2015) Vasopressors for the treatment of septic shock: systematic review and meta-analysis. *PLoS One*, **10** (8): e0129305.
Dellinger, R.P. (2013) Guidelines for management of severe sepsis and septic shock. *Intensive Care Medicine*, **39** (2), 165–228.

**14** *A 25-year-old woman is admitted to the ICU with 2 days of fever, vomiting, and increasing lethargy. She has a recent laceration on her leg with evidence of warmth and tenderness at the site. Her vitals are: temperature 103°F, heart rate 128 beats/minute, BP 74/45 mm Hg, RR 30 breaths/minute. She has cool extremities and diminished pulses. Which of the following statements is most accurate?*
  **A** *There is up-regulation of adrenergic receptors*
  **B** *Cytokines do not induce myocardial suppression*
  **C** *This patient suffers primarily from vasomotor paralysis*
  **D** *Sepsis induces abnormalities in the cardiomyocyte, leading to cardiovascular dysfunction*
  **E** *Albumin is better than NS as first line resuscitation*

This patient has evidence of septic shock, presenting primarily with "cold" shock, which typically indicates some degree of cardiovascular dysfunction. This is thought to be sepsis-induced and involves down-regulation of adrenergic pathways, cytokine mediated cardiomyocyte dysfunction, and impaired intracellular $Ca^{2+}$ trafficking.

**Answer: D**

Avni, T., Lador, A., Lev, S., *et al.* (2015) Vasopressors for the treatment of septic shock: systematic review and meta-analysis. *PLoS One*, **10** (8): e0129305.
Dellinger, R.P. (2013) Guidelines for management of severe sepsis and septic shock. *Intensive Care Medicine*, **39** (2), 165–228. February 2013, Volume 39, Issue 2, pp 165–228

**15** *Which of the following therapeutics has been found to be effective in improving outcomes with sepsis?*
  **A** *Activated protein C*
  **B** *Steroids*
  **C** *Early administration of antibiotics*
  **D** *Albumin boluses*
  **E** *Trendelenburg positioning*

Of the choices given, only early antibiotics (7% increased mortality per hour delay) has been shown to have a significant impact on outcomes with sepsis. PROWESS and RESOLVE demonstrated no significant improvement with activated protein C, CORTICUS showed no significant differences with use of hydrocortisone, and the SAFE study revealed no differences between albumin vs. normal saline (and may worsen outcomes in patients with TBI).

**Answer: C**

Dellinger, R.P. (2013) Guidelines for management of severe sepsis and septic shock. *Intensive Care Medicine*, **39** (2), 165–228.

de Groot, B., Ansems, A., Gerling, D.H., *et al.* (2015) The association between time to antibiotics and relevant clinical outcomes in emergency department patients with various stages of sepsis: a prospective multi-center study. *Critical Care*, **19** (1), 194.

**16** *A 67-year-old man with a history of chronic obstructive pulmonary disease (COPD), hypertension, and chronic renal failure is admitted to the ICU with community-acquired pneumonia. His treatment includes broad-spectrum antibiotics, corticosteroids, and inhaled β2 stimulants. Due to a severe ileus and gastric intolerance, total parenteral nutrition is commenced. The patient's temperature normalizes after the third day in ICU, and his oxygenation improves. However, on the ninth hospital day he develops a fever with an increase in the peripheral leukocyte count. Antibiotics are stopped; and blood, urine, and sputum cultures are performed. Candida krusei is isolated from a single blood culture, and 60 000 CFU/mL of C. krusei is isolated from the urine. Which of the following is the most appropriate next step in the management of this patient?*
  **A** *Remove, culture, and replace all vascular catheters*
  **B** *Remove, culture, and replace all vascular catheters and begin intravenous (IV) fluconazole*
  **C** *Remove, culture, and replace all vascular catheters and begin IV amphotericin*
  **D** *Remove, culture, and replace all vascular catheters; replace urinary catheter; and begin amphotericin bladder irrigations*
  **E** *Repeat the blood and urine cultures and observe the patient*

The risk factors for *Candida* intravascular infection include use of broad-spectrum antibiotics, total parenteral nutrition, and immunosuppressive therapy. Because a single positive blood culture is highly predictive of systemic candida infection, it should never be considered a contaminant. The initial treatment of *Candida* infections includes removal of all possible foci of infection, including removal of intravascular lines. Candidemia may resolve spontaneously after removal of intravascular catheters. However, increasing evidence suggests that metastatic foci of infection may develop in some patients even after catheter removal and may manifest as endophthalmitis, endocarditis, arthritis, or meningitis. Therefore, all critically ill patients with candidemia should be regarded as having systemic infection and should be treated accordingly. Fluconazole and amphotericin demonstrate similar effectiveness in treating candidemia in patients without neutropenia and without major immunodeficiency. However, both in vitro and clinical data have demonstrated *C. krusei* to be intrinsically resistant to fluconazole. Prolonged bladder catheterization in the critically ill patient is often accompanied by the appearance of candiduria. Candiduria usually reflects catheter colonization; however, rarely, *Candida* species may cause cystitis and/or retrograde renal parenchymal infection. The management of asymptomatic candiduria in the catheterized patient, in whom no suspicion of renal candidiasis or renal obstruction exists, requires change of the indwelling catheter only, followed by observation. No data suggest that amphotericin B bladder irrigations prevent infections in colonized patients.

**Answer: C**

Fisher, J.F., Newman, C.L., and Sobel, J.D. (1995) Yeast in the urine: solutions for a budding problem. *Clinical Infectious Diseases*, **20**, 183–189.

Rex, J.H., Bennett, J.E., Sugar, A.M., *et al.* (1994) A randomized trial comparing fluconazole with amphotericin B for the treatment of candidemia in patients without neutropenia. *New England Journal of Medicine*, **331**, 1325–1330.

Rex, J.H., Pfaller, M.A., Barry, A.L., *et al.* (1995) Antifungal susceptibility testing of isolates from a randomized, multicenter trial of fluconazole versus amphotericin B as treatment of nonneutropenic patients with candidemia. *Antimicrobial Agents and Chemotherapy*, **39**, 40–44.

**17** *Which of the following is true of vasopressin in septic shock?*
  **A** *Continuous infusion at low doses improves 28-day overall mortality*
  **B** *Continuous infusion at low doses improves mortality in patients with severe septic shock*

**C** *Continuous infusion at low doses increases cardiac output*

**D** *Continuous infusion at low doses reduces the catecholamine infusion requirement*

**E** *Is the first line vasopressor for septic shock*

Vasopressin is a peptide synthesized in the hypothalamus and released from the posterior pituitary. Vasopressin produces a wide range of physiologic effects, including blood pressure maintenance. Acting through vascular V1-receptors, the endogenous hormone directly induces vasoconstriction in hypotensive patients but does not significantly alter vascular smooth muscle constriction in humans with normal blood pressure. Landry and colleagues demonstrated that patients with septic shock had inappropriately low levels of serum vasopressin compared with patients with cardiogenic shock, who had normal or elevated levels of vasopressin. In addition, they demonstrated that supplementing a low-dose infusion of vasopressin in septic shock patients allowed for the reduction or removal of the other catecholamine vasopressors. This was seen despite a reduction in cardiac output. Although these results were duplicated in subsequent studies, none evaluated outcomes such as length of stay or mortality until recently. A randomized double-blind study comparing vasopressin versus norepinephrine for the treatment of septic shock demonstrated no difference in 28-day mortality between the two treatment groups. Subgroup analysis of patients with severe septic shock, defined as requiring 15 μg/min of norepinephrine or its equivalent, also did not demonstrate a mortality benefit. However, patients with less severe septic shock (i.e., requiring 5–15 μg/min of norepinephrine) experienced a trend toward lower mortality when treated with low-dose (0.01–0.03 U/min) vasopressin.

**Answer: D**

Landry, D.W., Levin, H.R., Gallant, E.M., *et al.* (1997) Vasopressin deficiency contributes to the vasodilation of septic shock. *Circulation*, **95**, 1122–1125.

Russell, J.A., Walley, K.R., Singer, J., *et al.* (2008) Vasopressin versus norepinephrine infusion in patients with septic shock. *New England Journal of Medicine*, **358**, 877–787.

**18** *The role of the coagulation system in the sepsis-induced inflammatory cascade includes:*

**A** *Up-regulating fibrinolysis.*

**B** *Blocking further inflammation.*

**C** *Down-regulating the anticoagulant system*

**D** *Up-regulating the anticoagulant system*

**E** *All of the above*

The coagulation system plays an important role in the sepsis-induced inflammatory cascade. Coagulation is activated by the inflammatory reaction to tissue injury and is activated independent of the type of microbe (e.g., gram-positive and gram-negative bacteria, viruses, fungi, or parasites). Increased coagulation contributes to mortality in sepsis by down-regulating fibrinolysis and the anticoagulant systems. The collaboration between clotting and inflammation, which works to wall off damaged and infected tissues, is an important host survival strategy. Coagulation induced by inflammation can in turn contribute to further inflammation. A key to determining survival in sepsis is to limit the damage while retaining the benefits of localized clotting and controlled clearance of pathogens.

A continuum of coagulopathy in sepsis has been suggested, extending from the appearance of mild coagulation abnormalities prior to the onset of any clinical signs of severe sepsis to consumption of anticoagulant proteins and suppression of the fibrinolytic system. Depletion of anticoagulant and fibrinolytic factors contributes to the microvascular deposition of fibrin that is associated with organ dysfunction. Coagulation abnormalities in sepsis contribute significantly to organ dysfunction and death.

**Answer: C**

Cinel, I. and Opal, S.M. (2009) Molecular biology of inflammation and sepsis: a primer. *Critical Care Medicine*, **37** (1), 291–304.

Dettenmeier, P., Swindell, B., Stroud, M., *et al.* (2003) Role of activated protein C in the pathophysiology of severe sepsis. *American Journal of Critical Care*, **12** (6), 518–524.

Dhainaut, J.F., Shorr, A.F., Macias, W.L., *et al.* (2005) Dynamic evolution of coagulopathy in the first day of severe sepsis: relationship with mortality and organ failure. *Critical Care Medicine*, **33** (2), 341–348.

**19** *The major cause of vasodilation in sepsis appears to be mediated by:*

**A** *ATP-sensitive potassium channels in smooth muscle*

**B** *ATP-sensitive calcium channels in smooth muscle*

**C** *L-arginine*

**D** *Interruption of sympathetic afferents endings*

**E** *None of the above*

The endothelium is an endocrine organ, capable of regulating the function of the microcirculation. The most important compound produced is nitric oxide (NO), an endogenous vasodilator (it is the mechanism by which nitrate drugs work). Its major effects are to cause local vasodilatation and inhibition of platelet aggregation. NO is produced from l-arginine by nitric oxide synthetase (NOS), and its actions are mediated by cGMP. NO is an essential to the normal functioning of the vascular system. There are two forms of the enzyme NOS, a constitutive form, produced as part of the normal regulatory mechanisms, and an inducible form, whose production appears to be pathologic. Inducible NOS (iNOS) is an offshoot of the inflammatory response, by TNF and other cytokines. It results in massive production of NO, causing widespread vasodilatation (due to loss of vasomotor tone) and hypotension, which is hyporeactive to adrenergic agents.

NO has a physiological antagonist, endothelin-1, a potent vasoconstrictor whose circulating level is increased in cardiogenic shock and following severe trauma.

The major cause of vasodilation in sepsis appears to be mediated by ATP-sensitive potassium channels in smooth muscle. The result of activation is increased permeability of vascular smooth muscle cells to potassium, and hyperpolarization of the cell membranes, preventing muscle contraction, leading to vasodilation.

In addition to potassium channels and inducible nitric oxide, there is a relative deficiency of vasopressin in early sepsis, the cause and significance of which is unknown.

**Answer: A**

Jackson, W.F. (2000) Ion channels and vascular tone. *Hypertension*, **35** (1 Pt 2), 173–178.

Quayle, J.M., Nelson, M.T., and Standen, N.B. (1997) ATP-sensitive and inwardly rectifying potassium channels in smooth muscle. *Physiological Reviews*, **77** (4), 1165–1232.

# 6

## Hemodynamic and Respiratory Monitoring
*Stephen M. Welch, DO, Christopher S. Nelson, MD and Stephen L. Barnes, MD*

1 *A 35-year-old woman is involved in a high-speed motor vehicle collision. Vital Signs: HR: 134, RR: 20, BP: 70/30, $O_2$ Sat: 95%. She complains of pain in her left upper quadrant. Two large-bore peripheral IV's are obtained. Two units of uncrossmatched packed red blood cells are ordered and started. Focused sonography was found to be grossly positive at the perisplenic space. She is taken emergently for an exploratory laparotomy. Which of the following hemodynamic profiles would you expect if a PA catheter were placed in this patient?*

Central venous pressure (CVP); Right ventricular pressure (RV); Pulmonary artery pressure (PA); Pulmonary artery wedge pressure (PAWP); Aortic Pressure (AO); Cardiac Index (CI); Systemic vascular resistance (SVR)

   A *CVP: 15, RV: 25/15, PA: 25/15, PAWP: 15, AO: 70/40, CI: 1.5, SVR: 1850*
   B *CVP: 2, RV: 25/2, PA 20/6, PAWP: 6, AO: 70/40, CI: 3.7, SVR 750*
   C *CVP: 15, RV: 30/15, PA: 25/10, PAWP 18, AO: 70/40, CI: 1.6, SVR: 1850*
   D *CVP 4, RV: 25/4, PA: 25/10, PAWP 10, AO: 130/80, CI: 3.5, SVR: 1000*
   E *CVP 2, RV: 20/2, PA: 20/4, PAWP: 4, AO: 70/40, CI: 1.8, SVR: 1850*

In hypovolemic shock there is a significant decrease in total blood volume which will decrease CVP, RV, PA, PAWP, AO, and CI. The body will attempt to increase the SVR to compensate for these changes to all of the hemodynamic parameters. Answer A is suggestive of cardiac tamponade. Answer B is suggestive of early septic shock. Answer C is suggestive of cardiogenic shock. Answer D is normal physiology. Understanding the physiologic changes that can be seen in various types of shock is essential to guide resuscitation efforts in the critically ill.

**Answer: E**

Rhodes, A. and Grounds, R.M. (2005) New technologies for measuring cardiac output: the future? *Current Opinion in Critical Care*, **11** (3), 224–226.

Richard, C., Warszawski, J., Anguel, N., *et al.* (2003) Early use of the pulmonary catheter and outcomes in patients with shock and acute respiratory distress syndrome: a randomized control trial. *Journal of the American Medical Association*, **290**, 2713–2720.

**2 and 3** *A 16-year-old cyanotic appearing man is brought to the trauma bay by the fire department. He was found to be unresponsive in his bedroom with an unknown down time during a house fire. GCS currently is 8. His mother is at bedside and reports that he has asthma for which he takes a rescue inhaler as needed. She denies any knowledge of him smoking or drinking. Rapid sequence intubation is performed and a cuffed 7-0 endotracheal tube is placed with no complications. Bronchoscopy is performed which shows moderate carbonaceous sputum and erythema in the distal and proximal bronchi. His oxygen saturation is 94% ($SpO_2$) measured by pulse oximetry. Laboratory data shows a carboxyhemoglobin (COHb) of 10%.*

2 *Which of the following is true in regards to this patient's oxygen saturation?*
   A *His $SpO_2$ can more accurately be measured with multi-wavelength CO-oximeter*
   B *His $SpO_2$ is falsely low secondary to carboxyhemoglobin*
   C *His $SpO_2$ saturation is normal for his bronchial findings*
   D *His $SpO_2$ saturation is falsely high secondary to his asthma history*
   E *His $SpO_2$ is appropriate at his time*

*Surgical Critical Care and Emergency Surgery: Clinical Questions and Answers*, Second Edition.
Edited by Forrest "Dell" Moore, Peter Rhee, and Gerard J. Fulda.
© 2018 John Wiley & Sons Ltd. Published 2018 by John Wiley & Sons Ltd.
Companion website: www.wiley.com/go/moore/surgical_criticalcare_and_emergency_surgery

**3** *Several factors cause peripheral pulse oximetry monitors to lose accuracy. Of all of the factors listed below, which would result in a falsely high reading?*
   **A** *Methemoglobin*
   **B** *Severe anemia*
   **C** *Glycohemoglobin A1c levels*
   **D** *Sulfhemoglobin*
   **E** *Venous congestion*

Pulse oximetry measures peripheral arterial oxygen saturation ($SpO_2$) as a surrogate marker for tissue oxygenation. It has become the standard for continuous, noninvasive assessment of oxygenation, such that it is now known as the "fifth vital sign." Conventional pulse oximeters use two light emitting diodes and a photodetector which measure oxygenated and deoxygenated hemoglobin and correlate a numeric value via the absorbance it detects. Deoxyhemoglobin absorbs light maximally in the red band spectrum (600–750 nm) while oxyhemoglobin absorbs the infrared band (850–1000 nm). Multiple factors can affect the accuracy of pulse oximetry monitors. Falsely elevated readings can be caused by carboxyhemoglobin, glycohemoglobin A1c, and sickle-cell anemia. Falsely low readings can be caused by methemoglobinemia, sulfhemoglobinemia, severe anemia, black/blue/green nail polish, motion artifact, and venous congestion. CO-oximetry is a four wavelength (or more) non-invasive monitoring system that allows additional measurements of blood constituents. It not only measures oxygenated and deoxygenated hemoglobin, as pulse oximetry does, but also dyshemoglobins. These include carboxyhemoglobin and methemoglobin.

**Answer 2: A**

**Answer 3: C**

Chan, E.D., Chan, M.M., and Chan, M.M. (2013) Pulse oximetry: understanding its basic principles facilitates appreciation of its limitations. *Respiratory Medicine*, **107** (6),789–799.

Jurban, A. (2004) Pulse oximetry. *Intensive Care Medicine*, **30** (11), 2017–2020.

**4** *A 28-year old woman is brought to the trauma bay after being kicked in the left flank by her horse. The incident happened approximately 30 minutes ago. She currently has a GCS of 15 and complains of severe left-sided back pain. Vital signs are as follows: BP: 87/61, HR: 122, RR: 28, $O_2$ SAT: 97% on room air. FAST exam showed no fluid. Two-large bore peripheral IV's were obtained during transport. She receives 1 unit of uncrossmatched packed red blood cells for initial resuscitation and her blood pressure normalizes. A Foley catheter is placed and 200 cc of frank blood returns. A CT scan is performed with grade V kidney injury being seen with active extravasation of contrast from the left renal hilum. As the scan is completed her blood pressure drops to 64/30 and her heart rate increased to 155. She is taken for emergent laparotomy and left nephrectomy is performed. Balanced transfusion is initiated, the patient remains mechanically ventilated postoperatively and is admitted to the SICU for postoperative resuscitation and monitoring. Advanced minimally invasive hemodynamic monitoring is being performed via radial arterial line catheter including measurements of stroke volume and stroke volume variability. What percentage of stroke volume variability corresponds to an adequate intravascular volume status?*
   **A** *5%*
   **B** *10%*
   **C** *20%*
   **D** *25%*
   **E** *30%*

Stroke volume variability (SVV) is a phenomenon that occurs naturally. Intrathoracic pressure changes during inspiration and expiration cause the arterial pressure to rise and fall due to changes in intrathoracic pressure. Studies have consistently found that SVV > 10% is associated with fluid responsiveness. The normal range of variation in spontaneously breathing patients have been reported between 5–10 mm Hg. Normal SVV values for patients that are mechanically ventilated ranged from 10 to 15%. When compared to traditional indicators of volume status (i.e., heart rate, central venous pressure, mean arterial pressure) SVV has been shown to have a higher sensitivity and specificity when assessing intravascular volume status.

**Answer: B**

Berkenstadt, H., Margalit, N. Hadani, M., *et al.* (2001) Stroke volume variation as a predictor of fluid responsiveness in patients undergoing brain surgery. *Anesthesia and Analgesia*, **92** (8), 984–989.

Hofer, C.K., Senn, A., Weiber, L., and Zollinger, A. (2008) Assessment of stroke volume variation for prediction of fluid responsiveness using the modified FloTrac and PiCCOplus system. *Critical Care*, **12** (3), R82.

Reuter, D.A., Kirchner, A., Felbinger, T.W., *et al.* (2003) Usefulness of left ventricular stroke volume variation to assess fluid responsiveness in patients with reduced cardiac function. *Critical Care Medicine*, **31** (5), 1399–1404.

**5** *A 71-year-old woman with coronary artery disease, diabetes mellitus, chronic obstructive pulmonary disease, peripheral vascular disease and a 60-pack year history of smoking is admitted to the ICU with severe shock from a diagnosis of a necrotizing soft tissue infection involving the left lower extremity. A wide local excision was performed to remove the affected area with application of a negative pressure dressing. Intravenous fluid resuscitation and appropriate IV antimicrobials are initiated. In relation to placement of an arterial line catheter, which of the following does not occur as the distance from the heart increases?*

**A** *The dicrotic notch becomes smaller*
**B** *The pulse pressure rises*
**C** *The systolic pressure rises*
**D** *The waveform narrows*
**E** *The diastolic pressure rises*

Arterial catheters are commonly placed in critically ill patients. In addition to continuous blood pressure analysis, other applications of an arterial catheter include assessment of fluid responsiveness and estimation of cardiac output. Pressure waves can vary depending on the site cannulated. As the arterial pressure wave is conducted away from multiple effects can be observed including: the wave appears narrower, the dicrotic notch becomes smaller, the perceived systolic and pulse pressure rise and the perceived diastolic pressure falls. The pulse pressure increases from the core to the periphery. As the diameter of the artery narrows, the systolic pressure becomes overestimated.

**Answer: E**

De Backer, D., Hennen, S., Piagnerelli, M., *et al.* (2005) Pulse pressure variations to predict volume responsiveness: influence of tidal volume. *Intensive Care Medicine*, **31** (4): 517–523.

McGee, W.T., Horswell, J.L., Calderon, J., *et al.* (2007) Validation of a continuous, arterial pressure-based cardiac output measurement: a multicenter, prospective clinical trial. *Critical Care.* **11**, R105

Parrillo, J. and Dellinger, R. (2007) *Critical Care Medicine: Principles of Diagnosis and Management in the Adult,* 3rd edn, Mosby/Elsevier, Philadelphia, PA.

**6** *A morbidly obese 68-year-old woman with atrial fibrillation, diabetes, and COPD presents to the Emergency Department with a 7-day history of right lower quadrant abdominal pain. Her medications include warfarin, glucophage, and a daily multi-vitamin. CT scan results are suggestive of perforated appendicitis with periappendiceal abscess and a mild amount of free intraperitoneal fluid. Her INR is 3.1 for* which she receives a dose of prothrombin complex concentrates (PCC) at 30 units/kg to facilitate normalization. After this, the patient is taken urgently to the operating room where open appendectomy is performed. On HD#4 she begins to develop hypotension, tachycardia along with oxygen desaturations. A chest x-ray is performed which suggests right lower lobe consolidation. The presumptive diagnosis of septic shock is made secondary to right lower lobe pneumonia. To guide resuscitation a pulmonary artery (PA) catheter is placed. As you are watching the catheter pass from the right ventricle and into the pulmonary artery which pressure do you expect to change the most?*

**A** *Left atrial pressure*
**B** *Central venous pressure*
**C** *Systolic pressure*
**D** *Diastolic pressure*
**E** *None of these*

As a PA catheter is being placed there are specific wave form recordings that a clinician should be familiar with. As the catheter is passed into the right atrium the pressure recording resembles the central venous pressure waveform. Next, the catheter will pass into the right ventricle which will result in higher systolic pressure waveforms. As you continue to pass the catheter from the ventricle and into the pulmonary artery a diastolic step-up occurs. Prothrombin complex concentrates (PCC) should be considered in patients who present with supratherapeutic INR and/or serious bleeding who require rapid reversal of INR for surgery, especially if they have cardiac disease. However, if the patient is hypovolemic from third spacing due to sepsis, the use of FFP as volume replacement would be ideal to reverse the induced coagulopathy as well as to treat hypovolemia with a natural colloid rather than crystalloid which does not stay intravascular for long. Normal dosing ranges between 25–50 units/kg with INR reduction that can be seen as early as 10 minutes after administration. Normalization of INR is much faster with PCC compared to FFP infusion. In this case where the patient has had this abscess for 7 days the urgency may not be present.

**Answer: D**

Chatterjee, K. (2009) The Swan-Ganz catheters: past, present, future. *Circulation*, **119**, 147–152.

Cruz, K. and Franklin, C. (2001) The pulmonary artery catheter: uses and controversies. *Critical Care Clinics*, **17** (2), 271–291.

Kelley, C.R. and Rabbani, L.E. (2013) Pulmonary-artery catheterization. *New England Journal of Medicine*, **369**, e35

Khorsand, N., Lisette, G., Meijer, K., *et al.* (2013) A low fixed dose of prothrombin complex concentrate is cost effective in emergency reversal of vitamin K antagonists. *Haematologica*, **98** (6), e65–e67.

**7** *The patient from the previous question begins to show signs of cardiac decompensation with depressed contractility. The patient is started on ionotropic support with dobutamine. What is the mechanism of action of the vasodilatory effects seen with this medication?*
  **A** *Alpha-1 stimulation*
  **B** *cAMP activation*
  **C** *Alpha-2 stimulation*
  **D** *Beta-1 stimulation*
  **E** *Beta-2 stimulation*

Dobutamine stimulates myocardial beta1-adrenergic receptors primarily by the (+) enantiomer and some alpha1 receptor agonism by the (-) enantiomer, resulting in increased contractility and heart rate, and stimulates both beta2- and alpha1-receptors in the vasculature. Although beta2 and alpha1 adrenergic receptors are also activated, the effects of beta2 receptor activation may equally offset or be slightly greater than the effects of alpha1 stimulation, resulting in some vasodilation in addition to the inotropic and chronotropic actions. Alpha1 receptor activation causes vasoconstriction of blood vessels of the skin, kidney, and brain while also causing contraction of smooth muscles of the ureter, vas deferens, urethral sphincter, and ciliary body. Alpha2 receptor activation causes insulin release and stimulates glucagon release. Beta1 receptors activation causes increased heart rate (+ chronotropic effect), increased contraction (+ inotropic effect), increased renin release, and ghrelin. Beta2 receptor activation causes vasodilation along with smooth muscle relaxation of the bronchus, bronchioles, detrusor and uterine muscles. Additionally, its activation inhibits insulin release while stimulating gluconeogenesis and glycolysis.

**Answer: E**

Leier, C.V. (1988) Regional blood flow responses to vasodilators and inotropes in congestive heart failure. *American Journal of Cardiology*, **62** (8), 86E–93E.
Puymirat, E., Fagon, J.Y., Aegerter, P., *et al.* (2016) Cardiogenic shock in intensive care units: evolution of prevalence, patient profile, management and outcomes, 1997–2012. *European Journal of Heart Failure*, **19** (2), 192–200.

**8** *A 73-year-old man is admitted to the SICU after open cholecystectomy secondary to gangrenous cholecystitis. He is becoming increasingly hypotensive with his* mean arterial pressures ranging between 40–45 mm Hg. Fluid resuscitation is initiated with only a transient response. It is decided to place a central venous catheter (CVC) to begin an infusion of vasoactive medication(s). Which of the following is associated with best practice guidelines for CVC placement?
  **A** *Chlorhexidine skin antisepsis before insertion and during dressing changes*
  **B** *Insertion with real-time ultrasound guidance when applicable*
  **C** *Time-out prior to procedure*
  **D** *Safe disposal of sharps*
  **E** *All of the above*

Catheter-related blood stream infections (CRBSI) are common with approximately 80 000 CRBSI per year. Guidelines for prevention of CRBSI were developed by the Centers for Disease Control and Prevention. The best practices guidelines include hand hygiene, use of full barrier precautions, sterile dressing placement, optimal catheter site selection, chlorhexidine skin antisepsis, insertion with real-time ultrasound guidance, maintenance of catheter site, and education of healthcare personnel.

**Answer: E**

Marschall, J., Mermel, L.A., Classen, K.M, *et al.* (2008) Strategies to prevent central line-associated bloodstream infections in acute care hospitals. *Infection Control and Hospital Epidemiology*, **29** (suppl 1), S22–S30. Erratum in: *Infection Control and Hospital Epidemiology*, **30** (8), 815.
O'Grady, N.P., Alexander, M., Burns, L.A., *et al.* (2011) Healthcare Infection Control Practices Advisory Committee (HICPAC). Guideline for the prevention of intravascular catheter-related infections. *Clinical Infectious Diseases*, **52** (9), 1087–1099.

**9** *A pulmonary artery catheter uses the thermodilution principle for determining cardiac output. Which cardiac abnormality may produce a falsely elevated cardiac output reading?*
  **A** *Mitral prolapse*
  **B** *Aortic stenosis*
  **C** *Left-to-right intracardiac shunt*
  **D** *Aortic regurgitation*
  **E** *Mitral stenosis*

The thermodilution principle predicts that, when an indicator substance is added to a stream of flowing blood, the rate of blood flow is inversely proportional to the mean concentration of the indicator at a downstream site. In the case of thermodilution, the indicator is approximately 10 mL of iced or room temperature saline or dextrose that is cooler than blood. The cold fluid mixes in the right heart chambers and the cooled blood flows into the pulmonary artery. The cooled blood flows past the thermistor on the distal end of the catheter which records the change in temperature over time. This is recorded as a temperature/time curve with the area under the curve being inversely proportional to the rate of blood flood in the pulmonary artery. This flow is equivalent to the cardiac output. Right-to-left and left-to-right intracardiac shunts can produce falsely decreased or elevated cardiac output measurements with this technique by attenuating the peak of the temperature-time curve. The blood going from the left heart through the septal defect will decrease the temperature gradient and make it seem that the cardiac output in the right ventricle is higher than what is seen past the aortic valve which is the true cardiac output.

**Answer: C**

Kovacs, G., Avian, A., Olschewski, A., and Olschewski, H. (2013) Zero reference level for right heart catheterization. *The European Respiratory Journal*, **42** (6), 1586–1594.

London, M.J., Moritz, T.E., Henderson, W.G., *et al.* (2002) Standard versus fiberoptic pulmonary artery catheterization for cardiac surgery in the Department of Veteran Affairs: a prospective, observational, multicenter analysis. *Anesthesiology*, **96** (4), 860–870.

Sandham, J.D., Hull, R.D., Brant, R.F., *et al.* (2003) A randomized, controlled trial of the use of pulmonary artery catheters in high-risk surgical patients. *New England Journal of Medicine*, **348**, 5–14.

10   A 41-year-old man was admitted to the ICU five days ago due to injuries sustained in a roll-over motor vehicle collision. He was intubated upon arrival due to a Glasgow Coma Scale (GCS) of 5. Injuries identified included a right mid-shaft femur fracture, bilateral pulmonary contusions, right sided superior/inferior pubic rami fractures and diffuse axonal injury with associated cerebral contusion. On HD#6 he begins to have elevated temperatures 38.8 °C. Blood, urine, sputum, and catheter cultures were obtained. He is found to have a catheter-related blood stream infections (CRBSI). In regards to CRBSI's which of the following is true?

A CRBSI is most commonly caused by Gram-positive cocci that are catalase-positive and coagulase-negative

B CRBSI is most commonly caused by Gram-positive cocci that are catalase-positive and coagulase-positive

C CRBSI is most commonly due to Gram-negative rods

D CRBSI is mostly commonly due to Gram-positive rods

E CRBSI is caused equally by gram-positive and gram-negative bacteria

CRBSI are an important cause of hospital-acquired infections associated with morbidity, mortality, and cost. The most common organism associated with catheter-related septicemia is *Staphylococcus epidermidis* (27%); *Staphylococcus aureus* (24%), *Candida* species (17%), *Klebsiellsa* (11%) or *Enterobacter* (11%), *Serratia* (5%), *Enterococcus* (5%), and others (10%). *Staphylococcus epidermidis* is catalase-positive and coagulase-negative, answer A. They often implant on catheters or other surgical implants due to their ability to form biofilms that grow on these devices. *Staphylococcus aureus* is catalase-positive and coagulase-positive, answer B. CRBSI is not commonly caused by rod-shaped bacteria or gram-negative bacteria.

**Answer: A**

Leonidu, L. and Gogos, C. (2010) Catheter-related bloodstream infections: catheter management according to pathogen. *International Journal of Antimicrobial Agents*, **36** (Suppl. 2), S26–S32.

O'Grady, N.P., Alexander, M., Burns, L.A., *et al.* (2011) Healthcare Infection Control Practices Advisory Committee (HICPAC). Guideline for the prevention of intravascular catheter-related infections. *Clinical Infectious Diseases*, **52** (9), 1087–1099.

Salyers, A.A. and Whitt, D.D. (2002). *Bacterial Pathogenesis: A Molecular Approach*, 2nd edn, ASM Press, Washington, DC.

11   A 67-year-old man is admitted to the ICU after an elective right hemicolectomy secondary to non-obstructing cecal adenocarcinoma found on routine colonoscopy 3 weeks prior. He has a history of congestive heart failure and has smoked a half of a pack of cigarettes every day for the past 30 years On HD#3 he begins to experience shortness of breath and confusion. An ECG is ordered and shows ST elevation in leads V4, V5, and V6 with reciprocal changes in lead II and aVF. He is taken to the cardiac catheterization lab where percutaneous coronary intervention (PIC) is performed. A PA catheter was also placed prior to return to the ICU. Which of the following is an absolute contraindication for PA catheter placement?

A Right atrial mass

B Coagulopathy

C Atrial fibrillation

D History of bilateral carotid endarterectomy

E Cardiac pacemaker

There are multiple indications and contraindications for PA catheter placement. Indications for placement include shock (cardiogenic, septic, traumatic), new-onset pulmonary hypertension, large scale fluid resuscitation, cardiovascular surgery, and acute MI just to name a few. Contraindications to PA catheter placement include both absolute and relative. Absolute contraindications include infection at insertion site, right atrial/ventricular mass, and Tetralogy of Fallot. Relative contraindications include arrhythmias, coagulopathy, and newly inserted pacemaker wires. Potential sites for insertion include internal jugular, subclavian, and femoral approaches. PA catheters provide useful information but studies have not shown it to be useful to improve outcomes because the interpretation of the information is not always correct.

**Answer: A**

Hadian, M. and Pinsky, M. (2006) Evidence-based review of the use of the pulmonary artery catheter: impact data and complications. *Critical Care*, **10** (Suppl 3), S8.

Koo, K.K., Sun, J.C., Zhou, Q., *et al.* (2011) Pulmonary artery catheters: evolving rates and reasons for use. *Critical Care Medicine*, **39** (7), 1613–1618.

12  Which of the following parameters is the most reliable indicator that an intubated patient will be successfully be liberated from the ventilator?
    **A** Patient following commands when sedation is held
    **B** Tidal Volume
    **C** Rapid Shallow Breathing Index
    **D** Negative Inspiratory Force
    **E** Respiratory Rate

The rapid shallow breathing index (RSBI) is the ratio of respiratory frequency to tidal volume ($f/V_T$). Patients who cannot tolerate independent breathing tend to breathe rapidly and shallow. RSBI scores less than 105 correlates with a patient having approximately an 80% chance of being successfully extubated, whereas an RSBI greater than 105 virtually guarantees weaning failure. The other parameters mentioned have not been shown alone to be a reliable marker for successful ventilator liberation. Though RSBI scoring has been shown as a useful tool when attempting to liberate a patient from ventilator support; a clinician should always use clinical judgment when extrapolating its data. If the RSBI is above 105 it will indeed predict failure but the clinician should understand what that means. As an example, to get a score of greater than 100; if the tidal volume is less than 250 cc, that means that the respiratory rate is greater than 25 and patients should not be extubated if the tidal volume is that low in most instances. In another example, if the patients' tidal volume is 500 cc, to result in a RSBI of 100, the patient has to be breathing more than 50 times a minute. 50/0.5 L equals 100. Obviously a patient should not be extubated if the RR is that high.

**Answer: C**

Esteban, A., Frutos, F., Tobin, M.J., *et al.* (1995) A comparison of four methods of weaning patients from mechanical ventilation. Spanish Lung Failure Collaborative Group. *New England Journal of Medicine*, **332** (6), 345–350.

McConville, J.F. and Kress, J.P. (2012) Weaning patients from the ventilator. *New England Journal of Medicine*, **367** (23), 2233–2239.

Tanios, M.A., Nevins, M.L., Hendra, K.P., *et al.* (2006) A randomized, controlled trial of the role of weaning predictors in clinical decision making. *Critical Care Medicine*, **34** (10), 2530–2535.

13  Emergency medical services (EMS) is called to the home of a 67-year old man who is experiencing a severe asthma exacerbation. He ultimately requires intubation on the way to the hospital. After intubation, the patient's oxygen saturation continues to decline, he suffers pulseless electrical activity (PEA), cardiac arrest, and expires despite aggressive resuscitation attempts. What is the likely cause of this patient's cardiac arrest?
    **A** Pulmonary Embolism
    **B** Myocardial Infarction
    **C** Cerebrovascular Event
    **D** Tension Pneumothorax
    **E** Misplaced Endotracheal Tube

Unrecognized misplaced intubation (UMI) is defined as the placement of an endotracheal tube in a location other than the trachea that is unrecognized by the clinician. UMI has been extensively documented in the emergency medical services (EMS) literature, with reported rates ranging from 7 to 25%. Whether an endotracheal tube is misplaced initially, dislodged enroute to the hospital or within the hospital can be of disastrous consequence. End-tidal $CO_2$ monitoring can help identify problems immediately after intubation and before critical hypoxemia becomes manifest. This gives the clinician an opportunity to rectify the problem before the patient suffers adverse consequences. Additionally, the concept of end-tidal $CO_2$ monitoring is easily taught and well understood by EMS personnel.

**Answer: E**

Gravenstein, J.S., Jaffe, M.B., and Paulus, D.A. (eds) (2011) *Capnography*, 2nd edn, Cambride University Press, New York City.

Silvestri, S., Ralls, G.A., Krauss, B., *et al.* (2005) The effectiveness of out-of-hospital use of continuous end-tidal carbon dioxide monitoring on the rate of unrecognized misplaced intubation within a regional emergency medical services system. *Annals of Emergency Medicine*, **45**, 497–503.

**14 and 15** *A 68-year-old woman presents to the emergency department with severe abdominal pain, obstipation, distension, and a 30-pound weight loss. CT scan reveals a distal colonic obstruction at the level of the rectosigmoid junction. She has no significant past medical history and has never undergone colonoscopic evaluation of her colon. She has diffuse distension and left lower quadrant focal peritonitis on physical examination. The patient is taken urgently for exploratory laparotomy at which time a left hemi-colectomy with end colostomy is performed. Laboratory analysis post-operatively is significant for a white blood cell count of 15.2, hemoglobin 9.6, albumin 2.9, INR 1.7 and creatinine of 2.4 mg/dL. Vitals signs reveal heart rate: 97, respiratory rate: 20, and blood pressure: 162/90. Cardiac output was 6 when measured by peripheral pulse wave evaluation. Arterial blood gas is performed which shows a pH: 7.37, $PaCO_2$: 42, $HCO_3$-: 22, $SaO_2$: 95%, $PaO_2$: 90, Base Deficit: -1.1.*

**14** Oxygen Delivery (mL/min/m):

**A** *Can be calculated by MAP × (1.34 × Hbg x $PaO_2$) + (.003 × $SaO_2$) × 10*

**B** *Can be calculated by MAP × (1.34 × Hbg x $SaO_2$) + (.003 × $PaO_2$) × 10*

**C** *Can be calculated by CO × (1.34 × Hbg x $SaO_2$) + (.003 × $PaO_2$) × 10*

**D** *Can be calculated by CO × (1.34 × Hbg x $PaO_2$) + (.003 × $SaO_2$) × 10*

**E** *Can be calculated by CO × (1.34 × Hbg x $PaO_2$) + (.003 × Hbg + $SaO_2$) x 10*

**15** What is the oxygen delivery ($DO_2$) for this patient?

**A** *450 mL/min*

**B** *550 mL/min*

**C** *690 mL/min*

**D** *760 mL/min*

**E** *1660 mL/min*

Oxygen delivery (DO) is the volume of oxygen delivered to the systemic vascular bed per minute and is the product of cardiac output (CO) and arterial oxygen concentration ($CaO_2$). $CaO_2$, or arterial oxygen content, can be defined as the volume (mL) of oxygen contained in 100 mL of blood. Three measurements are truly needed to calculate the $DO_2$: cardiac output (CO), hemoglobin concentration, and arterial $O_2$ saturation ($SaO_2$). Therefore, $DO_2 = CO × CaCO_2 × 10$ where $CaCO_2 = (1.34 × Hbg × SaO_2 + (0.003 × PaO_2)$. A multiplier of 10 is used to convert the $CaO_2$ from mL/dL to mL/L. A normal healthy adult at rest should have a $DO_2$ of 900–1000 mL/min. Another option is to calculate the oxygen delivery index ($DO_2I$) by substituting the cardiac index (CI) in place of cardiac output (CO). This takes into account the body surface area (BSA) of the individual. A normal $DO_2I$ ranges from 500–600 mL/min/m$^2$. The constant 1.34 represents the amount of oxygen bound to each gram of hemoglobin. The constant 0.003 represents the dissolved hemoglobin in the blood. Under normal atmospheric pressure, the addition of $(0.003 × PaO_2)$ is a small variable that is often ignored. The largest increase in the delivery of oxygen is achieved through increasing cardiac output (CO). It is essential for a practitioner to understand oxygen delivery and how it can be optimized when providing adequate hemodynamic support in the critically ill patient.

**Answer 14: C**

**Answer 15: D**

Marino, P. (2014) *The ICU Book*, 4th edn, KluwerHealth/ Lippincott Williams & Wilkins, Philadelphia, PA.

Parillo, J. and Dellinger, R. (2008) *Critical Care Medicine: Principles of Diagnosis and Management in the Adult*, 3rd edn, Mosby/Elsevier, Philadelphia, PA.

**16** *A 82-year-old woman is seen in the emergency department with a sudden onset of abdominal pain that began approximately three hours ago. She has a past medical history of peripheral vascular disease, coronary artery disease, hypertension, hyperlipidemia, and diabetes. Her BMI is calculated to be 37. A CT was performed which showed diffuse thickening of a large portion of her small bowel. On physical examination she has guarding and rebound tenderness diffusely. Her vital signs include blood pressure: 94/62, heart rate 122, respiratory rate: 37, and oxygen saturation: 94% on 2L nasal cannula. Her ABG values are as follows: pH 7.19, $CO_2$ 16, $PO_2$ 70, $HCO_3^-$ 11, BE: -18. A laparotomy is performed and 30 cm of distal ileum is resected due to full thickness ischemia. She requires two vasoactive medications intra-operatively to maintain a mean arterial pressure > 60. The patient has is transferred to the SICU. Normalization of which of the following parameters is most consistent with successful fluid resuscitation in the critically ill?*

A *Blood Pressure*
B *Hemoglobin*
C *Lactate*
D *Serum creatinine*
E *Respiratory Rate*

Lactic acid is a product of cellular metabolism that can accumulate when cells lack sufficient oxygen to undergo aerobic metabolism. Lactic acidosis may be caused by numerous underlying acute or chronic medical conditions. Adding lactate determinations to oxygen transport monitoring provides a more complete assessment of tissue oxygenation. Lactate clearance has been a highly studied topic as of recent to guide as a resuscitation endpoint. Studies have shown that patients who have a decrease by 20% (from the admission value) every 2 hours for the initial 8 hours required less inotropic support, less ventilator days, and ICU days than patients who did not meet the parameter. Additionally, lactate clearance early in the hospital course may indicate a resolution of global tissue hypoxia and is associated with decreased mortality rates.

**Answer: C**

Jansen, T., Bommel, J., Schoonderbeek, F., *et al.* (2010) Early lactate-guided therapy in intensive care unit patients: a multicenter, open-label, randomized controlled trial. *American Journal of Respiratory and Critical Care Medicine*, **182** (6), 752–761.

Jones, A. (2013) Lactate clearance for assessing response to resuscitation in severe sepsis. *Academic Emergency Medicine*, **20** (8), 844–847.

Marty, P., Roquilly, A., Vallée, F., *et al.* (2013) Lactate clearance for death prediction in severe sepsis or septic shock patients during the first 24 hours in intensive care unit: an observational study. *Annals of Intensive Care*, **3** (1), 1–7.

17  *A 27-year old man is injured after falling 18 feet off of a ladder. He suffers a grade 3 splenic laceration, a grade 2 liver laceration, multiple left sided rib fractures, a right femur fracture and a left-sided subdural hematoma without mass effect. Chest x-ray is negative. He is initially hypotensive but responds to resuscitation and has HR of 90, blood pressure 110/70, $SaO_2$ 95% with a respiratory rate of 16. He is admitted to the SICU. A left radial arterial catheter is placed along with a right subclavian central venous catheter. Central venous pressure (CVP) is transduced to help guide resuscitation. One hour after admission his CVP increases steadily increases from 4 to 20. What is the most likely cause?*
A *Hypovolemia*
B *Deep Inhalation*

C *Distributive shock*
D *Tension Pneumothorax*
E *Subclavian vein insertion site*

Central venous pressure (CVP) is the blood pressure in the vena cava and reflects the amount of blood returning to the heart. CVP provides a good approximation of right atrial pressure and to right ventricular end diastolic pressure. Thus, CVP is equivalent to the right-sided filling pressure. Normal values vary between 4 and 12 cm $H_2O$. In this scenario the patient has poly-trauma with increasing CVP. While there can be many reasons for high CVP the acute rapid rise is most likely due to a tension pneumothorax in this scenario and is the only choice that would cause a rise in CVP. The other choices provided, hypovolemia, deep inhalation and distributive shock are factors that cause a decrease in CVP. The insertion site will not impact CVP.

**Answer: D**

Magder, S. (2006) Central venous pressure monitoring. *Current Opinion in Critical Care*, **12** (3), 219–227.

Westphal, G.A., Silva, E., Caldeira, F.M., *et al.* (2006) Variation in amplitude of central venous pressure curve induced by respiration is a useful tool to reveal fluid responsiveness in postcardiac surgery patients. *Shock*, **26** (2), 140–145.

Weyland, A. and Grune, F. (2009) Cardiac preload and central venous pressure. *Anaesthesist*, **58** (5), 506–512.

18  *A 30-year old man is involved in a lateral impact motor vehicle collision. He suffers multiple orthopedic injuries and requires intubation due to decreased GCS. A right internal jugular central venous catheter is placed to assist in volume resuscitation and hemodynamic monitoring. The phlebostatic axis is correctly identified and the catheter is connected properly. When is the proper time during a normal breath cycle to accurately measure intravascular pressure?*
A *During breath holding*
B *End of expiration*
C *End of inspiration*
D *During spontaneous breating trial (SBT)*
E *It can be measured at any point in the breath cycle*

The phlebostatic axis corresponds to a point located by drawing an imaginary line from the fourth intercostal space at the sternum and finding its intersection with an imaginary line drawn down the center of the chest below the axilla. It corresponds to the position of the right and left atrium with the patient in a supine position. Changes in thoracic pressure can cause discrepancy between intravascular and transmural pressures. Intravascular pressures should be equivalent to transmural pressures at the end of expiration.

**Answer: B**

Kovacs, G., Avian, A., Pienn, M., *et al.* (2014) Reading pulmonary vascular pressure tracings: how to handle the problems of zero leveling and respiratory swings. *American Journal of Respiratory and Critical Care Medicine*, **190** (3), 252–257.

Marino, P. (2014) *The ICU Book*, 4th edn, KluwerHealth/ Lippincott Williams & Wilkins, Philadelphia, PA.

Parillo, J. and Dellinger, R. (2008) *Critical Care Medicine: Principles of Diagnosis and Management in the Adult*, 3rd edn, Mosby/Elsevier, Philadelphia, PA.

**19 and 20**   *A 75-year-old woman is in the surgical intensive care unit 12 hours after an emergent exploration and Hartmann procedure for perforated diverticulitis. She remains mechanically intubated, hemodynamically labile and oliguric despite aggressive administration of crystalloids. Non-invasive hemodynamic and laboratory data are as follows: Body surface area (BSA) 2 m², Temperature 37.8°C, heart rate 118, mean arterial pressure (MAP) 55, central venous pressure (CVP) 10, cardiac output (CO) 5 L/min, $FiO_2$ 70%, pH 7.34, $pCO_2$ 40 mm Hg, $pO_2$ 70 mm Hg, $SaO_2$ 95%, mixed venous oxygen saturation ($MVO_2$) 70%. (Assume 1.34 ml of $O_2$ per gram Hgb at 100% saturation.)*

**19**   *Systemic vascular resistance (SVR):*
  **A** *Can be calculated by (MAP – CVP/CO) × 80*
  **B** *Can be calculated by (MAP – CO/CVP) × 80*
  **C** *Can be calculated by (MAP – CVP/BSA) × 80*
  **D** *Can be calculated by (MAP – CO/BSA) × 80*
  **E** *Is a measurement that also includes pulmonary vascular resistance*

**20**   *What is the systemic vascular resistance (dyne sec/ cm⁵) of the patient?*
  **A** *400*
  **B** *640*
  **C** *720*
  **D** *1800*
  **E** *2000*

Systemic vascular resistance (SVR) is the resistance that must be overcome to push blood through the circulatory system and create flow. Peripheral resistance is determined by three main factors: autonomic activity, sympathetic activity, and blood viscosity. The total hydraulic force that opposes pulsatile flow is known as impedance. Vascular resistance is derived by assuming that hydraulic resistance is analogous to electrical resistance. Therefore, SVR can be calculated by rearrangement of Ohm's Law (V = IR). This relationship is applied to the systemic and pulmonary circulations, creating the following derivations:

$$PVR = 80 * (PAP - PCWP)/CO, \text{normal } 100 - 200 \, dyn - s/cm^5$$

$$SVR = 80 * (MAP - CVP)/CO, \text{normal } 900 - 1200 \, dyn - s/cm^5$$

**Answer 19: A**

**Answer 20: C**

Haft, J.W. (2011) Ischemic heart disease, in: *Greenfield's Surgery: Scientific Principles and Practice*, 5th edn (eds M.W. Mulholland, K.D. Lillemoe, G.M. Doherty, *et al.*), Philadelphia, PA: Lippincott Williams and Wilkins, pp. 149–157.

Marino, P. (2014) *The ICU Book*, 4th edn, KluwerHealth/ Lippincott Williams & Wilkins, Philadelphia, PA.

Parillo, J. and Dellinger, R. (2008) *Critical Care Medicine: Principles of Diagnosis and Management in the Adult*, 3rd edn, Mosby/Elsevier, Philadelphia, PA.

# 7

## Airway and Perioperative Management
*Stephen M. Welch, DO, Jeffrey P. Coughenour, MD and Stephen L. Barnes, MD*

1 *An obese 42-year-old woman present to anesthesia clinic for pre-operative evaluation. In a sitting position the patient is asked to open her mouth and protrude her tongue to which you see the base of the uvula and soft palate. What is her Modified Mallampati classification class?*
   A *Class 0*
   B *Class I*
   C *Class II*
   D *Class III*
   E *Class IV*

The Mallampati classification was first described in 1985 as a method to predict difficult endotracheal intubation using direct laryngoscopy. With the mouth wide open the patient is asked to protrude the tongue as much as possible. The visibility of the uvula, faucial pillars, and soft palate are assessed (see Figure 7.1 and Table 7.1).

**Answer: D**

Mallampati, S.R., Gatt, S.P., Gugino, L.D., *et al.* (1985) A clinical sign to predict difficult tracheal intubation: a prospective study. *Canadian Anesthetists Society Journal*, **32**, 429–434.
Walls, R.M. (2012) The emergency airway algorithms, in *Manual of Emergency Airway Management*, 4th edn (eds R.M. Walls and M.F. Murphy), Lippincott Williams and Wilkins, Philadelphia, PA, pp. 22–34.

2 *An edentulous 63-year-old woman is admitted to the ICU with inhalation injury after a house fire. As she is being observed she begins to have respiratory stridor. There is difficulty with bag mask ventilation and intubation attempts show generalized edema without visualization of the cord structures. Cricothyrotomy is attempted. What factors predict the difficulty of cricothyrotomy?*
   A *Previous thyroid surgery*
   B *Obesity*

   C *Previous neck irradiation*
   D *Poor visualization of anatomic landmarks*
   E *All of the above*

Assessment for difficult cricothyrotomy can be performed by patient history and physical examination. The mnemonic "SMART" is a tool that can used to assess for difficulties that may occur:

S: Surgery (recent or remote)
M: Mass (abscess, hematoma, other)
A: Access or Anatomy (obesity, poor landmarks)
R: Radiation (scarring, deformity)
T: Tumor (including intrinsic airway tumor)

Clinicians should be aware of identifiable factors in patients with difficult airways as these can dictate outcomes.

**Answer: E**

Aslani, A., Ng, S.C., Hurley, M., *et al.* (2012) Accuracy of identification of the cricothyroid membrane in female subjects using palpation: an observational study. *Anesthesia and Analgesia*, **114** (5), 987–992.
Murphy, M. and Walls, R.M. (2004) Identification of the difficult and failed airway, in *Manual of Emergency Airway Management* (eds R.M. Walls, M.F. Murphy, and R.C. Luten), Lippincott Williams & Wilkins, Philadelphia, PA, pp. 8–21.

3 *A 45-year old woman is scheduled to undergo an elective cholecystectomy. On physical examination you appreciate morbidly obese woman with a Mallampati IV airway classification. The use of which modality will improve her first-chance orotracheal intubation success rate?*
   A *Gum-Elastic Bougie*
   B *Direct Laryngoscopy*
   C *Video Laryngoscopy*
   D *Laryngeal Mask Airway*
   E *All choices have similar success rates*

*Surgical Critical Care and Emergency Surgery: Clinical Questions and Answers*, Second Edition.
Edited by Forrest "Dell" Moore, Peter Rhee, and Gerard J. Fulda.
© 2018 John Wiley & Sons Ltd. Published 2018 by John Wiley & Sons Ltd.
Companion website: www.wiley.com/go/moore/surgical_criticalcare_and_emergency_surgery

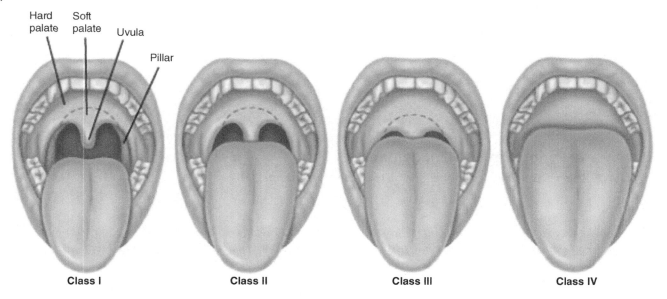

**Figure 7.1**

**Table 7.1** The Original and Modified Mallampati Classification classes.

| Original Scoring | Modified Scoring |
| --- | --- |
| Class I: Faucial pillars, soft palate and uvula could be visualized | Class I: Soft palate, uvula, fauces, pillars visible |
| Class II: Faucial pillars and soft palate could be visualized, but uvula was masked by the base of the tongue | Class II: Soft palate, uvula, fauces visible |
| Class III: Only soft palate visualized | Class III: Soft palate, base of uvula visible |
| | Class IV: Only hard palate visible |

It is important, to recognize possible pitfalls that a patient may encounter during a routine visit, elective surgery, or hospital admission. In recent literature there has been multiple studies that have compared video laryngoscopy (VL) versus direct laryngoscopy (DL) both in real-time and in simulation models. A recent article published by De Jong et al. in 2014 showed that VL reduces the risk of difficult orotracheal intubation, esophageal intubation, and first-attempt success rates. Moreover, studies have shown that simulation-based training is an effective way to teach VL skills. Also, VL allows for a higher success rate, faster response time, and a decrease in the number of attempts by health-care students and health-care professionals under the conditions. A Gum-Elastic Bougie (Eschman Introducer) can be used as an adjunct for intubation but does not necessarily increase first chance intubation rates. Laryngeal mask airway (LMA) is a devise that forms a seal on top of the glottis rather than passing through the glottis as an endotracheal tube does. It thus does not increase intubation success rate.

**Answer: C**

De Jong, A., Molinari, N., Conseil, M., *et al.* (2014) Video laryngoscopy versus direct laryngoscopy for orotracheal intubation in the intensive care unit: a systematic review and meta-analysis. *Intensive Care Medicine*, **40** (5), 629–639.

Silverberg, M.J., Li, N., Acquah, S.O., *et al.* (2015) Comparison of video laryngoscopy versus direct laryngoscopy during urgent endotracheal intubation: a randomized controlled trial. *Critical Care Medicine*, **43** (3), 636–641.

Vanderbilt, A., Mayglothling, J., Pastis, N.J., *et al.* (2014) A review of the literature: direct and video laryngoscopy with simulation as educational intervention. *Advances in Medical Education and Practice*, **5**, 15–23.

4 *A 64-year-old obese woman is being treated inpatient for a hospital acquired gram-negative urinary tract infection. She subsequently develops a refractory* Clostridium difficile *colitis requiring subtotal colectomy. After a successful operation you are informed by anesthesiologist that the patient has continued paralysis. What drug is the most likely the cause of this finding?*

A *Morphine*
B *Piperacillin-Tazobactam*
C *Flagyl*
D *Gentamicin*
E *Vancomycin*

Aminoglycoside antibiotics are known to potentiate the effects of neuromuscular blocking agents. Clindamycin causes end-plate ion channel blockade while Gentamicin reduces pre-junctional acetylcholine release and thereby potentiating the action of non-depolarizing neuromuscular blocking agents. Though this is a rare phenomenon, it is important to be familiar with drug interactions when presented with atypical findings presented by the surgical patient. The other drugs listed have not been shown to potentiate the effects of NMBA's.

**Answer: D**

Guzman, J. and Manimekalai, N. (2014) Potentiation of neuromuscular blockade effect of rocuronium for 4 hours due to perioperative gentamicin, clindamycin and magnesium sulfate. *Austin Journal of Anesthesia and Analgesia*, **2** (6), 1032.

Lee, J.H., Lee, S.I., Chung, C.J., *et al.* (2013) The synergistic effect of gentamicin and clindamycin on rocuronium-induced neuromuscular blockade. *Korean Journal of Anesthesiology*, **64** (2), 143–151.

**5** *A 52-year-old man is scheduled to undergo an elective laparoscopic cholecystectomy secondary to symptomatic cholelithiasis. The patient denies smoking and drinks occasionally. He states he has hypertension that is controlled with medication. His most recent HBA1C level checked one month ago was 12.3 although he does take his scheduled hypoglycemic he has been prescribed. What is the correct American Society of Anesthesiologists (ASA) classification for this patient?*

**A** *I*
**B** *II*
**C** *IIb*
**D** *III*
**E** *IV*

The ASA physical status classification system is used for assessing the fitness of patients before surgery. It provides a common language between providers for documentation and ease of data abstraction for research. There are limitations with the classification system (i.e. assuming that age has no relation to physical fitness), therefore it should not be used as the sole determinant of patient status and perioperative risk.

ASA I: A normal healthy patient; Non-smoking, no or minimal alcohol use

ASA II: A patient with mild system disease; Mild diseases without functional limitation. Examples include: Current smoker, social alcohol drinker, pregnancy, obesity (BMI > 30 but < 40), well-controlled DM/HTN, mild lung disease.

ASA III: A patient with severe systemic disease; Substantial functional limitations. One or more moderate to severe disease(s). Examples include poorly controlled DM or HTN, COPD, morbid obesity (BMI ≥ 40), active hepatitis, alcohol dependence or abuse, implanted pacemaker, moderate reduction in ejection fraction, ESRD, History > 3 months of MI, IA, or CAD/stents.

ASA IV: A patient with severe systemic disease that is a constant threat to life. Examples include recent < 3 month history of MI, CVA, TIA, or CAD/ stents, ongoing cardiac ischemia, severe valve dysfunction, DIC, ARD, or ESRD not undergoing regularly scheduled dialysis.

ASA V: A patient who is not expected to survive without the operation. Examples include Ruptured abdominal/ thoracic aneurysm, massive trauma, intracranial bleed with mass effect, ischemic bowel in the face of significant cardiac pathology or multi-organ dysfunction

ASA VI: A declared brain-dead patient whose organs are being removed for donor purposes.

The patient in our scenario has uncontrolled diabetes as shown by his recently checked HBA1C level >12.

**Answer: D**

ASA Physical Status Classification System, American Society of Anesthesiologists, www.asahq.org (accessed October 1, 2016).

Fitz-Henry, J. (2011) The ASA classification and perioperative risk. *Annals of the Royal College of Surgeons of England*, **93** (3), 185–187.

Daabiss, M. (2011) American Society of Anesthesiologists physical status classification. *Indian Journal of Anaesthesia*, **55** (2), 111–115.

**6** *A 22-year-old male presents to the trauma bay with a 6 cm laceration to his right forearm after punching through a window. His neurovascular exam is within normal limits. The incident happened approximately 45 minutes ago. You decide to give him prophylactic antibiotics. You want to examine the wound and close it in the trauma bay. Your intern asks you the mechanism of action of local anesthetics. You tell him that:*

**A** *The exact mechanism is unknown*
**B** *Anesthetics work by reversibly binding calcium channels along the nerve*
**C** *Anesthetics work by blocking acetylcholine release from the presynaptic cleft*
**D** *Anesthetics work by reversibly binding sodium channels within the nerve fibers*
**E** *Anesthetics work by competitively inhibiting potassium channels along the nerve*

The mechanism of local anesthetics are well known and it works by reversibly blocking sodium channels within nerve fibers, which prevents transmission of pain signals by disrupting depolarization of the nerve. Lidocaine is a local anesthetic in the amide class and is the most commonly used anesthetic for local infiltration. Lidocaine without epinephrine should not exceed 4 mg/kg (0.4 mL/kg of 1% lidocaine). On the other hand, lidocaine with epinephrine should not exceed 7 mg/kg (7 mL/kg of 1% lidocaine). For an added margin of safety 80% of the maximum allowable dose should be used in children under 8 years of age. The addition of epinephrine provides local vasoconstriction with prolongs the duration of action, decreases local bleeding during the procedure, and reduces systemic lidocaine absorption. In addition, lidocaine with epinephrine may be used in the face, digits, or penis as there is no convincing evidence of harm as traditional teachings have suggested; though it should be avoided in patients with peripheral artery disease. Lidocaine does not directly affect the calcium channels, acetylcholine release, nor the potassium channels. Another commonly used local anesthetic is Bupivacaine (Marcaine). Bupivacaine can also be used plain or mixed with epinephrine. Onset of action of Bupivacaine is approximately 15–30 minutes with its maximum dose ranging from 2.5 mg/kg without epinephrine and 3 mg/kg with epinephrine. Two classes of local anesthetics exist and can be grouped into the esters or the amides. An easy way to distinguish between an ester and an amide is to view the generic name of the drug being used. If the generic name has an "i" prior to the –caine, then it is an amide (Lidocaine, Bupivacaine, Prilocaine, Mepivacaine). But, if there is not an "i" prior to the –caine then it is an ester (Cocaine, Procaine, Tetracaine, Benzocaine). Remember this will not work with trade or commercial names.

**Answer: D**

Achar, S. and Kundu, S. (2002) Principle of office anesthesia: part I: infiltrative anesthesia. American Family Physician, **66** (1), 91–94.

McCreight, A. and Stephan, M. (2008) Local and regional anesthesia, in *Textbook of Pediatric Emergency Procedures*, 2nd edn (eds C. King and F.M. Henretig) Lippincott, Williams, & Wilkins, Philadelphia, PA, pp. 439–468.

Tetzlaff, J.E. (2000) The pharmacology of local anesthetics. Anesthesiology Clinics of North America, **18** (2), 217–233.

7 *A 72-year-old male presents to the Emergency Department and is found to have profound renal and hepatic toxicity. He is confused and thrashing around.*

*His vital signs show: BP: 95/60 mm Hg, RR: 18 breaths/min, Pulse: 112 beats/min, O₂ Sat: 97%. A decision is made to intubate the patient and the resident calls you to bedside to ask you which neuromuscular blocking agent (NMBA) would be the best choice for the procedure in this patient?*

**A** *Cisatricurium*
**B** *Rocuronium*
**C** *Pancuronium*
**D** *Vecuronium*
**E** *Tubocurarine*

Cisatricurium (Nimbex) is eliminated by the body via Hofmann degradation. This process is also known as exhaustive methylation. However, 5–10% is still metabolized through the liver and 10–15% is excreted unchanged by the kidneys. It is a non-depolarizing neuromuscular-blocking drug and is of intermediate duration of action with a biological half-life of 20–30 minutes. Rocuronium, Pancuronium, Vecuronium, and Tubocurarine all undergo liver metabolism and clearance. Cisatricurium is the best option. Of the listed drugs vecuronium has the shortest onset of 60 seconds whereas rocuronium and pancuronium has onset of 90 seconds. Tubocurarine has an onset of 300 seconds.

**Answer: A**

Elliot, J.M. and Bion, J.F. (1995) The use of neuromuscular blocking drugs in the intensive care practice. *Acta Anaesthesiologica Scandinavica*, **39**, 70–82.

Murray, M.J., Cowen, J., DeBlock, H., *et al.* (2002) Clinical practice guideline for sustained neuromuscular blockade in adult critically ill patient. *Critical Care Medicine*, **30** (1), 142–156.

8 *A middle-aged male is brought to the trauma bay after being found unresponsive on the side of the road with his motorcycle laying approximately 50 yards from him. He was un-helmeted per EMS report. The patient has visible bruising to the right side of his face and blood coming from his right ear. His Glasgow Coma Score is 7 (E = 2, V = 2, M = 3). Which drug(s) are you going to use during rapid-sequence intubation of this patient?*

**A** *Propofol*
**B** *Midazolam*
**C** *Ketamine*
**D** *Any of these*
**E** *None of these*

It is important to know the side effects of drugs that are used during rapid-sequence intubation, especially in the head-injured patient. Midazolam and propofol have both been used in head-injured patients, but are less favorable due to the risk of hypotension-induced secondary brain injury. It is important to prevent secondary brain injury by maintaining cerebral perfusion pressures (MAP-ICP) and also ensuring adequate oxygenation of the patient. Therefore, agents with less hemodynamic side effects are desired. Though historical teaching suggests that ketamine may cause increases in intracranial pressures, this has not been seen in more recent literature. Another good alternative once could consider for this patient is etomidate, but this drug has been associated with decreased corticosteroid synthesis. Induction dose of ketamine is 1–4.5 mg/kg IV. Approximately 100 mg is used often.

**Answer: C**

Bar-Joseph, G., Guilburd, Y., Tamir, A., and Guilburd, J.N. (2009) Effectiveness of ketamine in decreasing intracranial pressure in children with intracranial hypertension. *Journal of Neurosurgery: Pediatrics*, **4** (1), 40–46.

Zeiler, F.A., Teitelbaum, J., West, M., and Gillman, L.M. (2014) The ketamine effect on ICP in traumatic brain injury. Neurocritical Care, **21** (1), 163–173.

9  *Which factor is most associated with wrong-site surgical procedures?*
   A *Multiple surgical procedures*
   B *Multiple surgeons*
   C *Failures of communication*
   D *Emergency surgical procedures*
   E *Lack of procedural understanding by the patient*

In 2004 the Joint Commission developed and enacted a Universal Protocol that was set forth to prevent wrong-site, wrong-procedure, and wrong-person surgeries. This protocol at its simplest form consists of three steps: 1) A pre-procedural verification process; 2) Marking of the surgical site; and 3) A time out prior to the operative procedure. Although these events are rare they are still considered never-events, with a majority being related to communication failures between the surgical team, patient, and family members. The other choices including multiple surgical procedures, multiple surgeons, emergency surgeries as well as lack of procedural understanding by the patients all have an impact but the communication failures is the most associated problem with wrong-site surgical procedures.

**Answer: C**

Hampel, S., Booth, M.J., Shanman, R., *et al.* (2015) Wrong-site surgery, retained surgical items, and surgical fires—a systematic review of surgical never events. *Journal of the American Medical Association Surgery*, **150** (8), 796–805.

Hanchanale, V., Raj Rao, A., Motiwala, H., and Karim, O. (2014) Wrong site surgery! How can we stomp it? *Urology Annals*, **6** (1), 57–62.

10  *A 75-year-old male falls from a standing height at home and suffers a broken right hip. He has a past medical history of hyperlipidemia, diabetes, and angina. His is alert and oriented but is unable to give an accurate medication list. He is cleared for surgery and undergoes fixation of his right hip and suffers an acute MI postoperatively. Which of his home medications may have help prevent this event?*
   A *Lisinopril*
   B *Metoprolol*
   C *Vicodin*
   D *Metformin*
   E *Ibuprofen*

Beta Blockers have potential beneficial effects when taken perioperatively. In addition to helping prevent/control arrhythmias, beta blockade also helps reduce myocardial oxygen demand that is produced by catecholamine release during stress periods. Acute withdrawal of beta blockers pre- or postoperatively can lead to substantial morbidity and even mortality. Aspirin has not been shown to improve cardiovascular or mortality outcomes. Moreover, they have been found to increase bleeding risk in these groups. The other medications mentioned also have not shown a mortality risk when being held.

**Answer: B**

Kennedy, J.M., van Rij, A.M., Spears, G.F., *et al.* (2000) Polypharmacy in a general surgical unit and consequences of drug withdrawal. *British Journal of Clinical Parmacology*, **49**, 353–362.

Shammash, J.B., Trost, J.C., Gold, J.M., *et al.* (2001) Perioperative beta-blocker withdrawal and mortality in vascular surgical patients. *American Heart Journal*, **141** (1), 148–153.

Wallace, A.W., Au, S., and Cason, B.A. (2010) Association of the pattern of use of perioperative B-blockade and postoperative mortality. *Anesthesiology*, **113** (4), 794–805.

11  *In regards to perioperative statin therapy which of the following is true?*
   A *Statins should not be given during the perioperative period*
   B *Statins have been shown to increase thrombogenesis in the perioperative period*

C *Statins result in arterial constriction*

D *Statins are not associated with rhabdomyolysis*

E *Statins have been shown to be cardioprotective*

The most widely accepted theory of the continuation of statin therapy in the perioperative period is due to plaque stabilization. This is thought to occur secondary to the reduction of thrombin-induced expression and lipopolysaccharide induced expression of tissue factor, which results in anti-inflammatory properties that causes coronary plaque stabilization. Investigations have also shown that postoperative statin withdrawal was an independent predictor of myonecrosis. Complications of statin withdrawl have been shown to manifest as early as day 4 from cessation of the drug. Thus, statins should be resumed as early as possible if held during the perioperative period. Statins have not been shown to increase thrombogenesis, arterial vasoconstriction, nor rhabdomyolysis.

**Answer: E**

Biccard, B.M. (2008) A peri-operative statin update for non-cardia surgery. Part I: the effects of statin therapy on atherosclerotic disease and lessons learnt from statin therapy in medical (non-surgical) patients. *Anasthesia*, **63** (1), 52–64

Hindler, K., Shaw, A.D., Samuels, J., *et al.* (2006) Improved postoperative outcomes associated with preoperative statin therapy. *Anesthesiology*, **105** (6), 1260–1272.

Kapoor, A.S., Kanji, H., Buckingham, J., *et al.* (2006) Strength of evidence for perioperative use of statins to reduce cardiovascular risk: systemic review of controlled studies. *British Medical Journal*, **333**, 1149–1152

**12** *A 52-year-old otherwise healthy woman presents to the emergency department 8 days postoperatively from a right-sided laparoscopic hernia repair. CT of the abdomen and pelvis show a large intra-abdominal fluid collection in the right para-colic gutter with stigmata suggestive of abscess. She is hypotensive, tachypneic, and is confused. She is diagnosed with septic shock. Which of the following clinical manifestations would also likely be seen in early septic shock?*

A *Decreased urinary excretion of sodium (<20 mEq/L)*

B *Decreased cardiac output (CO)*

C *Increased gastric motility*

D *Multifactorial anemia*

E *Increased systemic vascular resistance (SVR)*

Manifestation of shock, severe shock, and septic shock can be seen in multiple organ systems throughout the body. The neurological manifestations can include confusion, irritability, or agitation. The cardiovascular effects can include hypotension, tachycardia, a decrease in systemic vascular resistance (SVR), and an increase in cardiac output (early) with a subsequent decrease in late shock. Pulmonary manifestations include tachypnea, hypoxemia, and marked respiratory alkalosis. Renal effects include oliguria and azotemia. Urinary excretion of sodium may be markedly reduced with urine osmolality being increased. This can lead to acute tubular necrosis or renal failure. Gastrointestinal manifestations include decreased motility and stress ulceration. Cardiac output may eventually be decreased but in the initial states of sepsis, due to the decreased SVR and tachycardia, cardiac output is increased. Multifactorial anemia is not initially caused by sepsis.

**Answer: A**

Blanco, J., Muriel-Bombin, A., Sagredo, V., *et al.* (2008) Incidence, organ dysfunction and mortality in severe sepsis: a Spanish multicentre study. *Critical Care*, **12** (6), 1–14.

Dellinger, R.P., Levy, M.M., Carlet, J., *et al.* (2008) Surviving Sepsis Campaign: international guideline for the management of severe sepsis and septic shock. *Intensive Care Medicine*, **34** (1), 17–60.

Singer, M., Deutschman, C.S., Seymour, C.W., *et al.* (2016) The third international consensus definitions for sepsis and septic shock (Sepsis–3). *Journal of the American Medical Association*, **315** (8), 801–810.

**13** *Which of the following is associated with an increased incidence for stress ulcers in high risk ICU patients?*

A *INR > 1.3*

B *Platelet count < 75 000*

C *Mechanical ventilation for > 48 hours*

D *PTT > 1.3 times the control value*

E *Antibiotic administration*

Stress ulcerations tend to be shallow and cause oozing from superficial capillary beds. Deeper lesions can occur leading to massive hemorrhage or perforation. Though ulcers can be categorized into both early and late, it is uncertain if they same pathophysiology applies to both. However, it is thought that they result from impaired mucosal protection and/or hypersecretion of acid. Though there are disagreements defining everyone who falls into the "high-risk" category, but patients with coagulopathy (INR > 1.5), platelet count < 50 000, PTT > 2, mechanical ventilation > 48 hours, history of GI ulceration/bleeding, TBI, burns, and spinal cord injuries are associated with increased incidence of stress ulcer formation.

**Answer: C**

Alhazzani, W., Alenezi, F., Jaeschke, R., *et al.* (2013) Proton pump ihibitors versus histamine 2 receptor antagonists for stress ulcer prophylaxis in critically ill patients: a systematic review and meta-analysis. *Critical Care Medicine*, **41** (3), 693–705.

Stollmann, N. and Metz, D. (2005) Pathophysiology and prophylaxis of stress ulcer in intensive care unit patients. *Journal of Critical Care*, **20** (1): 35–45.

**14** *A healthy 36-year-old man is scheduled to undergo an elective open ventral hernia repair. A detailed history and physical examination reveal no underlying medical conditions. Which of the following test(s) are indicated prior to his surgery?*
  A *No further workup is necessary*
  B *CBC*
  C *12-lead EKG*
  D *BUN/Creatinine and 12-lead EKG*
  E *Chest radiograph*

All patients undergoing non-cardiac surgery should have a detailed history and physical examination to stratify them for cardiovascular perioperative risk. Determining the functional capacity of a patient during perioperative testing is one way to avoid unnecessary surgical morbidity and mortality. Functional capacity is often expressed in terms of metabolic equivalents (METs), where 1 MET is the resting or basal oxygen consumption of a 40–year-old, 70-kg man. In the perioperative literature, functional capacity is classified as excellent (>10 METs), good (7–10 METs), moderate (4–6 METs), poor (<4 METs), or unknown. Perioperative cardiac and long-term risks are increased in patients unable to perform 4 METs of work during daily activities. Functional status can also be assessed more formally by activity scales, such as the Duke Activity Status Index (DASI) and the Specific Activity Scale. Certainly, further workup(s) and testing may be warranted if history and physical examination warrant and as calculated functional capacity dictates. The ACC/AHA guidelines were recently updated in 2014 and a step-wise approach is taken to determine the appropriate diagnostic workup.

**Answer: A**

Fleisher, L., Fleischmann, K., Auerback, A., *et al.* (2014) 2014 ACC/AHA Guideline on perioperative cardiovascular evaluation and management of patients undergoing noncardiac surgery. A report of the American College of Cardiology/American Heart Association Task Force on Practice Guidelines. *Journal of the American College of Cardiology*, **64** (22), 77–137.

Ford, M.K., Beattie, W.S., and Wijeysundera, D.N. (2010) Systematic review: prediction of perioperative cardiac complications and mortality by the revised cardiac risk index. *Annals of Internal Medicine*, **152** (1), 26–35.

Reilly, D.F., McNeely, M.J., Doerner, D., *et al.* (1999) Self-reported exercise tolerance and the risk of serious perioperative complications. *Archives of Internal Medicine*, **159** (18), 2185–2192.

**15** *A 72-year-old man underwent percutaneous coronary intervention (PCI) with placement of a bare metal stent. He was scheduled prior to the stent placement to be seen in your office regarding a bulge in his right groin that is causing a dull pain with exertion and intermittent constipation. In the office you diagnose an inguinal hernia on physical examination that is reducible with no associated skin changes. His stent was placed three weeks ago. What are the recommendations you should educate this patient in regards to the timing of his operation?*
  A *Repair of the hernia can be completed at any time if aspirin is continued*
  B *Deferring the surgery at least 18 months after stent placement is ideal*
  C *Deferring surgery at least 4–6 weeks is preferred in this case*
  D *Surgery should be performed at least 6 months after bare metal stent placement*
  E *He should only have his hernia repaired if it becomes incarcerated/strangulated*

Non-cardiac surgery is often needed in patients that have received PCI. It is important to know if a bare metal stent or a drug eluting stent was used as it dictates appropriate timing of surgery. Although it is preferable to defer surgery for at least 12 months irrespective of stent type (Grade 1C); this is often not feasible. This patient has a symptomatic inguinal hernia that should be repaired but only after appropriate timing. In patients who cannot wait at least 12 months for non-cardiac surgery, an attempt should be made to defer surgery for at least 30 days after bare metal stent placement and at least six months after drug-eluting stent placement (Grade 1B). Of course, patients whom have had recent PCI and present with urgent/emergent surgical procedures; relative risk and benefits are weighed as is the continuation of dual antiplatelet therapies (DAPT) in the perioperative period.

**Answer: C**

Cruden, N.L., Harding, S.A., Flapan, A.D., *et al.* (2010) Previous coronary stent implantation and cardiac events in patients undergoing noncardiac surgery. *Circulation: Cardiovascular Interventions*, **3** (3), 236–242.

Hawn, M.T., Graham, L.A., Richman, J.R., *et al.* (2012) The incidence and timing of noncardiac surgery after cardiac stent implantation. *Journal of the American College of Surgeons*, **214** (4), 658–666.

**16** *A 42-year-old woman is undergoing a diagnostic laparoscopy for suspected appendicitis. Insufflation of the abdomen is performed with carbon dioxide to 15 mm Hg. What physiologic changes may be seen during intraabdominal insufflation?*

**A** *Decreased cardiac output*
**B** *Bradycardia*
**C** *Increased systemic vascular resistance (SVR)*
**D** *Decreased cardiac index*
**E** *All of the above*

Laparoscopic procedures are increasing in number since they began over two decades ago, with the most common abdominal operation being performed in the United States by general surgeons being cholecystectomy. The rate of serious complications associated with a laparoscopic approach are relatively low with those being related to initial abdominal access during laparoscopy occurring in less than 1% of patients. Complications related to insufflation of gas include subcutaneous emphysema, cardiac arrhythmia, pain, and pneumothorax. Additionally, with most centers using 15 mm Hg pressure to produce pneumoperitoneum for appropriate visualization of intra-abdominal structures venous return to the heart can decrease causing all of the physiologic effects mentioned above.

**Answer: E**

Jiang, X., Anderson, C., and Schnatz, P.F. (2012) The safety of direct trocar versus Veress needle for laparoscopic entry: a meta-analysis of randomized clinical trials. *Journal of Laparoendoscopic and Advanced Surgical Techniques*, **22** (4), 362–370.

Koksoy, C., Kuzu, M.A., Kurt, I., *et al.* (1995) Haemodynamic effects of pneumoperitoneum during laparoscopic cholecystectomy: a prospective comparative study using bioimpedance cardiography. *British Journal of Surgery*, **82** (7), 972–974.

Trottier, D.C., Martel, G., and Boushey, R.P. (2009) Complications in laparoscopic intestinal surgery: prevention and management. *Minerva Chirurgica*, **64** (4), 339–354.

**17** *A 62-year-old woman is brought to the trauma bay secondary to a motor vehicle collision. She was a restrained passenger in a car that was involved in a head on collision at approximately 40 mph. Her past medical history is significant for diabetes, which is well controlled. Focused assessment with sonography was negative in the trauma bay. Vital signs show a HR: 104 beats/min, RR: 18 breaths/min, BP: 106/62 mm Hg. She complains of chest and abdominal pain for which she receives a CT of the* chest, abdomen, and pelvis with IV contrast. *A Grade II splenic laceration with no active extravasation of contrast and left sided pulmonary contusion were diagnosed. On hospital day 1 she begins to develop acute kidney injury. What is the most likely etiology?*

**A** *Poor oral intake due to pain*
**B** *Related to pain medication*
**C** *Under resuscitation with crystalloid in the trauma bay*
**D** *Contrast induced nephropathy*
**E** *This is an expected finding after trauma in her age group*

Contrast-induced nephropathy (CIN) occurs after the administration of radiocontrast media and can lead to acute kidney injury (AKI). CIN is defined as an acute decline in renal function after exposure to intravenous radiocontrast media. In most cases, the injury is reversible but there is some evidence that its development is associated with adverse outcomes. Clinical laboratory abnormalities that can be seen with this condition include a > 25% increase in baseline creatinine levels, fractional excretion of sodium > 1%, and granular brown casts on urinalysis. Oral intake due to pain, pain medications would not cause this on hospital day 1. A retrospective review of trauma patients showed the incidence of CIN to be as high as 5.1% in blunt trauma patients. Patient groups found to be predisposed to CIN where elderly patients along with those having low glomerular filtration rates.

**Answer: D**

Barrett, B.J. (1994) Contrast nephrotoxicity. *Journal of the American Society of Nephrology*, **5** (2), 125.

Hipp, A., Desai, S., Lopez, C., and Sinert, R. (2008) The incidence of contrast-induced nephropathy in trauma patients. *European Journal of Emergency Medicine*, **15** (3), 134–139.

Rudnick, M. and Feldman, H. (2008) Contrast-induced nephropathy: what are the true clinical consequences? *Clinical Journal of the American Society of Nephrology*, **3** (1), 263–272.

**18** *An 82-year-old cachectic appearing man with severe COPD presents to the emergency department with a large bowel obstruction verified by CT scan. A large colonic mass was noted distal to the splenic flexure. Upon further questioning, he has lost 40 pounds over the last six months and has never undergone colonoscopy. The patient was taken to operating room for left hemicolectomy with hand-sewn anastomosis. He has been unable to liberate from the ventilator since surgery.*

On hospital day 6 he begins to have bowel sounds and passes a small amount of maroon colored stool. You decide you want to begin nutritional support. What is the preferred nutritional route for this patient?

**A** *Peripheral parenteral nutrition*
**B** *Add dextrose to IV fluids*
**C** *Enteral nutrition*
**D** *Total parenteral nutrition*
**E** *Continue NPO*

Enteral nutrition is the preferred way to achieve nutritional support in the critically ill patient. Although this may not be achievable depending on the clinical scenario (i.e., high output fistula, malabsorption) therefore other forms of nutrition will need to be sought. Enteral nutrition is an active therapy that attenuates the metabolic response and favorably modulates the immune system. Additionally, it is less expensive than parenteral nutrition, is associated with less infectious complications and overall better patient outcomes. Originally, it had been thought that post-pyloric feeding would be superior to gastric feeding but recent studies have shown no overall benefit. Peripheral parenteral nutrition has not been shown to change outcomes. While in the fasting state the addition of dextrose would decrease nitrogen loss, it is not the preferred method as the calories from it would be minimal. While TPN provides calories starting it on postoperative day 6 has not yet been shown to be of any benefits and there are data to demonstrate its association with complications and increased use of resources. No nutrition has also been shown to be of worse outcome.

**Answer: C**

Seron-Arbeloa, C., Zamora-Elson, M., Labarta-Monzon, L., and Mallor-Bonet, T. (2013) Enteral nutrition in critical care. *Journal of Clinical Medicine Research*, **5** (1), 1–11.

White, H., Sosnowski, K., Tran, K.. *et al.* (2009) A randomized controlled comparison of early post-pyloric versus early gastric feeding to meet nutritional targets in ventilated intensive care patients. *Critical Care*, **13** (6), 1–8.

**19** *The patient in the above scenario is started on enteral tube feedings. 24-hours after the initiation of enteral nutrition he begins to have ectopy on continuous cardiac monitoring. What is the most common biochemical derangement seen with refeeding syndrome?*

**A** *Hypophosphatemia*
**B** *Hypomagnesemia*
**C** *Hypokalemia*
**D** *Hyponatremia*
**E** *Hyperkalemia*

Refeeding syndrome (RFS) can be defined as the potentially fatal shifts in fluids and electrolytes that may occur in malnourished patients receiving artificial nutrition (enteral or parenteral). These shifts are a result of hormonal and metabolic changes with the biochemical hallmark of RFS being hypophosphatemia. However, other metabolic derangements may occur including hypokalemia, hypomagnesemia, abnormal sodium and fluid balance, changes in glucose, protein, and fat metabolism. These disturbances usually occur within 12 to 72 hours of refeeding. RFS was first described during World War II as cardiac and neurologic dysfunction was seen.

**Answer: A**

Fuentebella, J. and Kerner, J.A. (2009) Refeeding syndrome. *The Pediatric Clinics of North America*, **56** (5), 1201.

Mehanna, H. (2008) Refeeding syndrome: what it is, and how to prevent and treat it. *British Medical Journal*, **336** (7659), 1495–1498.

Ornstein, R.M., Golden, N.H., Jacobson, M.S., and Shenker, I.R. (2003) Hypophosphatemia during nutritional rehabilitation in anorexia nervosa: implications for refeeding and monitoring. *Journal of Adolescent Health*, **32** (1), 83–88.

**20** *A 28-year-old woman with no past medical history presents to the emergency department with right lower quadrant abdominal pain. Ultrasound is performed and is suggestive of acute appendicitis. She is taken to the operative room for laparoscopic appendectomy. As you begin the case the anesthesiologist notes an acute rise in end tidal $CO_2$, masseter rigidity, and temperature elevation to 40.4 °C. What is the likely cause of this phenomenon?*

**A** *Ketamine*
**B** *Sevoflurane*
**C** *Propofol*
**D** *Etomidate*
**E** *Severe sepsis*

Malignant hyperthermia (MH) occurs when a patient is exposed to a volatile anesthetic (sevoflurane, isoflurane, succinylcholine, desflurane, halthothane, enflurane). The incidence of MH in the general population is estimated to be approximately 1:100 000 administered anesthetics, though this is thought to be an underestimation due to subclinical reactions. The majority of malignant hyperthermia-susceptible patients have mutations encoding for abnormal RYR1 or DHP receptors; with exposure to triggering agents leading to unregulated passage of calcium from the sarcoplasmic reticulum into the intracellular space, leading to an acute MH crisis. Dantrolene administration at 2.5 mg/kg IV is to be given rapidly if the diagnosis is made but subsequent bolus doses of 1 mg/kg (up to 10 mg/kg) if signs of MH have not abated. Ketamine, propofol and etomidate has not been found to cause MH and sepsis would not cause the other listed symptoms.

**Answer B**

Nelson, P. and Litman, R.S. (2014) Malignant hyperthermia in children: an analysis of the North American malignant hyperthermia registry. *Anesthesia and Analgesia*, **118** (2), 369–374.

Wappler, F. (2001) Malignant hyperthermia. *European Journal of Anaesthesiology*, **18** (10), 632–652.

# 8

## Acute Respiratory Failure and Mechanical Ventilation
*Adrian A. Maung, MD and Lewis J. Kaplan, MD*

**1** *In the immediate postoperative setting, noninvasive ventilation has been demonstrated to be most effective at:*
   **A** *Reversing atelectasis*
   **B** *Decreasing laryngeal edema*
   **C** *Improving cardiac performance*
   **D** *Reducing inspiratory stridor*
   **E** *Decreasing wheezing*

By applying positive pressure ventilation, noninvasive ventilation (NIV) is able to augment a patient's native respiratory efforts, overcoming critical closing pressures and volumes, and better match regional time constant variations, thereby moving the zero-pressure point more proximal in the airway. These effects help reverse atelectasis and therefore NIV has been used to great effect in the immediate postoperative setting in the PACU as well as on the general ward. NIV has no effect on laryngeal edema, inspiratory stridor or wheezing. NIV may augment cardiac performance by reversing hypoxic pulmonary vasoconstriction.

**Answer: A**

Jaber, S., Chanques, G., and Jung, B. (2010) Postoperative noninvasive ventilation. *Anesthesiology*, **112** (2), 453–461.
Papadakos, P.J., Karcz, M., and Lachmann, B. (2010) Mechanical ventilation in trauma. *Current Opinion in Anaesthesiology*, **23** (2), 228–232.

**2** *A 72-year-old, non-obese woman undergoes a laparoscopic ventral hernia repair without incident. She is extubated in the OR but is found to be hypoxic, hypercarbic, and acidotic in the PACU requiring reintubation. The most likely cause of her acute respiratory failure is:*
   **A** *Acute pulmonary edema from volume overload*
   **B** *Postoperative hemorrhage*
   **C** *Carbon dioxide gas embolism*
   **D** *Inadequate neuromuscular blocker reversal*
   **E** *Abdominal compartment syndrome*

Inadequate reversal of neuromuscular blocking (NMB) agents is an important cause for acute respiratory failure in the PACU, although it is less likely than intrinsic pulmonary disorders – an unlikely event in this healthy 72-year-old woman. The likelihood of NMB reversal inadequacy is increased in the elderly, the clinically severely obese, patients with hypoperfusion, and those whose procedure occurs more rapidly than anticipated after receiving a long-acting NMB agent. Uneventful OR cases are uncommonly associated with pulmonary edema in the relatively young, but are more frequently observed in those with preexisting significant cardiopulmonary disease. While a patient with obesity is likely to have pulmonary HTN, pulmonary edema is still less likely than inadequate NMB agent reversal. Postoperative hemorrhage is uncommonly associated with hypercarbia, and $CO_2$ embolism generally occurs while the abdomen in insufflated with $CO_2$—not after desufflation. Similarly, ventral hernia repair that is performed laparoscopically is unlikely to result in abdominal compartment syndrome as patients who are suitable for a laparoscopic repair generally do not demonstrate significant loss of domain.

**Answer: D**

Cobb, W.S., Fleishman, H.A., Kercher, K.W., *et al.* (2005) Gas embolism during laparoscopic cholecystectomy. *Journal of Laparoendoscopic and Advanced Surgical Techniques. Part A*, **15** (4), 387–390.
Lee, P.J., MacLennan, A., Naughton, N.N., and O'Reilly, M. (2003) An analysis of reintubations from a quality assurance database of 152 000 cases. *Journal of Clinical Anesthesia*, **15** (8), 575–581.

**3** *A 19-year-old man undergoes an uneventful laparoscopic appendectomy for microperforated appendicitis. The case goes more quickly than anticipated and he is transferred to the PACU still intubated. He is then extubated with a train-of-four of 4/4 twitches and*

*Surgical Critical Care and Emergency Surgery: Clinical Questions and Answers*, Second Edition.
Edited by Forrest "Dell" Moore, Peter Rhee, and Gerard J. Fulda.
© 2018 John Wiley & Sons Ltd. Published 2018 by John Wiley & Sons Ltd.
Companion website: www.wiley.com/go/moore/surgical_criticalcare_and_emergency_surgery

*shortly thereafter develops stridor as well as hypoxia despite vigorous respiratory efforts and gas movement. A portable CXR is most likely to demonstrate:*

A *Westermark sign*
B *Pneumothorax*
C *Pulmonary edema*
D *Diffuse atelectasis*
E *Clear lung fields*

This patient is demonstrating the classic presentation of negative pressure pulmonary edema. It primarily occurs in young, muscular patients who are able to move large volumes of gas using significant muscular effort. Hypoxia is common as is stridor as the patient tries to move gas through partly opposed cords. Westermark sign is consistent with pulmonary embolus and is inconsistent with this presentation. Pneumothorax should demonstrate asymmetric breath sounds. Atelectasis should demonstrate decreased air movement, especially at the bases in the postoperative patient, and a normal CXR would be unexpected in a patient with hypoxemia.

**Answer: C**

Krodel, D.J., Bittner, E.A., Abdulnour, R., *et al.* (2010) Case scenario: acute postoperative negative pressure pulmonary edema. *Anesthesiology*, **113** (1), 200–207.

4  *A 56-year-old man undergoes an urgent sigmoid colectomy and Hartmann's pouch for perforated diverticulitis eight hours prior. Due to a history of coronary disease he is monitored using telemetry. The patient has the acute onset of tachycardia to 146 beats/min and an ECG strip demonstrates p waves with three different morphologies. His respiratory rate is 34 breaths/min, BP is 146/88 mm Hg with a $S_aO_2$ of 94% on 40% $O_2$ by FM. The most appropriate and effective therapy for this condition is:*

A *Furosemide 40 mg IVP and KVO IVF*
B *100% oxygen via non-rebreather mask*
C *BiPAP at 15/7 cm $H_2O$ and $FIO_2$ 100%*
D *Amiodarone 150 mg IVP bolus*
E *Intubation and mechanical ventilation*

An ECG trace with tachycardia demonstrating p waves of three different morphologies is termed multifocal atrial tachycardia (MAT). MAT is unique among atrial dysrhythmias in that is it strongly associated with impending acute respiratory failure and as such represents a stress rhythm. Therapy hinges on addressing the patient's elevated work of breathing by providing immediate endotracheal intubation and mechanical ventilation. None of the other therapies provides definitive management and do not address the underlying cause of

MAT. BiPAP does provide some ventilatory support but is in general inadequate at relieving the patient of all of the work of breathing.

**Answer: E**

Biggs, F.D., Lefrak, S.S., Kleiger, R.E., *et al.* (1977) Disturbances of rhythm in chronic lung disease. *Heart and Lung*, **6** (2), 256–261.

5  *A 77-year-old woman is involved in a motor vehicle collision with rollover. She arrives on 100% by non-rebreather with a $SaO_2 = 96\%$. Her respirations are shallow and labored. She has a past medical history remarkable for COPD. Her CXR demonstrates rib fractures on the left of 2 through 7. The most appropriate step to manage her respiratory status is:*

A *Nebulized albuterol and atrovent*
B *Morphine bolus and PCA pump*
C *Bolus and scheduled IV ketorolac*
D *Fursoemide 40 mg IVP and Q day*
E *Paravertebral block placement*

Rib fracture management hinges on adequate analgesia to support coughing, deep breathing, and maintenance of ventilation of the segments of lung that are contused and underlie the fractured ribs. Inadequate ventilatory efforts lead to widespread atelectasis and eventually an unsupportable work of breathing. One must also balance analgesia with sedative effects of analgesic medications. In particular, this patient has COPD and may be more sensitive to reductions in respiratory drive with the potential for significant $CO_2$ retention and respiratory acidosis. Thus, an analgesic method that minimizes sedation is ideal, and placing a paravertebral block meets those needs. Ketorolac can do so as well but is generally an add-on medication to an opioid or block-based regimen, as NSAIDs are generally inadequate as stand-alone agents for multiple rib fracture management, and are generally contraindicated with those at high risk for hemorrhage. Inhaled agents designed to manage bronchoconstriction are useful adjuncts but not primary therapy for rib fracture management and diuresis is generally inappropriate immediately after acute injury because patients generally need fluid resuscitation to support macro- and micro-circulatory oxygen delivery.

**Answer: E**

Bulger, E.M., Edwards, T., Klotz, P., and Jurkovich, G.J. (2004) Epidural analgesia improves outcome after multiple rib fractures. *Surgery*, **136** (2), 426–430.
Mohta, M., Verma, P., Saxena, A.K., *et al.* (2009) Prospective, randomized comparison of continuous thoracic epidural and thoracic paravertebral infusion in

patients with unilateral multiple fractured ribs: a pilot study. *Journal of Trauma, Injury, Infection, and Critical Care,* **66** (4), 1096–1101.

**6** *A 42-year-old man remains in the SICU on post-injury day 2 after a fall from 20 feet. He sustained multiple axial skeletal injuries, a grade III splenic laceration (nonoperative management) and a small left-sided SDH. Since admission he has received 10 L crystalloids and two units of packed red blood cells. He is sedated and mechanically ventilated on AC/VCV and you are called for slowly rising peak airway pressures without a change in other parameters or SaO$_2$; he is readily suctioned for moderately bloody secretions. His INR is 2.2 and his urine output has decreased from 70 mL/hour to 18 mL/hour. The next most appropriate step in management is:*
   **A** *Magnesium sulfate 4 gm IVP*
   **B** *N-acetyl cysteine prior to suctioning*
   **C** *Neuromuscular blockade*
   **D** *Bladder pressure measurement*
   **E** *Change to pressure control ventilation*

The clinician must frequently assess rising peak airway pressures. In this scenario, slowly rising pressures indicate a different process than those that rise acutely. The bloody secretions provide a clue that the patient is likely coagulopathic. Given his multiple injuries he is likely to need large-volume fluid resuscitation and is at risk for clotting factor dilution and failure of nonoperative management of his splenic laceration as well. Each of these factors can lead to an increase in intra-abdominal pressure from visceral edema, hemorrhage, as well as acute ascites formation. Measuring the intra-abdominal pressure using the bladder pressure to assess for intra-abdominal HTN and abdominal compartment syndrome would readily assess for this possibility. The lack of change in other ventilator parameters is also suggestive of a process that is external to the pulmonary circuit. Thus, magnesium sulfate for bronchodilatation will not address the underlying condition. N-acetyl cysteine is proven to be ineffective at mucolysis and has been more recently supplanted with hypertonic saline nebulizers. Neuromuscular blockade may mask the underlying cause and should be used with caution. Changing the ventilator mode will also not address the intra-abdominal HTN.

**Answer: D**

Lui, F., Sangosanya, A., and Kaplan, L.J. (2007) Abdominal compartment syndrome: clinical aspects and monitoring. *Critical Care Clinics,* **23** (3), 415–433.

**7** *A 68-year-old woman remains intubated and ventilated on postoperative day 6 after a ruptured AAA repair. She is febrile to 101.8$^0$F, tachycardic to 104 beats/min, but not hypotensive. She has thick yellow secretions. A CXR demonstrates bibasilar atelectasis. Her WBC is 9.4 × 10$^3$/microL with 72% neutrophils. The next most appropriate step is management is to:*
   **A** *Begin empiric vancomycin and piperacillin-tazobactam*
   **B** *Obtain an urgent CT scan of the abdomen and pelvic area*
   **C** *Obtain a bronchoalveolar lavage*
   **D** *Administer acetaminophen and a cooling blanket*
   **E** *Send stool sample for C. difficile*

This patient's presentation may be consistent with new onset ventilator-associated pneumonia with signs and symptoms that include fever, tachycardia, yellow secretions, and > 3 days of mechanical ventilation. The CXR does not describe a new infiltrate and therefore, the diagnosis of ventilator-associated infection (VAI) is not clear. Current data identify that the invasive diagnosis of pneumonia is more cost effective than an empiric therapeutic course of antimicrobial management. Therefore, the best choice is to perform a flexible bronchoscopy and bronchoalveolar lavage to investigate for airway inflammation and to obtain a specimen for culture. This method allows one to culture directly from the involved airway segment, and to avoid culturing tracheal secretions that may be colonized with bacteria resident in the omnipresent biofilm that accompanies indwelling devices.

**Answer: C**

Fagon, J.Y. (2006) Diagnosis and treatment of ventilator-associated pneumonia: fiberoptic bronchoscopy with bronchoalveolar lavage is essential. *Seminars in Respiratory and Critical Care Medicine,* **27** (1), 34–44.
Porzecanski, I. and Bowton, D.L. (2006) Diagnosis and treatment of ventilator-associated pneumonia. *Chest,* **130** (2), 597–604.

**8** *Which of the following interventions will prolong the inspiratory time in volume-cycled ventilation:*
   **A** *Decreasing the respiratory rate*
   **B** *Increasing the PEEP*
   **C** *Changing to a square waveform*
   **D** *Decreasing the flow rate*
   **E** *Neuromuscular blockade*

Prolonging the inspiratory time (Ti) in volume-cycled ventilation (VCV) may be accomplished by any of the following interventions: increasing the tidal volume (increased time to deliver more gas), decreasing the flow rate (longer time to deliver the same volume of gas), or changing to a decelerating waveform (progressive decrease in gas flow requires a longer tome to deliver the same volume of gas). Neuromuscular blockade, increased PEEP and a change in respiratory rate will not alter the Ti at all. Changing to a square waveform will provide a constant gas flow and will shorten Ti. Thus, the only intervention that will prolong Ti is decreasing the flow rate.

**Answer: D**

Bailey, H. and Kaplan, L.J. (2009) Mechanical ventilation, in *Clinical Procedures in Emergency Medicine*, 5th edn (eds J. Hedges and J. Roberts), W.B. Saunders, Philadelphia, PA, pp. 138–159.

**9** *A 72-year-old patient remains ventilated after a low anterior resection for malignancy. On body weight and habitus-appropriate AC/VCV, the patient remains hypoxic. Which of the following interventions is most likely to improve oxygenation?*
   **A** *Decrease in peak airway pressure*
   **B** *Increase in expiratory time*
   **C** *Increase in mean airway pressure*
   **D** *Increase in respiratory rate*
   **E** *Increase in dead space: tidal volume*

Oxygenation most closely correlates with mean airway pressure and is a reflection of the area under the curve described by the gas-flow waveform. Decreasing peak airway pressure will not change $pO_2$. Increases in expiratory time may increase $CO_2$ clearance if the patient has difficulty with expiratory flow (as in COPD) as may an increase in respiratory rate if minute ventilation is inadequate. An increase in the dead space to tidal volume ratio is associated with an increase in $pCO_2$ and a decrease in $pO_2$, and when the ratio approaches 70% it generally indicates an unsupportable work of breathing.

**Answer: C**

Bailey, H. and Kaplan, L.J. (2009) Mechanical ventilation, in *Clinical Procedures in Emergency Medicine*, 5th edn (eds J. Hedges and J. Roberts), W.B. Saunders, Philadelphia, PA, pp. 138–159.

**10** *A 24-year-old man is S/P MVC with persistent large volume air leaks via bilateral chest tubes placed for the management of traumatic pneumothoraces. He is currently managed on AC/VCV with a delivered VT of 750 mL and recovered volume of 400 mL. Which is the next most appropriate intervention?*
   **A** *Initiation of high-frequency oscillation ventilation*
   **B** *Increase in delivered tidal volume on AC/VCV*

   **C** *VATS for stapled lung repair using bovine pericardium*
   **D** *Initiation of extracorporeal membrane oxygenation*
   **E** *Change to inverse ratio pressure control ventilation*

This patient demonstrates a parenchymal-pleural fistula (PPF) with a net loss of 350 cc of tidal volume out through the chest tubes. The management of such injuries relies in part on excluding a fistula from a major bronchus (bronchopleural fistula; BPF) that would prompt surgical repair. Once a major bronchial disruption is excluded, one may manage the PPF by reducing peak airway pressure and minimizing intratidal shear forces. One effective management strategy is to change from AC/VCV to high-frequency oscillation ventilation, a strategy that uses very small quantities of gas delivered at a very high frequency by a driving pressure to create a central column of standing gas that moves by laminar flow in major airways, and more turbulent but relatively static waves in more distal airways. Gas returns more proximally along the lateral aspects of the central jet of high-frequency and a small volume of machine-delivered gas is generated. In this way HFOV is more effective at oxygenation than it is $CO_2$ clearance. The small volumes and the lack of intratidal shear help PFF to heal. Increasing the delivered tidal volume, or prolonging the inspiratory time as in inverse ratio PCV will drive more gas out through the PFF and impede healing. ECMO is not supported for this condition as first-line therapy (but may serve as a bridge), and VATS is generally not indicated as there are typically multiple areas of leak that are not amenable to surgical stapling. Another useful technique is simultaneous independent lung ventilation that allows the clinician to use two different modes of ventilation and very different airway pressures and gas flow rates.

**Answer: A**

Cheatham, M.L. and Promes, J.T. (2006) Independent lung ventilation in the management of traumatic bronchopleural fistula. *American Surgeon*, **72** (6), 530–533.

Ha, D.V. and Johnson, D. (2004) High frequency oscillatory ventilation in the management of a high output bronchopleural fistula: a case report. *Canadian Journal of Anaesthesia*, **51** (1), 78–83.

**11** *A 54-year-old patient is s/p abdominal wall reconstruction and is changed from AC/VCV to airway pressure release ventilation (APRV) for hypoxemic rescue. Which of the following observations is expected?*
   **A** *Lower mean airway pressures*
   **B** *Increased need for sedation for comfort*

**C** *Uncoupling of oxygenation and ventilation*
**D** *Increased minute ventilation requirement*
**E** *Higher central venous pressures*

Airway pressure release ventilation (APRV) is a modified form of high-pressure CPAP that is periodically turned off for a very short time to allow gas egress and $CO_2$ clearance. It is a superior recruitment mode and relies on a significant increase in mean airway pressure to match regional time constant variations, recruit atelectatic alveoli, and improve oxygenation. Airway pressure release ventilation's effect on $p_aO_2$ may occur independent from its effect on $CO_2$ clearance, and maximal change in $CO_2$ often lags behind the maximal change in $pO_2$; in this way oxygenation and ventilation are uncoupled. Airway pressure release ventilation generally requires less sedation, is more efficient than traditional AC/VCV and requires lower minute ventilation for equivalent $CO_2$ clearance. Due to the effects of abrogation of hypoxic pulmonary vasconstriction and the subsequent reduction in downstream pressures, the measured CVP typically decreases.

**Answer: C**

Bailey, H. and Kaplan, L.J. (2009) Mechanical ventilation, in *Clinical Procedures in Emergency Medicine*, 5th edn (eds J. Hedges and J. Roberts), W.B. Saunders, Philadelphia, PA, pp. 138–159.
Kaplan, L.J., Bailey, H., and Formosa, V. (2001) APRV increases cardiac performance in patients with acute lung injury/adult respiratory distress syndrome. *Critical Care*, **5** (4), 221–226.

**12** *A 62-year-old woman is immediately s/p right hepatic lobectomy for malignancy. She sustained a large volume blood loss and was resuscitated and therefore left on mechanical ventilation. She is placed on the same ventilator settings that were used in the OR. Which of the following findings is expected before the patient begins to take spontaneous breaths?*
 **A** *Higher $p_aCO_2$*
 **B** *Higher $p_aO_2$*
 **C** *Auto-PEEP*
 **D** *Decreased inspiratory time*
 **E** *Increased expiratory time*

Intraoperative ventilator settings generally reflect neuromuscular blockade or deep sedation as well as the reduction in metabolic rate that accompanies inhalational or intravenous general anesthesia. Thus, the minute ventilation required for maintaining a normal $CO_2$ clearance will be less than that required in the SICU where the patient generally has a normal or elevated metabolic rate by comparison to that present in the OR under anesthesia. Thus, if the patient is placed on the same settings used in the OR, only a higher $pCO_2$ is expected before spontaneous respiratory efforts may adjust the minute ventilation to meet $CO_2$ production needs.

**Answer: A**

Bailey, H. and Kaplan, L.J. (2009) Mechanical ventilation, in *Clinical Procedures in Emergency Medicine*, 5th edn (eds J. Hedges and J. Roberts), W.B. Saunders, Philadelphia, PA, pp. 138–159.

**13** *You are called to the bedside of a patient on body weight and habitus-appropriate AC/VCV settings with high peak airway pressures; she is postoperative day 2 after a Hartmann's procedure for perforated diverticulitis. $SaO_2$ is 97% on $FIO_2$ of 0.4. The most appropriate investigation is:*
 **A** *Pulmonary artery catheter assessment*
 **B** *Lower inflection point assessment*
 **C** *Pressure versus volume tracing assessment*
 **D** *Flow versus time tracing assessment*
 **E** *CT scan to assess for pulmonary embolus*

High peak airway pressures on a body weight and habitus-appropriate AC/VCV settings may be a reflection of increased airway resistance, or inappropriate gas delivery for the volume of available lung. The latter may be especially true in the patient with perforated diverticulitis who may have received significant fluid resuscitation to help manage her peritonitis-associated capillary leak syndrome. Thus, some evaluation of how gas delivery is being received by the patient's lung is appropriate. Bedside assessment may be readily accomplished by using the dynamic pressure-volume curve and assessing for increases in airway pressure without a corresponding increase in pulmonary volume, producing a characteristic curve trace known as the "bird's beak phenomenon" which reflects alveolar overdistension. Placing a pulmonary artery catheter will not help in investigating peak airway pressures, nor will a CT to evaluate for pulmonary embolus be appropriate in the absence of hypoxemia. The flow-over-time trace is useful to assess for auto-PEEP. Determination of the lower inflection point in the dynamic or static pressure volume curve assesses for inadequate PEEP, not the presence or absence of alveolar overdistension.

**Answer: C**

Pestana, D., Hernandez-Gancedo, C., Royo, C., *et al.* (2005) Pressure-volume curve variations after a recruitment manoeuvre in acute lung injury/ARDS patients:

implications for the understanding of the inflection points of the curve. *European Journal of Anaesthesiology*, **22** (3), 175–180.

Vieillard-Baron, A. and Jardin, F. (2003) The issue of dynamic hyperinflation in acute respiratory distress syndrome patients. *European Respiratory Journal— Supplement* **42**, 43s–47s.

**14** *A 35-year-old man is postinjury day 2 following a collision with an automobile and remains mechanically ventilated on inverse-ratio pressure control ventilation for the management of severe bilateral pulmonary contusions. He is hemodynamically appropriate on low-dose norepinephrine. He has the following ABG: 7.18/$P_aCO_2$: 63/ $P_aO_2$: 72 on AC 8/PCV 30/Ti 4.0/80%/PEEP: +10, decelerating waveform. The next most appropriate intervention is:*

**A** *CT scan to rule out pulmonary embolus*
**B** *$D_5W$ + 75 mEq/L $NaHCO_3$ at maintenance rate*
**C** *Increase in AC rate to 12 breaths/min*
**D** *Decrease PEEP to 5 cm $H_2O$ pressure*
**E** *Decrease inspiratory time ($T_i$) to 3.2 seconds*

This patient demonstrates a respiratory acidosis and is only marginally oxygenated on high-level airway pressure ventilator settings to manage his severe bilateral pulmonary contusions. This would suggest that his ventilator settings may be optimally adjusted for his pulmonary mechanics, and he requires pressor support to help manage pulmonary flow. In such circumstances, allowing the patient to have a higher than normal $pCO_2$ provided there is adequate oxygenation may be ideal to avoid inducing ventilator-induced lung injury in an effort to clear additional $CO_2$. This strategy is termed "permissive hypercapnia" and may require buffering of the associated respiratory acidosis as suggested by using a sodium bicarbonate-containing infusion. There is no need to perform a CT scan for pulmonary embolus as the underlying cause of respiratory failure is identified as pulmonary contusion. Increasing the respiratory rate in fixed inspiratory time PCV will decrease $CO_2$ clearance and increase $pCO_2$. Decreasing PEEP will move the zero pressure point more distally and lead to worsened oxygenation. Decreasing the inspiratory time may increase $CO_2$ clearance by increasing the available expiratory time but will also decrease oxygenation and is counterproductive.

**Answer: B**

Hemmila, M.R and Napolitan, L.M. (2006) Severe respiratory failure: advanced treatment options. *Critical Care Medicine*, **34** (9 Suppl), S278–S290.

**15** *A 68-year-old clinically severely obese woman is two days s/p an extensive head and neck resection with radial forearm free flap and tracheostomy. While in the SICU she becomes agitated and her tracheostomy is dislodged. She is acutely hypoxic. The most appropriate management is:*

**A** *Initiation of heliox (80/20) therapy*
**B** *Oral endotracheal intubation*
**C** *Tracheostomy tube replacement*
**D** *100% $O_2$ via tracheostomy mask*
**E** *Nebulized albuterol and IV furosemide*

The standard and safe approach to a dislodged tracheostomy tube prior to a well-formed track forming (generally postoperative day 7) is to place a standard oral endotracheal tube to secure airway control. The surgeon's finger may need to cover the trachesotomy site to help keep the orally placed tube from egressing via the tracheotomy site. Once the airway is secured from above, the tracheostomy tube may be safely replaced in a controlled fashion. Many surgeons will place tracheal stay sutures to facilitate pulling up on the trachea and easing replacement should the tube become dislodged, although there is little- to-no strong data supporting this practice. In this case, the patient's body habitus will likely render replacement via the stoma site more difficult, especially since her neck was dissected and many planes that would help guide the tube into the trachea have been disturbed – increasing the likelihood of extratracheal placement. Heliox has some role in reducing airway gas passage in patients with stidor. One hundred percent $O_2$ via tracheostomy mask requires a tube to be present to be efficacious, and albuterol and a diuretic are not effective management strategies for a dislodged tracheostomy tube.

**Answer: B**

Barbetti, J.K., Nichol, A.D., and Choate, K.R., *et al.* (2009) Prospective observational study of postoperative complications after percutaneous dilatational or surgical tracheostomy in critically ill patients. *Critical Care and Resuscitation*, **11** (4), 244–249.

Colman, K.L., Mandell, D.L., and Simons, J.P. (2010) Impact of stoma maturation on pediatric tracheostomy-related complications. *Archives of Otolaryngology Head and Neck Surgery*, **136** (5), 471–474.

Engels, P.T., Bagshaw, S.M., Meier, M., and Brindley, P.G. (2009) Tracheostomy: from insertion to decannulation. *Canadian Journal of Surgery*, **52** (5), 427–433.

**16** *A 16-year-old patient is shot in the left chest, arrives with agonal vital signs, undergoes a transverse thoracotomy for resuscitation, and undergoes nonanatomic* *lingual resection, repair of a thoracic aortic tangential injury and bi-ventricular lacerations, as well as a nonanatomic right middle lobe resection. On attempts at closure, he becomes tachycardia and hypotensive. The next most appropriate step in management is:*

**A** *Exploratory laparotomy for abdominal decompression*
**B** *Intraoperative mannitol for diuresis*
**C** *Intraoperative CVVH for solute and water removal*
**D** *Thoracic closure with pressor agent BP support*
**E** *Thoracic packing and open chest management*

Compartment syndrome is not limited to an extremity or the abdomen as it may also occur in the chest. Treatment paradigms are similar in that the cavity to be closed is instead temporarily expanded to allow for visceral edema. More often described after cardiac surgery, thoracic compartment syndrome is also reported after extensive thoracic injury. While abdominal decompression addresses abdominal compartment syndrome and may address refractory intracranial HTN as well, it does not as effectively address thoracic pressures as does leaving the chest open. Diuresis is not acutely effective in reducing visceral edema immediately after injury and is generally contraindicated during resuscitation from hemorrhagic shock. Similarly, renal support therapies are ineffective and not supported during resuscitation for total body salt and water removal. Pressor support is inappropriate when a simple maneuver like leaving the chest open is performed, which will more directly support perfusion without increasing myocardial consumption of oxygen.

**Answer: E**

Kaplan, L.J., Trooskin, S.Z., and Santora, T.A. (1996) Thoracic compartment syndrome. *Journal of Trauma*, **40** (2), 291–293.
Rizzo, A.G. and Sample, G.A. (2003) Thoracic compartment syndrome secondary to a thoracic procedure: a case report. *Chest*, **124** (3), 1164–1168.

**17** *A 32-year-old woman is admitted to the burn ICU with 60% total BSA third-degree burns to the torso and lower extremities, including a circumferential chest burn. She is intubated in the ED and placed on pressure control ventilation with settings of AC 12/PCV 20/T<sub>i</sub> 2.0 sec/FIO₂ 100%/+5 generating a VT of 550 mL with an initial ABG = 7.41/42/350. Twelve hours later, after fluid resuscitation, her resultant tidal volumes are in the 200s and a subsequent ABG = 7.20/60/280. Over the next six hours, she requires a progressive increase in PC to recover the*

*desired tidal volume. Bladder pressure is 10 mm Hg. Chest x-ray is clear. The next step in management should be to:*

**A** *Change to volume cycled ventilation*
**B** *Increased pressure control*
**C** *Increase PEEP to 10 cm H₂O pressure*
**D** *Bilateral thoracic escharotomies*
**E** *Decompressive laparotomy*

Full-thickness circumferential burns over the torso can result in significant compromise of chest wall movement and hinder ventilation. This is manifested either with decreasing tidal volumes in pressure-cycled ventilation (and increasing pCO₂) or increasing peak airway pressures in volume-cycled ventilation (with high airway pressure limited gas delivery and rising pCO₂). The definitive treatment is to incise the thick eschar that is limiting chest-wall excursion. Abdominal compartment syndrome may present similarly but would be associated with an elevated bladder pressure and an attributable organ failure. Increasing PEEP, increasing the pressure control limit, and changing to volume-cycle ventilation will not address the circumferential thoracic eschar.

**Answer: D**

Foot, C., Host, D., Campher, D., et al. (2008) Moulage in high-fidelity simulation: a chest wall burn escharotomy model for visual realism and as an educational tool. *Simulation in Healthcare: The Journal of The Society for Medical Simulation*, **3** (3), 183–185.
Orgill, D.P. and Piccolo, N. (2009) Escharotomy and decompressive therapies in burns. *Journal of Burn Care and Research*, **30** (5), 759–768.

**18** *A 54-year-old, 70 kg man is postoperative day 2 following an orthotopic hepatic transplantation. He has been maintained on AC/VCV and has just completed a 30-minute spontaneous breathing trial on pressure support of 5 cm H₂O and PEEP of 5 cm H₂O with the following parameters obtained: negative inspiratory force 15 cm H₂O, minute ventilation 12 L/min, SaO₂ at completion 95% on FIO₂ 0.4, and a respiratory rate that started at 16 breaths/min and ended at 24 breaths/min with a spontaneous tidal volume of 500 mL. He is net negative by 1200 mL over the last 12 hours. The next most appropriate course of action is to:*

**A** *Resume the prior AC/VCV settings*
**B** *Extubate to 40% O₂ via face mask*
**C** *Repeat the trial 12 hours later*
**D** *Change to flow-by and reevaluate*
**E** *Obtain a CXR to rule out pulmonary edema*

This question assesses the appropriate determinants for safe extubation. Weaning parameters are commonly obtained but perhaps the most useful is the rapid shallow breathing index (RSBI; aka. Tobin index), obtained by dividing the frequency of respiration by the tidal volume. Here the RSBI is 24 breaths/min divided by 0.5 L yielding an index of 48; an index less than 105 is generally believed to be supportive of the ability of a patient to support their own work of breathing without mechanical ventilatory support. Since negative inspiratory force is effort dependent its validity is readily questioned. In this case, the NIF is less than 25 (normal value) and would mitigate against extubation. However, the acceptable total minute ventilation, respiratory rate, oxygen saturation, and net negative fluid balance, and the low RSBI readily supports extubation. Repeating the trial, changing to flow-by or obtaining a CXR are all argued against by the excellent spontaneous breathing trial performance.

**Answer: B**

Lessard, M.R. and Brochard, L.J. (1996) Weaning from ventilatory support. *Clinics in Chest Medicine*, **17** (3), 475–489.

19  Which statement regarding non-invasive positive pressure ventilation (NIPPV) is most accurate?
    A  Level I evidence in patients with COPD exacerbations
    B  Level I evidence in postoperative patients to prevent reintubation
    C  NIPPV is ineffective in cardiogenic pulmonary edema patients
    D  NIPPV can provide patients a mandatory respiratory rate
    E  NIPPV effectively clears secretions in cystic fibrosis patients

NIPPV utilizes pressure-cycled modes that assist respiration and provide a PEEP equivalent to help retard alveolar collapse and assist in alveolar recruitment. The clinician sets the amount of pressure during inspiration and expiration while the patient controls the respiratory rate and inspiratory and expiratory times. Level I evidence supports the use of NIPPV in patients with COPD exacerbations, maintaining extubation in COPD patients and as an adjunct in treatment of cardiogenic pulmonary edema. Its use in postoperative patients is not as well defined, although CPAP by helmet has been demonstrated to be effective in managing atelectasis. Two multicenter randomized trials have failed to show benefit in established respiratory distress although other smaller trials have demonstrated some benefit. Only negative pressure ventilation has been proven effective in enhancing expectoration of secretions in the cystic fibrosis patient population.

**Answer: A**

Jhanji, S. and Pearse, R.M. (2009) The use of early intervention to prevent postoperative complications. *Current Opinion in Critical Care*, **15** (4), 349–354.
Osthoff, M. and Leuppi, J.D. (2010) Management of chronic obstructive pulmonary disease patients after hospitalization for acute exacerbation. *Respiration*, **79** (3), 255–261.

20  Contraindications for noninvasive positive pressure ventilation (NIPPV) include:
    A  Hemodynamic instability
    B  Excessive secretions
    C  Inability to protect the airway
    D  Respiratory arrest
    E  All of the above

Contraindications for NIPPV include inability to protect the airway, respiratory arrest, hemodynamic instability, agitation, uncooperative patient, excessive secretions or significant upper GI bleeding. There is a theoretical but unproven concern regarding the use of NIPPV in patients with recent upper GI anastomosis.

**Answer: E**

Jaber, S., Chanques, G., and Jung, B. (2010) Postoperative noninvasive ventilation. *Anesthesiology*, **112** (2), 453–461.
Papadakos, P.J., Karcz, M., and Lachmann, B. (2010) Mechanical ventilation in trauma. *Current Opinion in Anaesthesiology*, **23** (2), 228–132.

21  A 58-year-old woman is admitted to the SICU after undergoing exploratory laparotomy and Hartmann's procedure for Hinchey Class IV diverticulitis. She is mechanically ventilated on 60% FiO2. Her PaO2 on ABG is 78 mm Hg. Chest x-ray demonstrates bilateral opacities. She is placed on low-tidal volume ARDSnet ventilation. Additional therapy that has been demonstrated to reduce mortality includes:
    A  Inhaled nitric oxide
    B  Early initiation of prone ventilation
    C  Prone ventilation for refractory hypoxemia
    D  High dose steroids if unimproved at 2 weeks
    E  All of the above

A number of therapies have been tried to decrease the significant mortality associated with Acute Respiratory Distress Syndrome (ARDS). Low tidal volume ventilation was the first intervention demonstrated to improve mortality. Inhaled nitric oxide improves oxygenation but has not been shown to decrease morbidity and mortality and has been associated with risk of acute kidney injury.

The role of early steroids remains controversial but there is no benefit to late (after 14 days) steroids administration. The PROSEVA trial reported improved mortality with early prone ventilation in patients with severe ARDS.

**Answer B**

Guérin, C., Reignier, J., Richard, J.C., *et al.* (2013) Prone positioning in severe acute respiratory distress syndrome. *New England Journal of Medicine*, **368** (23), 2159–2167.

Petrucci, N. and De Feo, C. (2013) Lung protective ventilation strategy for the acute respiratory distress syndrome. *Cochrane Database Systematic Reviews*, **28** (2).

**22** *A 19-year-old man is admitted to the intensive care unit with respiratory failure after a fall. He has multiple bilateral rib fractures and pulmonary contusions. Over the next 24 hours, he develops progressive hypoxemia despite multiple ventilator adjustments including airway pressure release ventilation, low tidal volume ventilation, and prone positioning. The team is considering extracorporeal membrane oxygenation (ECMO). Which of the following is true regarding the role of ECMO for respiratory failure management?*
  **A** *ECMO is only proven beneficial in neonates.*
  **B** *A specialized center is not required to provide ECMO therapy*
  **C** *ECMO rescue has survival benefit in adult and pediatric patients*
  **D** *ECMO is only indicated as an adult lung or heart transplant bridge*
  **E** *None of the above*

Initial studies done in 1970s and 1990s examining the use of ECMO in adults with acute respiratory failure demonstrated no survival advantage with increased rate of complications. However, more recent controlled studies have demonstrated survival benefit in neonatal, pediatric, and adult patients with respiratory failure. Indications for ECMO in adults include hypoxic and/or hypercapneic respiratory failure in patients with predicated risk of death > 50% after the failure of other conventional therapies. Cardiac failure is also an indication for ECMO.

**Answer: C**

Kulkarni, T., Sharma, N.S., and Diaz-Guzman, E. (2016) Extracorporeal membrane oxygenation in adults: a practical guide for internists. *Cleveland Clinic Journal of Medicine*, **83** (5), 373–384.

Tramm, R., Ilic, D., Davies, E.R., *et al.* (2015) Extracorporeal membrane oxygenation for critically ill adults. Cochrane Database Systematic Reviews, Jan 22.

**23** *Which of the following interventions is most likely to repair the condition depicted in the waveform in Figure 8.1 for a patient on AC/VCV?*
  **A** *No change is required*
  **B** *Increase flow rate*
  **C** *Increase tidal volume*
  **D** *Increase PEEP*
  **E** *Decrease sedation*

The flow-over-time waveform depicts the classic appearance of auto-PEEP where the next breath begins before the exhalation trace (below the horizontal black line) returns to baseline. Therefore, the tracing identifies that there is gas trapping from the prior breath that creates auto-PEEP. Many interventions may address this potentially destabilizing condition and the one selected depends on the clinical circumstance. However, all interventions aim to increase the available time for exhalation. Therefore, A is wrong as the condition can lead to cardiovascular collapse much like tension pneumothorax. C increases the tidal volume and in VCV lead to an increase in inspiratory time and a decrease in expiratory time – the exact opposite of the desired repair strategy. D worsens the PEEP effect. E would increase the level of alertness and in general leads to an increase in respiratory rate. With a fixed inspiratory time determined by the waveform and the flow rate, this will also decrease the available time for gas exodus. Only B leads to a decreased inspiratory time and therefore an increased expiratory time.

**Answer: B**

Maung, A.A. and Kaplan, L.J. (2013) Waveform analysis during mechanical ventilation. *Current Problems in Surgery*, **50** (10), 438–446.

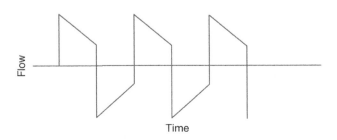

**Figure 8.1**

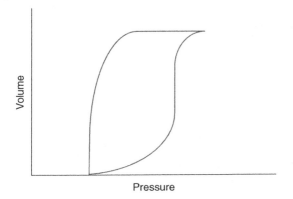

**Figure 8.2**

24 *Which of the following maneuvers would best address the abnormality depicted in Figure 8.2 in a patient on AC/VCV?*
   **A** *Inhaled nitric oxide*
   **B** *Increase PEEP*
   **C** *Change to square waveform*
   **D** *Decrease tidal volume*
   **E** *Increase respiratory rate*

Figure 8.2 is a pressure-volume curve and depicts the findings of pressure-volume dysregulation with alveolar over distension known as the "bird's beak" phenomenon. This indicates that the volume being provided is greater than the available lung to accommodate the prescribed volume. Therefore, option D is the best as it will decrease the total volume. A will change vascular volumes but not alveolar volume. Increased PEEP (B) will worsen the over distension by increasing the volume of unexhaled gas. Changing to a square waveform (C) will also exacerbate the problem by shortening the inspiratory time forcing the same volume to be delivered over a shorter period of time. E will potentially worsen the problem by creating auto-PEEP and will certainly do nothing to decrease the delivered volume or the rate at which it is delivered to the lung.

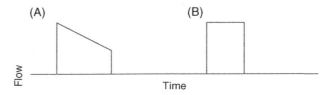

**Figure 8.3**

**Answer: D**

Maung, A.A. and Kaplan, L.J. (2013) Waveform analysis during mechanical ventilation. *Current Problems in Surgery*, **50** (10), 438–446.

25 *Which statement best characterizes the flow-over-time waveform A compared to B in Figure 8.3 for a patient receiving AC/VCV, assuming that the peak flow is identical?*
   **A** *Shorter inspiratory time*
   **B** *Higher plateau pressure*
   **C** *Increased PEEP*
   **D** *Lower peak airway pressure*
   **E** *Higher mean airway pressure*

The waveform in A is a decelerating curve while B is a square waveform. Decelerating delivery profiles have lower peak, higher mean, and lower plateau pressures as well as longer inspiratory times and shorter expiratory times compared to gas delivery using a square waveform. Unless there is auto-PEEP, neither waveform is typically associated with an increase in PEEP. Therefore, only E is correct.

**Answer: E**

Maung, A.A. and Kaplan, L.J. (2015) Ventilator gas delivery wave form substantially impacts plateau pressure and peak-to-plateau pressure gradient determination. *Journal of Trauma and Acute Care Surgery*, **78** (5), 976–979.

# 9

## Infectious Disease
Yousef Abuhakmeh, DO, John Watt, MD and Courtney McKinney, PharmD

**1** *A 64-year-old diabetic man is postoperative day seven after coronary artery bypass surgery. Over the past 48 hours, he has developed increasing chest pain, fevers, and an increasing insulin requirement. His white count is $16 \times 10^3$/microL, heart rate is 104 beats/min and his temperature is 38.9 °C. A CT scan of the chest reveals pneumomediastinum and a distinct fluid collection.*

*What is the most appropriate initial management of this patient?*

**A** *Surgical debridement of the sternum and mediastinum*
**B** *Initiate broad-spectrum antibiotic coverage with vancomycin and ciprofloxacin*
**C** *Initiation of broad-spectrum antibiotic coverage with piperacillin/tazobactam and vancomycin*
**D** *Obtain blood cultures, initiate broad-spectrum antibiotic coverage with piperacillin/tazobactam and vancomycin and drain the fluid collection*
**E** *Substernal aspiration for gram stain and culture, followed by initiation of broad-spectrum antibiotic coverage with piperacillin/tazobactam and vancomycin*

Nearly all patients with postoperative mediastinitis will have fever, tachycardia, signs of wound infection, and signs of systemic infection. Bacteremia may be the first sign of mediastinitis. Blood cultures should be obtained and empiric antibiotic therapy initiated with coverage against Gram-positive cocci and Gram-negative bacilli. The most common microorganism isolated is methicillin-susceptible *Staphylococcus aureus* (MSSA).

**Answer: D**

Fariñas, M.C., Galo Peralta, F., Bernal, J.M., *et al.* (1995) Suppurative mediastinitis after open-heart surgery: a case-control study covering a seven-year period in Santander, Spain. *Clinical Infectious Diseases*, **20** (2), 272–279.

Fowler, V.G., Jr, Kaye, K.S., Simel, D.L., *et al.* (2003) Staphylococcus aureus bacteremia after median sternotomy: clinical utility of blood culture results in the identification of postoperative mediastinitis. *Circulation*, **108** (1), 73–78.

Trouillet, J.L., Vuagnat, A., Combes, A., *et al.* (2005) Acute poststernotomy mediastinitis managed with debridement and closed-drainage aspiration: factors associated with death in the intensive care unit. *Journal of Thoracic and Cardiovascular Surgery*, **129** (3), 518–524.

**2** *A 71-year-old man, in the ICU after a lower extremity amputation for gangrenous limb ischemia, develops frequent watery bowel movements on postoperative day three. Stool studies confirm presence of C.* difficile *toxins, and he is started on oral metronidazole and vancomycin regimens, with which he has been treated previously for several prior episodes of C.* difficile *colitis. After three days of treatment, his abdomen remains mildly distended, he continues to have more than three bowel movements per day and is suspected to have an ileus with a high nasogastric tube output. His white count has increased to $29 \times 10^3$/microL and has been advanced to rectal vancomycin and IV metronidazole.*

*The most appropriate management of this patient includes:*

**A** *Fecal microbiota transplant*
**B** *Initiation of fidaxomicin*
**C** *Conversion from IV to rectal metronidazole*
**D** *Addition of IV Vancomycin*
**E** *Subtotal colectomy*

Standard treatment of *C. difficile* infection consists of metronidazole and oral vancomycin up to four times daily. Intracolonic administration of vancomycin is appropriate in the setting of profound ileus. *C. Diff* colitis can be classified as severe in the setting of white blood

*Surgical Critical Care and Emergency Surgery: Clinical Questions and Answers*, Second Edition.
Edited by Forrest "Dell" Moore, Peter Rhee, and Gerard J. Fulda.
© 2018 John Wiley & Sons Ltd. Published 2018 by John Wiley & Sons Ltd.
Companion website: www.wiley.com/go/moore/surgical_criticalcare_and_emergency_surgery

cell count >15 000 cells/microL, serum albumin < 3 g/dL, and/or a serum creatinine level ≥ 1.5 times the premorbid level. Meta-analyses have shown efficacy of fecal microbiota transplant in the treatment of severe or recurrent *C. difficile* infections. Donor fecal material may be administered via enema, colonoscope, nasogastric tube, or orally via frozen capsules. Administration via colonoscope has been shown to be superior to upper GI administration. Fidaxomicin (answer B) is an alternative agent for the treatment of recurrent *C. difficile* colitis and has demonstrated similar cure rates to oral vancomycin with a lower incidence of subsequent recurrence. However, fidaxomicin is only available for administration via the enteral route – in a patient with severe ileus, fidaxomicin may not be effective. Rectal metronidazole and IV vancomycin are not effective for treatment of *C. difficile* colitis. Subtotal would only be indicated if the patient were displaying signs of toxic megacolon.

**Answer: A**

Cohen, S.H., Gerding, D.N., Johnson, S., *et al.* (2010) Clinical practice guidelines for Clostridium difficile infection in adults: 2010 update by the society for healthcare epidemiology of America (SHEA) and the infectious diseases society of America (IDSA). *Infection Control and Hospital Epidemiology*, **31** (5), 431–455.

Cornely, O.A., Miller, M.A., Louie, T.J., *et al.* (2012) Treatment of first recurrence of Clostridium difficile infection: fidaxomicin versus vancomycin. *Clinical Infectious Diseases*, **55** (2), 154–161.

Furuya-Kanamori, L., Doi, S.A.R., Paterson, D. L., *et al.* (2016). Upper versus lower gastrointestinal delivery for transplantation of fecal microbiota in recurrent or refractory clostridium difficile infection: a collaborative analysis of individual patient data from 14 studies. *Journal of Clinical Gastroenterology*, **51** (2), 145–150.

Surawicz, C.M., Brandt, L.J., Binion, D.G., *et al.* (2013) Guidelines for diagnosis, treatment, and prevention of Clostridium difficile infections. *American Journal of Gastroenterology*, **108** (4), 478–498.

**3** *A 74-year-old man is mechanically ventilated for the sixth day after craniotomy for traumatic epidural hematoma. Over the past 48 hours he has developed intermittent fevers, along with a localized right lower lobe infiltrate on chest X-ray, and a leukocytosis. He is diagnosed with ventilator-associated pneumonia and started on appropriate empiric therapy. Culture results are positive for a* Pseudomonas aeruginosa *isolate that was susceptible to the initial antibiotic regimen. What is the appropriate duration of therapy?*
**A** *5 days*
**B** *7 days*
**C** *10 days*
**D** *14 days*
**E** *Duration based on clinical course and CPIS score*

Though some data demonstrated an increased risk of recurrent VAP when infections caused by resistance-prone isolates (MRSA, Pseudomonas, Acinetobacter) were treated with a shorter course of antibiotics (seven to eight days) versus a longer course (14–15 days), more recent meta-analyses have not shown an increased risk of recurrence associated with shorter durations of treatment. Shorter treatment courses reduce antibiotic exposure and recurrent pneumonia due to MDR organisms. Duration of antibiotic therapy has not been shown to influence outcomes such as mortality, duration of mechanical ventilation, or length of ICU stay. The current Infectious Disease Society of America (IDSA) and American Thoracic Society (ATS) guidelines recommend a shorter (7 day) treatment course for VAP with the important caveat that duration may be influenced by patient-specific factors such as rate of clinical improvement in conjunction with radiologic and laboratory findings.

The use of clinical criteria alone, rather than the combined use of clinical criteria and semi-objective measures such as the Clinical Pulmonary Infection Score (CPIS), is recommended for use to determine the need for initiation or discontinuation of treatment for VAP. Analysis of trials using CPIS as a diagnostic aid for VAP demonstrated unacceptably low sensitivity and specificity. Evaluation of data regarding CPIS-informed antibiotic de-escalation demonstrated no effect on clinical outcomes, and therefore its use is not recommended.

**Answer: B**

Chastre, J., Wolff, M., Fagon, J.Y., *et al.* (2003) Comparison of 8 vs 15 days of antibiotic therapy for ventilator-associated pneumonia in adults: a randomized trial. *Journal of the American Medical Association*, **290** (19), 2588–2598.

Kalil, A.C., Metersky, M.L., Klompas, M., *et al.* (2016) Management of adults with hospital-acquired and ventilator-associated pneumonia: 2016 clinical practice guidelines by the Infectious Diseases Society of America and the American Thoracic Society. *Clinical Infectious Diseases*, **63** (5), 61–111.

**4** *A 62-year-old diabetic man is admitted to the ICU postoperatively, following laparotomy and washout for perforated diverticulitis. Overnight, his heart rate ranges from 110 to 128 beats/min and his MAP ranges from 50 to 68 mm Hg, despite resuscitation* *with Lactated Ringer's solution. His urine output has decreased to < 15 ml/hr, his white count is $19 \times 10^3$/microL, his hemoglobin is 6.8 g/dL, and his lactate is 4.7 mmol/L. His oxygen saturation is 94% on 2 L $O_2$ via nasal cannula. Empiric antibiotics were initiated preoperatively. Over the next 24 hours his oxygen saturations drop slightly, his MAP remains less than 65 and his lactate continues to rise. His stroke volume variation is less than 10%. What is the appropriate next step in the management of this patient?*

**A** *1-2 L bolus of additional crystalloid solution*
**B** *Initiation of IV hydrocortisone*
**C** *Infusion of albumin instead of Lactated Ringer's*
**D** *Placement of pulmonary artery catheter for hemodynamic monitoring*
**E** *Transfusion of 1 unit packed red blood cells*

The patient in this scenario is showing signs of continued hypoperfusion after adequate volume resuscitation and is likely suffering from a component of cardiac insufficiency. The international Surviving Sepsis Guidelines recommend that during the acute resuscitation phase, if resuscitation goals (MAP > 65, Urine output > 0.5 mL/kg/hr, central venous pressure 8–12 cm $H_2O$, mixed venous oxygen saturation < 70%) are not met, packed red blood cell transfusion is warranted. The most recent guidelines suggest transfusion to a goal hemoglobin level of 7–8 g/dL. It is also recommended that transfusion be initiated with 1 unit of blood, rather than 2 units. Steroids are indicated for shock refractory to vasopressor support or for patients with known or suspected adrenal insufficiency. Pulmonary artery catheters have failed to show mortality benefit in multiple studies.

**Answer: E**

Carson, J. L., Guyatt, G., Heddle, N.M., et al. (2016). Clinical practice guidelines from the AABB: red blood cell transfusion thresholds and storage. *Journal of the American Medical Association*, **316** (19), 2025–2035.

Dellinger, R.P., Levy, M.M., Rhodes, A., et al. (2013) Surviving Sepsis campaign: international guidelines for management of severe sepsis and septic shock. *Intensive Care Medicine*, **39** (2), 165–228 and *Critical Care Medicine*, **41** (2), 580–637.

Marik, P.E. (2009) Critical illness-related corticosteroid insufficiency. *Chest*, **135** (1), 181–193.

Shah, M.R., Hasselblad, V., Stevenson, L.W., et al. (2005) Impact of the pulmonary artery catheter in critically ill patients: meta-analysis of randomized clinical trials. *Journal of the American Medical Association*, **294** (13), 1664–1670.

**5** *All of the following practices should be included in a standard ventilator-associated pneumonia (VAP) prevention bundle, EXCEPT:*

**A** *Early mobility*
**B** *Surveillance cultures obtained every 72 hrs*
**C** *Head of bed elevation to 30 degrees*
**D** *Daily sedation interruption*
**E** *Daily spontaneous breathing trials*

Ventilated patients who develop pneumonia suffer from a mortality of up to 46%, and VAP is the second most common health care-associated infection in the United States. VAP prevention bundles have been created in an effort to decrease rates of VAP, and their associated sequelae. Bundles commonly include daily sedation medication holiday with spontaneous breathing trials, daily oral hygiene, head of bed elevation, facilitation of early mobility, use of endotracheal tubes with subglottic suctioning and judicious use of sedation. Surveillance cultures are not recommended as they may prompt treatment of colonization and unnecessary antibiotic exposure which may lead to increased rates of infection with MDR organisms.

**Answer: B**

American Thoracic Society and Infectious Diseases Society of America (2005) Guidelines for the management of adults with hospital-acquired, ventilator-associated, and healthcare-associated pneumonia. *American Journal of Respiratory and Critical Care Medicine*, **171** (4), 388–416.

Ferreira, C.R., de Souza, D.F., Cunha, T.M., et al. (2016) The effectiveness of a bundle in the prevention of ventilator-associated pneumonia. *Brazilian Journal of Infectious Diseases*, **20** (3), 267–271.

Klompas, M., Branson, R., Eichenwald, E.C., et al. (2014) Strategies to prevent ventilator-associated pneumonia in acute care hospitals: 2014 update. *Infection Control and Hospital Epidemiology*, **35** (8), 915–936.

**6** *A 67-year old diabetic man is in the surgical ICU after undergoing exploratory laparotomy for mesenteric ischemia. He is in septic shock, with persistent hypotension, refractory to IV crystalloid and high-dose norepinephrine infusion. Which of the following vasoactive agents is most appropriate to initiate in addition to the patient's norepinephrine infusion?*

**A** *Vasopressin*
**B** *Dobutamine*
**C** *Dopamine*
**D** *Phenylephrine*
**E** *Milrinone*

For the patient in septic shock, the Surviving Sepsis Guidelines recommend norepinephrine as the initial vasopressor of choice, however the guidelines do not make a firm recommendation about which agent should be initiated if the response to norepinephrine is inadequate. Clinicians may consider addition of vasopressin at a dose of 0.03 Units/min to either aid in raising MAP or allowing for a reduction in the dose of norepinephrine, but vasopressin should not be used as the initial vasopressor. Epinephrine may also be added to or substituted for norepinephrine in patients for whom an additional agent is needed. Dopamine should only be considered as an alternative to norepinephrine in a small subset of patients who have bradycardia and are at low risk for a development of a tachyarrhythmia. Phenylephrine should be reserved for patients who develop severe arrhythmias due to norepinephrine, those with low MAPs and a known high cardiac output, or as salvage therapy. Ionotropes such as dobutamine and milrinone may be considered in the setting of myocardial dysfunction and evidence of continued tissue hypoperfusion despite adequate MAPs.

**Answer: A**

Dellinger, R.P., Levy, M.M., Rhodes, A., *et al.* (2013) Surviving Sepsis campaign: international guidelines for management of severe sepsis and septic shock. *Intensive Care Medicine*, **39** (2), 165-228 and *Critical Care Medicine*, **41** (2), 580–637.

Russell, J.A., Walley, K.R., Singer, J., *et al.* (2008) Vasopressin versus norepinephrine infusion in patients with septic shock. *New England Journal of Medicine*, **358** (9), 877–887.

7  *A 31-year-old patient is in the SICU after a motorcycle crash and subsequent craniotomy with ventriculostomy placement for intracranial pressure (ICP) monitoring. The patient has continued bloody drainage from the catheter, elevated ICP, and continued fevers. CSF analysis confirms ventriculitis. The appropriate empiric IV antibiotic regimen may include all of the following except:*

   A *Vancomycin plus cefepime*
   B *Vancomycin plus gentamicin*
   C *Vancomycin plus meropenem*
   D *Vancomycin plus ceftazidime*
   E *Vancomycin plus piperacillin/tazobactam*

Approximately 64% of ventriculostomy-associated CSF infections are caused by gram-positive bacteria, predominantly *S. epidermidis* and *S. aureus*. 35% are caused by gram-negative organisms, which include *Acinetobacter* spp. (9.3%), *Pseudomonas* spp. (6%), and enteric organisms.

About 1% of infections are due to *Candida* spp. Initial empiric coverage should include vancomycin combined with an anti-pseudomonal cephalosporin (cefepime or ceftazidime), or meropenem plus vancomycin. Aminoglycosides are an acceptable alternative to anti-pseudomonal beta-lactams. Piperacillin/tazobactam should be avoided due to its poor CNS penetration. In addition, any infected indwelling devices should be removed, replaced, or externalized.

**Answer: E**

Ramanan, M., Lipman, J., Shorr, A., *et al.* (2015) A meta-analysis of ventriculostomy-associated cerebrospinal fluid infections. *BMC Infectious Diseases*, **15** (1), 1–12.

Ziai, W.C. and Lewin, J.J. (2008). Update in the diagnosis and management of central nervous system infections. *Neurologic Clinics*, **26** (2), 427–468.

8  *A patient is admitted to the burn unit after sustaining > 40% BSA burn of varying degrees. He is treated with early debridement where necessary, in addition to topical therapies. On hospital day three the patient develops a fever to 102 °F, along with decreased urine output and tachypnea. He is also requiring norepinephrine and vasopressin infusion to maintain a MAP > 65 mm Hg. Blood cultures are drawn and initial gram stain reveals gram-negative rods. The most appropriate empiric antibiotic regimen consists of:*

   A *Gentamicin + piperacillin/tazobactam*
   B *Gentamicin + ertapenem*
   C *Ciprofloxacin + clindamycin*
   D *Meropenem + piperacillin/tazobactam*
   E *Imipenem/cilastatin + cefepime*

Patients with severe sepsis, septic shock, or immune suppression with risk factors for *P. aeruginosa* should be treated with combination therapy consisting of a parenteral aminoglycoside (gentamicin, tobramycin, amikacin) plus one of the following: anti-pseudomonal cephalosporin, beta-lactam/beta-lactamase inhibitor (piperacillin/tazobactam), or an anti-pseudomonal carbapenem (imipenem, doripenem, or meropenem). Of note, it should be emphasized that higher anti-pseudomonal dosing or extended infusion be used for piperacillin/tazobactam. Ertapenem has no activity against *P. aeruginosa*. Ciprofloxacin may be considered once sensitivities have confirmed susceptibility, but is not appropriate for empiric therapy. Clindamycin lacks activity against gram-negative organisms.

**Answer: A**

Dellinger, R.P., Levy, M.M., Rhodes, A., *et al.* (2013) Surviving Sepsis campaign: international guidelines for management of severe sepsis and septic shock. *Intensive Care Medicine*, **39** (2), 165–228 and *Critical Care Medicine*, **41** (2), 580–637.

Micek, S.T., Welch, E.C., Khan, J., *et al.* (2010) Empiric combination antibiotic therapy is associated with improved outcome against sepsis due to Gram-negative bacteria: a retrospective analysis. *Antimicrobial Agents and Chemotherapy*, **54** (5), 1742–1748.

9    *A patient is recovering in the SICU after undergoing thoracotomy, washout and intercostal muscle flap for repair of a distal esophageal tear from repetitive vomiting due to severe diabetic gastroparesis. The patient is receiving total parenteral nutrition. Which of the following medications is most likely to decrease this patient's risk of post-operative mortality?*

     **A** *Cefazolin*
     **B** *Esomeprazole*
     **C** *Regular insulin*
     **D** *Fluconazole*
     **E** *Vancomycin*

Invasive candidiasis has a known mortality of > 50%. Risk factors include neutropenia, central venous catheters, known colonization, hemodialysis, parenteral nutrition, broad-spectrum antibiotic exposure, trauma, and recent surgery (gastrointestinal perforation, anastomotic leakage, transplant patients). Meta-analyses have shown that prophylaxis with fluconazole in non-neutropenic critically ill patients with risk factors for candidiasis reduces invasive fungal infections and improves mortality.

**Answer: D**

Cortegiani, A., Russotto, V., Maggiore, A., *et al.* (2016) Antifungal agents for preventing fungal infections in non-neutropenic critically ill patients. *Cochrane Database Systematic Review* **16** (1).

Koehler, P. (2016) Contemporary strategies in the prevention and management of fungal infections. *Infectious Disease Clinics of North America*, **30** (1), 265–275.

Playford, E.G., Webster, A.C., Sorrell, T.C., *et al.* (2006) Antifungal agents for preventing fungal infections in non-neutropenic critically ill and surgical patients: systematic review and meta-analysis of randomized clinical trials. *Journal of Antimicrobial Chemotherapy*, **57** (4), 628–638.

10    *A 55-year-old patient is admitted to the hospital for RLQ abdominal pain, presumed to be a recurrent bout of diverticulitis. Empiric antibiotics for intra-abdominal infection are initiated. Laboratory analysis reveals profound leukopenia. The patient reveals to you that he has a history of HIV, and is non-compliant with his antiretroviral (ART) regimen. His CD4 count is 40 cells/mm$^3$. What is the most likely opportunistic infectious agent causing this patient's symptoms?*

     **A** *Toxoplasma gondii*
     **B** *Cytomegalovirus*
     **C** *Coccidioides immitis*
     **D** *Candida glabrata*
     **E** *Mycobacterium avium intracellulare*

Cytomegalovirus (CMV) is uncommon in the ART era, but may occur in up to 5% of patients with advanced immunosuppression and a CD4 count of < 50 cells/mm$^3$ who are either not receiving or not responding to ART. CMV causes an ischemic colitis, usually near the terminal ileum and proximal colon. There is a risk of bowel perforation along with peritonitis. Approximately 10–15% of HIV/AIDS patients with abdominal pain will have etiologies related to their underlying immunosuppression.

**Answer: B**

Kaplan, J.E., Benson, C.A., Holmes, K.K., *et al.* (2009) Guidelines for prevention and treatment of opportunistic infections in HIV-infected adults and adolescents. *Morbidity and Mortality Weekly Report*, **58** (4), 1–207.

Yoganathan, K.T., Morgan, A.R., and Yoganathan, K.G. (2016) Perforation of the bowel due to cytomegalovirus infection in a man with AIDS: surgery is not always necessary!. *BMJ Case Reports*, bcr2015214196.

11    *Which of the following is TRUE regarding prevention of catheter-associated urinary tract infection (CAUTI) in hospitalized patients?*

     **A** *The catheter drainage bag should always be kept below the level of the bladder.*
     **B** *Daily irrigation of bladder catheter to prevent blockage*
     **C** *Removal of catheter 48 hours postoperatively*
     **D** *Routine catheter changes*
     **E** *Routine bacteriologic monitoring for early UTI detection and treatment*

Duration of catheterization is the most important risk factor for developing CAUTI, and catheters should ideally be removed within 24 hours postoperatively, if not contraindicated. Urinary catheters are responsible for 80% of hospital-acquired UTIs. Guidelines are in place at most institutions, and usually include the following: The use of urinary catheters should be minimized where possible, the need for the catheter should be reviewed daily, insertion should be performed with aseptic technique and sterile equipment, and drainage systems should be closed and sterile, kept below the level of the bladder. Routine irrigation, catheter changes, bacteriologic monitoring, and systemic antimicrobial prophylaxis should be avoided.

**Answer: A**

Chenoweth, C. and Sanjay, S. (2013) Preventing catheter-associated urinary tract infections in the intensive care unit. *Critical Care Clinics*, **29** (1), 19–32.

Hooton, T.M., Bradley, S.F., Cardenas, D.D., *et al.* (2009) Diagnosis, prevention, and treatment of catheter-associated urinary tract infections in adults: 2009 international clinical practice guidelines from the Infectious Disease Society of America. *Clinical Infectious Diseases*, **50** (5), 625–663.

**12** *Which of the following practices is NOT in accordance with catheter-related infection prevention practices?*

  **A** *Avoid routine or scheduled replacement of central venous access devices*

  **B** *Prepare skin with > 0.5% chlorhexidine with alcohol before CVC insertion and during dressing changes*

  **C** *Designate trained personnel who demonstrate competence for the insertion and maintenance of peripheral and central intravascular catheters*

  **D** *Avoid using the jugular or femoral insertion sites in adult patients to minimize infection risk for non-tunneled CVCs.*

  **E** *Apply topical antibiotic preparations to all central venous catheter insertion sites during dressing changes in order to minimize incidence of blood-stream infections*

Intravascular catheter-related infections in the ICU increase hospital length of stay, and are responsible for roughly 80 000 bloodstream infections in the United States each year. With the exception of choice D, the above practices are category 1A recommendations for the prevention of catheter-related bloodstream infections. Femoral vein line insertions should be avoided if possible, as they have been shown to have high colonization rates and higher rates of central line-associated bloodstream infections. Topical antibiotics are recommended only for hemodialysis catheters at the time of insertion and with each hemodialysis session. Routine use of topical antibiotics on other type of CV access devices may promote fungal infection and anti-microbial resistance.

**Answer: E**

O'Grady, N.P., Alexander, M., Burns, L.A., *et al.* (2011) Guidelines for the prevention of intravascular catheter-related infections. *Clinical Infectious Diseases*, **52** (9), 162–193.

**13** *A 68-year-old woman with multiple bilateral rib fractures after a ground-level fall has been in the SICU for five days. Her respiratory function has steadily declined. On hospital day six, she develops fevers and the morning CXR shows a developing RLL infiltrate, concerning for pneumonia. All of the following factors are associated with an increased risk of developing pneumonia in trauma patients EXCEPT for?*

  **A** *Failed pre-hospital intubation*

  **B** *Long bone fracture*

  **C** *Pulmonary contusion*

  **D** *Rib fractures*

  **E** *Traumatic brain injury*

Trauma patients are at a higher risk for developing pneumonia in comparison to medical ICU patients. There are several traumatic injuries that have been associated with an increased risk of developing pneumonia: pulmonary contusions, rib fractures, sternal fractures, spinal cord injury, and traumatic brain injury. Furthermore, failed pre-hospital intubation is associated with development of VAP in trauma patients. Patients who sustain chest trauma are three times more likely to develop pneumonia than patients without chest injuries.

**Answer: B**

Hui, X., Haider, A., Hashmi, Z., *et al.* (2013) Increased risk of pneumonia among ventilated patients with traumatic brain injury: every day counts! *Journal of Surgical Research*, **184** (1), 438–443.

Mangram, A.J., Sohn, J., Zhou, N., *et al.* (2015) Trauma-associated pneumonia: time to redefine ventilator-associated pneumonia in trauma patients. *The American Journal of Surgery*, **210** (6), 1056–1062.

**14** *A 44-year old man arrives to the trauma bay by EMS after sustaining an injury to his forearm with a circulating saw. He has exposed muscle, with minimal bleeding. His wound is copiously irrigated and sutured closed. He is admitted for observation and on hospital day one he complains of worsening pain and swelling at the site. You notice spreading erythema and extreme tenderness on physical exam. The most likely causative organism in this patient's infection is:*

A Staphylococcus aureus
B Vibrio vulnificus
C Clostridium perfringens
D *Polymicrobial*
E Streptococcus pyogenes

This patient is suffering from a necrotizing soft tissue infection (NSTI), which carries a mortality of > 20%. This rapidly progressing infection typically involves the underlying fat, muscle, and fascia. Bacteria track subcutaneously, producing endo- and exotoxins that cause tissue ischemia (via thrombosis of perforating vessels to the skin), liquefactive necrosis, and systemic illness. Non-specific, early signs are erythema, pain, and swelling. Late findings include bullae, crepitus, and skin ischemia. NSTIs are classified as Type I (polymicrobial), Type II (Group A Streptoccus with or without *Staphylococcus aureus*) and Type III (*Vibrio vulnificus*). Polymicrobial infections account for approximately 55–75% of NSTIs, followed by monomicrobial infections (15%) with *Streptococcus pyogenes* and/or *Staphylococcus aureus*. Clostridial infections are now rare, accounting for less than 5% of occurrences. The gold standard modality for diagnosis of NSTI is operative exploration.

**Answer: D**

Sarani, B., Strong, M., Pascual, J., *et al.* (2009) Necrotizing fasciitis: current concepts and review of the literature. *Journal of the American College of Surgeons*, **208** (2), 279–288.

Sartelli, M., Malangoni, M.A., May, A.K., *et al.* (2014) World Society of Emergency Surgery guidelines for management of skin and soft tissue infections. *World Journal of Emergency Surgery*, **9** (1), 57.

15 *The patient in the previous question is taken to the operating room for wide debridement of his arm. At exploration, the surgeon notes there to be "dishwater" fluid and liquefactive necrosis of the fat, fascia, and underlying muscle, confirming the diagnosis of necrotizing soft tissue infection (NSTI).*

*In addition to repeat exploration and debridement, what is the most appropriate empiric antibiotic regimen for this patient?*
A *Piperacillin/tazobactam + clindamycin + metronidazole*
B *Vancomycin + meropenem*
C *Ciprofloxacin + vancomycin + ertapenem*
D *Clindamycin + vancomycin + imipenem/cilastatin*
E *Meropenem + ampicillin/sulbactam*

Recommended empiric antibiotic coverage for NSTI should include coverage of gram-positive, gram-negative, and anaerobic organisms. Acceptable regimens include a carbapenem (imipenem, meropenem, ertapenem) or broad-spectrum penicillin with beta-lactamase inhibitor (piperacillin/tazobactam) with coverage against MRSA (vancomycin, daptomycin, linezolid) plus clindamycin (for its antitoxin effects against certain strains of *Staphylococcus* and *Streptococcus*, particularly in the setting of shock).

**Answer: D**

Sarani, B., Strong, M., Pascual, J., *et al.* (2009) Necrotizing fasciitis: current concepts and review of the literature. *Journal of the American College of Surgeons*, **208** (2), 279–288.

Stevens, D.L., Bisno, A.L., Chambers, H.F., *et al.* (2014) Practice guidelines for the diagnosis and management of skin and soft tissue infections: 2014 update by the Infectious Diseases Society of America. *Clinical Infectious Diseases*, **59** (2), 10–52.

16 *A 68-year-old woman is postoperative day 3 following left hemicolectomy with colostomy and Hartmann's pouch due to perforated diverticulitis with feculent peritonitis. Her postoperative course is complicated by fever and worsening abdominal pain. Intra-abdominal cultures taken at the time of the operation grew ESBL (extended-spectrum β-lactamase) Escherichia coli. The appropriate antibiotic regimen for this organism is:*
A *Vancomycin*
B *Cefepime*
C *Piperacillin-tazobactam*
D *Ceftaroline*
E *Meropenem*

Increasing antimicrobial resistance is a major concern. ESBLs are gram-negative bacteria, such as *Escherichia coli* and *Klebsiella pneumoniae*, that break open the β-lactam ring of penicillins, cephalosporins, and aztreonam. Enterobacteriaceae and *Pseudomonas aeruginosa* are other frequently encountered resistant pathogens. Examples of beta-lactam antibiotics vulnerable to ESBsL are: piperacillin-tazobactam, cefepime, and ceftaroline. Vancomycin only treats gram-positive organisms. Carbapenems are much more resistant to beta-lactamases than the other β-lactams, although there has been an emergence of carbapenem-resistant species, such as *Acinetobacter baumannii*. Current treatment for ESBL gram-negative infections is carbapenems.

**Answer: E**

Mehrad, B., Clark, N.M., Zhanel, G.G., *et al.* (2015) Antimicrobial resistance in hospital-acquired gram-negative bacterial infections. *Chest*, **147** (5), 1413–1421.

Paterson, D.L. and Bonomo, R.A. (2005) Extended-spectrum β-lactamases: a clinical update. *Clinical Microbiology Reviews*, **18** (4), 657–686.

Wong-Beringer, A. (2001) Therapeutic challenges associated with extended spectrum, β-Lactamase-producing *Escherichia coli* and *Klebsiella pneumoniae*. *Pharmacotherapy*, **21** (5), 583–592.

**17** *A 71-year-old man is in the ICU for five days after colon resection for ischemic colitis. He is ventilated and persistently febrile, with a white count of $17.1 \times 10^3$/microL. He is also receiving TPN via PICC line. The patient was previously in septic shock and steroids are currently being weaned. Urine cultures have grown* Candida glabrata, *resistant to fluconazole and caspofungin. The most appropriate antifungal is:*

**A** *Griseofulvin*
**B** *Traconazole*
**C** *Micafungin*
**D** *Voriconazole*
**E** *Amphotericin B deoxycholate*

*Candida glabrata* has high rates of resistance to the azoles (fluconazole, itraconazole, voriconazole). Risk factors for systemic infection include prior antibiotic exposure, Candida from other sites, central venous catheter, TPN, and immunocompromised state. The appropriate treatment is conventional amphotericin B deoxycholate.

**Answer: E**

Pappas, P.G., Kauffman, C.A., Andes, D.R., *et al.* (2016) Clinical practice guideline for the management of candidiasis: 2016 update by the Infectious Diseases Society of America. *Clinical Infectious Diseases*, **62** (4), 1–50.

**18** *Empiric therapy for VAP for a patient who has been intubated in the hospital for 72 hours should cover all of the following EXCEPT:*

**A** Streptococcus pneumoniae
**B** Haemophilus influenzae
**C** *Vancomycin-resistant* Enterococcus *(VRE)*
**D** *Methicillin-susceptible* Staphylococcus aureus *(MSSA)*
**E** Pseudomonas aeruginosa

In patients without risk factors for MDR organisms, the most common pathogens responsible for VAP are *Streptococcus*, *Haemophilus*, MSSA, and Moraxella species. Appropriate initial antibiotics are quinolones, ceftriaxone, or ampicillin/sulbactam.

Risk factors for developing MDR pneumonia include: prior antibiotic exposure (within 90 days), septic shock at the time of VAP, five or more days of hospitalization prior to the development of VAP and acute renal replacement therapy prior to VAP. When the possibility of MDR exists, treatment should be expanded to include *Pseudomonas aeruginosa*, Enterobacter, Serratia, Klebsiella, and MRSA. Appropriate antibiotic choices are vancomycin or linezolid for MRSA, and piperacillin-tazobactam (beta-lactam/beta lactamase inhibitor), fluoroquinolones, or aminoglycosides for Pseudomonas coverage. VRE is not a common causative pathogen of VAP. It is mainly born out of selection from antibiotic administration.

**Answer: C**

Guillamet, C.V. and Kollef, M.H. (2015) Update on ventilator-associated pneumonia. *Current Opinion in Critical Care*, **21** (5), 430–438.

Kalil, A.C., Metersky, M.L., Klompas, M., *et al.* (2016) Management of adults with hospital-acquired and ventilator-associated pneumonia: 2016 clinical practice guidelines by the Infectious Diseases Society of America and the American Thoracic Society. *Clinical Infectious Disease*, **63** (5), 61–111.

Kollef, M.H. (1993) Ventilator-associated pneumonia: a multivariate analysis. *Journal of the American Medical Association*, **270** (16), 1965–1970.

# 10

## Pharmacology and Antibiotics
*Michelle Strong, MD and CPT Clay M. Merritt, DO*

**1** *A 48-year-old female presents to the emergency room for severe abdominal pain and fever. A CT scan shows significant pneumoperitoneum most consistent with a perforated duodenal ulcer, small volume ascites, and a cirrhotic appearing liver. You are consulted as the Acute Care Surgeon on call. The patient is a poor historian, and you gain very little information about her medical problems. On physical exam, you notice she has a loop graft arteriovenous fistula in her left arm, a large distended abdomen, and severe epigastric pain. What is the main mechanism of metabolism and elimination for the neuromuscular blocking agent best suited for this patient during surgery?*

**A** *Hydrolysis of the drug by plasma cholinesterase and elimination in the urine*

**B** *Metabolized and eliminated via spontaneous, enzyme independent, chemical degradation*

**C** *No metabolism subsequently the drug is elimin Cated unchanged in urine*

**D** *Metabolized by liver to less active metabolite and mostly eliminated through the liver*

**E** *Metabolism by spontaneous degradation but elimination is primarily in the urine*

The patient described above has significant hepatic and renal dysfunction. Most of the commonly used neuromuscular blocking agents (paralytics) require either hepatic and/or renal function to effectively eliminate the paralytic drug from the body; except cisatracurium (Table 10.1). Cisatracurium, an isomer of atracurium, undergoes spontaneous chemical degradation (not an enzymatic process) in a process known as Hofmann elimination. Cisatracurium is unique from atracurium in that both metabolism and elimination occur by Hofmann elimination. In this process, cisatracurium degrades to two metabolites that do not possess paralytic potential. Cisatracurium is often the paralytic of choice in patients with severe hepatic and renal dysfunction. Hofmann elimination is a temperature- and

pH-dependent process, and therefore the rate of degradation is highly influenced by body pH and temperature: An increase in body pH favors the elimination process, whereas a decrease in temperature slows down the process. Atracurium undergoes Hoffman elimination as well, however, unlike cisatracurium, it has an active metabolite which is then mostly excreted in the urine.

**Answer: B**

Hull, C.J. (1995) Pharmacokinetics and pharmacodynamics of the *benzylisoquinolinium* muscle relaxants. *Acta Anaesthesiologica Scandinavica*, **39** (s106), 13–17.

Sparr, H.J., Beaufort, T.M., and Fuchs-Buder, T. (2001) Newer neuromuscular blocking agents: how they compare with established agents? *Drugs*, **61**, 919–942.

**2** *A 70-year-old man has been admitted to the ICU after colectomy because of his history of the end-stage renal disease, respiratory failure, and pain management. The procedure was uncomplicated, and the patient is extubated 2 hours after admission to the ICU. On examination, the patient's RR is 18 breaths/min, and he rates his pain on a 0–10 scale as 7. He is currently doing well, receiving oxygen at 4L/min by nasal cannula.*

*Which one of the following analgesics for postoperative pain management is most appropriate for this patient?*

**A** *Fentanyl*

**B** *Morphine*

**C** *Oxycodone*

**D** *Hydromorphone*

**E** *Meperidine*

Morphine should be used cautiously. Morphine metabolites can accumulate increasing therapeutic and adverse effects in patients with renal failure. Both parent and metabolite can be removed by dialysis. Hydromorphone

**Table 10.1** Method of elimination of neuromuscular blocking agents.

| Neuromuscular blocking agent | Metabolism | Primary route of elimination |
|---|---|---|
| Succinylcholine (Answer A) | Plasma cholinesterase | Urine |
| Cisatracurium (Answer B) | Hofmann Elimination | Hofmann Elimination (77–80%) |
| Pancuronium (Answer C) | Not metabolized | Urine |
| Vecuronium | Liver | Liver |
| Rocuronium (Answer D) | Liver | Liver |
| Atracurium (Answer E) | Hofmann Elimination | Urine |

should be used cautiously and the dose adjusted as appropriate in patients with renal failure. The 3-glucuronide metabolite of hydromorphone can accumulate and cause neuro-excitatory effects in these patients. The parent drug can be removed by dialysis, but metabolite accumulation remains a risk. Oxycodone should not be used in patients with renal failure. Metabolites and oxycodone itself can accumulate causing toxic and CNS-depressant effects. There is no data on oxycodone and its metabolites' removal with dialysis. Meperidine should not be used. Metabolites can accumulate causing increased risk of adverse effects. There are few data on meperidine and its metabolites in dialysis. Fentanyl appears safe, but dose adjustment is necessary. There are no active metabolites to add a risk of adverse effects. Use some caution because fentanyl is poorly dialyzable.

**Answer: A**

Davison, S.N. (2003) Pain in hemodialysis patients: prevalence, cause, severity, and management. *American Journal of Kidney Disorders*, **42**, 1239–1247.

Foral, P.A., Ineck, J.R., and Nystrom, K.K. (2007) Oxycodone accumulation in a hemodialysis patient. *Southern Medical Journal*, **100**, 212–214.

Kurella, M. (2003) Analgesia in patients with ESRD: a review of available evidence. *American Journal of Kidney Disorder*, **42**, 217–228.

3   *You have just started your surgical practice at a new level 3 trauma center. Much of your practice will focus on gastrointestinal surgery. You would like to use the drug alvimopan (Entereg) in your practice. The clinical pharmacist reminds you about the prescribing limitations for alvimopan. Which of the following options best describes the prescription limitations of alvimopan?*

   A  Max of 15 days of therapy, must start after surgery, surgery must include bowel resection and anastomosis
   B  Max of 15 doses of therapy, must start after surgery, surgery must include bowel resection and colostomy creation
   C  Max of 15 days of therapy, must start before surgery, surgery must include bowel resection
   D  Max of 15 doses of therapy, must start before surgery, surgery must include bowel resection and anastomosis
   E  No max number of days or doses must start after surgery, surgery must include bowel resection and colostomy creation

Alvimopan (Brand name: Entereg) is a μ-opiate receptor antagonist that specifically targets peripheral μ receptors in the GI tract. Alvimopan has a boxed warning for an association with increased incidence of myocardial infarction when the drug is used for more than one week (>15 doses). The Food and Drug Administration (FDA), through the Food and Drug Administration Amendments Act of 2007 approved a Risk Evaluation and Mitigation Strategy (REMS) for alvimopan's association with increased myocardial infarction incidence. The REMS for Alvimopan requires hospitals to enroll in the Entereg Access Support and Education (EASE) program. The EASE program helps ensure proper usage of Alvimopan. Alvimopan prescription limitations include those shown in Table 10.2.

Alvimopan has been shown to decrease time to return to bowel function and length of hospital stay after open abdominal surgery. One contraindication for use is a patient taking opiates at therapeutic doses for greater than seven days before starting alvimopan.

**Answer: D**

**Table 10.2** Alvimopan prescription limitations.

| Indication for use | Inpatient undergoing partial bowel resection with primary anastomosis |
|---|---|
| First dose | 12 mg PO given 30 minutes to 5 hours before surgery |
| Subsequent dosing | 12 mg PO given twice daily (BID) starting the day after surgery |
| Max dosing | 15 doses |
| Patient status | Patient must be an inpatient while taking alvimopan |

Vaughan-Shaw, P.G., Fecher, I.C., Harris, S., *et. al.* (2012) A meta-analysis of the effectiveness of the opioid receptor antagonist alvimopan in reducing hospital length of stay and time of GI recovery in patients enrolled in a standardized accelerated recovery program after abdominal surgery. *Diseases of the Colon and Rectum*, **55**, 611–620.

Xu, L.L., Zhou, X.Q., Yi, P.S., et. al. (2016) Alvimopan combined with enhanced recovery strategy for managing postoperative ileus after open abdominal surgery: a systematic review and meta-analysis. *Journal of Surgical Research*, **203**, 211–221.

4 *A 64-year-old woman was on continuous electrocardiographic monitoring because of a history of coronary artery disease following an open cholecystectomy. On postoperative day 1, she developed nausea and vomiting. She was treated with multiple doses of an antiemetic. She had a rhythm strip showing QT-prolongation and then torsade de pointes. She was successfully resuscitated.*

   *Which one of the following antiemetics was most likely used to treat her nausea and vomiting?*

  **A** *Famotidine*
  **B** *Prochlorperazine*
  **C** *Metoclopramide*
  **D** *Ondansetron*
  **E** *Dexamethasone*

Some drugs can lead to QT prolongation and torsade de pointes. Phenothiazines, such as prochlorperazine, used for nausea and vomiting have the potential of prolonging the QT interval. Droperidol may also cause QT prolongation. Fortunately, it rarely produces this phenomenon at recommended doses. Ondansetron (serotonin antagonist) and metoclopramide (antidopaminergic and antiserotonergic) are *not* known to cause QT prolongation. H2 blockers and steroids are also *not* known to cause QT prolongation.

Postoperative nausea and vomiting are often multifactorial in origin. Drugs, physical stimuli, or emotional stress can cause the release of neurotransmitters that stimulate serotoninergic (5-HT3), dopaminergic (d2), histaminergic (H1), and muscarinic (M1) receptors. The vomiting center, rather than a discrete area, is a neural network comprised of the chemoreceptor trigger zone, area postrema, and nucleus tractus solitarius.

Phenothiazines and butyrophenones act on D2, H1, and M1 receptors. Benzamides, such as metoclopramide and domperidone, affect 5-HT3 and 5-HT4 receptors; scopolamine is an M1-receptor antagonist, and diphenhydramine and cyclizine are H1-antagonists. Specific 5-HT3-receptor antagonists, such as ondansetron and granisetron, represent the most recently developed class of antiemetics.

**Answer: B**

Sung, Y.F. (1996) Risks and benefits of drugs used in the management of postoperative nausea and vomiting. *Drug Safety*, **14**, 181–197.

Yap, G.Y. and Camm, A.J. (2003) Drug induced QT prolongation and torsades de pointes. *Heart*, **89**, 1363–1372.

5 *A 53-year-old woman who weighs 100 kg and is 5 ft tall fell down several stairs and sustained an anterior right hip dislocation. Her past medical history was positive for chronic alcoholism. She underwent operative reduction. Preoperatively, her blood urea nitrogen is 32 mg/dL; serum creatinine is 3.3 mg/dL; serum glucose was 155 mg/dL, aspartate aminotransaminase 315 U/L, and international normalized ratio (INR) was 1.4. The following day, she developed sudden onset of shortness of breath. Pulmonary embolism diagnosis was made. Enoxaparin 100 mg q 12 h subcutaneously was begun.*

   *Which one of the following statements about the current enoxaparin dose is most correct?*

  **A** *She is excessively anticoagulated because dosing should be based on ideal body, not actual body weight*
  **B** *She is inadequately anticoagulated, because of morbid obesity and increased volume of distribution*
  **C** *She is inadequately anticoagulated, because of hepatic dysfunction*
  **D** *She is excessively anticoagulated, because of renal dysfunction*
  **E** *She is inadequately anticoagulated, because of increased cytochrome P450 activity*

Low-molecular-weight heparins (LMWHs) do not undergo hepatic metabolism and primarily undergo renal elimination. Thus, answer C is not correct. Generally, dosing of LMWH is based on *actual body weight*. However, if a patient weighs more than 140 kg (this patient is only 100 kg), using standard dosing may cause excessive anticoagulation. This patient is likely to be over anticoagulated from LMWH accumulation due to her renal dysfunction, not from excessive LMWH dose.

The primary advantages of LMWH, compared with unfractionated heparin (UFH), are better bioavailability and consistency of action. Dose-independent renal clearance of LMWHs results in predictable antithrombotic activity; thus, anticoagulation monitoring is typically not needed.

**Answer: D**

Hirsch, J., Warkentin, T.E., Shaughnessy, S.G., *et al.* (2001) Heparin and low-molecular-weight heparin: mechanisms of action, pharmacokinetics, dosing, monitoring, efficacy, and safety. *Chest*, **119**, 64S–94S.

6  *A 52-year-old woman with diabetes was treated 10 days ago for a urinary tract infection by the medical service. She was readmitted 3 days ago with diarrhea, abdominal pain, and fever. She had stool samples sent for* Clostridium difficile *toxin and then was started empirically on Flagyl 500 mg orally every 8 hours. She was transferred to the ICU for confusion, hypotension, abdominal distention, and continued severe diarrhea.*

*All of the following would be appropriate treatment considerations except:*

A  *Vancomycin PO*
B  *Surgical consultation*
C  *Intravenous immunoglobulin*
D  *Tigecycline IV*
E  *Vancomycin IV*

*Clostridium difficile* infection (CDI) has become more refractory to standard therapy. Recent data showed severe refractory CDI successfully treated with tigecycline. Oral vancomycin is now advocated as the therapy of choice for severe CDI. Vancomycin administered intravenously does not reach therapeutic levels in the colonic lumen. Metronidazole, administered either orally or intravenously, only reaches low therapeutic levels in the colon. Therefore, even a slightly elevated minimal inhibitory concentration (MIC) of *C. difficile* for metronidazole may lead to therapy failure. Recently, *C. difficile* was reported to have low MIC values for tigecycline.

Because *C. difficile* colitis is a toxin-mediated disease, it has been assumed that immune globulin acts by binding and neutralizing toxin. Off-label use of pooled IVIG from healthy donors has been used in cases of severe refractory *C. difficile* infection and in patients with recurrent disease.

Surgical management should be considered in patients with severe CDI who fail to respond to medical therapy or have signs of systemic toxicity, organ failure, or peritonitis.

**Answer: E**

Herpers, B.J., Vlaminckx, B., Burkhardt, O., *et al.* (2009) Intravenous tigecycline as adjunctive or alternative therapy for severe refractory Clostridium difficile infection. *Clinical Infectious Diseases*, **48**, 1732–1735.

McPherson, S., Rees, C.J., Ellis, R., *et al.* (2006) Intravenous immunoglobulin for the treatment of severe, refractory and recurrent Clostridium difficile diarrhea. *Diseases of the Colon and Rectum*, **49**, 640–645.

Synnott, K., Mealy, K., Merry, C., *et al.* (1998) Timing of surgery for fulminating pseudomembranous colitis. *British Journal of Surgery*, **85**, 229–231.

The next paragraph relates to questions 7 and 8.

7  *A 62-year-old female is being treated with continuous unfractionated heparin infusion for the last five days. She has a mechanical mitral valve and is three days postoperative from a difficult laparoscopic converted to open cholecystectomy and has already required one unexpected takeback to the OR. Her platelet count has dropped by 60% over the last two days. What is the best immediate option for her anticoagulation management?*

A  *Stop heparin infusion and wait for platelets to return to normal before restarting heparin*
B  *Stop heparin infusion and start low molecular weight heparin injections*
C  *Continue heparin infusion and start coumadin until INR is in therapeutic range*
D  *Continue heparin infusion and start rivaroxaban*
E  *Stop heparin infusion and start argatroban infusion*

Heparin-induced thrombocytopenia (HIT) occurs when antibodies bind to platelet factor 4 (PF4). The PF4-heparin-antibody complex binds to and causes platelet activation which promotes thrombosis. Hence when considering this reaction, it is of no surprise that HIT does not always present as thrombocytopenia in the face of current heparin use. It can also present as life and limb threatening thrombosis. The diagnosis of HIT is often made clinically. A platelet drop of > 50% of the patient's baseline platelet value in the face of current or past heparin administration should raise suspicion for HIT. HIT has been found to occur in patients that have stopped heparin use nearly 3 weeks prior. There are laboratory tests available to diagnosis HIT. ELISA can be used to test for antibodies against PF4. Functional assay testing crosses patient serum with healthy donor platelets and looks for subsequent platelet activation and aggregation. ELISA testing is more sensitive than functional assay testing with regards to identifying PF4 antibodies.

When HIT is suspected the first line treatment is to stop heparin administration. Patients with HIT are not just at risk for thrombocytopenia (and possible related bleeding), but they are also at risk for significant thrombosis and thus require anticoagulation even after the offending agent is stopped. By this rationale, answer choices A, C, and D are wrong. This patient has a mechanical mitral valve and therefore requires lifelong anticoagulation. Though rivaroxaban (Factor-Xa inhibitor) provides anti-coagulation, it is not an ideal agent for this patient, who has already returned to the OR once, because of its longer half-life (5–9 hours) and has no specific reversal agent available. For this reason answer choice D is again not the best answer. Answer choice B is wrong because low molecular weight heparin can also cause and perpetuate HIT. Argatroban (direct thrombin inhibitor) has a half-life of approximately 40 min in patients with normal liver function and of the available answer choices is the best choice for anticoagulation in this patient.

**Answer: E**

**8** *The above patient has a rise in her platelet count to normal levels and has stabilized from a surgical standpoint. You would like to transition her from argatroban to coumadin. Which of the following is the best anticoagulation management for this patient?*

  **A** *Start coumadin, continue argatroban until INR is 4 and then proceed with coumadin alone*
  **B** *Start coumadin, continue argatroban until INR is 2 and then proceed with coumadin alone*
  **C** *Stop argatroban and begin Coumadin once argatroban has been metabolized and cleared from patient*
  **D** *Stop argatroban and begin coumadin only if platelets do not return to a normal level*
  **E** *Start Coumadin, do not stop argatroban until the patient is discharged from the hospital and her INR is between 2 and 3*

Patients with HIT remain in a thrombotic state even after platelet counts return to normal. Stopping continuous anticoagulation therapy abruptly (without transitioning to warfarin with a therapeutic INR) has been associated with limb gangrene secondary to thrombosis (why answers C and D are incorrect). Argatroban can also elevate INR. Therefore, anticoagulating the patient to a mildly supratherapeutic range (INR of 4) and then rechecking INR 4–6 hours after stopping the argatroban infusion is recommended (why answers B and E are incorrect). Because of the thrombotic state associated with HIT, patients require anticoagulation for 3 months, though this patient will require lifelong anticoagulation because of her mechanical mitral valve. The decision to transition from continuous infusion based anticoagulation to oral coumadin anticoagulation is patient specific but usually occurs when the platelet count is clearly on the rise or close to normal. In surgical patients specifically, the decision to transition also includes the stability of the patient and the likelihood that the patient would require re-operation or intervention. An anticoagulant with a short half-life would be preferred in the patient likely requiring operative intervention.

**Answer: A**

Alving, B.M. (2003) How I treat heparin-induced thrombocytopenia and thrombosis. *Blood*, **101**, 31–37.

**9** *Which one of the following statements is not true as it relates to the use of benzodiazepines in the ICU for sedation?*

  **A** *Benzodiazepines have anxiolytic, sedative-hypnotic, muscle relaxant, and anticonvulsant properties*
  **B** *Benzodiazepines are effectively removed with hemodialysis, which is recommended for management of overdose*
  **C** *The mechanism of action of benzodiazepines is to modulate the subunits of the gamma amino butyric acid (GABA$_A$) receptor*
  **D** *Midazolam has rapid onset of action and a short half-life of 1.5–3.5 hours*
  **E** *When used for prolonged periods, the solvent used for lorazepam infusion has been reported to cause acute tubular necrosis and lactic acidosis*

The benzodiazepines are the most common sedative medications used in the ICU. They have anxiolytic, sedative-hypnotic, muscle relaxant, and anticonvulsant properties. Their mechanism of action is to modulate the benzodiazepine receptor (subunits of GABA$_A$ receptor). The binding of benzodiazepines to the GABA$_A$ receptor increases the affinity of GABA and its receptor, thereby increasing the opening frequency of GABA$_A$ receptor. As a consequence of this, benzodiazepines potentiate GABAergic neurotransmission. Most benzodiazepines are metabolized by the liver, and the metabolites are excreted by the kidneys. Thus, benzodiazepines are *not* effectively removed by hemodialysis. Midazolam is a short-acting benzodiazepine that has a half-life between 1.5 and 3.5 hours. Midazolam has properties that make it useful for continuous infusion because it has a rapid onset of effects, it is potent, and patients are usually awakened rapidly after discontinuation of the infusion. Midazolam elimination may be decreased in critically ill patients with low albumin, decreased renal function, or obesity. Lorazepam is recommended in the ICU for patients requiring sedation for longer than 24 hours. However, the solvent used for lorazepam infusion contains propylene glycol and with prolonged use or high dosage has been reported to cause acute tubular necrosis, lactic acidosis, and a hyperosmolar state.

Flumazenil is used as an antidote in the treatment of benzodiazepine overdoses. It reverses the effects of benzodiazepines by competitive inhibition at the benzodiazepine binding site on the GABA$_A$ receptor.

**Answer: B**

Murray, M.J., Oyen, L.J., and Browne, W.T. (2008) Use of sedative, analgesics, and neuromuscular blockers, in *Critical Care Medicine: Principles of Diagnosis and Management in the Adult*, 3rd edn (eds J.E. Parrillo and R.P. Dellinger), Mosby, Philadelphia, PA, pp. 327–342.

**10** *Which one of the following is the correct mechanism of action of dexmedetomidine?*
  **A** *It has been proposed to act as a sodium channel blocker*
  **B** *It inhibits dopamine-mediated neurotransmission in the cerebrum and basal ganglia*
  **C** *It acts to modulate subunits of the $GABA_A$ receptor in the limbic system of the brain*
  **D** *It acts by binding to $\alpha_2$-adrenoreceptors located in the locus coeruleus, subsequently releasing norepinephrine and decreasing sympathetic activity*
  **E** *Its effects are mediated by the activation of the $\mu_1$ receptor*

Dexmedetomidine is a new sedative agent that acts by binding to $\alpha_2$-adrenoreceptors located in the locus coeruleus with an affinity of 1620:1 compared with the affinity of the $\alpha_1$-receptor. At this site, it releases norepinephrine and decreases sympathetic activity. It has sedative, analgesic, and amnestic properties.

**Answer: D**

Murray, M.J., Oyen, L.J., and Browne, W.T. (2008) Use of sedative, analgesics, and neuromuscular blockers, in *Critical Care Medicine: Principles of Diagnosis and Management in the Adult*, 3rd edn (eds J.E. Parrillo and R.P. Dellinger), Mosby, Philadelphia, PA, pp. 327–342.

**11** *A distinct advantage of lipid amphotericin B formulations over traditional amphotericin B deoxycholate is:*
  **A** *Lipid formulations are much less expensive*
  **B** *Lipid formulations have higher clinical efficacy with candidiasis infections*
  **C** *Lipid formulations are better suited to treat urinary tract fungal infections*
  **D** *Lipid formulations are less renal toxic*
  **E** *Lipid formulations can be used in pregnant patients*

Amphotericin B is an antibiotic by class. It is a member of the polyene antibiotic family along with nystatin and natamycin. However, it is the only one used for the treatment of systemic fungal infections. Polyene antibiotics bind to ergosterol, the fungal version of cholesterol, in the fungal cell membrane. As a result of this binding, fungal cell membrane permeability increases and the cell dies.

Amphotericin B comes in two broad types: lipid based and traditional. There are three distinct lipid formulas. The most important advantage of the lipid formulations over amphotericin B deoxycholate is less renal toxicity (Answer D). Amphotericin B deoxycholate has been found to cause acute kidney injury in up to 50% of patients. Lipid formulations, in general, are more expensive (Answer A). There is no literature to support lipid amphotericin B for candidiasis infections with regards to clinical efficacy (Answer B). Amphotericin B deoxycholate is metabolized in the liver and eliminated from the body via excretion in the urine. Lipid formulations undergo less renal elimination than non-lipid amphotericin and therefore are not ideal for treating urinary fungal infections (Answer C). Both lipid formulations and amphotericin B deoxycholate can be used safely in pregnant patients (both are Class B medications) (Answer E).

**Answer: D**

Moen, M.D., Lyseng-Williamson, K.A., and Scott, L.J. (2009) Liposomal amphotericin B: a review of its use as empirical therapy in febrile neutropenia and in the treatment of invasive fungal infections. *Drugs*, **69**, 361–392.
Pappas, P.G., Kauffman, C.A., Andes, D.R., *et al.* (2015) Clinical practice guideline for the management of candidiasis: 2016 update by the Infectious Diseases Society of America. *Clinical Infectious Diseases*, **62**, e1–e50.

**12** *Which one of the following definitions of pharmacokinetic and pharmacodynamic principles in the critically ill patient is incorrect?*
  **A** *Drug absorption is altered by gut wall edema, changes in gastric or intestinal blood flow, concurrent administration of enteral nutrition and incomplete oral medication dissolution*
  **B** *The volume of distribution is altered by fluid shifts, hypoalbuminemia, and mechanical ventilation*
  **C** *Metabolic clearance by the liver, mostly via the cytochrome $P_{450}$ system, may be compromised in the critically ill patient by decreases in hepatic blood flow, intracellular oxygen tension, and cofactor availability*
  **D** *Alterations in renal function increase the half-life of medications cleared via the kidney and result in accumulation of drugs or their metabolites*
  **E** *The response to antibiotics that have time-dependent killing pharmacodynamics would be improved by administering a higher dose of the drug to increase the area under the inhibitory curve.*

Critically ill patients have alterations in both pharmacokinetics and pharmacodynamics of medications. Pharmacokinetics characterizes what the body does to a drug – the absorption, distribution, metabolism, and elimination of the drug. Pharmacodynamics is what the drug does to the body and describes the relationship between the concentration of drug at the site of action and the clinical response observed. Many factors affect drug absorption, distribution, and clearance in the critically ill patient. Failure to recognize these variations may result in unpredictable serum concentrations that may lead to therapeutic failure or drug toxicity. Drug absorption is altered by gut wall edema and stasis, changes in gastric and intestinal blood flow, concurrent medications, and therapies such as enteral nutrition and incomplete disintegration or dissolution of oral medications. The volume of distribution describes the relationship between the amount of drug in the body and concentration in the plasma. Fluid shifts, particularly after fluid resuscitation, and protein binding changes that occur during critical illness alter drug distribution. Plasma protein concentrations may change significantly during critical illness and may affect the volume of distribution by altering the amount of the active unbound or free drug. Metabolic clearance by the liver is the predominant route of drug detoxification and elimination. With the hepatic dysfunction that may occur in the critically ill patient, drug clearance may be decreased secondary to reduced hepatic blood flow, decreased hepatocellular enzyme activity, or decreased bile flow. A common pathway for drug metabolism is the cytochrome $P_{450}$ system. Critical illness may compromise this system by decreasing hepatic blood flow, intracellular oxygen or cofactor availability. Antibiotics are usually categorized as having either concentration dependent or time-dependent killing. The activity of concentration-dependent antibiotics increases as the peak serum concentrations of drug increase. Time-dependent antibiotics kill at the same rate regardless of the peak serum concentration that is attained above the MIC (minimum inhibitory concentration). Thus, an increase in dose is *not* associated with improved AUIC (area under the inhibitory concentration curve). Instead, increasing dosing frequency would improve antibiotic killing.

**Answer: E**

Devlin, J.W. and Barletta, J.F. (2008) Principles of drug dosing in criticaly ill patients, in *Critical Care Medicine: Principles of Diagnosis and Management in the Adult*, 3rd edn (eds J.E. Parrillo and R.P. Dellinger), Mosby, Philadelphia, PA, pp. 343–376.

**13** *Antibiotic resistance is a world crisis. Most nosocomial outbreaks caused by antibiotic-resistant microorganisms have occurred in patients hospitalized in an ICU. Which of the following statements is an incorrect principle of antimicrobial therapy?*
  **A** *Fever without other indications of infection should mandate antimicrobial therapy in an ICU patient*
  **B** *Unless antimicrobial therapy is being given for surgical prophylaxis, gram-stain smears, cultures, and other appropriate diagnostic tests should be obtained before starting antimicrobial therapy for treatment of presumed infection in an ICU patient*
  **C** *The need for continued antimicrobial therapy should be reassessed daily. If diagnostic studies are negative after 72 hours and the patient is not exhibiting signs of sepsis, antibiotic therapy should be discontinued*
  **D** *Surgical antimicrobial prophylaxis should not extend beyond 24 hours postoperatively*
  **E** *If cultures identify the infecting microorganism(s), therapy should be modified to the most narrow-spectrum drug(s) likely to be effective*

Antimicrobials are widely misused and overused. Methods of controlling antimicrobial use include restricted formularies, policies on clinical microbiology laboratory on reporting of susceptibility testing, and automatic stop orders for surgical prophylaxis. Several principles can reduce unnecessary antimicrobial therapy and improve the use of the drugs that are given. Fever without indications of infection should *not* mandate automatically beginning antimicrobial therapy in an ICU patient. Fever is not uncommon in the postoperative patient, especially in the early postoperative period. Appropriate cultures should be obtained, and empiric antibiotics started if indicated, especially if the patient is exhibiting signs and symptoms consistent with sepsis. The need for continued antibiotic therapy should be reassessed *daily*, and if diagnostic tests are negative in 48–72 hours without signs of sepsis, antimicrobial therapy should be stopped. Surgical antimicrobial *prophylaxis* should not extend beyond 24 hours postoperatively and, in most cases, can be limited to one postoperative dose. If cultures identify the infecting micro-organism or micro-organisms, antimicrobial therapy should be modified as soon as possible to the most narrow-spectrum drug or drugs likely to be effective.

**Answer: A**

Dellit, T.H., Owens, R.C., McGowan, J.E., Jr, *et al.* (2007) Infectious Diseases Society of America and the Society of Healthcare Epidemiology of America guidelines for developing and institutional program to enhance stewardship. *Clinical Infectious Diseases*, **44**, 159–177.

Maki, D.G., Crnich, C.J., and Safdar, N. (2008) Nosocomial infection in the intensive care unit, in *Critical Care Medicine: Principles of Diagnosis and Management in the Adult*, 3rd edn (eds J.E. Parrillo and R.P. Dellinger), Mosby, Philadelphia, PA, pp. 1003–1069.

**14** *A 76-year-old obese woman (100 kg) with diabetes and a history of methicillin-resistant* staph aureus *(MRSA) soft-tissue skin infection develops ventilator-associated pneumonia following sigmoid colon resection with colostomy and Hartmann's procedure for perforation from diverticulitis. Broncho-alveolar lavage gram-stain shows many gram-positive cocci.*

*From microbial sensitivity, pharmacokinetic, and pharmacodynamic perspectives, which one of the following antimicrobial agents is likely to give optimal empiric treatment?*

**A** *Cefepime 1 gm IV q 12 hours*
**B** *Vancomycin 1 gm IV q 12 hours*
**C** *Linezolid 600 mg IV q 12 hours*
**D** *Daptomycin 500 mg IV q 24 hours*
**E** *Quinupristin/dalfopristin 500 mg IV q 12 hours*

This patient is at increased risk for, and likely has, a MRSA ventilator-associated pneumonia (VAP). Cefepime has activity against most Gram-negative bacilli, but poor activity against methicillin-resistant *S. aureus* and *enterococci*. Vancomycin is still the standard antibiotic for the treatment of nosocomial pneumonia. Vancomycin has *very poor lung tissue penetration*. Thus, among the choices listed, vancomycin would *not* be the best choice. Specifically, the dose suggested here is not likely to result in adequate lung penetration. There are great concerns about the inactivation of daptomycin by pulmonary surfactants, and thus it is not recommended for treatment of MRSA pneumonia. Linezolid has been shown in several studies to have excellent lung penetration. Quinupristin-dalfopristin (Synercid) is bactericidal for clindamycin-susceptible isolates of MRSA. However, clinical response rates of MRSA pneumonia were only 19% for quinupristin-dalfopristin when compared with a 40% response rate for vancomycin.

**Answer: C**

American Thoracic Society/Infectious Diseases Society of America (2005) Guidelines for the management of adults with hospital-acquired, ventilator-associated, and health care-associated pneumonia. *American Journal of Respiratory Critical Care Medicine*, **171**, 388–416.

**15** *A 55-year-old male with a history of severe COPD was admitted with a diagnosis of septic shock from perforated diverticulitis. He has no known drug allergies. On hospital day 10 and ventilator day 9, he* develops a fever, purulent tracheal secretions and requires more ventilator support. He is currently receiving IV ciprofloxacin and metronidazole with a good clinical response until now. He has also been on CRRT for the last week. Which of the following represents the best course of action for this patient's antibiotic regimen?*

**A** *Continue metronidazole, continue ciprofloxacin, add levofloxacin*
**B** *Continue metronidazole, stop ciprofloxacin, add piperacillin-tazobactam*
**C** *Continue ciprofloxacin, stop metronidazole, add vancomycin*
**D** *Continue ciprofloxacin, stop metronidazole, add piperacillin-tazobactam and vancomycin*
**E** *Continue metronidazole, stop ciprofloxacin, add linezolid*

The concern for this patient is the development of ventilator-associated pneumonia (VAP). The Infectious Disease Society of America (IDSA) released new guidelines for the management of VAP in 2016. Hospital antibiograms should be used to guide VAP treatment decisions when at all possible. The antibiotic choices for VAP are based on facility antibiograms and the probability of multidrug resistant (MDR) organisms causing VAP. The goal is to tailor empiric antibiotic coverage to the most likely organism(s) causing infection. Several risk factors for MDR pathogens are provided by the most recent guidelines (see Table 10.3).

This patient has at least three risk factors for MRSA and MDR *Pseudomonas* VAP. Current guidelines advocate two antipseudomonal antibiotics from two separate classes (β-Lactam and non- β-Lactam) when patients exhibit any risk factor for MDR *Pseudomonas* VAP. The

**Table 10.3** Risk factors for MDR pathogens.

| Risk Factors for MDR VAP | Risk Factors for MRSA VAP | Risk Factors for MDR Pseudomonas VAP |
|---|---|---|
| Prior IV antibiotic use within 90 days | Prior IV antibiotic use within 90 days | Prior antibiotic use within 90 days |
| Septic shock at time of VAP | | |
| ARDS preceding VAP | | |
| Five or more days of hospitalization before the occurrence of VAP | | |
| Acute renal replacement therapy before VAP onset | | |

guidelines also recommend the addition of vancomycin or linezolid for MRSA coverage, when risk factors are present. Answer A is incorrect because ciprofloxacin and levofloxacin are in the same class (antipseudomonal, non-β-Lactam) and metronidazole offers no MRSA coverage. Answer B is incorrect because there is no MRSA coverage and only one agent is available for *pseudomonas* coverage (piperacillin-tazobactam). Answer C is incorrect because it only offers one antibiotic for Pseudomonas (ciprofloxacin). Answer E is incorrect because it offers no coverage for *Pseudomonas*.

**Answer: D**

Kalil, A.C., Metersky, M.L., Klompas, M., *et al.* (2016) Management of adults with hospital-acquired and ventilator-associated pneumonia: 2016 clinical practice guidelines by the Infectious Diseases Society of America and the American Thoracic Society. *Clinical Infectious Diseases*, **63**, e61–e111.

16  A 65-year-old man has been in the ICU for one week following an open cholecystectomy secondary to gangrenous cholecystitis with bacteremia. Intravenous ceftazidime was started empirically perioperatively. The blood culture was positive for Escherichia coli sensitive to ceftazidime, cefepime, and meropenem, but resistant to aztreonam and piperacillin.

   On day 2 of treatment, the patient continues to have fever and tachycardia. Which one of the following interventions is the best antimicrobial treatment strategy for this patient?
   A  Discontinue ceftazidime, and start cefepime
   B  Add gentamicin
   C  Add fluoroquinolone
   D  Discontinue ceftazidime, and start meropenem
   E  Continue ceftazidime and add fluconazole

Despite the susceptibility results, the organism is not sensitive to ceftazidime. Ceftazidime is a potent inducer of chromosomal β-lactamase expression. Extended spectrum β-lactamases (ESBLs) are plasmid-mediated enzymes that inactivate all β-lactam antibiotics, except for cephamycins (cefoxitin) and carbapenems. Detection of ESBLs is often difficult. Some microbiology laboratories do not employ reliable methods, which may result in false susceptible reporting of ESBL strains to cefotaxime, ceftazidime, and ceftriaxone. Cefepime, a fourth-generation cephalosporin, does not appear to induce this type of chromosomal-mediated resistance to the same degree as ceftazidime but is susceptible to the action of ESBLs. Most ESBLs also co-express resistance to other agents including aminoglycosides and fluoroquinolones.

Carbapenems (specifically meropenem) are the most effective agents against ESBLs. An ESBL E-test should be performed for this isolate, and the patient should be started on meropenem pending the results.

**Answer: D**

Pfaller, M.A. and Segreti, J. (2006) Overview of the epidemiological profile and laboratory detection of extended-spectrum beta-lactamases. *Clinical Infectious Disorders*, **42**, S153–S163.

17  An 18-year-old boy sustained multiple gunshot wounds to the abdomen. He underwent multiple laparotomies with resection of multiple enterotomies and delayed abdominal closure. He received antibiotic prophylaxis with cefoxitin for his laparotomies. On postoperative day 10, he developed pneumonia. He had a bronchoalveolar lavage that grew P. aeruginosa.

   Which one of the following antimicrobial medications would be least likely to successfully treat this patient?
   A  Levaquin 750 mg IV q 24 hr
   B  Piperacillin/tazobactam 4.5 gm IV q 6 hr
   C  Ceftriaxone 1 gm IV q 24 hr
   D  Meropenem 500 mg IV q 6 hr
   E  Amikacin 15 mg/kg IV q24 hr

*P. aeruginosa* is a ubiquitous, avirulent opportunist organism. Its virulence is enhanced in critically ill patients. Therapy is complicated by both intrinsic and acquired resistance to a diverse spectrum of antimicrobials. Although antibiotic resistance in gram-negative bacilli may occur from several mechanisms, one that provides a foundation for understanding resistance is related to β-lactamase production in gram-negative organisms. These enzymes can be divided into categories of type I and nontype I enzymes. Type I β-lactamases are chromosomally mediated, with production controlled by the *ampC* gene. The microorganisms that produce these enzymes are Serratia, *P. aeruginosa*, Acinetobacter, Citrobacter, and Enterobacter. The mnemonic "SPACE bugs" may be used to remember these organisms. Nosocomial infections of lung, skin, urine, or blood are caused by one of these pathogens 20% of the time. The four classes of antibiotics that have the most predictable stability in the presence of the Type I β-lactamases are aminoglycosides, carbapenems, fluoroquinolones, and fourth generation cephalosporins (i.e., cefepime). Type I β-lactamases have an affinity for cephalosporins and thus, third-generation cephalosporins are *not* stable in the presence of these enzymes (i.e., ceftriaxone). Also, β-lactamase inhibitors, clavulanic acid, sulbactam, and tazobactam also lack stability against these enzymes; however, tazobactam is the most likely to resist their destruction. Thus, piperacillin/tazobactam is effective against this micro-organism and is considered an antipseudomonal penicillin.

**Answer: C**

Chastre, J., Wolff, M., Fagon, J.Y., *et al.* (2003) Comparison of 8 vs. 15 days of antibiotic therapy for ventilator-associated pneumonia in adults: a randomized trial. *Journal of the American Medical Association,* **290**, 2588–2598.

Godke, J. and Karam, G. (2008) Principles governing antimicrobial therapy in the intensive care unit in *Critical Care Medicine: Principles of Diagnosis and Management in the Adult,* 3rd edn (eds J.E. Parrillo and R.P. Dellinger) Mosby, Philadelphia, PA, pp. 1071–1088.

18 *A 58-year-old male was struck by a motor vehicle and had multiple significant injuries including bilateral rib fractures with a flail segment on the right and right pulmonary contusion. He was admitted to the surgical/trauma ICU 10 days ago. He was intubated during his initial assessment in the trauma bay and has been difficult to wean from the ventilator. He has had a central line in place since admission. He began spiking fevers 2 days ago and is now requiring vasopressors. He was placed on piperacillin/tazobactam and vancomycin empirically, but clinically he has not improved. His blood cultures come back positive for candida species pending. What is the best treatment choice for this patient with the current information?*
   A *Fluconazole 200 mg IV daily*
   B *Amphotericin B deoxycholate 3–5 mg/kg IV daily*
   C *Micafungin 100 mg IV daily*
   D *Flucytosine 25 mg/kg IV every 6 hours*
   E *Voriconazole 2 mg/kg IV daily*

Empiric antifungal therapy should be considered in critically ill patients with risk factors for invasive candidiasis and no other known cause of fever. It should be based on clinical assessments of risk factors, surrogate markers for invasive candidiasis, and/or culture data from nonsterile sites. Empiric antifungal therapy should be started as soon as possible in patients with risk factors and who have clinical signs of septic shock. The preferred empiric therapy for suspected candidiasis in nonneutropenic patients in the ICU is an echinocandin (micafungin 100 mg IV daily, caspofungin 70 mg IV × 1 followed by 50 mg IV daily, anidulafungin 200 mg IV × 1 followed by 100 mg IV daily). Thus, answer C is correct. Fluconazole at higher doses 800 mg IV × 1 followed by 400 mg IV daily

is an acceptable alternative for patients who have not had recent azole exposure. A is incorrect because the dose is subtherapeutic. Lipid formulation of amphotericin B 3–5 mg/kg IV daily is an alternative if there is an intolerance to other antifungals. Amphotericin B deoxycholate 1 mg/kg is the treatment of choice in neonatal candidiasis. Thus, B is incorrect since the lipid formulation would be appropriate, also, the dose is too high for the deoxycholate and likely toxic. Voriconazole is used in much higher doses (6 mg/kg) BID × 2 then 3 mg/kg BID but offers little advantage over fluconazole as initial therapy. It is recommended as step-down therapy for selected cases of candidemia due to *C. krusei*, for additional mold coverage and for neutropenic patients. Flucytosine is usually used in combination with other antifungals and reserved for very severe infections. It is used more commonly in combination with Amphotericin B for central nervous system candidiasis.

**Answer: C**

Pappas, P.G., Kauffman, C.A., Andes, A.R., *et al.* (2016) Clinical practice guidelines for the management of candidiasis: 2016 update by the Infectious Diseases Society of America. *Clinical Infectious Diseases,* **62**, e1–e50.

19 *A 43-year-old diabetic woman who is found to have a fever of 39.0 °C and blood pressure 81/43 mm Hg 18 hours after exploratory laparotomy for lysis of adhesions. She is transferred to the ICU, and her examination is notable for acute distress with erythema and bullous lesions near the surgical wound. Aspiration of one of the lesions reveals numerous white blood cells with Gram-positive cocci in chains. What is the antibiotic that would be most helpful in reducing toxin production in this patient?*
   A *Clindamycin*
   B *Ciprofloxacin*
   C *Aztreonam*
   D *Cefepime*
   E *Gentamicin*

Necrotizing soft tissue infection is an uncommon, severe infection that causes necrosis of the subcutaneous tissue and fascia with sparing of the underlying muscle. Two types, based on microbiology, are described. In type, I, at least one anaerobic species is isolated along with one or more facultative anaerobes and members of Enterobacteriaceae. In type II, group A streptococci (GAS) are isolated alone (also known as hemolytic streptococcal gangrene). Predisposing factors include blunt and penetrating trauma, varicella infection, intravenous drug abuse, surgical procedures, childbirth, and possibly nonsteroidal anti-inflammatory drug use, but necrotizing soft tissue infections may occur in the absence of an obvious portal of entry. Type II necrotizing fasciitis is commonly associated with Streptococcal toxic shock syndrome. The involved area is extremely painful, erythematous, and edematous. The infection spreads widely in deep fascial planes with relative sparing of the overlying skin and therefore may be unrecognized. This form of necrotizing fasciitis is present in approximately 50% of cases of streptococcal toxic shock syndrome. The skin becomes dusky, and bullae develop. Streptococci can usually be cultured from the fluid in the early bullae or from the blood. Mortality from this infection is high. Treatment consists of penicillin and clindamycin. Intravenous immunoglobulin administration may also be considered.

Recent studies suggest clindamycin is superior to penicillin in the treatment of necrotizing fasciitis due to GAS. Penicillin failure is probably due to a reduction in bacterial expression of critical penicillin binding proteins during the stationary growth phase of these bacteria. Clindamycin is likely more effective because it is not affected by inoculum size or stage of growth, suppresses toxin production, facilitates phagocytosis of *S. pyogenes* by inhibiting M-protein synthesis, suppresses production of regulatory elements controlling cell wall synthesis, and has a long post-antibiotic effect.

**Answer: A**

Sarani, B., Strong, M., Pascual, J., *et al.* (2009) Necrotizing fasciitis: current concepts and review of the literature. *Journal of the American College of Surgeons*, **208**, 279–288.

**20** *As the Acute Care Surgeon on-call, you have taken a patient with an incarcerated ventral hernia to the operating room for open surgical repair. You have requested that the CRNA paralyze the patient during the operation to ease your surgical approach. The case goes well, and you alert the CRNA that you will be finished much faster than anticipated, however, the patient has just received another dose of Rocuronium. What drug will reverse the paralytic action of Rocuronium the fastest?*

**A** *Atropine*

**B** *Edrophonium*

**C** *Glycopyrrolate*

**D** *Neostigmine bn*

**E** *Sugammadex*

Neuromuscular blocking agents (NMBAs) can be broken into two main classes: depolarizing and nondepolarizing agents. Succinylcholine is the only member of the depolarizing class of NMBAs, and there is no reversal agent available. The nondepolarizing NMBAs are Rocuronium, Pancuronium, Vecuronium, Atracurium, and its isomer, Cisatracurium. Neostigmine and other acetylcholinesterase inhibitors (choices B and D) were long the only reversal agents available for depolarizing NMBAs. These agents increase the endogenous amount of acetylcholine available for binding at the neuromuscular junction thus, competitively counteract the NMBAs effect. Sugammadex (Choice E) was approved for use in Europe in 2008 but not approved by the FDA for use in the United States until December 2015. Sugammadex is a novel class of drugs called Selective Relaxant Binding Agents (SRBAs). The mechanism of action is twofold: 1) encapsulating (chelating) steroid backboned NMBAs (Rocuronium, Pancuronium, Vecuronium) making them inactive and removing them from the neuromuscular junction thus, restoring muscle function; 2) the NMBAs that are already bound to nicotinic receptors will dissociate from the receptor. Sugammadex exerts its effect by forming very tight complexes at a 1:1 ratio with aminosteroid muscle relaxants (rocuronium > vecuronium >> pancuronium). The intermolecular (van der Waals') forces, thermodynamic (hydrogen) bonds, and hydrophobic interactions make the sugammadex–rocuronium complex very tight (Figure 10.1). The resulting reduction in free rocuronium plasma concentration creates a gradient

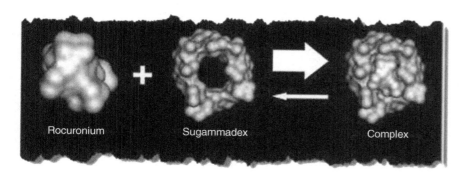

**Figure 10.1**

between the tissue compartment (including the NMJ) and plasma; free rocuronium moves from tissue to plasma, with a reduction in nicotinic receptor occupancy at the NMJ. Multiple trials have found Sugammadex is faster at reversing Rocuronium and Vecuronium-induced paralysis than both Neostigmine and Edrophonium (choices B and D) while having similar adverse event profiles as the traditional cholinesterase inhibitors. Atropine and Glycopyrrolate (Choices A and C) are both anticholinergic drugs that are often used in conjunction with cholinesterase inhibitors (Neostigmine and Edrophonium) to help offset their cholinergic effects such as bradycardia and excessive salivation. They have no role in NMBA reversal when used by themselves.

**Answer: E**

Abrishami, A., Ho, J., Wong, J., *et al.* (2009) Sugammadex, a selective reversal medication for preventing postoperative residual neuromuscular blockade. *Cochrane Database of Systematic Reviews*, **4**.

Keating, G.M. (2016) Sugammadex: a review of neuromuscular blockade reversal. *Drugs*, **76** (10), 1041–1052.

Welliver, M., McDonough, J., Kalynych, N., and Redfern, R. (2009) Discovery, development, and clinical application of sugammadex sodium, a selective relaxant binding agent. *Drug Design Development and Therapy*, **2**, 49–59.

**21** *The FDA issued a black box warning for increased risk of death for which antibiotic when compared to other antibiotics?*

**A** *Daptomycin*
**B** *Tigecycline*
**C** *Colistin*
**D** *Linezolid*
**E** *Caspofungin*

On the basis of noninferiority trials, tigecycline received FDA approval in 2005. In 2010, the FDA warned in a safety communication that tigecycline was associated with an increased risk of death. Tigecycline versus active comparators demonstrated a significant increase in mortality and noncore rates. Overall, tigecycline was associated with a 0.7% absolute or 30% relative increase in mortality and a 2.9% absolute or 12% relative increase in noncore rates. In subgroup analysis, this effect was independent of infection type, trial design, and study size. Of importance, unfavorable outcomes were similarly associated with tigecycline therapy for approved and nonapproved indications. Although the underlying cause of death in trials of tigecycline are uncertain, the corresponding elevated risk of noncore suggests the possibility of inadequate antimicrobial activity. Tigecycline should not be used when other effective antibiotic choices are available.

**Answer: B**

Prasad, P., Sun, J., Danner, R.L., *et al.* (2015) Excess deaths associated with tigecycline after approval based on noninferiority trails. *Clinical Infectious Diseases*, **54**, 1699–1709.

# 11

# Transfusion, Hemostasis, and Coagulation

*Erin Palm, MD and Kenji Inaba, MD*

**1** *A 22-year-old man sustained a gunshot wound to the right upper quadrant. He arrives in the emergency department 20 minutes after injury. Blood pressure is 70/0 mm Hg, heart rate 140 beats/min. Focused Abdominal Sonography for Trauma (FAST) is positive for intra-abdominal hemorrhage and the patient is taken directly to the operating room. In the operating room, he is found to have a laceration of the right lobe of the liver and inferior vena cava with ongoing massive hemorrhage.*

*Current evidence most strongly supports the following approach to blood component therapy for this patient:*

**A** *Early use of prothrombin complex concentrate (PCC)*

**B** *Goal directed component transfusion based on PT/ PTT and platelet count*

**C** *Avoidance of un-crossmatched blood transfusion*

**D** *Transfusion of blood components in a fixed ratio*

**E** *Minimizing transfusion of fresh frozen plasma*

In patients receiving massive transfusion, studies have shown a survival advantage in patients who received a high ratio of FFP to PRBC during initial resuscitation. Retrospective studies originating from the military and civilian experience found that the optimal ratio of FFP:PRBC transfusion may be as high as 1:1. A prospective, randomized controlled trial comparing a transfusion ratio of 1:1:1 FFP:platelet:PRBC versus a 1:1:2 ratio demonstrated improved hemostasis and fewer deaths from hemorrhage by 24 hours in the 1:1:1 group. There was no increase in respiratory complications in the 1:1:1 group, despite prior retrospective associations between increased FFP transfusion and acute respiratory distress syndrome (ARDS). However, the study did not demonstrate a difference in overall mortality between the two arms. The preponderance of evidence currently supports a balanced transfusion strategy that targets an FFP:PRBC ratio approaching 1:1.

PCC is effective for rapid reversal of oral anticoagulants such as warfarin. Outside of this special population, the role of PCC in trauma remains unproven.

Component therapy based on traditional lab results will result in a marked delay in administration of FFP and platelets. In addition, laboratory studies may not accurately represent in vivo clotting activity.

Although crossmatched blood minimizes the risk of transfusion reaction, performing crossmatch may take too long in a bleeding patient. Initial resuscitation with un-crossmatched type-specific or type O blood may be necessary.

**Answer: D**

Holcomb, J.B., Tilley, B.C., Baraniuk, S., *et al.* (2015) Transfusion of plasma, platelets, and red blood cells in a 1:1:1 vs a 1:1:2 ratio and mortality in patients with severe trauma: the PROPPR randomized clinical trial. *Journal of the American Medical Association*, **313** (5), 471–482.

**2** *A 45-year-old man was admitted to the ICU five days ago after a motorcycle crash in which he suffered a severe left pulmonary contusion, pneumothorax, cardiac contusion, humerus fracture, clavicle fracture, and brachial plexus injury. Blood pressure is 130/85 mm Hg. He is currently undergoing a spontaneous breathing trial. The patient's hemoglobin is 8.1 g/dL from 8.0 yesterday, platelets 30 000/mm$^3$ from 31 000/mm$^3$, prothrombin time 18 s from 18 s, and partial thromboplastin time 42 s from 20 s. The patient has not been transfused any blood products during this admission.*

*Which blood products should be transfused at this time?*

**A** *Red blood cells, platelets, and fresh-frozen plasma*

**B** *Red blood cells and platelets*

**C** *Red blood cells*

**D** *Platelets*

**E** *No blood products*

*Surgical Critical Care and Emergency Surgery: Clinical Questions and Answers*, Second Edition.
Edited by Forrest "Dell" Moore, Peter Rhee, and Gerard J. Fulda.
© 2018 John Wiley & Sons Ltd. Published 2018 by John Wiley & Sons Ltd.
Companion website: www.wiley.com/go/moore/surgical_criticalcare_and_emergency_surgery

In this stable trauma patient without evidence of active bleeding, no blood products are needed at this time. A restrictive transfusion strategy maintaining hemoglobin at 7.0–9.0 g/dL has been shown to be as effective as a liberal transfusion strategy maintaining hemoglobin concentration at 10.0–12.0 g/dL. For those with an APACHE II score ≤ 20, 30-day mortality is significantly less with a restrictive strategy.

In the absence of clinical bleeding, FFP transfusion may be associated with an increased incidence of acute lung injury.

Evidence to support prophylactic platelet transfusion in critically ill patients without active bleeding is conflicting. Several authors have recommended avoidance of prophylactic platelet transfusion altogether, while others have recommended thresholds ranging from 10 000/mm$^3$ to 100 000/mm$^3$ for patients at risk of bleeding.

**Answer: E**

Hébert, P., Wells, B., Blajchman, M., *et al*. (1999) A multicenter, randomized, controlled clinical trial of transfusion requirements in critical care. *New England Journal of Medicine*, **340** (6), 409–417.

Napolitano, L., Kurek, S., and Luchette, F. (2009) Clinical practice guideline: red blood cell transfusion in adult trauma and critical care. *Critical Care Medicine*, **37** (11), 3124–3157.

3 *A 68-year-old woman is admitted to the surgical intensive care unit after a fall resulting in a right femoral neck fracture. The patient's home medications include warfarin for atrial fibrillation. On admission, her laboratory tests are Hg 10.4 g/dL, Hct 32%, platelet count 155 000/mm$^3$, prothrombin time 32 s, INR 3.1, and activated thromboplastin time 33 s. In preparation for surgery, six units of FFP are ordered to reverse her anticoagulation. After transfusion of two units FFP, the patient complains of shortness of breath, and develops a fever of 38.5 °C, heart rate of 115 beats/min, and SaO$_2$ 85%. Respiratory status deteriorates rapidly, requiring intubation and mechanical ventilation. A chest X-ray demonstrates diffuse bilateral infiltrates. CVP is 10 mm Hg.*

*What is the most appropriate intervention?*

A *Administer diuretics*
B *Administer corticosteroids*
C *Administer heparin bolus followed by continuous infusion*
D *Administer antibiotics*
E *Aggressive respiratory support*

Early fever, hypoxia, and pulmonary infiltrates associated with transfusion are most typical of transfusion-associated acute lung injury (TRALI). TRALI is a serious complication of transfusion defined as hypoxia (PaO$_2$/FiO$_2$ ≤ 300 or SpO$_2$ > 90%), bilateral infiltrates on chest X-ray, and pulmonary artery occlusion pressure ≤ 18 mm Hg or no clinical evidence of left atrial hypertension. Additional criteria include: acute lung injury developing during or within six hours of transfusion, no acute lung injury present before transfusion, or a clinical course that suggests acute lung injury worsening as a result of transfusion. Symptoms include dyspnea, hypotension and fever. The treatment of TRALI is respiratory support, including measures to avoid worsening of lung injury.

Transfusion of all types of blood products can cause TRALI. Pathogenesis is related to donor antibodies in the transfused blood, and may also be related to modifications of stored blood. Measures to prevent TRALI include a restrictive transfusion policy, as well as blood bank measures such as predominant use of plasma from male donors.

The differential diagnosis of respiratory distress during or after transfusion includes TRALI, transfusion-associated circulatory overload (TACO), anaphylactic reaction, and bacterial contamination of blood products. The patient presented is unlikely to have TACO as evidenced by associated fever and relatively low CVP.

Corticosteroids, antibiotics, and heparin are not indicated in the treatment of TRALI. The role of diuretics is unclear and their use should be individualized.

**Answer: E**

Benson, A., Moss, M., and Silliman, C. (2009) Transfusion-related acute lung injury (TRALI): a clinical review with emphasis on the critically ill. *British Journal of Haematology*, **147**, 431–443.

Lin, Y., Saw, C.L., Hannach, B., and Goldman, M. (2012) Transfusion-related acute lung injury prevention measures and their impact at Canadian Blood Services. *Transfusion*, **52** (3), 567–574.

4 *A 32-year-old woman involved in a high-speed motor vehicle collision, sustained an open book pelvic fracture. CT of the pelvis shows active extravasation of contrast. She becomes hypotensive and massive transfusion protocol is activated. Which of the following is true regarding use of tranexamic acid (TXA) in trauma patients?*

A *TXA is effective if administered within 24 hours of presentation*
B *TXA is an inhibitor of fibrinolysis*
C *Patients who receive TXA are at increased risk of vascular occlusive events such as stroke and MI*
D *There is no data to support a mortality benefit in trauma patients who receive TXA*
E *TXA reduces hemorrhage, but is not cost effective due to the high price of the drug*

The activation of the clotting cascade in surgery and trauma also activates the pathway for clot breakdown, fibrinolysis. Hemorrhaging patients may develop pathologic hyper-fibrinolysis, contributing to coagulopathic bleeding. Tranexamic acid (TXA) is a synthetic derivative of the amino acid lysine that inhibits fibrinolysis by blocking the lysine binding site on plasminogen. In elective surgery patients, TXA has been shown to reduce the need for blood transfusion.

The CRASH-II trial was a randomized, placebo-controlled trial of TXA in trauma patients with significant bleeding. CRASH-II demonstrated a significant reduction in all-cause mortality, as well as deaths due to hemorrhage, in the patients who received TXA. There was no increase in vascular occlusive events in patients receiving TXA.

TXA should be administered within 3 hours of presentation for greatest benefit. The dosing used in the trial was 1 gram infused over 10 minutes, followed by a second dose of 1 gram over 8 hours.

Multiple studies demonstrate that TXA is cost effective, including trauma patients. It is available as an inexpensive generic medication.

**Answer: B**

The CRASH-2 Collaborators (2010) Effects of tranexamic acid on death, vascular occlusive events, and blood transfusion in trauma patients with significant hemorrhage (CRASH-2): a randomized, placebo-controlled trial. *Lancet*, **376**, 23–32.

5 *Liberal transfusion of packed red blood cells (PRBCs) in stable ICU patients is associated with:*
   A *Improved oxygen consumption*
   B *Increased incidence of nosocomial pneumonia*
   C *Decreased incidence of acute respiratory distress syndrome (ARDS)*
   D *Decreased mortality*
   E *Decreased incidence of multi-organ failure*

Contemporary evidence-based guidelines discourage liberally transfusing PRBCs in most non-bleeding patients. Although transfusion of PRBCs was traditionally used to improve oxygen delivery, multiple studies have failed to demonstrate an improvement in end-organ oxygen consumption with transfusion. This may be partially explained by the decreased deformability and adverse microcirculatory effects of stored red blood cells.

Risks associated with PRBC transfusion include fluid overload, fever, acute transfusion reaction, increased rate of multi-organ failure, increased infection rates, transfusion-associated immunomodulation, human error with incorrect blood administration, TRALI, and viral transmission.

**Answer: B**

Hebert, P., Wells, G., Blajchman, M., *et al.* (1999) A multicenter, randomized, controlled clinical trial of transfusion requirements in critical care. *New England Journal of Medicine*, **340** (6), 409–417.

Mirski, M.A., Frank, S.M., Kor, D.J., *et al.* (2015) Restrictive and liberal red cell transfusion strategies in adult patients: reconciling clinical data with best practice. *Critical Care Medicine*, **19** (1), 1–11.

6 *A hospital's massive transfusion protocol should be immediately activated for which of the following patients?*
   A *A 63-year-old man with grade IV liver laceration who has received 4 units of packed red blood cells over the last 12 hours in the intensive care unit*
   B *A 23-year-old man with a gunshot wound to the right chest, who had 500 cc of blood drained on initial chest tube placement*
   C *A 31-year-old man with gunshot wound to the epigastrium who has fluid on abdominal ultrasound and has received 8 units of uncrossmatched blood for hypotension in the emergency department*
   D *A 55-year-old man with grade IV splenic laceration and active contrast extravasation on abdominal CT scan*
   E *A 71-year-old woman taking warfarin for atrial fibrillation who sustained a loss of consciousness after falling down a flight of stairs*

Massive transfusion has been variably defined as $\geq 10$ units PRBC in the first 6–24 hours. Definitions may also include a rate of transfusion such as $\geq 3$ units PRBC per hour. Survival in trauma patients who require massive transfusion can be improved by timely administration of blood products in proper ratios. In several major trauma centers, implementation of a massive transfusion protocol (MTP) to streamline the rapid and continued delivery of appropriate blood products has been shown to improve outcomes.

When activated, the MTP should result in rapid delivery of PRBCs and FFP. The goal is to achieve balanced FFP:PRBC transfusion ratios of between 1:1 and 1:2. Some MTPs also provide platelets in a balanced ratio.

There are no uniformly accepted criteria for activating an MTP. Clinical factors that have been validated as individual predictors of massive transfusion when measured at the time of presentation are: systolic blood pressure $\leq 90$ mm Hg, heart rate $\geq 120$ beats/min, positive fluid on abdominal FAST, INR > 1.5, and arterial base deficit > 6. Emergency department transfusion of uncrossmatched PRBC is also associated with massive transfusion. Alternatively, protocols can be initiated when a specific threshold such as 6–10 PRBC has been transfused, to ensure subsequent transfusion of one unit of FFP for each unit PRBC.

Of the above patients, only patient C has a clear indication for initiation of MTP.

**Answer: C**

Callcut, R.A., Cotton, B.A., Muskat, P., *et al.* (2013) Defining when to initiate massive transfusion: a validation study of individual massive transfusion triggers in PROMMTT patients. *Journal of Trauma and Acute Care Surgery*, **74** (1), 59–65.

Riskin, D.J., Tsai, T.C., Hernandez-Boussard, T., *et al.* (2009) Massive transfusion protocols: the role of aggressive resuscitation versus product ratio in mortality reduction. *Journal of the American College of Surgeons*, **209** (2), 198–205.

7 *A 33-year-old man is undergoing exploratory laparotomy for a gunshot wound to the liver with massive hemorrhage and hemorrhagic shock. Rapid thrombelastography (TEG) demonstrates a prolonged activated clotting time (ACT), prolonged K time, decreased angle (TEG α) and normal maximum amplitude (MA).*

*Using goal-directed component replacement based on the above rapid TEG results, this patient should receive:*

A *Fresh frozen plasma*
B *Platelets*
C *Fresh frozen plasma and platelets*
D *Aminocaproic acid*
E *Cryoprecipitate*

Thrombelastography has been used as a guide to blood product replacement for acutely bleeding patients, and has been studied as an alternative to ratio-based mass transfusion protocols. TEG offers the advantage of real-time point of care testing of coagulation function in whole blood. A rapid TEG differs from conventional TEG because tissue factor is added to the whole blood specimen, resulting in accelerated reaction and subsequent analysis.

The R value, which is recorded as activated clotting time (ACT) in the rapid TEG specimen, reflects clotting factor activation and the time to onset of clot formation (Figure 11.1). A deficiency of clotting factors will result in a prolonged ACT, which can be treated by FFP transfusion.

The K value is the interval from the beginning of clot formation to a fixed level of clot firmness measured at a standard 20 mm amplitude. It reflects the activity of thrombin which cleaves fibrinogen. Similarly, the α angle reflects the rate of clot formation and is another measure of fibrinogen activity. A prolonged K value and a decreased α angle represent a fibrinogen deficit which can be treated by transfusion of FFP or cryoprecipitate.

The maximum amplitude (MA) measures the final clot strength, reflecting the end result of platelet-fibrin interaction. If the MA is decreased after transfusion of FFP, then platelet transfusion should be considered.

The patient described has a prolonged ACT as well as prolonged K time and decreased α angle. This is best treated by FFP transfusion to replace both the clotting factor deficiency and fibrinogen deficiency. If the K time remains prolonged after correction of the ACT, then cryoprecipitate can be given.

**Answer: A**

Inaba, K., Rizoli, S., Veigas, P.V., *et al.* (2015) 2014 consensus conference on viscoelastic test-based transfusion guidelines for early trauma resuscitation: report of the panel. *Journal of Trauma and Acute Care Surgery*, **78** (6), 1220–1229.

Johansson, P.I., Stensballe, J., Oliveri, R., *et al.* (2014) How I treat patients with massive hemorrhage. *Blood*, **124** (20), 3052–3058.

8 *A 53-year-old man with hepatitis C cirrhosis presents with massive hematemesis. He has a history of portal*

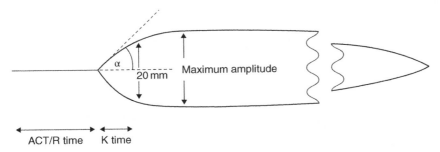

**Figure 11.1**

*hypertension and esophageal varices. He is intubated in the ER. An NG tube is placed with ongoing bloody output, and his blood pressure is 70/50 mm Hg. Massive transfusion protocol is activated. The patient's blood type is unknown and crossmatch is pending. In addition to type O packed red blood cells (PRBCs), what type of plasma should be transfused?*

**A** *Blood group O plasma only*
**B** *Blood group AB plasma only*
**C** *Blood group B plasma only*
**D** *Blood group AB plasma, or low titer anti-B group A plasma*
**E** *Blood group O plasma, or low titer anti-B group A plasma*

In massively bleeding patients, plasma should be transfused with PRBCs in a roughly equal ratio. This cirrhotic patient also has increased risk of coagulopathy due to poor liver synthesis of clotting factors.

Blood group AB is the "universal plasma donor." Group AB plasma lacks anti-A and anti-B isohemagglutinins. To avoid an ABO-incompatible transfusion in a patient whose blood type is unknown, type AB plasma should be used. Plasma does not need to be Rh-compatible.

One drawback of making thawed plasma available for MTP is plasma wastage. Most plasma is frozen shortly after collection and stored as fresh frozen plasma (FFP). When thawed, plasma must be used within 5 days. An alternative is to use liquid plasma (i.e., never frozen plasma), which has a shelf life of weeks rather than days.

Donors with blood group AB are rare. To conserve AB plasma, some institutions have implemented protocols that use thawed group A plasma for emergency release.

**Answer: D**

Novak, D.J., Bai, Y., Cooke, R.K., *et al.* (2015) Making thawed universal donor plasma available rapidly for massively bleeding trauma patients: experience from the Pragmatic, Randomized Optimal Platelets and Plasma Ratios (PROPPR) trial. *Transfusion*, **55** (6), 1331–1339.
Zielinski, M.D., Johnson, P.M., Jenkins, D., *et al.* (2013) Emergency use of prethawed Group A plasma in trauma patients. *Journal of Trauma and Acute Care Surgery*, **74** (1), 69–74.

**9** *Which of the following is true regarding platelets in massive transfusion?*
**A** *Platelets should be transfused empirically in a high ratio*
**B** *Platelet transfusion is unnecessary in a massive transfusion if sufficient FFP is transfused*
**C** *Apheresis platelets are more effective than pooled donor platelets*
**D** *Platelet transfusion should only be given for actively bleeding patients with a platelet count less than 50 000/mm³*
**E** *Apheresis platelets are associated with an increased rate of bacterial contamination compared to pooled donor platelets*

Retrospective studies show improved survival in trauma patients who receive a high ratio of platelets to packed red blood cells during massive transfusion. A high ratio of platelets to PRBC is defined variably in these studies as approximately one unit of apheresis platelets for every 6–10 units of PRBC transfused. Additionally, the randomized controlled PROPPR trial showed faster hemostasis and fewer deaths from hemorrhage in the group treated with a higher ratio of FFP and platelets to PRBC. During a massive transfusion, platelets should be transfused in an appropriate ratio without waiting for clinical laboratory results to confirm low platelet counts.

No study has definitively compared outcomes between apheresis and pooled donor platelets in trauma patients. One unit of apheresis platelets is obtained from a single donor, while pooled platelets are combined from six to eight donors. As a result, pooled platelets have a higher risk of bacterial contamination as well as viral transmission, however there is no difference in transfusion-related lung injury.

**Answer: A**

Holcomb, J.B., Tilley, B.C., Baraniuk, S., *et al.* (2015) Transfusion of plasma, platelets, and red blood cells in a 1:1:1 vs a 1:1:2 ratio and mortality in patients with severe trauma: The PROPPR randomized clinical trial. *Journal of the American Medical Association*, **313** (5), 471–482.
Inaba, K., Lustenberger, T., Rhee, P., *et al.* (2011) The impact of platelet transfusion in massively transfused trauma patients. *Journal of the American College of Surgeons*, **211**, 573–579.

**10** *A 35-year-old man is admitted to the intensive care unit following an emergency splenectomy and nephrectomy for injuries sustained in a motorcycle crash. He required a total of 12 units packed red blood cells intraoperatively. What electrolyte abnormality is most likely to occur?*
**A** *Hypokalemia*
**B** *Hyperkalemia*
**C** *Hypocalcemia*
**D** *Hypomagnesemia*
**E** *Respiratory acidosis*

Hypocalcemia is the most common abnormality associated with massive transfusion, occurring in >90% of patients receiving a massive blood transfusion. Stored blood is anticoagulated with citrate, which binds calcium and causes hypocalcemia after large-volume blood transfusion. Complications of hypocalcemia include prolonged QT, decreased myocardial contractility, hypotension, muscle tremors, pulseless electrical activity and ventricular fibrillation.

Hyper- and hypokalemia are both common electrolyte abnormalities following massive transfusion, with each occurring in approximately 20% of patients. The potassium concentration of plasma increases in stored blood, becoming higher with increased duration of PRBC storage. Rapid transfusion through a central venous catheter has been associated with cardiac arrest in vulnerable populations, including critically ill adults.

Hypomagnesemia may also result from dilution, or from the binding of magnesium to citrate.

Acidosis occurs in approximately 80% of massive transfusion patients, however it is most commonly metabolic acidosis.

**Answer: C**

Giancarelli, A., Birrer, K.L., Alban, R.F., *et al.* (2016) Hypocalcemia in trauma patients receiving massive transfusion. *Journal of Surgical Research*, **202** (1), 182–187.

Sihler, K. and Napolitano, L. (2010) Complications of massive transfusion. *Chest*, **137**, 209–220.

11 *A 71-year-old woman taking warfarin for chronic atrial fibrillation arrives in the emergency department after a fall down a flight of stairs at home. She is awake and able to follow commands, but a large scalp hematoma is noted. A CT head shows a sub-durdal hematoma.*

*What is the fastest way to reverse her coagulopathy?*

A *Activate the massive transfusion protocol*
B *Administer 4-factor prothrombin complex concentrate*
C *Transfuse fresh frozen plasma*
D *Transfuse fresh frozen plasma and administer vitamin K*
E *No reversal is needed because her GCS is 15*

A protocol for the rapid evaluation, diagnosis, and treatment of anticoagulated trauma patients reduces the mortality of warfarin-anticoagulated trauma patients with intracranial hemorrhage. Protocols include emergent CT head and rapid reversal of coagulopathy.

Historically, warfarin reversal was achieved with rapid administration of FFP. In 2013, the US FDA approved Kcentra, a 4-factor prothrombin complex concentrate

(PCC). A randomized controlled trial comparing 4-factor PCC to FFP for treatment of major bleeding in patients on vitamin K antagonists showed 4-factor PCC achieved rapid reversal of the INR more effectively than FFP. The safety profile in the two groups was the same.

Since its approval in the US, experience with Kcentra in trauma settings has been favorable. However, access to Kcentra may still be limited at some institutions, so it is important to consider including PCC in hospital protocols for rapid reversal of anticoagulation to ensure its timely availability.

**Answer: B**

Berndtson, A.E., Huang, W.T., Box, K., *et al.* (2015) A new kid on the block: outcomes with Kcentra 1 year after approval. *Journal of Trauma and Acute Care Surgery*, **79** (6), 1004–1008.

Sarode, R., Milling, T.J., Jr, Refaai, M.A., *et al.* (2013) Efficacy and safety of a 4-factor prothrombin complex concentrate in patients on vitamin K antagonists presenting with major bleeding: a randomized, plasma-controlled, phase IIIb study. *Circulation*, **128** (11), 1234–1243.

12 *A 26-year-old previously healthy woman is admitted to the surgical ICU after appendectomy for perforated appendicitis with peritonitis. Post-operatively she required reintubation for progressive shortness of breath and hypoxia. A chest X-ray demonstrates diffuse bilateral infiltrates. On the first postoperative day, platelet count is 75 000/mm³, PT 19 s, PTT 50 s, oozing is noted from IV sites, and blood is suctioned from her endotracheal tube. Which of the following test results would be consistent with the diagnosis of disseminated intravascular coagulation?*

A *Increased antithrombin level*
B *Elevated fibrin degradation products*
C *Decreased bleeding time*
D *Elevated fibrinogen level*
E *Decreased D-dimer*

Disseminated intravascular coagulation (DIC) is characterized by widespread microvascular thrombosis with activation of the coagulation system and impaired protein synthesis, leading to exhaustion of clotting factors and platelets. The end result is organ failure and profuse bleeding from various sites. DIC is always associated with an underlying condition that triggers diffuse activation of coagulation, most commonly sepsis, trauma with soft tissue injury, head injury, fat embolism, cancer, amniotic fluid embolism, toxins, immunologic disorders, or transfusion reaction.

There is no single laboratory test that can confirm or rule out a diagnosis of DIC. A combination of tests in a patient with an appropriate clinical condition can be used to make the diagnosis. Low platelet count, elevated fibrin degradation products or D-dimer, prolonged prothrombin time, and low fibrinogen level are all consistent with a diagnosis of DIC.

**Answer: B**

Levi, M. (2007) Disseminated intravascular coagulation. *Critical Care Medicine*, **35** (9), 2191–2195.

**13** *A 23-year-old man was involved in a bicycle-versus-auto accident, sustaining a large, complex laceration to the right anterior tibial region. No other injuries were identified. Dorsal pedal and posterior tibial pulses were normal. Admission laboratory studies showed hemoglobin of 11.3 g/dL, platelet count 210 000/mm$^3$, prothrombin time of 12.8 s, and activated partial thromboplastin time of 65 s. He underwent irrigation and debridement in the operating room with no vascular injury identified. Throughout the operation, the surgeons noted significant ongoing bleeding from the exposed soft tissues, saturating through multiple dressings. Dorsal pedal and posterior tibial pulses remained intact.*

*Which one of the following is the most likely etiology of this patient's bleeding?*

**A** *Disseminated intravascular coagulation*
**B** *Hemophilia A*
**C** *Hypothermia*
**D** *Von Willebrand disease*
**E** *Arterial injury*

Hemophilia may present as excessive bleeding after trauma or surgery. Frequently the bleeding is delayed. An alternative presentation is a large subcutaneous or soft tissue hematoma after an invasive procedure.

Patients with mild or moderate hemophilia A have a factor VIII level that is 1–50% of normal. These patients may have no history of spontaneous bleeding into joints or soft tissues, yet may develop significant bleeding complications after trauma or surgery. Laboratory abnormalities in hemophilia are characterized by a normal prothrombin time, variable prolongation of partial thromboplastin time, and a normal platelet count. The diagnosis can be confirmed with a Factor VIII assay and treated with concentrated Factor VIII. Hemophilia B (Factor IX deficiency) has a similar presentation and treatment. In an emergency, if specific clotting factors are not available, FFP or prothrombin complex concentrate can be used to treat hemophiliac bleeding.

In contrast to clotting factor deficiencies, platelet defects including Von Willebrand disease are typically characterized by spontaneous mucocutaneous bleeding and epistaxis, or immediate bleeding and diffuse oozing at the surgical site.

Disseminated intravascular coagulation may occur after severe trauma, however this patient's injury was not extensive and he had an elevated partial thromboplastin time at presentation.

Arterial injury is unlikely given the delayed presentation of bleeding and normal distal pulses.

**Answer: B**

Cohen, A. (1995) Treatment of inherited coagulation disorders. *American Journal of Medicine*, **99**, 675–62.
Mensah, P.K. and Gooding, R. (2015) Surgery in patients with inherited bleeding disorders. *Anaesthesia*, **70** (Suppl 1), 112–120.

**14** *A 61-year-old woman with a history of aortic stenosis and chronic renal insufficiency underwent aortic valve replacement. Unfractionated heparin was started 6 hours after surgery. On post-operative day 5, she developed pain in the right lower extremity. Examination demonstrated a cool extremity with absent distal pulses. Platelet count fell from 220 000/mm$^3$ on day 3 to 90 000/mm$^3$ on day 5, and creatinine increased from 1.8 mg/dL on day 3 to 2.9 mg/dL on day 5. She was taken to the operating room where she underwent thrombectomy of the right femoral artery. Intraoperatively, extensive white clot was present in the superficial femoral artery.*

*Which therapeutic option is most appropriate at this time?*

**A** *Discontinue unfractionated heparin and start argatroban*
**B** *Discontinue unfractionated heparin and start enoxaparin*
**C** *Discontinue unfractionated heparin and start lepirudin*
**D** *Increase unfractionated heparin*
**E** *Discontinue anticoagulation*

The patient likely has heparin-induced thrombocytopenia (HIT). HIT is a life-threatening disorder that occurs after exposure to unfractionated, or less commonly, low molecular weight heparin. HIT usually occurs after 5–10 days of heparin therapy and is caused by antibodies against the heparin-platelet factor 4 complex. Thrombotic complications occur in 20–50% of patients. The thrombus associated with HIT has been described as "white clot" with predominantly fibrin platelet aggregates and few red blood cells.

Thrrombocytopenia is common in the critically ill, and diagnosis of HIT can be difficult. Laboratory confirmation includes immunoassay for the detection of PF4-heparin antibodies and a confirmatory functional assay measuring serotonin release from activated platelets. Delays in obtaining test results often mean that management decisions must be made on the basis of clinical suspicion. Clinical findings that imply a diagnosis HIT are:

- Platelet fall of more than 50% from baseline, with platelet nadir > 20,000. Profound thrombocytopenia suggests a cause other than HIT
- Onset on day 5–10 of heparin exposure
- Thrombosis, skin necrosis, or an anaphylactoid reaction after heparin bolus
- No other cause for the thrombocytopenia is present.

Treatment of HIT includes discontinuation of all sources of heparin and if anticoagulation is clinically warranted, use of a direct thrombin inhibitor such as lepirudin, argatroban, or bivalirudin. Lepirudin requires renal clearance and should be avoided in renal insufficiency. Therefore, treatment with argatroban is the best answer in this case.

**Answer: A**

Greinacher, A. (2015) Heparin-induced thrombocytopenia. *New England Journal of Medicine*, **373** (3), 252–261.

15  *A 55-year-old homeless man is admitted to the ICU after being found down in a local park. He is lethargic, hypoxic, mildly hypotensive, and tachycardic. Chest X-ray demonstrates multiple right rib fractures with a large right pleural effusion. Laboratory data include white blood cell count 15 000/mm³, hemoglobin 9 g/dL, platelet count 90 000/mm³, prothrombin time 13 s, partial thromboplastin time 35 s, sodium 145 meq/L, blood urea nitrogen 140 mg/dL, and creatinine 8 mg/dL. Prolonged bleeding is noted from venipuncture sites.*

*Which therapy should be administered prior to chest tube placement?*

**A** *Conjugated estrogens*
**B** *Platelet transfusion*
**C** *Fresh frozen plasma*
**D** *Desmopressin acetate*
**E** *Hemodialysis*

This patient is profoundly uremic with clinical evidence of bleeding. Coagulopathy in uremic patients is multifactorial and includes platelet dysfunction. It results in mucocutaneous bleeding, and bleeding in response to injury or invasive procedures. Prothrombin time and partial thromboplastin time may be normal, and platelet counts are normal to slightly low. Bleeding from surgical procedures may be difficult to control.

Desmopressin acetate (dDAVP) is the simplest way to rapidly improve platelet function in the uremic patient. The dose of dDAVP is 0.3–0.4 µg/kg administered either intravenously or subcutaneously. Desmopressin acts by increasing the release of Factor VIII and von Willebrand Factor (vWF) from the endothelium and will cause improvement in bleeding time within one hour. Unfortunately, the effect is short lived, lasting 4–24 hours, and tachyphylaxis may develop with repeated doses.

Cryoprecipitate is a source of Factor VIII, vWF and fibrinogen. It acts rapidly and can be used to treat coagulopathic bleeding. However, its effect may be unpredictable in uremic patients.

Hemodialysis can correct the bleeding time in uremic patients, but is time consuming and may acutely prolong bleeding through platelet activation on artificial surfaces.

Administering conjugated estrogens can achieve more sustained control of uremic bleeding, with peak efficacy reached after five to seven days.

A platelet transfusion should be given if the effusion is found to be a hemothorax, or if there is evidence of ongoing bleeding at any site.

**Answer: D**

Hedges, S., Dehoney, S., Hooper, J., *et al.* (2007) Evidence-based treatment recommendations for uremic bleeding. *Nature Clinical Practice Nephrologyi*, **3** (3), 138–153.

Mannucci, P., Remuzzi, G., Pusineri, F., *et al.* (1983) Deamino-8-d-arginine vasopressin shortens the bleeding time in uremia. *New England Journal of Medicine*, **308** (1), 8–12.

16  *A 58-year-old man presents to clinic with a new diagnosis of colovesical fistula secondary to diverticulitis. A colonoscopy reveals no evidence of malignancy. His past medical history is significant for coronary artery disease for which he underwent coronary stenting of the left anterior descending artery with a drug-eluting stent 3 months ago. His current medications include aspirin and clopidogrel.*

*He is being evaluated for sigmoid colectomy. What is the best perioperative strategy with regard to his platelet inhibitors?*

**A** *Transfuse platelets and proceed with surgery immediately*
**B** *Stop aspirin and clopidogrel immediately, then proceed with surgery in seven days*

C *Continue aspirin, stop clopidogrel immediately, then proceed with surgery in seven days*

D *Wait 3 months, then stop clopidogrel for five days and proceed with surgery*

E *Wait 9 months, then stop clopidogrel for five days and proceed with surgery*

The combination of aspirin and clopidogrel is commonly used following coronary stent placement. For patients with coronary artery stents undergoing elective non-cardiac surgery, it is recommended that surgery be delayed for at least 4 weeks following bare metal stent placement, and at least 6 months following placement of a drug-eluting stent. Premature interruption in antiplatelet therapy confers a risk of stent thrombosis and myocardial infarction.

Perioperative management of antiplatelet agents should balance the risk of surgical bleeding with the risk of stent thrombosis. It is important to know the indication for stenting, the date of implant, the type of stent used, as well as the proposed duration of current antiplatelet therapy. When possible, surgery should be delayed until after the recommended period of dual antiplatelet therapy. This stable patient with colovesical fistula and recent drug-eluting stent can safely defer surgery until he reaches the 6-month interval.

If urgent surgery must be performed, the risk and consequences of surgical bleeding must be assessed. For procedures with a low bleeding risk, dual antiplatelet agents should be continued through the surgery. If surgical bleeding risk requires cessation of clopidogrel, aspirin alone should be continued if possible.

Guidelines vary with regard to the length of time antiplatelet therapy should be held pre-operatively. Recommendations range from 5 to 10 days.

When long-acting anti-platelet agents must be stopped for urgent operations, there is evidence to support bridging with a short-acting intravenous antiplatelet agent such as tirofiban or abciximab. These medications can be stopped 4–6 hours prior to the procedure with normalization of the bleeding time.

**Answer: D**

Darvish-Kazem, S., Gandhi, M., Marcucci, M., and Douketis, J.D. (2013) Perioperative management of antiplatelet therapy in patients with a coronary stent who need noncardiac surgery: a systematic review of clinical practice guidelines. *Chest*, **144** (6), 1848–1856.

**17** *An 18-year-old man is admitted to the surgical ICU following a right thoracotomy and right upper lobe non-anatomic lobectomy for bleeding near the pulmonary hilum after a gunshot wound to the chest.*

*A wound to the thoracic spine was difficult to control and was packed with sponges. He received 12 units of packed red blood cells, 10 units of fresh frozen plasma, and 1 unit of apheresis platelets in the operating room. Vital signs: BP 100/60mm Hg, HR 120 beats/min, temperature 32.5°C. Laboratory studies: hemoglobin 8.5g/dL, platelets 100 000/mm³, prothrombin time 14s, partial thromboplastin time 40s. Chest tube output is 150mL for the first hour in the ICU.*

*What is the most appropriate treatment for his bleeding?*

A *Transfuse FFP*

B *Transfuse platelets*

C *Transfuse cryoprecipitate*

D *External warming*

E *Return to the operating room*

Following surgical control of bleeding and massive resuscitation, ongoing aggressive resuscitation is required to reverse the "lethal triad" of coagulopathy, acidosis, and hypothermia.

Clotting factor and platelet deficiencies have been addressed early during this resuscitation by maintaining a high ratio of FFP and platelets to red blood cell transfusion. A platelet count of 100 000/mm³ and slightly prolonged PT and PTT demonstrate adequate platelets and clotting factors.

Hypothermia < 35°C is a strong independent risk factor for mortality in trauma patients, with more severe hypothermia conveying greater risk of mortality. Hypothermia contributes to coagulopathy through platelet and clotting factor dysfunction. Notably, clotting assays performed in the laboratory are warmed to 35°C. Therefore, laboratory values may not represent the patient's actual clotting activity in vivo.

Recommended measures for re-warming a patient with body temperature 32.5°C include forced air warming, infusion of warmed fluids, under-body heating pads, radiant warmers, and humidified ventilation. If bleeding continues after aggressive warming and correction of clotting abnormalities, the patient must return to the operating room without further delay.

**Answer: D**

Inaba, K., Teixeira, P., Rhee, P., *et al.* (2009) Mortality impact of hypothermia after cavitary explorations in trauma. *World Journal of Surgery*, **33** (4), 864–869.

Perlman, R., Callum, J., Laflamme, C., *et al.* (2016) A recommended early goal-directed management guideline for the prevention of hypothermia-related transfusion, morbidity, and mortality in severely injured trauma patients. *Critical Care*, **20** (1), 1–11.

**18** A 29-year-old man was involved in a motorcycle crash. He now has a distended abdomen that is diffusely tender. Blood pressure is 80/60 mm Hg. What fluid should be administered?
  **A** Lactated ringers
  **B** Hypertonic saline
  **C** O positive blood
  **D** Type specific blood
  **E** Crossmatched blood

The described patient has hemoperitoneum and should be taken to the operating room for control of any surgically correctable sources of bleeding. Crystalloid resuscitation should be minimized and type O blood transfused without delay. O positive blood can be used for male patients and women beyond childbearing age. If uncrossmatched blood resources are limited, O negative blood is reserved for woman of child-bearing age to avoid the risk of Rh isoimmunization. O positive blood has been shown to be safe for transfusion in hemorrhaging trauma patients, with a very low rate of transfusion reaction.

Advantages of using uncrossmatched type O blood include immediate availability before type specific blood becomes available and avoidance of errors in multi-casualty situations. The safety of type O blood has been improved by prescreening donor blood for anti-A and anti-B antibodies, which can lead to hemolysis of native red blood cells.

**Answer: C**

Ball, C.G., Salomone, J.P., Shaz, B., *et al.* (2010) Uncrossmatched blood transfusions for trauma patients in the emergency department: incidence, outcomes and recommendations. *Canadian Journal of Surgery*, **54** (2), 111–115.

Dutton, R., Shih, D., Edelman, B., *et al.* (2005) Safety of uncrossmatched type-O red cells for resuscitation from hemorrhagic shock. *Journal of Trauma*, **59** (6), 1445–1449.

**19** A 78-year-old man presents after a ground-level fall. He has a history of atrial fibrillation and his medications include rivaroxaban (Xarelto), which his family confirms he took this morning. On physical exam, he is withdrawing to pain and mumbling incomprehensible sounds. He has a parietal scalp hematoma. CT of the head shows a large subdural hematoma with 2 mm midline shift. Neurosurgery plans to perform craniotomy. The best strategy for reversing the patient's anticoagulation is:
  **A** No reversal is required if the INR is < 2
  **B** Administer the specific FDA-approved reversal agent idarucizumab
  **C** Administer platelets
  **D** Administer platelets and FFP
  **E** Administer 4-factor prothrombin complex concentrate (PCC)

Since 2010, three new oral anticoagulant medications have been approved in the United States as alternatives to warfarin and low molecular weight heparin: rivaroxaban, abixaban, and dabigatran (Table 11.1) Rivaroxaban (brand name Xarelto) acts by inhibiting factor Xa, as does apixaban (Eliquis). Their introduction is an improvement over LWMH, which also inhibitis factor Xa, because patients can take pills rather than injections. The third drug, dabigatran (Pradaxa), is a direct thrombin inhibitor.

The major advantage of these medications is, in contrast to warfarin, they do not require INR monitoring. In clinical trials, bleeding events on these medications were comparable to, or lower than, bleeding events in patients receiving warfarin or low molecular weight heparin for similar indications.

The major drawbacks of these agents are 1) their anticoagulation effect is not reliably measured by common laboratory tests, and 2) effects can be difficult to reverse. In 2016, the FDA approved idarucizumab as a specific reversal agent for dabigatran. However at this time, the two oral anti-Xa inhibitors have no specific reversal agent.

FFP can be used to resuscitate patients on these medications who suffer low- to moderate-risk bleeding events. However, FFP is not a specific reversal agent. It takes time infuse and cannot rapidly reverse coagulopathy. Administration of FFP can also lead to volume overload and transfusion reactions. For all of these reasons, FFP is not an ideal therapy.

**Table 11.1**

| Medication | Brand name (US) | Mechanism | Specific reversal agent | Renal excretion (%) | Half life |
| --- | --- | --- | --- | --- | --- |
| Dabigatran | Pradaxa | Direct thrombin inhibitor | idarucizumab | 80–85 | 7–17 hours |
| Rivaroxaban | Xarelto | Factor Xa inhibitor | – | 36 | 6–17 hours |
| Apixaban | Eliquis | Factor Xa inhibitor | – | 25 | 8–14 hours |

This patient has a life-threatening intracranial hemorrhage that requires rapid reversal of rivaroxaban. For emergency reversal of rivaroxaban or apixaban, 4-factor prothrombin complex concentrate (PCC) should be used. PCC can also be used to reverse dabigatran if idarucizumab is unavailable. Finally, for dabigatran specifically, hemodialysis can also be helpful because its excretion is primarily renal.

**Answer: E**

Faraoni, D., Levy, J.H., Albaladejo, P., *et al.* (2015) Updates in the perioperative and emergency management of non-vitamin K antagonist oral anticoagulants. *Critical Care*, **19**, 1–6.

Siegal, D.M., Garcia, D.A., and Crowther, M.A. (2014) How I treat target-specific oral anticoagulant-associated bleeding. *Blood*, **123** (8), 1152–1158.

# 12

# Analgesia and Anesthesia

*Marquinn D. Duke, MD and Juan C. Duchesne, MD*

**1** *A 28-year-old man underwent a laparoscopic appendectomy. He was induced with propofol for the surgery. What is the mechanism of action for propofol?*
   **A** *GABA (gamma-aminobutyric acid) agonist*
   **B** *GABA (gamma-aminobutyric acid) antagonist*
   **C** *Alpha-2 adrenergic agonist*
   **D** *Alpha-2 adrenergic antagonist*
   **E** *Mu receptor antagonist*

Benzodiazepines and propofol are GABA agonists. Propofol is often used for short-term sedation, because it has a fast onset and clearance. The common side effects of propofol are hypotension, respiratory depression, hypertriglyceridemia, pancreatitis, and propofol infusion syndrome. Propofol can be used in patients with neurologic injury. It can decrease intracranial pressure, cerebral blood flow, and cerebral metabolism. Since it has a short half-life, it can allow for sedation holidays for assessment of neurologic function, which has translated to shorter vent dependent days when compared to benzodiazepines. However, Propofol can cause hypotension and respiratory suppression, so it must be used with caution. Flumazenil is an example of a GABA antagonist. Opioids have an effect on mu receptors. Naloxone, a reversal agent for opioids, is a mu receptor antagonist. Dexmedetomidine is an example of an alpha-2 agonist. Mirtazapine is an example of an alpha-2 antagonist.

**Answer: A**

Jacobi, J., Fraser, G.L., Coursin, D.B., *et al.* (2002) Clinical practices guidelines for the sustained use of sedatives and analgesics in the critically ill adult. *Critical Care Medicine*, **30** (1), 119–141.

Mehta, S., McCullagh, I., and Burry, L. (2009) Current sedation practices: Lessons learned from international surveys. *Critical Care Clinics*, **25**, 471–488.

Riker, R.R. and Fraser, G.L. (2009) Altering intensive care sedation paradigms to improve patient outcomes. *Critical Care Clinics*, **25**, 527–538.

Sakata, R.K. (2010). Analgesia and sedation in intensive care unit. *Revista Brasileira de Anestesiologia*, **60** (6), 648–658.

**2** *A 58-year-old woman has had a sigmoidectomy for perforated diverticulitis, which failed medical management. The surgery was uncomplicated, but she was left intubated overnight. On attempts to extubate the patient in the SICU the next morning, she became very agitated. The best option for weaning sedation in preparation would be?*
   **A** *Weaning the propofol more slowly*
   **B** *Changing the patient to dexmedetomidine*
   **C** *Changing the patient to midazolam*
   **D** *Leave the patient intubated, and aim for extubation the next day*
   **E** *Changing the patient to lorazepam*

Dexmedetomidine is a sedative, analgesic, and anxiolytic that is an agonist on the central alpha-2 adrenergic receptors. It does not cause respiratory depression, and can be used in patients who are not intubated. Propofol has a fast onset and clearance, with clearance generally in less than 6 minutes. It is eliminated by hepatic conjugation. Weaning more slowly is unlikely to have a different outcome. Midazolam and lorazepam are benzodiazepines, are powerful amnestics and can cause respiratory depression. In addition midazolam has an active metabolite that causes toxicity and results in severe confusion and agitation. The half-life of these benzodiazepines are extremely long and since they are fat soluble they can leach from the fatty store for days. If benzodiazepines are used they should not be used as drips due to the long plasma half live. Leaving the patient intubated, without attempting additional routes of weaning would not be the correct action in this patient, as the patient would have a prolonged ventilator period and increased associated risks, such as an increased risk of pneumonia.

**Answer: B**

Jacobi, J., Fraser, G.L., Coursin, D.B., *et al.* (2002) Clinical practices guidelines for the sustained use of sedatives and analgesics in the critically ill adult. *Critical Care Medicine*, **30** (1), 119–141.

Karol, M.D. and Maze, M. (2000) Pharmacokinetics and interaction pharmacodynamics of dexmedetomidine in humans. *Best Practice & Research Clinical Anesthaesiology*, **14**, 261–269.

Riker, R.R., Shehabi, Y., Bokesch, P.M. *et al.* (2009) Dexmedetomidine versus midazolam for sedation of critically ill patients: a randomized trial. *Journal of the American Medical Association*, **301**, 489–499.

3   A 45-year-old woman was admitted to the SICU with > 60% BSA burn after being pulled rescued from a burning house. Two days after admission, she went into respiratory distress, requiring intubation. Which medication should not be used during intubation?
   A *Pancuronium*
   B *Cisatracurium*
   C *Rocuronium*
   D *Vecuronium*
   E *Succinylcholine*

Neuromuscular blockers and sedatives are often used in rapid sequence intubation. The neuromuscular blockers can be categorized as depolarizing or non-depolarizing. Succinylcholine is a depolarizing agent. Pancuronium, cisatracurium, rocuronium, and vecuronium are non-depolarizing agents. Depolarizing agents stimulate all cholinergic receptors by binding to the acetylcholine receptors. This causes stimulation, followed by muscular paralysis. The depolarization by succinylcholine and its metabolites leads to a potassium efflux from the muscle. This can lead to hyperkalemia, precipitating an arrhythmia. Burn victims are at risk of developing severe hyperkalemia, due to tissue injury. In this population, succinylcholine should not be used, to minimize the risk of the development of hyperkalemia.

**Answer: E**

Gronert, G.A. (2001) Cardiac arrest after succinylcholine: mortality greater with rhabdomyolysis than receptor upregulation. *Anesthesiology*, **94**, 523–529.

Li, J., Murphy-Lavoie, H., Bugas, C., *et al.* (1999) Complications of emergency intubation with and without paralysis. *American Journal of Emergency Medicine*, **17**, 141–143.

Martyn, J.A. and Richtsfeld, M. (2006) Succinylcholine-induced hyperkalemia in acquired pathologic states: etiologic factors and molecular mechanisms. *Anesthesiology*, **104**, 158–169.

4   A 62-year-old man with stage 3 chronic kidney disease had a left hemicolectomy for colon cancer. On postoperative day 2, he becomes oliguric, with an increasing serum creatinine. He only complains of incisional pain. Which medication would be the best to manage his pain?
   A *Dilaudid*
   B *Morphine*
   C *Fentanyl*
   D *Meperidine*
   E *Ketorolac*

Dilaudid, morphine, and meperidine are narcotics that undergo hepatic metabolism, but renal excretion. They may have accumulation of their metabolites in renal failure. The half-life of dilaudid is approximately 2.3 hours, the half-life of morphine is 2.5–3 hours, and the half-life of meperidine is 2–5 hours. These would be prolonged further in patients with renal failure. Ketorolac is a non-steroidal anti-inflammatory drug (NSAID). Its use is contraindicated in renal failure. Fentanyl is metabolized by the liver into inactive metabolites. The half-life of fentanyl is approximately 2–5 hours. The active metabolite of fentanyl is extremely short and is minutes. Due to the short half life of the active metabolite it is ideal to be given in the form of a continuous dose. However, since it is metabolized in the liver, this would be the most appropriate choice.

**Answer: C**

American Pain Society (2003) *Principles of Analgesic Use in the Treatment of Acute Pain and Cancer Pain*, 5th edn, American Pain Society, Glenview, IL.

Ball, M., McQuay, H.J., Moore, R.A., *et al.* (1985) Renal failure and the use of morphine in intensive care. *Lancet*, **325** (8432), 784–786.

Haragsim, L., Dalal, R., Bagga, H., and Bastani, B. (1994) Ketorolac-induced acute renal failure and hyperkalemia: report of three cases. *American Journal of Kidney Disease*, **24** (4), 578–580.

King, S., Forbes, K., Hanks, G.W., *et al.* (2011) A systematic review of the use of opioid medication for those with moderate to severe cancer pain and renal impairment: A European Palliative Care Research Collaborative opioid guidelines project. *Palliative Medicine*, **25** (5), 525–552.

5   A 75-year-old man is in a motor vehicle collision. One week later, the patient develops sepsis and multiple organ failure with severe ARDS, liver insufficiency, and acute kidney injury. He is on maximal support on the ventilator and needs to be paralyzed to optimize

*the ventilator requirements. Which medication would be the best choice for neuromuscular blockade for this patient?*

**A** *Cisatracurium*
**B** *Succinylcholine*
**C** *Vecuronium*
**D** *Pancuronium*
**E** *Rocuronium*

Neuromuscular blockade can be either depolarizing or non-depolarizing. Succinylcholine is a depolarizing agent, and is not suggested for long-term neuromuscular blockage. Vecuronium, pancuronium, and rocuronium are non-depolarizing neuromuscular blocking agents. They are degraded in the liver, but have active metabolites. They are eliminated by urine. In hepatic or renal insufficiency, the effect of the blockade may be significantly prolonged. Cisatracurium goes through Hofmann elimination, which is an organ-independent degradation process. There is minimal risk in patients with liver or renal disease.

**Answer: A**

De Laet, I., Hoste, E., Verholen, E., *et al.* (2007) The effect of neuromuscular blockers in patients with intra-abdominal hypertension. *Intensive Care Medicine*, **33**, 1811–1814.

Society of Critical Care Medicine, American Society of Health-System Pharmacists (2002) Sedative, analgesia, and neuromuscular blockade of the critically ill adult: revised clinical practice guidelines for 2002. *Critical Care Medicine*, **30**, 117–118.

6 *Which neuromuscular blocking agent would be the preferred choice for rapid sequence intubation in a patient with a contraindication to succinylcholine?*

**A** *No paralytic agent should be used*
**B** *Pancuronium*
**C** *Vecuronium*
**D** *Atracurium*
**E** *Rocuronium*

Giving a paralytic should be used if there is any rigidity in the patient, in order to ease the process. Pancuronium has a slower onset and longer duration (60–90 minutes). This would not be ideal in rapid sequence intubation. Vecuronium undergoes rapid hepatic uptake, with a shorter duration of action than pancuronium. However, its elimination and half-live are increased in hepatic insufficiency. Atracurium may cause a histamine release and transient cardiac effects (e.g., tachycardia, decreased mean arterial pressure). The effects are not prolonged, but would not be ideal in rapid sequence intubation. Rocuronium causes a neuromuscular blockade that is

sufficient for intubation in 60–90 seconds. There is not any histamine release. The half-life is 20–35 minutes.

**Answer: E**

Feldman, S.A. and Fauvel, N. (1994) Onset of neuromuscular block, in Applied Neuromuscular Pharmacology (ed. B.J. Pollard), Oxford University Press, Oxford and New York, pp. 69–84.

Murray, M.D., Cowen, J., DeBlock, H., *et al.* (2002) Clinical practice guidelines for sustained neuromuscular blockade in the adult critically ill patient. *Critical Care Medicine*, **30**, 142–156.

7 *A 60-year-old woman underwent a bronchoscopy and transbronchial biopsy for suspected lung cancer. The procedure was performed by a pulmonologist, who used midazolam and fentanyl for sedation and topical benzocaine for local analgesia. After the start of the procedure, she developed cyanosis and became hypoxic. The oxygen monitor noted a saturation of 83%. She was admitted to the intensive care unit due to persistent cyanosis and hypoxemia. She had equal, but coarse breath sounds, which was noted prior to the procedure. She was place on 100% supplemental oxygen, with only a small improvement of her oxygen saturation, to 87%. An ABG demonstrated a $PaCO_2$ of 35 mm Hg and a $PaO_2$ of 400 mm Hg. What is the most likely etiology of the patient's current condition?*

**A** *Hypoventilation due to over sedation*
**B** *Iatrogenic pneumothorax*
**C** *Intracardiac shunt*
**D** *Aspiration pneumonitis*
**E** *Topical benzocaine*

The patient is suffering from methemeglobinemia. This condition causes a disparity between $PaO_2$ on an ABG and pulse oximetry readings. Clues to the diagnosis are the presence of central cyanosis with normal $PaO_2$ on ABG and low saturation on pulse oximetry. When methemoglobin levels rise above 10%, cyanosis is frequently present, and at higher levels, hypoxemia and metabolic acidosis can occur. The recommended treatment is IV methylene blue (1–2 mg/kg over 3–5 minutes). Local anesthetic agents, such as benzocaine are some of the common drugs implicated in the etiology of acquired methemoglobinemia. A minimal decrease in $PaCO_2$ would rule out hypoventilation, as hypoventilation would be associated with an elevated $PaCO_2$. Breath sounds were equal bilaterally, making a pneumothorax less likely. There is no evidence of an intracardiac shunt. Aspiration pneumonitis would not be likely, given the rapid decline and discrepancy in ABG findings.

**Answer: E**

Moore, T.J., Walsh, C.S., Cohen, M.R., *et al.* (2004) Report adverse event cases of methemoglobinemia associated with benzocaine products. *Archives of Internal Medicine,* **164**, 1192–1196.

Umbreit, J. (2007) Methemoglobinemia: it's not just blue – a concise review. *American Journal of Hematology,* **82**, 134–144.

**8** *A 63-year-old woman is undergoing an elective right hemicolectomy for cancer. She has moderate cirrhosis from a prolonged history of alcohol use and stage 2 renal failure due to hypertension. Additionally, she is taking theophylline for COPD. Which anesthetic agent should be avoided?*

**A** *Sevoflurane*
**B** *Isoflurane*
**C** *Desflurane*
**D** *Halothane*
**E** *Propofol*

Sevoflurane can react with material in carbon dioxide and lead to renal tubular necrosis in laboratory animals. This has not been demonstrated in human studies. It is not associated with hepatic failure. The metabolism of isoflurane and desflurane has little potential for nephrotoxicity and has not been implicated in liver failure. Halothane has been associated with liver damage. This can come in two forms: 1. Mild hepatic damage with moderately increased transaminase levels, transient jaundice, and low morbidity, 2. Or, more rarely, fulminant hepatic failure with high mortality. The second usually occurs after repeated exposure. Additionally, theophylline can cause arrhythmias in the presence of halothane. The potential for liver damage and the patient's use of theophylline would make halothane the medication to avoid. While propofol is metabolized in the liver, it is tolerated well in those with liver failure.

**Answer: D**

Conzen, P.F., Kharasch, E.D., Czerner, S.F., *et al.* (2002) Low-flow sevoflurane compared with low-flow isoflurane anesthesia in patients with stable renal insufficiency. *Anesthesiology* [comment], **97** (3), 578–584.

Elliott, R.H. and Strunin, L. (1993) Hepatotoxicity of volatile anaesthetics. *British Journal of Anaesthesia,* **70** (3), 339–348.

Kenna, J.G. and Jones, R.M. (1995) The organ toxicity of inhaled anesthetics. *Anesthesia & Analgesia,* **81** (Suppl. 6), 51–66.

Vaja, R., McNicol, L., and Sisley, I. (2010) Anaesthesia for patients with liver disease. *Continuing Education in Anaesthesia, Critical Care & Pain,* **10**(1), 15–19.

**9** *A 58-year-old man with a previous gastrectomy is undergoing an exploratory laparotomy for small bowel obstruction. He does not have any history of an adverse reaction to anesthesia during his first surgery. Which medication should be used with particular caution for this surgery?*

**A** *Succinylcholine*
**B** *Halothane*
**C** *Propofol*
**D** *Nitrous oxide*
**E** *Etomidate*

Nitrous oxide inactivates vitamin B12. Patients can develop megaloblastic anemia, bone marrow depression, and neurologic difficulties after prolonged exposure or chronic inhalation of nitrous oxide. Those with a vitamin B12 deficiency, which can occur after a gastrectomy, are at risk of a neurologic deterioration after a single dose. The neurologic effects can be reversed with vitamin B12 therapy.

**Answer: D**

Flippo, T.S. and Holder, W.D., Jr. (1993) Neurologic degeneration associated with nitrous oxide anesthesia in patients with vitamin B12 deficiency. *Archives of Surgery,* **128** (12), 1391–1395.

Louis-Ferdinand, R.T. (1994) Myelotoxic, neurotoxic and reproductive adverse effects of nitrous oxide. *Adverse Drug Reaction Toxicology Review,* **13** (4), 193–206.

**10** *An 89-year-old woman is intubated in the SICU due to decline of mental status while being monitored after a fall. Rapid sequence intubation was used, where the intubating physician used etomidate and succinylcholine. Her sedation is maintained with propofol and fentanyl throughout the night. She becomes hypotensive and is started on vasopressin. After 2 days, the patient is more alert, but has sustained low blood pressure, unable to be weaned off of vasopressors. The most likely cause of the patient's hypotension is because of which of the following?*

**A** *Insufficient fluid resuscitation*
**B** *Succinylcholine*
**C** *Etomidate*
**D** *Propofol*
**E** *Fentanyl*

A major disadvantage of etomidate is its inhibition of cortisol and mineralocorticoids synthesis in the adrenal glands. A single dose, or continuous infusion can lead to decreased adrenal steroid production. It is the likely causative factor in this patient. It is less likely that her hypotension is due to insufficient fluid resuscitation after two days of therapy. Propofol can cause hypotension, but would be held to evaluate for her mental status. It is less likely that propofol would cause such hypotension if it were at low enough levels for the patient to be alert. Succinylcholine was used for induction, and would have been metabolized. Fentanyl is less likely to cause hypotension.

**Answer: C**

Crozier, T.A., Beck, D., Schlaeger, M., *et al.* (1987) Endocrinological changes following etomidate, midazolam, or methohexital for minor surgery. *Anesthesiology*, **66** (5), 628–635.
Wagner, R.L. and White, P.F. (1984) Etomidate inhibits adrenocortical function in surgical patients. *Anesthesiology*, **61** (6), 647–651.

11 *A 21-year-old man has sustained polytrauma after being involved in a motorcycle crash. His injuries include a subdural hematoma, multiple long bone fractures, rib fractures, pulmonary contusions, and a splenic laceration. He has required multiple surgeries in the subsequent days. During his course, he has been maintained on high doses of propofol for sedation, fentanyl for pain, and vasopressin for blood pressure stabilization. On postoperative day 4, he is weaned off of pressors. However, on postoperative day 5, he begins to develop metabolic acidosis, renal failure, and electrolyte abnormalities. What is the likely cause of the patient's current condition?*
A *Propofol*
B *Fentanyl*
C *Vasopressin*
D *The discontinuation of vasopressin*
E *Multi-organ failure due to sepsis*

Propofol infusion syndrome has been used to describe the negative effects of long term, high dose use of propofol. It can be associated with cardiac failure, rhabdomyolysis, severe metabolic acidosis, renal failure, and electrolyte abnormalities.

**Answer: A**

Kam, P. and Cardone, D. (2007) Propofol infusion syndrome. *Anaesthesia*, **62** (7), 690–701.
Vasile, B., Rasulo, F., Candiani, A., *et al.* (2003) The pathophysiology of propofol infusion syndrome: a simple name for a complex syndrome. *Intensive Care Medicine*, **29** (9), 1417–1425.

12 *The early clinical manifestations of central nervous system toxicity of local analgesics are:*

A *Tachycardia and hypotension*
B *Tachycardia and hypertension*
C *Bradycardia and hypotension*
D *Bradycardia and hypertension*
E *No physical effect*

The manifestations of local analgesia toxicity start with tachycardia and hypertension. As blood levels continue to rise, symptoms can continue to progress to myocardial depression, hypertension, and decreased cardiac output. Severely elevated levels can lead to peripheral vasodilation, profound hypotension, conduction abnormalities, sinus bradycardia, and ventricular arrhythmias.

**Answer: B**

Brown, D.L., Ransom, D.M., and Hall, J.A. (1995) Regional anesthesia and local anesthetic-induced systemic toxicity: seizure frequency and accompanying cardiovascular changes. *Anesthesia & Analgesia*, **81** (2), 321–328.
Morishima, H.O., Pedersen, H., Finster, M., *et al.* (1985) Bupivicaine toxicity in pregnant and nonpregnant ewes. *Anesthesiology*, **63** (2), 134–139.
Mulroy, M.F. (2002) Systemic toxicity and cardiotoxicity from local anesthetics: incidence and preventive measures. *Regional Anesthesia & Pain Medicine*, **27** (6), 556–561.

13 *A 37-year-old woman underwent epidural anesthesia during her paniculectomy. Postoperatively, she was diagnosed with a postdural puncture headache. The most common symptoms include which of the following?*
A *Bilateral, frontal headache with relief when standing*
B *Bilateral, frontal headache with relief when supine*
C *Headaches associated with light sensitivity*
D *Headaches associated with loud sounds*
E *Headache with severe nausea and vomiting*

Postdural puncture headaches are associated with cerebrospinal fluid leak and decreased intracranial pressure after dural puncture. It can have associated ocular disturbances and auditory difficulties. The most common symptom is bilateral, frontal, or occipital headache that is relieved when supine. It is usually benign and self-limited. The most effective treatment is an epidural blood patch.

**Answer: B**

Liu, S.S. and McDonald, S.B. (2001) Current issues in spinal anesthesia [comment]. *Anesthesiology*, **94** (5), 888–906.

Safa-Tisseront, V., Thormann, F., Malassine, P., *et al.* (2001) Effectiveness of epidural blood patch in the management of post-dural puncture headache [comment]. *Anesthesiology*, **95** (2), 334–339.

Vercauteren, M.P., Hoffmann, V.H., Mertens, E., *et al.* (1999) Seven-year review of requests for epidural blood patches for headache after dural puncture: referral patterns and the effectiveness of blood patches. *European Journal of Anaesthesiology*, **16** (5), 298–303.

**14** *Hypothermia has been suggested as a factor in which perioperative complication?*
   **A** *Coagulopathy*
   **B** *Surgical wound infection*
   **C** *Cardiac morbidity*
   **D** *All of the above*
   **E** *None of the above*

Coagulopathy, wound infection, and cardiac morbidity are all implicated the effects of hypothermia perioperatively. Studies have demonstrated that hypothermia can be deleterious in the function of the proteins in the coagulopathy cascade. Perioperative hypothermia has been associated with an increased risk of wound infections. Maintenance of normothermia in non-cardiac surgery is associated with reduced incidence of cardiac events.

**Answer: D**

Flores-Maldonado, A., Medina-Escobedo, C.E., Rios-Rodriguez, H.M., and Fernandez-Dominguez, R. (2001) Mild perioperative hypothermia and the risk of wound infection. *Archives of Medical Research*, **32** (3), 227–231.

Frank, S.M., Fleisher, L.A., Breslow, M.J., *et al.* (1997) Perioperative maintenance of normothermia reduces the incidence of morbid cardiac events: a randomized clinical trial. *Journal of the American Medical Association*, **227** (14), 1127–1134.

Krause, K.R., Howells, G.A., Buhs, C.L., *et al.* (2000) Hypothermia-induced coagulopathy during hemorrhagic shock. *The American Surgeon*, **66** (4), 348–354.

Melling, A.C., Ali, B., Scott, E.M., and Leaper, D.J. (2001) Effects of preoperative warming on the incidence of wound infection after clean surgery: a randomized controlled trial. *The Lancet*, **358** (9285), 876–880.

Mitrophanov, A.Y., Rosendaal, F.R., and Reifman, J. (2013) Computational analysis of the effects of reduced temperature on thrombin generation: the contributions of hypothermia to coagulopathy. *Anesthesia & Analgesia*, **117** (3), 565–574.

Sessler, D.I. (2001) Complications and treatment of mild hypothermia. *Anesthesiology*, **95** (2), 531–543.

**15** *A 33-year-old woman is undergoing a laparoscopic cholecystectomy. After induction of anesthesia, where succinylcholine was used, the patient developed malignant hyperthermia. What is the most sensitive indicator of malignant hyperthermia?*
   **A** *Tachycardia*
   **B** *Tachypnea*
   **C** *Diaphoresis*
   **D** *Skeletal muscle rigidity*
   **E** *Increase in end tidal $CO_2$*

All of the above symptoms can be seen in a patient with malignant hyperthermia. Additionally, patients can have diaphoresis, myoglobinuria, myoglobinemia, hyperkalemia, hypercalcemia, and mixed acidosis. The most sensitive indicator is an unanticipated increase of the end-tidal $CO_2$ concentration. The specific cause of malignant hypertension is not known, but the role of increased intracellular calcium is implicated.

**Answer: E**

MacLennan, D.H. and Phillips, M.S. (1992) Malignant hyperthermia. *Science*, **256** (5058), 789–794.

Rosenberg, H. and Frank, S.M. (1999) Causes and consequences of hypothermia and hyperthermia, in *Anesthesia and Perioperative Complications*, 2nd edn (eds J.L. Benumof and L.J. Saidman), Mosby, St. Louis, MO, pp. 338–356.

**16** *Which of the following local anesthetics is classified as an ester?*
   **A** *Procaine*
   **B** *Lidocaine*
   **C** *Bupivacaine*
   **D** *Mepivacaine*
   **E** *Prilocaine*

Local anesthetics may be classified as amino esters or amino amides. Ester-linked local anesthetics are readily hydrolyzed in aqueous solution. Amide-linked anesthetics are relatively resistant to hydrolysis. The important difference between amides and esters, clinically, is that amides are metabolized in the liver. Esters are metabolized by plasma. Also, esters tend to have metabolites with a higher allergenic potential.

**Answer: A**

Dorian, R.S. (2005) Anesthesia of the surgical patient, in *Schwartz's Principles of Surgery* (ed. F.C. Brunicardi), McGraw-Hill, New York, pp. 1851–1873.

**17** *The development of hypotension during moderate sedation requires which of the following?*
  **A** *Aggressive volume and blood replacement*
  **B** *Vasodilating drugs*
  **C** *Vasopressors*
  **D** *Continuous monitoring to ensure that sedation is maintained*
  **E** *All of the above*

Hemodynamic instability is the most common cardiovascular complication occurring during moderate sedation. The direct cardiodepressant effect of many of the sedating drugs causes hypotension in the patient. A patient with pre-existing compromised circulatory volume is at the greatest risk for this complication. Hypotension may require aggressive volume and blood replacement to prevent low circulating pressures. In acute cases, vasoactive drugs may be required to supplement the patient's hemodynamic status. Other causes of hypotension could be pain histamine release. It is important that the cause of hypotension be identified so that proper therapy can be instituted to correct the problem.

**Answer: A**

Waston, D. (1998) *Conscious Sedation/Analgesia*, Mosby, St. Louis, MO.

**18** *The target level of sedation for a patient not expected to require mechanical ventilation for greater than 48 hours is:*
  **A** *RASS +4 (combative)*
  **B** *RASS +2 (agitated)*
  **C** *RASS -2 (light sedation)*
  **D** *RASS -4 (deep sedation)*
  **E** *RASS -5 (unarousable)*

Unless contraindicated, the optimal level of sedation is where the patient is alert, not agitated, able to maintain brief contact, and follow simple commands. This correlates to RASS 0 to -2 (see Table 12.1). A higher RASS score would lead to behavior that could be detrimental to their care. A lower RASS score would be preferred if long-term sedation is expected.

**Answer: C**

Robinson, B.R., Meuller, E.W., Henson, K., *et al.* (2008) An analgesia-delirium-sedation protocol for critically ill trauma patients reduces ventilator days and hospital length of stay. *Journal of Trauma: Injury, Infection, & Critical Care*, **65** (3), 517–526.

Sessler, C.N., Gosnell, M., Grap, M.J., *et al.* (2002) The Richmond Agitation-Sedation Scale: validity and

**Table 12.1** Richmond Agitation and Sedation Scale (RASS).

| +4 | Combative | Violent, immediate danger to staff |
|---|---|---|
| +3 | Very Agitated | Pulls or removes tubes(s) or catheters(s); aggressive |
| +2 | Agitated | Frequent non-purposeful movement, fights ventilator |
| +1 | Restless | Anxious, apprehensive but movements not aggressive or vigorous |
| 0 | Alert and calm | |
| −1 | Drowsy | Not fully alert, but has sustained awakening to voice (eye opening and contact ≥ 10 sec) |
| −2 | Light sedation | Briefly awakens to voice (eye opening and contact < 10 sec) |
| −3 | Moderate sedation | Movement or eye opening to voice (but no eye contact) |
| −4 | Deep sedation | No response to voice, but movement or eye opening to physical stimulation |
| −5 | Unarousable | No response to voice or physical stimulation |

reliability in adult intensive care patients. *American Journal of Respiratory and Critical Care Medicine*, **166**, 1338–1344.

Shapiro, M.B., West, M.A., Nathens, A.B., *et al.* (2007) Guidelines for sedation and analgesia during mechanical ventilation general overview. *The Journal of Trauma: Injury, Infection, and Critical Care*, **63** (4), 945–950.

**19** *Which of the following induction agents also has analgesic properties?*
  **A** *Midazolam*
  **B** *Lorazepam*
  **C** *Ketamine*
  **D** *Propofol*
  **E** *Thiopental*

Ketamine is classified as a dissociative anesthetic. It produces amnesia and analgesia. The other agents have amnestic properties, but provide no analgesia. Using a benzodiazepine in conjunction with ketamine can decrease the side effect of delirium and hallucinations, which is associated with ketamine.

**Answer: C**

Haas, D.A. and Harper, D.G. (1992) Ketamine: a review of its pharmacologic properties and use in ambulatory anesthesia. *Anesthesia Progress: A Journal for Pain and Anxiety Control in Dentistry*, **39** (3), 61–68.

Himmelseher, S. and Durieux, M.E. (2005) Ketamine for perioperative pain management. *Anesthesiology*, **102** (1), 211–220.

Kwok, R.F., Lim, J., Chan, M., *et al.* (2004) Preoperative ketamine improves postoperative analgesia after gynecologic laparoscopic surgery. *Anesthesia & Analgesia*, **98** (4), 1044–1049.

**20** *Which of the following medications provides anesthesia without decreasing respiratory drive?*
   **A** *Thiopental*
   **B** *Propofol*
   **C** *Midazolam*
   **D** *Diazepam*
   **E** *Dexmedetomidine*

Dexmedetomidine (i.e., Precedex) provides anesthesia without decreasing respiratory drive. It works through the CNS, as an alpha-2 receptor agonist. The other medications provide anesthesia, but are also associated with a depression in respiratory drive. Thiopental is categorized as a barbiturate. It is a GABA agonist, and can cause respiratory depression. Its use has been decreased, due to more recently developed medication regimens. Propofol is a hypnotic agent, with only partially understood mechanism of action. While it has a rapid onset and short half-life, it has a common effect of respiratory depression. Midazolam and Diazepam are benzodiazepines. They are often used as anxiolytics, but both have a historic association with a decrease in respiratory drive.

**Answer: E**

Bhana, N., Goa, K.L., and McClellan, K.J. (2000) Dexmedetomidine. *Drugs*, **59** (2), 263–268.

Eames, W.O., Rooke, G.A., Wu, R.S., and Bishop, M.J. (1996) Comparison of the effects of etomidate, propofol, and thiopental on respiratory resistance after tracheal intubation. *Anesthesiology*, **84** (6), 1307–1311.

Venn, R.M. and Grounds, R.M. (2001) Comparison between dexmedetomidine and propofol for sedation in the intensive care unit: Patient and clinician perceptions. *British Journal of Anaesthesia*, **87** (5), 684–690.

# 13

# Delirium, Alcohol Withdrawal, and Psychiatric Disorders
*Peter Bendix, MD and Ali Salim, MD*

**1** Which of the following is true regarding delirium?
  **A** *It is a diagnosis that requires formal psychiatric evaluation*
  **B** *It is uncommon in elderly, frail, postoperative patients*
  **C** *It is not associated with higher mortality*
  **D** *Decreased acetylcholine is associated with delirium*
  **E** *Dementia is a prerequisite for the development of delirium*

Delirium is an acute illness frequently found in the intensive care unit. It is often diagnosed and treated by the medical and surgical ICU treatments teams and does not require formal psychiatric consultation. Any physician familiar with the clinical signs and symptoms, as defined by the DSM-V, can make the diagnosis:

1) Disturbance in attention (inability to direct, focus, sustain, and shift attention) and awareness
2) Acute onset – hours to days – as a change from baseline, and has a waxing and waning character
3) Disturbance in cognition (memory deficit, disorientation, language, visuospatial ability, or perception)
4) Disturbance is not better explained by preexisting neurocognitive disorder or in the setting of coma
5) Evidence from the formal evaluation that the disorder is caused by a medical condition, intoxication or withdrawal, or medication side effect

It is a very common condition in the hospital and the ICU, with its incidence higher in the more acutely ill, more frail and elderly, and in postoperative patients. Elderly surgical patients are at high risk of developing delirium, with some estimates from the literature suggesting an incidence of 50%. High rates are seen in intensive care units, with as many as 70% of patients experiencing delirium. Worse short- and long-term outcomes have been measured in patients with severe delirium in the ICU.

Acetylcholine is the neurotransmitter which has been proposed as the final common pathway for the development of delirium. It has been observed that anticholinergic drugs can potentiate the development of delirium. Medications, inflammatory states, and the underlying absence of cholinergic neurons in conditions like Alzheimer's disease can all lead to insufficient acetylcholine and the development of delirium.

Risk factors associated with delirium are broad, but one group of patients is at much higher risk than all others; those with underlying degenerative brain disease such as dementia. And although dementia is not a prerequisite for the development of delirium and cannot be diagnosed during an episode of delirium, some studies have shown high rates of dementia diagnosis in the five years following an episode of delirium.

**Answer: D**

American Psychiatric Association (2013) *Diagnostic and Statistical Manual*, 5th edn, APA Press, Washington, DC.

Campbell, N., Boustani, M., Limbil, T., *et al.* (2009) The cognitive impact of anticholinergics: a clinical review. *Clinical Interventions in Aging*, **24**, 225–233.

Ely, E.W., Shintani, A., Truman, B., *et al.* (2004) Delirium as a predictor of mortality in mechanically ventilated patients in the intensive care unit. *Journal of the Amweican Medical Association*, **291** (14), 1753–1762.

Fick, D.M., Agostini, J.V., and Inouye, S.K. (2002) Delirium superimposed on dementia: a systematic review. *Journal of the American Geriatrics Society*, **50** (10), 1723–1732.

Francis, J. (1992) Delirium in older patients. *Journal of the American Geriatrics Society*, **40** (8), 829–838.

Lat, I., McMillian, W., Taylor, S., *et al.* (2009) The impact of delirium on clinical outcomes in mechanically ventilated surgical and trauma patients. *Critical Care Medicine*, **37** (6), 1898–1905.

Lundstrom, M., Edlund, A., Bucht, G., *et al.* (2003) Dementia after delirium in patients with femoral neck

*Surgical Critical Care and Emergency Surgery: Clinical Questions and Answers*, Second Edition.
Edited by Forrest "Dell" Moore, Peter Rhee, and Gerard J. Fulda.
© 2018 John Wiley & Sons Ltd. Published 2018 by John Wiley & Sons Ltd.
Companion website: www.wiley.com/go/moore/surgical_criticalcare_and_emergency_surgery

fractures. *Journal of the American Geriatrics Society*, **51** (7), 1002–1006.

**2** *A 75-year-old patient is admitted to the ICU following an emergent sigmoid resection for acute perforated diverticulitis. He has early dementia per the medical record. Which intervention would not reduce his risk of developing delirium in the ICU?*
   **A** *Use of his home hearing aids*
   **B** *Daily spontaneous awakening trial*
   **C** *Exercise with physical therapy on postoperative day 1*
   **D** *Exclusive use of opioid pain medication*

Several considerations in the ICU may reduce the incidence of delirium. Behavioral and care interventions such as orientation, cognitive stimulation, the establishment of sleep and wake cycles, early mobilization, use of glasses and hearing aids may all reduce the incidence of delirium in the ICU.

The management of ventilation and sedation in the ICU may impact the incidence of delirium. An ABCDE strategy has been proposed as a strategy to prevent the development of delirium:

a) Awakening: Daily awakening.
b) Breathing: Daily spontaneous breathing trial.
c) Coordination of awakening and spontaneous breathing trial
d) Delirium management according to the Society of Critical Care Medicine guidelines, 2013
e) Exercise and early mobility

The choice of sedative medication has been shown to impact the development of delirium in the ICU. Benzodiazepines – frequently the cornerstones of sedation regimens in the ICU – have now been shown to be more likely to cause delirium than alternatives such as dexmedetomidine.

Pain control is also central to the primary prevention of delirium, although certain populations and medications interact poorly. Nonopioid pain medications such as acetaminophen should be used preferentially, and alternatives such as ketamine may be effective for delirium prevention.

**Answer: D**

Barr, J., Fraser, G.L., Puntillo, K., *et al.* (2013) Clinical practice guidelines for the management of pain, agitation, and delirium in adult patients in the Intensive Care Unit: executive summary. *American Journal of Health-System Pharmacy*, **70** (1), 53–58.

Clegg, A. and Young, J.B. (2011) Which medications to avoid in people at risk of delirium: a systematic review. *Age and Ageing*, **40** (1), 23–29.

Deutschman, C.S.N. and Patrick, J. (2015) *Evidence-Based Practice of Critical Care*, Elsevier Health Sciences, Saint Louis.

Inouye, S.K., Bogardus, S.T., Jr., Charpentier, P.A., *et al.* (1999) A multicomponent intervention to prevent delirium in hospitalized older patients. *The New England Journal of Medicine*, **340** (9), 669–676.

Pandharipande, P.P., Pun, B.T., Herr, D.L., *et al.* (2007) Effect of sedation with dexmedetomidine vs. lorazepam on acute brain dysfunction in mechanically ventilated patients: the MENDS randomized controlled trial. *Journal of the American Medical Association*, **298** (22), 2644–2653.

Schweickert, W.D., Pohlman, M.C., Pohlman, A.S., *et al.* (2009) Early physical and occupational therapy in mechanically ventilated, critically ill patients: a randomized controlled trial. *Lancet*, **373** (9678), 1874–1882.

**3** *A 67-year-old patient is admitted to the ICU follow a motor vehicle collision with a subdural hemorrhage, bilateral rib fractures with hemopneumothorax, and a right femur fracture. On post-injury day 7, the patient is extubated. He is transferred out of the ICU. On post-injury day 10, he becomes agitated with his nurse, almost pulling out his left chest tube. Which feature would not be part of her CAM evaluation of the patient?*
   **A** *The acute onset of his mental status change*
   **B** *His distractability and lack of attention*
   **C** *His violent swings at the patient care assistant*
   **D** *His hypervigilant stare*

The evaluation of delirium should begin with clinical suspicion informed by the definition supplied above from the DSM-V. This should be weighed in relation to the patient's clinical history and presentation.

Suspicion for delirium should then prompt the use of the Confusion Assessment Method (CAM) tool (Table 13.1). This tool has a high sensitivity and specificity for the diagnosis of delirium. For patients in the ICU who are ventilated and sedated, the CAM-ICU can be used.

**Answer: C**

Deutschman, C.S.N. and Patrick, J. (2015) *Evidence-Based Practice of Critical Care*, Elsevier Health Sciences, Saint Louis.

Inouye, S.K., van Dyck, C.H., Alessi, C.A., *et al.* (1990) Clarifying confusion: the confusion assessment method. A new method for detection of delirium. *Annals of Internal Medicine*, **113** (12), 941–948.

**4** *An 87-year-old woman without alcohol use or other medication use history who is hospitalized for a recurrent small bowel obstruction has a nasogastric tube, a triple lumen central catheter, and is on telemetry.*

**Table 13.1** Confusion assessment method to assess delirium (CAM).

| Feature | Assessment |
| --- | --- |
| Acute onset and fluctuating course | Based on change from patient's baseline. Positive response to: "Is this mental status change acute?" "Is this mental status change fluctuating during the course of the day?" |
| Inattention | Positive response to: "Is there difficulty focusing attention, distractibility, or difficulty keeping track of what is being said?" |
| Disorganized thinking | Positive response to: Are there rambling, irrelevant conversation, unclear, illogical thoughts, frequent and unpredictable switching from subject to subject." |
| Altered level of consciousness | Positive response if other than "alert" |
| | Normal = alert |
| | Hyper alert = vigilant |
| | Drowsy, easily aroused = lethargic |
| | Difficult to arouse = stupor |
| | Unarousable = coma |
| *Delirium =* | Features 1 AND 2 + either 3 OR 4 |

*She is in a double bed room, without a window, near the nursing station. On hospital day five she becomes tachycardic, hypertensive, and agitated, striking her nurse. The intern is called to the bedside. Which of the following would be inappropriate?*

**A** *Review of MAR and recent labs*
**B** *Haloperidol*
**C** *Benzodiazepine*
**D** *Moving the patient to a different room*
**E** *Restraints*

The primary evaluation of the delirious patient should include a review of their medical and social history. This should include an investigation for the use of prior psychotropic medications, drugs, and alcohol. It should also include a review of the patient's current medications and the search for signs of metabolic derangements such as liver failure. Medications are a frequent cause of delirium.

Haloperidol is a traditional antipsychotic. Its mechanism of action is blocking dopamine receptors in the CNS. Side-effects of administration include extrapyramidal reactions, neuroleptic malignant syndrome, and QT prolongation/torsade de pointes. It is the current first-line therapy for the management of acute agitated delirium, although recent meta-analysis has shed doubt on its efficacy as a method of prevention.

Multicomponent therapy with behavioral interventions such as exposure to natural light and sleep cycle modifications of nursing care are important components of delirium management, both in primary prevention and treatment. This is discussed earlier in question 2.

It may be necessary to protect both the staff and the patient from the consequences of acute agitated delirium. This may require restraints to avoid the dislodgement of lines and to allow the administration of medical therapy. It is important to document the application of such interventions and adhere to clinical protocols with frequent reassessment for cessation.

There is no role for routine benzodiazepine administration in the treatment of delirium. In fact, these medications may potentiate delirium. Acutely agitated patients who are not candidates for antipsychotic medications may require emergent benzodiazepine treatment, but current evidence suggests less potentiation of delirium with the use of dexmedetomidine.

**Answer: C**

Baron, R., Binder, A., Biniek, R., *et al.* (2015) Evidence and consensus-based guideline for the management of delirium, analgesia, and sedation in intensive care medicine. Revision 2015 (DAS-Guideline 2015) – short version. *German Medical Science: GMS e-journal.* **13**, Doc19.

Lacasse, H., Perreault, M.M., and Williamson, D.R. (2006) Systematic review of antipsychotics for the treatment of hospital-associated delirium in medically or surgically ill patients. *The Annals of Pharmacotherapy*, **40** (11), 1966–1973.

Neufeld, K.J., Yue, J., Robinson, T.N., *et al.* (2016) Inouye SK, Needham DM. Antipsychotic medication for prevention and treatment of delirium in hospitalized adults: a systematic review and meta-analysis. *Journal of the American Geriatrics Society*, **64** (4), 705–714.

Siddiqi, N., Harrison, J.K., Clegg, A., *et al.* (2016) Interventions for preventing delirium in hospitalized non-ICU patients. *The Cochrane Database of Systematic Reviews*, **3**, Cd005563.

**5** *A 72-year-old woman is discharged from the hospital after a one-month stay following an incarcerated ventral hernia repair. During her admission she had a week- long episode of delirium follow extubation in the intensive care unit. What statement accurately reflects her long-term risks given her episode of delirium?*

**A** *Each additional day of delirium may have conferred additional risk of mortality*
**B** *She is at no long-term risk of cognitive impairment*

**C** *She is at no long-term risk of mortality given her episode of delirium*

**D** *If she had preexisting Alzheimer's disease, the episode of delirium will not impact her dementia progression*

This patient's episode of delirium is very significant to her long-term prognosis and recovery. It is a key component of her prolonged critical illness and conveys a significant risk to her long-term survival and cognitive prognosis.

Studies have shown that patients with delirium during their hospitalization are at double the risk of death in the first month and at six months after discharge. It is also known that the duration of the episode of delirium directly impacts long-term survival, with more days of delirium associated with shorter survival. In hospital, delirium has also been shown to be predictive of long-term cognitive impairment and to accelerate cognitive decline in dementia patients.

**Answer: A**

Fong, T.G., Jones, R.N., Shi, P., *et al.* (2009) Delirium accelerates cognitive decline in Alzheimer disease. *Neurology*, **72** (18). 1570–1575.

Girard, T.D., Jackson, J.C., Pandharipande, P.P., *et al.* (2010) Delirium as a predictor of long-term cognitive impairment in survivors of critical illness. *Critical Care Medicine*, **38** (7), 1513–1520.

McAvay, G.J., Van Ness, P.H., Bogardus, S.T., Jr., *et al.* (2006) Older adults discharged from the hospital with delirium: 1-year outcomes. *Journal of the American Geriatrics Society*, **54** (8), 1245–1250.

Pisani, M.A., Kong, S.Y., Kasl, S.V., *et al.* (2009) Days of delirium are associated with 1-year mortality in an older intensive care unit population. *American Journal of Respiratory and Critical Care Medicine*, **180** (11), 1092–1097.

Robinson, T.N., Raeburn, C.D., Tran, Z.V., *et al.* (2009) Postoperative delirium in the elderly: risk factors and outcomes. *Annals of Surgery*, **249** (1), 173–178.

**6** *A 37-year-old man is admitted following a motorcycle crash, with a right open femur fracture. On postinjury day three, he becomes tachycardic and hypertensive and is oriented only to himself. What are the two central neurotransmitters responsible for the physiology of his current presentation?*

**A** *Dopamine and Gamma-aminobutyric acid*

**B** *Glutamate and Gamma-aminobutyric acid*

**C** *Glutamate and Dopamine*

**D** *Serotonin and Gamma-aminobutyric acid*

The two central neurotransmitters responsible for the pathophysiology of alcohol withdrawal are gamma-aminobutyric acid (GABA) and glutamate. As an inhibitory neurotransmitter, GABA functions to suppress arousal. Chronic alcohol use induces the creation of greater numbers of GABA receptors, and the absence of the alcohol stimulation at the GABA receptors leads the absence of the chronic inhibitory signals to which the individual has become habituated. This underlies the treatment of alcohol withdrawal with benzodiazepine medications, which also function at the GABA receptor.

Glutamate functions in the opposite manner from GABA, as it is an excitatory neurotransmitter. Chronic alcohol use dampens glutamate action at its receptor, leading to increased receptor expression. When alcohol is abruptly taken away from the habituated person, these receptors lead to over excitation.

**Answer: B**

Mihic, S.J., Ye, Q., Wick, M.J., *et al.* (1997) Sites of alcohol and volatile anesthetic action on GABA(A) and glycine receptors. *Nature*, **389** (6649), 385–389.

Tsai, G., Gastfriend, D.R., and Coyle, J.T. (1995) The glutamatergic basis of human alcoholism. *American Journal of Psychiatry*, **152** (3), 332–340.

**7** *The same man in the question above is now diagnosed with delirium tremens. Which of the below medications is not part of the current standard of care for treatment of severe alcohol withdrawal?*

**A** *Alcohol*

**B** *Thiamine*

**C** *Diazepam*

**D** *Chlordiazepoxide*

Delirium tremens may begin between 48 and 96 hours after the patient's last drink. It is a clinical diagnosis based on the presence of a constellation of signs and symptoms:

- Hallucinations
- Disorientation
- Tachycardia
- Tachypnea
- Hypertension
- Hyperthermia
- Agitation and diaphoresis

The metabolic derangements of delirium tremens can include alkalosis from the tachypnea, hyponatremia, and hypokalemia with attendant dehydration. Supportive care to attend to these metabolic derangements is essential for the treatment of alcohol withdrawal. Thiamine and folate should be given to counteract Wernicke's encephalopathy.

**Table 13.2** Richmond Agitation Sedation Score (RASS).

| Score | Term |
| --- | --- |
| +4 | Combative |
| +3 | Very agitated |
| +2 | Agitated |
| +1 | Restless |
| 0 | Alert and calm |
| −1 | Drowsy |
| −2 | Light sedation |
| −3 | Moderate sedation |
| −4 | Deep sedation |
| −5 | Unarousable |

The current standard of care for the treatment of acute alcohol withdrawal is to use a symptom-triggered strategy following the Clinical Institute Withdrawal Assessment for Alcohol Scale (CIWA-Ar). Both IV and oral benzodiazepine regimens have been used to treat in response to positive scores on the CIWA-Ar scale. Calculators are available online for CIWA-Ar use. For intubated patients unable to verbalize, the Richmond Agitation Sedation Score (Table 13.2) may be used to assess for sedation.

Benzodiazepine therapy guided by the CIWA-Ar or RASS evaluations are the central therapy for the psychomotor agitation. Diazepam, lorazepam, oxazepam, and chlordiazepoxide are all used in response to positive scoring on the assessments.

Alternative therapies have not been shown to be superior to benzodiazepines in the treatment of alcohol withdrawal in the intensive care unit. Alcohol has been studied and found inferior.

**Answer: A**

Hodges, B. and Mazur, J.E. (2004) Intravenous ethanol for the treatment of alcohol withdrawal syndrome in critically ill patients. *Pharmacotherapy*, **24** (11), 1578–1585.

Mayo-Smith, M.F., Beecher, L.H., Fischer, T.L., *et al.* (2004) Management of alcohol withdrawal delirium. An evidence-based practice guideline. *Archives of Internal Medicine*, **164** (13), 1405–1412.

Ntais, C., Pakos, E., Kyzas, P., *et al.* (2005) Benzodiazepines for alcohol withdrawal. Cochrane Database Systematic Reviews, **5**(3).

Sessler, C.N., Gosnell, M.S., Grap, M.J., *et al.* (2002) The Richmond Agitation-Sedation Scale: validity and reliability in adult intensive care unit patients. *American Journal of Respiratory and Critical Care Medicine*, **166** (10), 1338–1344.

8 *A 45-year-old woman is admitted to the medical ICU after being found down outside the city's shopping mall, with a stab wound to her flank. She has a negative emergent exploratory laparotomy. Her medical history is unknown. On her first day in the intensive care unit, she is stable, is extubated, and admits to drinking a case of beer per day, along with a large bottle of wine each night. She begins to withdraw from alcohol at 48h. What is she not at higher risk for, given her alcohol use and withdrawal?*
   **A** *Sepsis*
   **B** *Hospital Mortality*
   **C** *Organ Failure*
   **D** *Short hospitalization*
   **E** *Liver failure*

Patients with alcohol dependence who have sepsis or liver failure have more than twice the risk for hospital mortality. A 2007 study published in *Critical Care Medicine* demonstrated that ICU patients with alcohol dependence had higher rates of sepsis (12.9% versus 7.6%, p .001), organ failure (67.3% versus 45.8%, p .001), septic shock (3.6% versus 2.1%, p = .001), and hospital mortality (9.4% versus 7.5%, p = .022), with fewer hospital-free days. Also, among patients with sepsis and liver failure, alcohol dependence increased the likelihood for hospital mortality by more than twofold. Patients with alcohol dependence may have a predilection to infection due to abnormalities in their immune systems (many such abnormalities have been demonstrated in animal models). Also, patients with chronic excessive use of alcohol have complicating medical conditions resulting from the substance abuse, such as cardiomyopathy, dysrhythmias, and cirrhosis.

**Answer: D**

O'Brien, J.M., Jr., Lu, B., Ali, N.A., *et al.* (2007) Alcohol dependence is independently associated with sepsis, septic shock, and hospital mortality among adult intensive care unit patients. *Critical Care Medicine*, **35** (2), 345–350.

9 *A 23-year-old man is admitted to the trauma service after he jumped off a footbridge in the local park. He has bilateral ankle fractures and an L4 compression fracture. On morning rounds he stares intently at the computer in his room and states that the machine is reading his thoughts. What are some of the initial management strategies for his presentation?*
   **A** *Emergent evaluation by the psychiatry service*
   **B** *Administration of an antipsychotic medication*
   **C** *Legal hold in the hospital with involuntary treatment*
   **D** *Medical evaluation for alternative etiology*
   **E** *All of the above*

Psychosis is characterized by some constellation of the following: delusions, hallucinations, disorganized thinking, and/or agitation and aggression. Acute primary psychoses are often familial in nature, with initial insidious presentations of the condition in the patient's teens and young adulthood. Medically induced psychoses often do not fit this pattern and instead are seen in patients with significant medical comorbidities, polypharmacy, and often present acutely, with little prodrome of behavior change.

The initial management of a patient exhibiting psychosis should be done in conjunction with the psychiatry service. Primary psychoses are chronic, life-threatening illnesses that will require consistent management in the outpatient setting. The establishment of clinical stability with the initial administration of an antipsychotic medication should be performed with an understanding of the frequent adverse effects of these medications. These can range in severity, from weight gain to sedation and extrapyramidal effects.

Ruling out medical etiologies is essential in most initial presentations of psychosis. Common etiologies are listed below:

- Delirium
- Endocrinopathies
- Hepatic/uremic encephalopathy
- Infectious diseases (HIV)
- Inflammatory disorders and demyelinating disorders, neurodegenerative conditions
- Metabolic disorders, vitamin deficiencies

Patients at risk to themselves or others are subject to involuntary hospitalization in most legal jurisdictions. Understanding the local laws regarding involuntary hospitalization and treatment are essential to any critical care provider.

**Answer: E**

American Psychiatric Association (2013) *Diagnostic and Statistical Manual*, 5th edn, APA Press, Washington, DC.

Sheitman, B.B., Lee, H., Strauss, R., *et al.* (1997) The evaluation and treatment of first-episode psychosis. *Schizophrenia Bulletin*, **23** (4), 653–661.

Webster, R. and Holroyd, S. (2000) Prevalence of psychotic symptoms in delirium. *Psychosomatics*, **41** (6), 519–522.

# 14

## Acid-Base, Fluid, and Electrolytes

*Joshua Dilday, DO, Asser Youssef, MD and Nicholas Thiessen, MD*

1   *A 50-year old, 70 kg man presents as a trauma after a motor vehicle accident. He is diagnosed with a traumatic brain injury and was admitted to the hospital. On hospital day 3, he is arousable but disoriented and complaining of thirst. On examination, he has clear lung sounds bilaterally, heart rate of 70 beats/min, and a blood pressure of 140/80 mm Hg. With IV normal saline set at 100 mL/hr, his urine output is 300 mL/hr for the past 12 hours. His laboratory values include: Na 160 mEq/L, K 4.3 mEq/L, Cl 105 mEq/L, $HCO_3$ 25 mEq/L, BUN 30 mg/dL, Cr 1.2 mg/dL, CVP is 3 mm Hg, Uosm is 160 mOsm/L.*

   *What is the most likely pathophysiology of the above scenario?*
   A   *Lack of renal response to anti-diuretic hormone*
   B   *Lack of anterior pituitary gland release of anti-diuretic hormone*
   C   *Overstimulation and release of anti-diuretic hormone*
   D   *Lack of posterior pituitary gland release of anti-diuretic hormone*
   E   *Excess resuscitation with saline*

Central diabetes insipidus (DI) is a failure of anti-diuretic hormone (ADH) released from the posterior pituitary gland. Causes include head trauma, encephalopathy, and meningitis. Central DI differs from nephrogenic DI; nephrogenic DI is a lack of end-organ responsiveness while central DI is a lack of ADH release. Central DI manifests as polyuria with dilute urine in setting of hypertonic plasma. Urine osmolarity is often < 200 mosm/L. Failure of the urine osmolarity to increase after fluid restriction is diagnostic confirmation. Treatment is aimed at replacing free water deficits and vasopressin, an ADH analogue.

**Answer: D**

Geheb, M.A. (1987) Clinical approach to the hyperosmolar patient. *Critical Care Clinics,* **3** (4), 797–815.
Makaryus, A.N. and McFarlane, S.I. (2006) Diabetes insipidus: diagnosis and treatment of a complex disease. *Cleveland Clinic Journal of Medicine,* **73** (1), 65–71.
Robertson, G.L. (2016) Diabetes insipidus: differential diagnosis and management. *Best Practice & Research Clinical Endocrinology & Metabolism,* **30** (2), 205–218.

2   *In the above patient, what is the free water deficit?*
   A   *4.5 L*
   B   *3.5 L*
   C   *6 L*
   D   *2 L*
   E   *3 L*

The above patient has central diabetes insipidus, leading to a hypernatremic state. The patient is unable to concentrate urine due to decreased ADH. Hypernatremia due to free water loss is managed by free water replacement. The free water deficit must first be calculated to determine the amount of replacement.

   Free water deficit formula = 0.6 (kg) x (Current Na/140 − 1) → 0.6 (70) x (160/140 − 1) = 6 L

**Answer: C**

Adrogué, H.J. and Madias, N.E. (2000) Hyponatremia. *New England Journal of Medicine,* **342** (21), 1581–1589.
Marino, P.L. and Sutin, K.M. (2014) *The ICU Book,* 4th edn, Lippincot Williams & Wilkins, Philadelphia, PA.
Pokaharel, M. and Block, C.A. (2011) Dysnatremia in the ICU. *Current Opinion in Critical Care,* **17** (6), 581–593.

3   *Your patient is postoperative day 1 from a pancreaticoduodenectomy for a tumor in the head of the pancreas. His serum sodium is 133 mEq/L. Currently the*

*patient is receiving an intravenous infusion of normal saline at 150 ml/hr. The urine output has been about 55 ml/hr. The patient appears warm, with mild edema in the lower extremities. Regarding fluid management, what should you do next?*

**A** *Increase normal saline rate to 175 ml/hr*
**B** *Change IV fluids to D5 ½ NS at 100 mL/hr*
**C** *Change IV fluids to lactated Ringers at 150 mL/hr*
**D** *Maintain current IV fluid and decrease rate to 100 mL/hr*
**E** *Maintain current IV fluid and rate*

Hypotonic hyponatremia results from either massive water intake, exceeding the capacity to excrete free water, or impaired water excretion. There are multiple causes of acute hyponatremia such as the syndrome of inappropriate antidiuretic hormone release, psychogenic self-induced water intoxication, excessive sweating, or use of cyclophosphamide, ecstasy (MDMA), or oxytocin. Non-hypotonic causes of hyponatremia include IgG therapy, irrigant absorption for prostate or intrauterine surgery, hyperglycemia and hyperlipidemia. In the above scenario, postoperative hyponatremia is caused by vasopressin secretion in response to surgical stress. Vasopressin could be secreted for two or more days postoperatively. Free water is retained. Sodium and potassium are excreted in the urine at high concentrations. As a result, isotonic fluids are "desalinated" and can lower the plasma sodium concentration. The treatment in this case is to avoid hypotonic fluid and excessive volume of isotonic fluids (NS, LR) after surgery. If symptoms of hyponatremia occur, hypertonic saline and diuretics are used.

**Answer: D**

Gowrishankar, M., Lin, S.H., Mallie, J.P., *et al.* (1998) Acute hyponatremia in the perioperative period: insights into its pathophysiology and recommendations for management. *Clinical Nephrology*, **50**, 352–360.
Steele, A., Gowrishankar, M., Abrahamson, S., *et al.* (1997) Postoperative hyponatremia despite near-isotonic saline infusion: a phenomenon of desalination. *Annals of Internal Medicine*, **126**, 20–25.

**4** *A 60-year-old man with an extensive abdominal surgical history presents with multiple days of colicky abdominal pain, significant nausea and vomiting, and inability to tolerate oral food intake. The patient states that his current symptoms are consistent with his previous episodes of small bowel obstruction. He states that he has vomited 10 times per day for the last four days. Which of the following would most fit in this scenario?*

**A** *Metabolic acidosis, hypokalemia, hyperchloremia, acidic urine*
**B** *Respiratory alkalosis, hypokalemia, hyperchloremia, acidic urine*
**C** *Metabolic alkalosis, hypokalemia, hypochloremia, acidic urine*
**D** *Metabolic alkalosis, hypokalemia, hyperchloremia, alkaline urine*
**E** *Metabolic acidosis, hypokalemia, hypochloremia, acidic urine*
**F** *Respiratory acidosis, hypokalemia, hyperchloremia, alkaline urine*

The above patient is presenting with a small bowel obstruction, likely related to his previous abdominal surgeries. If the vomiting from a small bowel obstruction is significant, it can lead to acid/base and electrolyte abnormalities. Proximal GI losses can cause a contraction metabolic alkalosis. During volume contraction, bicarbonate and sodium are reabsorbed to maintain electrical balance as there is insufficient chloride. The distal convoluted tubules will compensate sodium reabsorption by exchanging hydrogen and potassium. Thus, the kidney will excrete more hydrogen and potassium than usual. The metabolic alkalosis is caused by reabsorption of bicarbonate and loss of hydrogen. Renal potassium loss causes hypokalemia. The chloride is lost from GI losses but compensated by sodium and chloride reabsorption. Paradoxical aciduria is caused by hydrogen loss in exchange for sodium reabsorption.

**Answer: C**

Khanna, A. and Kurtzman, N.A. (2001) Metabolic alkalosis. *Respiratory Care*, **46** (4), 354–365.
Galla, J.H. (2000) Metabolic alkalosis. *Journal of the American Society of Nephrology*, **11** (2), 369–375.
Luke, R.G. and Galla, J.H. (2012) It is chloride depletion alkalosis, not contraction alkalosis. *Journal of the American Society of Nephrology*, **23** (2), 204–207.

**5** *A 58-year-old man is now postoperative day 4 after a colon resection for cancer. On examination, he has mild edema in his lower extremities. His chest x-ray shows mild congestive heart failure. He is receiving normal saline at 125 ml/hr and his serum sodium level is 132 mEq/L. His urine output is 40–50 ml/hr. The patient states he takes diuretics at home on occasion when he develops edema in his legs. How would you treat his serum sodium?*

**A** *Increase IV fluids to 150 ml/hr*
**B** *Decrease IV fluids to 75 ml/hr*
**C** *Treat with thiazide diuretics*

**D** *Change his IV fluids to hypertonic saline*
**E** *Treat with loop diuretics and ACE inhibitors*

One liter of normal saline will increase plasma sodium concentration by 1 mEq/L. Thus treating hyponatremia in edematous patients with saline will only exacerbate the problem. Thiazide diuretics are contraindicated since they block reabsorption of sodium and chloride in the distal tubules and prevent the generation of maximally dilute urine. Loop diuretics are the mainstay of treatment in this case as they improve free water excretion. With the addition of ACE inhibitors, congestive heart failure is treated and vasopressing secretion is reduced.

**Answer: E**

Adrogue, H.J. and Madias, N.E. (2000) Hyponatremia. *New England Journal of Medicine*, **342**, 1581–1589.

Sonnenblick, M., Friedlander, Y., and Rosin, A.J. (1993) Diuretic-induced severe hyponatremia: review and analysis of 129 reported patients. *Chest*, **103**, 601–606.

Sterns, R.H., Silver, S.M., and Spital, A. (2000) *Hyponatremia. The Kidney: Physiology and Pathophysiology*, Lippincott Williams & Wilkins, Philadelphia, PA.

6 *A 60-year-old man is admitted to the ICU after being involved in a multi-car collision. He is found to have multiple long bone fractures, a mesenteric hematoma, and a splenic laceration. He is managed nonoperatively at first, due to the low grade nature of his splenic laceration. However, the patient begins to require multiple infusions of saline boluses to maintain normal blood pressure. Despite multiple boluses, the patient is still hypotensive. Operative intervention is planned due to the persistent hypotension. On the way to the OR, an ABG is drawn and reveals: pH 7.21, $pCO_2$ 34, $pO_2$ 70 mm Hg, $HCO_3$ 18 mEq/L. Which of the following best describes his acid-base status?*
**A** *Primary metabolic alkalosis with respiratory compensation*
**B** *Primary metabolic acidosis with combined respiratory alkalosis*
**C** *Primary metabolic acidosis with respiratory compensation*
**D** *Primary metabolic acidosis with combined respiratory acidosis*
**E** *Primary respiratory alkalosis with metabolic compensation*

The patient has a metabolic acidosis likely from multiple saline boluses in an attempt to control his hypotension. Excessive saline infusion can cause a hyperchloremic non-gap metabolic acidosis. The diagnosis of primary metabolic acidosis is made by the low pH and low plasma $HCO_3$. Once the determination of metabolic acidosis is made, it should be determined if a gap acidosis is present. However, since no electrolytes were given to determine a gap, the next determination should be appropriate respiratory compensation. This can be done utilizing Winters' formula [$pCO_2 = (1.5 \times HCO_3) + 8 \pm 2$]. The formula predicts the expected $pCO_2$ in a primary metabolic acidosis. If the measured $pCO_2$ is greater than expected, a superimposed respiratory acidosis is present. If the measured $pCO_2$ is less than expected, a combined respiratory alkalosis is present. In the case above, the expected $pCO_2 = (1.5 \times 18) + 8 \pm 2 = 35 \pm 2$. The measured $pCO_2$ in the above patient (34) is an expected respiratory compensation for primary metabolic acidosis.

**Answer: C**

Emmett, M. and Narins, R.G. (1977) Clinical use of the anion gap. *Medicine*, **56** (1), 38–54.

Kellum, J.A. (2007) Disorders of acid-base balance. *Critical Care Medicine*, **35** (11), 2630–2636

Winter, S.D., Pearson, J.R., Gabow, P.A., *et al.* (1990) The fall of the serum anion gap. *Archives of Internal Medicine*, **150** (2), 311–313.

7 *A 36-year-old woman is brought to the trauma bay after a fall from a 3rd floor window. In addition to multiple long-bone fractures she is suspected of having a spinal cord injury based on physical exam findings. During the course of her trauma survey and resuscitation, she shows signs of respiratory compromise. Rapid sequence intubation is performed with etomidate and succinylcholine. Shortly after intubation, ECG readings show cardiac arrest. What is the most likely electrolyte abnormality affecting the above situation?*
**A** *Hyperkalemia*
**B** *Hypercalcemia*
**C** *Hypokalemia*
**D** *Hypomagnesia*
**E** *Hypocalcemia*

Succinylcholine is a short acting, depolarizing neuromuscular blocking agent that inhibits the Na-K exchange pump. This effect causes a minor increase in serum potassium. The vast majority of the time, this effect is minimal with no adverse reactions. However, denervation of the skeletal muscle and spinal cord injuries have been associated with life-threatening hyperkalemia after succinylcholine use. This has been attributed to an exaggerated response of depolarization in denervation injuries. Long-bone fractures have also been associated with hyperkalemia due to local tissue damage and release of intracellular potassium. ECG manifestations of hyperkalemia usually began as the serum potassium approaches 7 mEq/L. The earliest changes involve peaked T waves and PR interval lengthening. Hyperkalemia can eventually cause a widened QRS complex, heart block, ventricular fibrillation, and asystole.

**Answer: A**

Gronert, G. A. (2001) Cardiac arrest after succinylcholine: mortality greater with rhabdomyolysis than receptor upregulation. *The Journal of the American Society of Anesthesiologists*, **94** (3), 523–529.

Huggins, R.M., Kennedy, W.K., Melroy, M.J., and Tollerton, D.G. (2003) Cardiac arrest from succinylcholine-induced hyperkalemia. *American Journal of Health-System Pharmacy: AJHP: Official Journal of the American Society of Health-System Pharmacists*, **60** (7), 694–697.

Ponce, S.P., Jennings, A.E., Madias, N.E., and Harrington, J.T. (1985) Drug-induced hyperkalemia. *Medicine*, **64** (6), 357–370.

8   *A 70-year-old man with a long history of alcohol abuse and congestive heart failure is recently admitted for symptoms of altered mental status. The patient is found to be thiamine deficient and is treated with thiamine for suspected alcohol-related altered sensorium. During his hospital stay, the patient complains of vision changes and "changes in colors." An ECG is obtained (Figure 14.1) which shows evidence of digitalis toxicity.*

*In the above patient, what electrolyte abnormality is likely to be seen?*
A  *Hypochloremia*
B  *Hypomagnesemia*
C  *Hypercalcemia*
D  *Hypernatremia*
E  *Hyperchloremia*

Hypomagnesemia can exacerbate digitalis toxicity. While hypokalemia is commonly known to exacerbate digitalis toxicity as well, it is not the only electrolyte abnormality associated. The patient has a known history of alcohol abuse, which has been shown to cause hypomagnesemia in 30% of patients. Since hypokalemia is not an answer choice, hypomagnesemia is the best answer since it is both seen in alcohol abuse and associated with digitalis toxicity.

**Answer: B**

Cohen, L. and Kitzes, R. (1983) Magnesium sulfate and digitalis-toxic arrhythmias. *Journal of the American Medical Association*, **249** (20), 2808–2810.

Seller, R.H., Cangiano, J., Kim, K.E., *et al.* (1970) Digitalis toxicity and hypomagnesemia. *American Heart Journal*, **79** (1), 57–68.

Tong, G.M. and Rude, R.K. (2005) Magnesium deficiency in critical illness. *Journal of Intensive Care Medicine*, **20** (1), 3–17.

9   *A 47-year-old man presents with lower extremity numbness and tingling sensation that has been going*

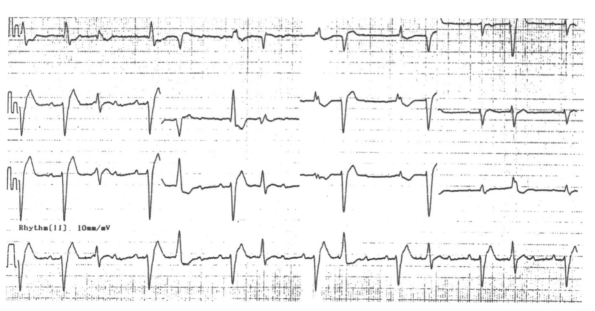

**Figure 14.1**

on for about 2 weeks. Recently, he states that he has developed some weakness in his muscles. His past medical history is unremarkable except for kidney stones. His metabolic panel reveals a potassium level of 6.8 mEq/dL, BUN 35 mg/dL, and Cr 1.5 mg/dL. Other values are within normal limits. A 12-lead EKG reveals elevated T waves and slight widening of QRS complexes. You diagnose him with hyperkalemia from Type 1 renal tubular acidosis (RTA). What is your next plan of action?

A Calcium chloride, glucose infusion with insulin, cation exchange resins
B Glucose infusion with insulin then cation exchange resins
C Glucose infusion with insulin, sodium bicarbonate, then lasix
D Thiazide diuretics, glucose infusion with insulin, then cation exchange resin
E Calcium chloride then dialysis

Multiple disorders are associated with impairment of renal potassium elimination. Most common etiologies are renal failure (impaired distal nephron excretion), severe dehydration, metabolic acidosis (loss of bicarbonate, diarrhea), rhabdomyolysis, RTA (Type 4, hyperkalemic type 1), increased dietary intake, or medication induced (succinylcholine, Beta$_2$-adrenergic blockade, insulin deficiency).

Aggressive treatment to lower serum potassium and to stabilize the cell membrane should be started for high levels of potassium, especially when EKG changes are present. Infusion of calcium raises the threshold excitability potential. Bicarbonate, glucose with insulin, and beta$_2$-adrenergic receptor stimulation lowers serum potassium by promoting potassium movement intracellularly. These measures are temporary, however. For severe or refractory cases, dialysis is warranted.

**Answer: A**

Allon, M. (1995) Hyperkalemia in end-stage renal disease: mechanisms and management. *Journal of the American Society of Nephrology*, **6**, 1134–1142.

Perazella, M.A. (2000) Drug-induced hyperkalemia: old culprits and new offenders. *American Journal of Medicine*, **109**, 307–314.

10 A 70-year-old man was involved in an auto versus pedestrian accident three days ago. He suffered a traumatic brain injury and has been complaining of headaches and hallucinations. Laboratory data: Na 120 mEq/L, K 4.0 mEq/L, Cl 96 mEq/L, bicarbonate 25 mEq/L, BUN 30 mg/dL, Cr 1.8 mg/dL, glucose 160 mg/dL. Urine osmolality 475 mOsm/kg, urine

sodium 196 mEq/L. CVP 4 mm Hg. Physical exam: cervical collar in place, spinal precautions, arousable but disoriented, lungs clear bilaterally with respiratory rate of 8 breaths/min, heart rate 50 beats/min. What would be the appropriate next step in his management?

A Initiation of intravenous normal saline at 150 mL/hr
B Demeclocycline 600 mg × 1 now and twice daily
C Conivaptan 40 mg IV × 1 now and daily for 3 days
D 150 mL/hour of 3% saline infusion × 2 hours
E Fluid restriction and furosemide 20 mg IV × 1 now

The patient is exhibiting symptoms of acute hyponatremia. The laboratory and clinical findings suggest a possible cerebral salt wasting syndrome (CSW), with hypovolemia and high urinary sodium. From a metabolic stand point, 3% saline infusion is administered for hyponatremia to increase serum sodium by 2 mEq/L/hr but not more than 12 mEq/L in the first 24 hours to avoid central pontine myelinolysis. Central pontine and extrapontine myelinolysis begins with lethargy and affective changes (generally after initial improvement of neurologic symptoms with treatment), followed by mutism or dysarthria, spastic quadriparesis, and pseudobulbar palsy. Once 3% saline infusion has started, symptoms should improve.

**Answer: D**

Ellison, D.H. and Berl, T. (2007) The syndrome of inappropriate antidiuresis. *New England Journal of Medicine*, **356** (20), 2064–2072.

Rivkees, S.A. (2008) Differentiating appropriate antidiuretic hormone secretion, inappropriate antidiuretic hormone secretion and cerebral salt wasting: the common, uncommon, and misnamed. *Current Opinion in Pediatrics*, **20** (4), 448–452.

Sterns, R.H. and Silver, S.M. (2008) Cerebral salt wasting versus SIADH: what difference? *Journal of the American Society of Nephrology*, **19** (2), 194–196.

11 A 60-year-old woman underwent an upper endoscopy for GI bleeding, which was readily controlled. The patient was given benzocaine prior to the procedure to anesthetize the posterior oropharynx. Postprocedure, the patient's oxygen saturation is 75% on 2 L nasal cannula. Blood gas reveals pH 7.40, PaCO$_2$ 40 mm Hg, PaO$_2$ 115 mm Hg, HCO$_3$ 24 mEq/L, base excess 0.6 mmol/L; Hgb is 8 g/dl. Electrolytes are normal. Her temperature is 37.0 °C, heart rate 120 beats/min, RR 22 breaths/min and BP 100/80 mm Hg. The patient is dizzy and confused. What is the most appropriate next step in management?

**A** *Place the patient on facemask 10 L/min $O_2$*
**B** *Give flumazenil 0.2 mg IV q1min × 1–5 doses prn*
**C** *Obtain stat CT chest with pulmonary embolism protocol*
**D** *Give naloxone 0.4 mg IV q2min prn*
**E** *Give methylene blue, 1 mg/kg IV × 1*

The clinical scenario is methemoglobinemia, given the discrepancy in the $PaO_2$ and $SaO_2$, and the use of the oxidizing agent benzocaine. Methemoglobinemia is a condition caused by oxidation of iron within the hemoglobin molecule from the ferrous ($Fe_2+$) to the ferric ($Fe_3+$) state. This oxidation significantly diminishes the oxygen-carrying capacity of hemoglobin and can lead to central and peripheral cyanosis, metabolic acidosis due to inability of the cells to carry out aerobic metabolism, and eventually coma and death if left untreated. The enzyme, NADH-methemoglobin reductase maintains methemoglobin at very low levels. The leading cause of methemoglobinemia is drug toxicity caused by an oxidizing toxin. The agents most frequently associated with methemoglobinemia are aniline, benzocaine, dapsone, pyridium, nitrites, nitrates, and naphthalene. When these drugs are metabolized by the cytochrome P-450 system in the liver, oxygen radicals are produced which can lead to oxidation of the hemoglobin iron.

**Answer: E**

Kane, G.C., Hoehn, S.M., Behrenbeck, T.R., and Mulvagh, S.L. (2007) Benzocaine-induced methemoglobinemia based on the Mayo Clinic experience from 28,478 transesophageal echocardiograms: incidence, outcomes, and predisposing factors. *Archives of Internal Medicine*, **167** (18), 1977–1982.

Moore, T.J., Walsh, C.S., and Cohen, M.R. (2004) Reported adverse event cases of methemoglobinemia associated with benzocaine products. *Archives of Internal Medicine*, **164** (11), 1192–1196.

**12** *After damage-control laparotomy for a gunshot wound to the abdomen, a patient developed a small bowel high-output enterocutaneous fistula. Which acid-base disturbance would be expected?*
**A** *Metabolic acidosis. Hyperchloremia. Wide anion gap.*
**B** *Metabolic acidosis. Hyperchloremia. Normal anion gap.*
**C** *Metabolic acidosis. Hypochloremia. Normal anion gap.*
**D** *Metabolic alkalosis. Hyperkalemia.*
**E** *Metabolic alkalosis. Hypokalemia.*

High output from the gastrointestinal tract causes loss of bicarbonate. Non-anion gap metabolic acidosis can be expected from bicarbonate losses. Since the acidosis is from the loss of bicarbonate and not the addition of an acid (e.g., lactate), a normal anion gap is expected. A widened anion gap would be expected from an etiology that caused the addition of an acid. The loss of bicarbonate causes a gain of chloride ions to maintain electrical neutrality. Because of this, normal gap metabolic acidosis has also been referenced as "hyperchloremic metabolic acidosis." The treatment in this setting would be to replace fluids and electrolytes.

**Answer: B**

DuBose, T.D. and Finkel, K.W. (2002) Metabolic acidosis, in *Acid-Base and Electrolyte Disorders* (eds T.D. DuBose and L.L. Hamm), W.B. Saunders & Co., Philadelphia, PA, pp. 55–66.

Rose, B.D. and Post, T.W. (2001) Introduction to simple and mixed acid-base disorders, in *Clinical Physiology of Acid-Base and Electrolyte Disorders*, McGraw-Hill, New York, pp. 535–550.

**13** *A 55-year-old man comes to the emergency room with complaints of nausea, constipation, and fatigue. He has a history of kidney stones. His serum calcium level is 12 mg/dL. What is the most appropriate initial treatment for his current condition?*
**A** *Hydration with normal saline*
**B** *Administration of bisphosphonates*
**C** *Infusion of calcitonin*
**D** *Dialysis*
**E** *Administration of steroids*

Hypercalcemia is defined as $[Ca_2+] > 10.4$ mg/dL. The most common cause is hyperparathyroidism. Other causes are malignancy, renal failure, or the use of thiazide diuretics. Symptoms of hypercalcemia are fatigue, depression, mental status changes, nausea, and vomiting. Signs are typically nephrolithiasis and arrhythmias (short QT interval). Patients are frequently hypovolemic. Restoring normal volume status can help with renal excretion of calcium. Forcing a diuresis with a loop diuretic may be the next step. Using hydration for hypercalcemia, the onset is typically hours to maintain adequate urine output. For bisphosphonates and calcitonin, the effect takes a day or two. Dialysis can be effective but it is very rarely needed.

**Answer: A**

Kapoor, M. and Chan, G.Z. (2001) Fluid and electrolytes abnormalities. *Critical Care Clinics*, **17** (3), 503–529.

Reilly, R.F. and Perazella, M.A. (2007) *Acid-Base, Fluid Electrolytes*, McGraw-Hill, New York.

**14** *A 17-year-old girl presents as a trauma after a minor single-vehicle crash. She was found to be* *confused and somnolent on scene. Laboratory analysis shows that the patient is in diabetic ketoacidosis. The patient is treated aggressively with IV normal saline and insulin. The patient is admitted and monitored. Two hours after admission, the patient's laboratory analysis shows the following: pH 7.2, Na 140 mEq/L, K 4.6 mEq/L, Cl 105 mEq/L, $HCO_3$ 20, $PaCO_2$ 38 mm Hg.*

*What is the correct acid-base status of the above patient?*

**A** *Anion gap metabolic acidosis with combined normal gap acidosis*

**B** *Anion gap metabolic acidosis*

**C** *Hyperchloremic metabolic acidosis*

**D** *Anion gap metabolic acidosis with superimposed respiratory acidosis*

**E** *Respiratory alkalosis*

The above patient has diabetic ketoacidosis upon presentation. The first step in management of acidemia is determining whether it is respiratory or metabolic in nature. Since the bicarbonate level is low and in the same direction as the pH, a metabolic acidosis is present. The next step is to determine if an anion gap (AG) is present. This can be determined by the equation $AG = Na - (Cl + HCO_3)$. Normal AG ranges are 3–12 mEq/L. The above patient has an AG of 15 mEq/L, thus leading to an anion gap metabolic acidosis. Diabetic ketoacidosis commonly presents with an anion gap. The treatment is aimed at fluid resuscitation and insulin for treatment of the acidosis. However, multiple saline fluid boluses can also cause a hyperchloremic non-gap metabolic acidosis. These two processes can occur simultaneously. If a non-gap metabolic acidosis is superimposed on an anion gap metabolic acidosis the measured bicarbonate will be less than expected. This can be delineated by measuring the gap-gap ratio.

$$\text{Gap-gap ratio} = AG\, \text{Excess}/HCO_3\, \text{Deficit}$$
$$= (AG - 12)/(24 - HCO_3).$$

In an anion gap metabolic acidosis the decrease in serum bicarbonate is equivalent to the increase in anion gap; thus, the ratio is equal to 1. However, if there is a second acidosis without an anion gap the decrease in bicarbonate is greater than the decrease in anion gap; thus, the ratio falls below 1. In the above patient, the measured bicarbonate is lower than expected, creating a ratio less than 1. The aggressive saline fluid hydration has caused a non-anion gap acidosis coexisting with the anion gap metabolic acidosis.

The utilization of Winter's formula, [expected $pCO_2 = (1.5 \times HCO_3) + 8 \pm 2$], determined that there is an appropriate respiratory response.

**Answer: A**

Emmett, M. and Narins, R.G. (1977) Clinical use of the anion gap. *Medicine*, **56** (1), 38–54.

Kellum, J.A. (2007) Disorders of acid-base balance. *Critical Care Medicine*, **35** (11), 2630–2636

Winter, S.D., Pearson, J.R., Gabow, P.A., *et al.* (1990) The fall of the serum anion gap. *Archives of internal medicine*, **150** (2), 311–313.

**15** *A 56-year-old woman with a history of chronic pancreatitis is admitted to the intensive care unit for a flare of severe pancreatitis. The patient is treated nonoperatively with IV fluids, bowel rest, and pain control. On hospital day 3, the patient begins to complain of perioral numbness and intermittent spasms of her hands and feet.*

*Treatment should be aimed at which of the following?*

**A** *Sodium replacement and increase in IV fluids*

**B** *Calcium and magnesium replacement*

**C** *Potassium and calcium replacement*

**D** *Sodium replacement and decrease in IV fluids.*

**E** *Potassium replacement and increase IV fluids*

The patient is suffering from an acute flare up of severe pancreatitis. While rare, it is well-documented that severe pancreatitis in the setting of chronic pancreatitis can cause hypocalcemia. The effects of hypocalcemia can present with perioral numbness and tingling, carpopedal spasms, tetany, seizures, hypotension, and ventricular ectopy. Decreases in serum magnesium also promote hypocalcemia by both inhibiting parathyroid hormone secretion and reducing end-organ responsiveness. Hypocalcemia with hypomagnesemia is refractory to calcium replacement alone. Therefore, both calcium and magnesium replacement are necessary.

**Answer: B**

Marino, P.L. and Sutin, K.M. (2014) *The ICU Book*, 4th edn. Lippincot Williams & Wilkins, Philadelphia, PA.

Scolapio, J.S., Malhi-Chowla, N., and Ukleja, A. (1999) Nutrition supplementation in patients with acute and chronic pancreatitis. *Gastroenterology Clinics of North America*, **28** (3), 695–707.

Worthley, L.I. and Baker, S.B. (2002) The essentials of calcium, magnesium and phosphate metabolism: part I. Physiology. *Critical Care and Resuscitation*, **4** (4), 301–308.

**16** *A 45-year-old homeless, alcoholic man is being treated at the hospital after an unknown traumatic event. The patient is intubated due to respiratory compromise and altered mental status. On hospital day 5, parental nutrition is started due to prolonged intubation and inability to pass an NG/OG tube* *secondary to facial trauma. After day 6 of parental nutrition, the patient begins to have new-onset anemia and a reduction in cardiac output.*

*Which of the following abnormalities is likely contributing to the above scenario?*

**A** *Hyperglycemia*
**B** *Hypernatremia*
**C** *Hypophosphatemia*
**D** *Hypomagnesemia*
**E** *Hypoglycemia*

Inorganic phosphate is an intercellular ion that participates in glycolysis and ATP production. Hypophosphatemia has been reported in up to 20% of critically ill patients and is usually a result of movement intracellularly. Glucose loading has been cited as the most common cause of hypophosphatemia in critically ill patients. This effect is commonly seen in alcoholic and malnourished patients. A common cause is seen in prolonged use of total parental nutrition. This form of "refeeding syndrome" can manifest as a decrease in cardiac output, hemolytic anemia, decreased energy availability, and increased oxygen disassociation. The risk of hypophosphatemia can be minimized with gradual advancements of initial total parental nutrition.

**Answer: C**

Bellomo, R. and French, C. (2004) A rapid intravenous phosphate replacement protocol for critically ill patients. *Critical Care and Resuscitation*, **6** (3), 175–179.
Knochel, J.P. (1977) The pathophysiology and clinical characteristics of severe hypophosphatemia. *Archives of Internal Medicine*, **137** (2), 203–220.

**17** *A 22-year-old man is treated with IV fluids during initial resuscitation in the trauma bay. There is some disagreement between the trauma staff regarding fluids of choice.*

*Comparing the difference between 0.9% saline and Plasma-Lyte, which of the following is true?*

**A** *0.9% saline can be infused with blood while Plasma-Lyte cannot*
**B** *Plasma-Lyte has a lower concentration of potassium*
**C** *Plasma-Lyte can decrease the likelihood of infusion-based metabolic acidosis*
**D** *0.9% saline has a higher concentration of calcium*
**E** *Plasma-Lyte has the same concentration of potassium as 0.9% saline*

Compared to normal saline and lactated Ringer's, Plasma-Lyte is a newer fluid choice. It is closer to physiologic pH due to its included buffers (acetate and gluconate) and physiologic chloride content. Saline and Plasma-Lyte can be infused with blood as they both lack calcium. Plasma-Lyte has a higher concentration of potassium compared to both normal saline and lactated Ringer's. Recent literature has shown that infusion-related metabolic acidosis is significantly decreased when using Plasma-Lyte compared to normal saline.

**Answer: C**

Chua, H.R., Venkatesh, B., Stachowski, E., *et al.* (2012). Plasma-Lyte 148 vs 0.9% saline for fluid resuscitation in diabetic ketoacidosis. *Journal of Critical Care*, **27** (2), 138–145.
Young, J.B., Utter, G.H., Schermer, C.R., *et al.* (2014). Saline versus Plasma-Lyte A in initial resuscitation of trauma patients: a randomized trial. *Annals of Surgery*, **259** (2), 255–262.

**18** *An 80-year-old COPD patient with a significant smoking history and suboptimal COPD control is admitted to the ICU after suffering a hip fracture in a motor vehicle accident. Respiratory therapy obtains an ABG and is concerned with the results. pH 7.31; $PaCO_2$ 60 mm Hg; $PaO_2$ 80 mm Hg; $HCO_3$ 32 mEq/L; $SpO_2$ 88%.*

*Which of the following is true regarding the acid-base status?*

**A** *Primary respiratory acidosis with metabolic acidosis*
**B** *Primary respiratory acidosis with metabolic compensation*
**C** *Primary metabolic acidosis with respiratory acidosis*
**D** *Primary respiratory acidosis without metabolic compensation*
**E** *Primary metabolic acidosis with respiratory compensation*

The above patient has a respiratory acidosis as evidenced by his decrease in pH and increase in $PaCO_2$. Given the information that he has suboptimal COPD control, it can be assumed that he likely has a chronic respiratory acidosis. The adequate metabolic compensation in a chronic respiratory acidosis can be determined by the following equation

$$HCO_3 = 24 + \left[ 0.4 \times \left( PaCO_2 - 40 \right) \right]$$

Thus, the expected bicarbonate level is within the correct range for compensation. If the patient were to have a metabolic acidosis or lack of compensation, the bicarbonate would be lower than expected.

**Answer: B**

Emmett, M. and Narins, R.G. (1977) Clinical use of the anion gap. *Medicine*, **56** (1), 38–54.

Kellum, J.A. (2007) Disorders of acid-base balance. *Critical Care Medicine*, **35** (11), 2630–2636

Winter, S.D., Pearson, J.R., Gabow, P.A., *et al.* (1990) The fall of the serum anion gap. *Archives of Internal Medicine*, **150** (2), 311–313.

**19** *During the course of her ICU stay, a 45-year-old diabetic woman was initially found to have an anion gap metabolic acidosis. She is malnourished and she has profound hypoalbuminemia at 1.9 g/dL.*

*Which of the following is true regarding the effect of albumin on metabolic acidosis?*

**A** *Hypoalbuminemia can mask an underlying anion gap*

**B** *Hypoalbuminemia will inflate the calculated anion gap*

**C** *Hyperalbuminemia can mask an underlying anion gap*

**D** *Albumin has no effect on the calculated anion gap*

**E** *Albumin is a measured anion in the anion gap calculation*

Albumin is the principle unmeasured ion and the principle determinant of the anion gap. A low albumin level will lower the anion gap and can mask the presence of other unmeasured anions (e.g., lactate). Hypoalbuminemia is present in the vast majority of ICU patients. Although calculating a new anion gap based upon a corrected albumin level has been proposed, this calculation is still controversial. However, it is important to realize that a decrease in albumin can potentially mask the anion gap in a metabolic acidosis.

**Answer: A**

Figge, J., Jabor, A., Kazda, A., and Fencl, V. (1998) Anion gap and hypoalbuminemia. *Critical Care Medicine*, **26** (11), 1807–1810.

**20** *A 22-year-old man is admitted to the ICU following a suicide attempt. The patient ingested an unknown substance that he "found in his garage." As part of his workup, the following laboratory analysis was made: pH 7.3; Na 140 mEq/L, K 4.6 mEq/L, Cl 104 mEq/L, $HCO_3$ 21, $PaCO_2$ 39 mm Hg.*

*Which of the following is true regarding the acid-base status?*

**A** *Non-anion gap metabolic acidosis*

**B** *Anion gap metabolic acidosis*

**C** *Combined metabolic acidosis and respiratory acidosis*

**D** *Respiratory acidosis*

**E** *Hypochloremic metabolic acidosis*

The above patient has an anion gap metabolic acidosis. The first step in management of acidemia is determining whether it is respiratory or metabolic in nature. Since the bicarbonate level is low and in the same direction as the pH, a metabolic acidosis is present. The next step is to determine if an anion gap (AG) is present. This can be determined by the equation $AG = Na - (Cl + HCO_3)$. Normal AG ranges are 3–12 mEq/L. The above patient has an AG of 15 mEq/L, thus causing an anion gap metabolic acidosis.

The utilization of Winter's formula, [expected $pCO_2 = (1.5 \times HCO_3) + 8 \pm 2$], determined that there is an appropriate respiratory response.

**Answer: B**

Emmett, M. and Narins, R.G. (1977) Clinical use of the anion gap. *Medicine*, **56** (1), 38–54.

Kellum, J.A. (2007) Disorders of acid-base balance. *Critical Care Medicine*, **35** (11), 2630–2636.

Winter, S.D., Pearson, J.R., Gabow, P.A., *et al.* (1990) The fall of the serum anion gap. *Archives of Internal Medicine*, **150** (2), 311–313.

**21** *If given one liter of fluid, which of the following fluid choices would promote the most edema?*

**A** *0.9% NaCl*

**B** *Plasma-Lyte*

**C** *Lactated Ringer's*

**D** *5% albumin*

**E** *Edema formation is only a factor of infusion rate*

Infusions of 0.9% NaCl promote interstitial edema formation. 0.9% NaCl has higher sodium concentration than other crystalloid solutions, as well as a higher sodium concentration than physiologic serum. Sodium is the main determinant of extracellular volume and is distributed uniformly in extracellular fluid. Plasma volume is only 25% of the extracelluar fluid. Since sodium in a cystalloid solution will distribute equally, 75% of the fluid administered will fill the interstitial fluid and promote edema. Plasma-Lyte, lactated Ringer's, and albumin solutions have lower sodium concentrations, thus leading to less edema and more plasma volume.

**Answer: A**

Awad, S., Allison, S.P., and Lobo, D.N. (2008) The history of 0.9% saline. *Clinical Nutrition*, **27** (2), 179–188.

Chowdhury, A.H., Cox, E.F., Francis, S.T., and Lobo, D.N. (2012) A randomized, controlled, double-blind crossover study on the effects of 2-L infusions of 0.9% saline and plasma-lyte® 148 on renal blood flow velocity and renal cortical tissue perfusion in healthy volunteers. *Annals of Surgery*, **256** (1), 18–24.

Marino, P.L. and Sutin, K.M. (2014) *The ICU Book*, 4th edn, Lippincot Williams & Wilkins, Philadelphia, PA.

**22** *If one liter of 0.9% NaCl solution is given, what is the expected increase in plasma volume?*
A *1 L*
B *225 mL*
C *275 mL*
D *775 mL*
E *1100 mL*

Because 0.9% NaCl is a sodium-heavy fluid, it will disseminate equally among all extracellular fluid compartments. Since plasma is only 25% of the extracellular fluid, it can be assumed that 25% of an added isotonic fluid will fill the plasma volume. However, despite the term "normal saline," 0.9% NaCl is actually slightly hypertonic compared to extracelluar fluid (308 mOsm/L vs. 290 mOsm/L). This hypertonicity causes a slight fluid shift from intracellular to the extracellular space. For every 1000 mL of 0.9% NaCl added, 1,100 mL of fluid is added to the extracellular fluid. Thus, 275 mL (25% of 1,100 mL) is added to the plasma.

**Answer: C**

Imm, A. and Carlson, R.W. (1993) Fluid resuscitation in circulatory shock. *Critical Care Clinics*, **9** (2), 313–333.

# 15

# Metabolic Illness and Endocrinopathies
*Andrew J. Young, MD and Therese M. Duane, MD*

**1** *A 67-year-old woman is admitted to the intensive care unit following a four-node parathyroidectomy with reimplantation for secondary hyperparathyroidism due to renal failure. She has a calcium level of 7.2 mg/dL 12 hours postoperatively. She is asymptomatic, but an ECG is obtained which shows a QT interval of 560 msec. Which of the following is the best treatment option for this patient?*
  **A** *Proceed urgently to the operating room for removal of the implanted parathyroid*
  **B** *Give 2 gm intravenous calcium gluconate*
  **C** *Electively re-explore the patient in the morning for a missed parathyroid gland*
  **D** *Double her calcitriol dose from 0.25 mcg to 0.5 mcg twice daily*
  **E** *Continue observation with no intervention at this time*

While several studies have tried to identify which factors predispose a patient to hypocalcemia after a parathyroidectomy, it is important to remember that all patients undergoing a parathroidectomy need frequent calcium level checks postoperatively as there is a high incidence of hypocalcemia. Patients undergoing subtotal parathyroidectomy may only require oral calcium and vitamin D supplementation, while those patients undergoing total parathyroidectomy with/without reimplantation usually require more aggressive calcium replacement therapy (i.e., intravenous calcium replacement). Patients with symptomatic hypocalcemia may exhibit peri-oral paresthesias, Trousseau sign (occlude blood flow to arm using a blood pressure cuff to induce muscle spasm of the hand and forearm), Chvostek's sign (tapping of the facial nerve to induce facial spasm on the ipsilateral side), hyper-reflexia, and ECG changes including prolonged QT interval. Intravenous calcium should be initiated if a patient exhibits any of these signs or symptoms.

**Answer: B**

Mittendorf, E.A., Merlino, J.I., and McHenry, C.R. (2004) Post-parathyroidectomy hypocalcemia: incidence, risk factors, and management. *The American Surgeon*, **70** (2), 114–119; discussion 119–120.

Torer, N., Torun, D., Torer, N., *et al.* (2009) Predictors of early postoperative hypocalcemia in hemodialysis patients with secondary hyperparathyroidism. *Transplantation Proceedings*, **41** (9), 3642–3646.

**2** *A 32-year-old man was admitted to the intensive care unit following a motor vehicle crash in which he suffered several small intracranial hemorrhages. A ventriculostomy catheter was placed to monitor his intracranial pressures. The patient has been receiving iso-osmotic intravenous fluids. On post-trauma day 5, his plasma mOsm is now > 320 mOsm, and his urine mOsm is 130 mOsm. He remains intubated with a feeding nasogastric tube in place and is hemodynamically normal. What is the best course of action?*
  **A** *Increase the amount of free water administration via his nasogastric feeding tube*
  **B** *Change his parenteral fluids to normal saline*
  **C** *Check placement of the venticulostomy tube to ensure the patient's intracranial pressures are not rising despite the improved readings*
  **D** *Begin low dose, twice daily dexamethasone*
  **E** *Check serum magnesium and correct if abnormal*

This patient has diabetes insipidus (DI), a deficiency of antidiuretic hormone (ADH) which can be seen following traumatic brain injury. There are two types of DI – central (associated with traumatic brain injury) and nephrogenic. Administration of exogenous ADH helps differentiate between the two types of DI. If the patient responds to the exogenous ADH then the cause is central, but if there is no response then the cause is nephrogenic. DI is characterized by high plasma osmolarity

*Surgical Critical Care and Emergency Surgery: Clinical Questions and Answers*, Second Edition.
Edited by Forrest "Dell" Moore, Peter Rhee, and Gerard J. Fulda.
© 2018 John Wiley & Sons Ltd. Published 2018 by John Wiley & Sons Ltd.
Companion website: www.wiley.com/go/moore/surgical_criticalcare_and_emergency_surgery

with a paradoxical low urine osmolarity. Initial treatment consists of increasing free water to try to correct hyperosmolarity as well as correcting any serum calcium or potassium abnormalities (thus E is incorrect). B is incorrect because the patient is hemodynamically normal and this action may worsen the hypernatremia. Patients with more severe DI will require desmopressin injection, but not dexamethasone (answer D).

**Answer: A**

Capatina, C., Paluzzi, A., Mitchell, R., and Karavitaki, N. (2015) Diabetes insipidus after traumatic brain injury. *Journal of Clinical Medicine*, **4** (7), 1448–1462.

Agha, A., Sherlock, M., Phillips, J., *et al.* (2005) The natural history of post-traumatic neurohypophysial dysfunction. *European Journal of Endocrinology*, **152** (3), 371–377.

3 *A 52-year-old man is septic in the ICU following a transthoracic esophagectomy. Despite fluid resuscitation and high-dose vasopressor support, he remains hypotensive. The Surviving Sepsis Campaign recommends which of the following as an additional step?*
   A *Empirically adding double coverage of anaerobes*
   B *High dose steroids (>300 mg hydrocortisone per day)*
   C *Waiting until speciation of cultures before beginning antibiotics so as not to increase the likelihood of resistance*
   D *Low-dose steroids (200 mg hydrocortisone per day)*
   E *Begin high dose synthetic thyroid hormone*

The Surviving Sepsis Campaign recommends the use of intravenous hydrocortisone (200 mg) for septic patients who do not respond to adequate fluid and vasopressor support. There are studies that both support and refute the benefit of steroids in sepsis, and thus the emphasis should be on maintaining adequate fluid resuscitation and vasopressor support. There is not a recommendation to perform an ACTH stimulation test. Double-coverage of anaerobes is not a recommendation, neither is waiting for culture results before starting antibiotics nor beginning high-dose synthetic thyroid hormone.

**Answer: D**

Annane, D., Bellissant, E., Bollaert, P.E., *et al.* (2015) Corticosteroids for treating sepsis. Cochrane Database Systematic Reviews. **12**, CD002243.

Dellinger, R.P., Levy, M.M., Rhodes, A., *et al.* (2013) Surviving Sepsis Campaign Guidelines Committee including the Pediatric Subgroup. Surviving sepsis campaign: international guidelines for management of severe sepsis and septic shock: 2012. *Critical Care Medicine*, **41**, 580–637.

4 *A 19-year-old man has been in the intensive care unit for the last two days following an all-terrain vehicle crash in which he sustained multiple orthopedic injuries and a T2 spinal cord injury. In the last 24 hours his blood glucose has started to increase, and the last two readings were 190 and 210 mg/dL respectively. You decide to begin a sliding scale insulin regimen. What is the best target blood glucose range for this patient?*
   A *70–90 mg/dL*
   B *81–110 mg/dL*
   C *120–140 mg/dL*
   D *<180 mg/dL*
   E *<200 mg/dL*

This multiply-injured trauma patient with a spinal cord injury and several orthopedic injuries will require blood glucose control with intravenously administered insulin. While this patient may not have been diabetic prior to his injuries, there will be changes in metabolism throughout the body that will contribute to higher blood sugar levels. In 2009, the NICE SUGAR trial suggested that trauma patients were found to be in a subgroup of critically ill patients that benefited from tight glucose control with a range of 81 to 108 mg/dL. However, several smaller studies and an update to the NICE SUGAR study in 2012 found that overall mortality *increased* when lower blood glucose levels were targeted. They could not determine a causal relationship, however the American Diabetes Association recommends a target blood glucose concentration of 140 to 180 mg/dL.

**Answer: D**

Standards of Medical Care in Diabetes–2012. (2012). Standards of medical care in diabetes–2012. *Diabetes Care*, **35** (Supplement_1), S11–S63.

The NICE-SUGAR Study Investigators (2012). Hypoglycemia and risk of death in critically ill patients. *New England Journal of Medicine*, **367** (12), 1108–1118.

5 *A 32-year-old woman is admitted to the ICU following a right laparoscopic adrenalectomy for an adrenal adenoma. The tumor was an active glucocorticoid-secreting tumor and she requires post-operative steroids. What constellation of signs and/or symptoms would suggest that the patient is having acute adrenal dysfunction?*
   A *Hypertension, emesis, hypokalemia, paresthesias*
   B *Hypertension, nausea without emesis, hyperkalemia, hypocalcemia*
   C *Hypotension, emesis, hyperkalemia, hypercalcemia, hypoglycemia, confusion*
   D *Hypotension, low fibrin split products, bleeding from the incision and venipuncture sites.*
   E *Hypertension, diabetes mellitus, muscle and bone weakness, osteoporosis, and rapid weight gain.*

An Addisonian crisis, or hypocortisolism, consists of hypotension, vomiting and diarrhea, hyperkalemia, hypercalcemia, hypoglycemia, fever, syncope, lethargy, and possible abdominal pain. This can be due to the removal of a glucocorticoid-producing adrenal adenoma. The over-production of glucocorticoids by the adenoma causes Cushing's Syndrome (answer E) with the subsequent atrophy of the contralateral adrenal gland. Patients should be placed on replacement therapy prior to adrenalectomy and continue with therapy afterwards to prevent hypocortisolism.

**Answer: C**

Brunt, L.M. and Moley, J. (2004) The pituitary and adrenal glands, in *Sabiston Textbook of Surgery*, 17th edn (ed. C.M. Townsend), Elsevier, Philadelphia, PA, pp. 1042–1044.

**6** *A 52-year-old man has been admitted to the ICU following emergent operation for a strangulated inguinal hernia. He is hypertensive despite adequate pain control. He has a history of hypertension and takes lisinopril at home. What is the mechanism of action of lisinopril?*
**A** *Breaks down bradykinin*
**B** *Prevents conversion of angiotensinogen to angiotensin I*
**C** *Prevents conversion of angiotensin I to angiotensin II*
**D** *Blocks renin synthesis in the juxtaglomerular complex.*
**E** *AT1-receptor antagonist*

The renin-angiotensin-aldosterone system begins with renin production in the juxtaglomerular complex after decreased blood pressure is sensed. Renin cleaves angiotensinogen to angiotensin I. Angiotensin I is then cleaved by angiotensin-converting enzyme (ACE) to create angiotensin II. ACE also breaks down bradykinin into its inactive form. Angiotensin II has multiple effects across a range of tissues. Angiotensin II supports the circulatory system by causing release of aldosterone, stimulating thirst, increasing sympathetic tone, and causing release of antidiuretic hormone. Aldosterone is a mineralocorticoid secreted by the adrenal glands that causes increased sodium absorption and potassium secretion in the kidney.

Lisinopril inhibits ACE thus answers A, B, D, and E are incorrect. Answer E is a different class of medications called Angiotensin Receptor Blockers (ARB). Lisinopril prevents the body's natural mechanism for volume retention. This is an important point especially in this particular case since the patient had a significant operation and his volume status is labile. While it is important

to restart home medications in patients admitted to the hospital, the clinical situation should be considered. For this particular patient, a shorter acting anti-hypertensive medication from a different class should be chosen.

**Answer C**

Corry, D.B. and Tuck, M.L. (2001) Renin-angiotensin system and aldosterone, in *Principles and Practice of Endocrinology and Metabolism*, 3rd edn (ed. K. Becker), Lippincott Williams & Wilkins, Philadelphia, PA, pp. 764–772.
Haas, C.E. and LeBlanc, J.M. (2004) Acute postoperative hypertension: a review of therapeutic options. *American Journal of Health System Pharmacy*, **61** (16), 1661–1673; quiz 1674–1675.

**7** *A 47-year-old woman underwent left adrenalectomy for a pheochromocytoma. In the ICU, she has been requiring low-dose vasopressor support to maintain an adequate blood pressure. The proper order of medications she should have received preoperatively for control of her hypertension is:*
**A** *metoprolol, phenoxybenzamine*
**B** *prazosin, phenoxybenzamine*
**C** *prazosin, metoprolol*
**D** *metoprolol, potassium chloride*
**E** *phenoxybenzamine, prazosin*

Pheochromocytomas produce excess catecholamines causing hypertension, headaches, sweats and sometimes a feeling of impending doom. It is also useful to remember the *rule of tens*: 10% are bilateral, 10% occur in children, 10% are extra-adrenal, and 10% are familial. Patients must be treated preoperatively to prevent hypertensive crisis due to tumor manipulation as well as circulatory collapse perioperatively. Preoperative treatment includes alpha-blockade (with phenoxybenzamine or prazosin) followed by beta-blockade. In addition, patients must be given adequate volume in order to tolerate the sudden cessation of high amounts of circulating catecholamines once the tumor has been removed. Patients may require vasopressor or inotropic support postoperatively. Answers A and D are incorrect and potentially life threatening since starting a beta-blocking medication without alpha-blockade first may cause unopposed alpha stimulation (and possibly a hypertensive crisis) from the catecholamines produced by the pheochromocytoma. Answers B and E are incorrect because both sets of medication are alpha-blockers.

**Answer: C**

Allen, C.T.B. and Imrie, D. (1977) Hypoglycaemia as a complication of removal of a pheochromocytoma. *Canadian Medical Association Journal*, **116**, 363.

Williams, D.T., Dann, S., and Wheeler, M.H. (2003) Phaeochromocytoma – views on current management. *European Journal of Surgical Oncology*, **29** (6), 483–490.

**8** *A 35-year-old woman underwent an uncomplicated celiotomy for a tubo-ovarian abscess. Three hours post-operatively, she began to have chest pain, confusion, and hypertension that has been difficult to control. Cardiac enzymes were ordered, her ECG shows sinus tachycardia and her chest x-ray appears normal. She has a past medical history of Graves disease for which she takes methimazole although she had not been able to tolerate anything by mouth prior to her presentation. The most appropriate medication to give at this time is:*

**A** *Methimazole 25 mg PO*
**B** *Potassium iodide 5 drops PO*
**C** *Aspirin 325 mg PO*
**D** *Hydrocortisone 100 mg IV*
**E** *Oxygen 2 L/min*

This patient is experiencing thyroid storm given her history of Graves disease and operative stress. While four of the above answers may be correct, it is important to give them in the proper order as follows: stop new thyroid gland synthesis with anti-thyroid medication (methimazole or propylthiouracil), then treatment with iodine therapy to stop thyroid hormone release (potassium iodide or Lugol's solution), followed by treatment of adrenergic symptoms (hydrocortisone and/or beta-blockers). Giving iodine therapy prior to anti-thyroid therapy may exacerbate a thyroid storm. Furthermore, there should be a delay of 30 to 60 minutes prior to giving iodine therapy. She had been taking methimazole for her Graves disease, but she may have missed doses secondary to her disease process or perhaps her maintenance dose is not enough given this new stress. The safe course of action is to give the methimazole first, then wait 30 to 60 minutes to give the potassium iodide.

Patients with Graves disease can be treated with either propylthiouracil or methimazole, although the FDA has issued a warning against propylthiouracil as it may cause hepatotoxicity. The cardiovascular effects of thyrotoxicosis can be severe and are treated with a beta-blocker. Propranolol is preferred as it also blocks T4 to T3 conversion at higher doses. Thyroid storm, while rare, can occur in patients with clinical or subclinical hyperthyroid disease following a precipitating event (e.g., infection, trauma). Mortality from thyroid storm ranges from 20 to 30%.

**Answer: A**

Kayak, B. and Burman, K. (2006) Thyrotoxicosis and thyroid storm. *Endocrinology and Metabolism Clinics of North America*, **35** (4), 663–686.

Klein, I. and Ojamaa, K. (2001) Thyroid hormone and the cardiovascular system. *New England Journal of Medicine*, **344** (7), 501–509.

**9** *A 28-year-old man suffered a severe traumatic brain injury from a motorcycle crash. There is concern for diffuse axonal injury. His current Glasgow Coma Scale is 6 and he requires vasopressors to maintain an adequate cerebral perfusion pressure. A morning cortisol level is drawn and is 10 μg/dL. This patient most likely has:*

**A** *Sheehan's syndrome*
**B** *A normal ACTH*
**C** *A normal cortisol level*
**D** *Adrenal Insufficiency*
**E** *Sepsis*

While the determination of adrenal insufficiency (AI) can be difficult in the traumatic brain injury (TBI) population, studies suggest that a morning cortisol level of less than 15 μg/dL in a TBI patient indicates AI. Given his TBI and possible disruption of the hypothalamic-pituitary-adrenal (HPA) axis, it is unclear what his ACTH may be (thus B is incorrect). It is important to note the low level of cortisol in this patient and stress-dose glucocorticoids should be considered given this patient's vasopressor requirement. Sheehan's syndrome is hypopituitarism caused by ischemic necrosis during hemorrhagic shock experienced by the mother in childbirth. While this patient may have sepsis, there is not enough information to make this diagnosis.

**Answer: D**

Blair, J.C. (2010) Prevalence, natural history and consequences of posttraumatic hypopituitarism: a case for endocrine surveillance. *British Journal of Neurosurgery*, **24** (1), 10–17.
Cohan, P., Wang, C., McArthur, D.L., *et al.* (2005) Acute secondary adrenal insufficiency after traumatic brain injury: a prospective study. *Critical Care Medicine*, **33** (10), 2358–2366.

**10** *A 19-year-old man has been in the intensive care unit for the last 14 days following an assault for which he sustained a right occipital skull fracture and associated subarachnoid hemorrhage. Over the past 5 days he has become progressively more hyponatremic despite free water restriction. Today his serum sodium level is 118 mmol/L, plasma osmolarity 241 mOsm/kg and urine osmolarity 500 mOsm/kg water. What key test(s) need to be done before making the diagnosis of the Syndrome of Inappropriate Antidiuretic Hormone (SIADH)?*

A *Demeclocycline challenge*
B *Thyroid and adrenal function tests*
C *Urine creatinine*
D *Desmopressin challenge (desmopressin)*
E *Corticotropin stimulation test*

This patient most likely has SIADH, however there are certain criteria that must be met prior to diagnosis: plasma osmolarity < 275 mOsm/kg, urine osmolarity > 100 mOsm/kg water, normal renal function, clinical euvolemia, elevated urinary sodium excretion, and absence of other potential causes – namely hypothyroidism, hypocortisolism or recent diuretic use. SIADH is essentially a diagnosis of exclusion. Treatment begins with free water restriction, but can include salt tablets and/or hypertonic saline administration coupled with loop diuretics. Neurological effects are usually seen when plasma sodium decreases below 120 mmol/L. It is important to begin correction at a relatively slow rate if that patient has been experiencing hyponatremia for > 48 hours to prevent central pontine myelinolysis. Demeclocycline is used in the treatment of SIADH and is not used to make the diagnosis of SIADH. Urine creatinine, desmopressin challenge, or a corticotropin stimulation test will not aid in making the diagnosis of SIADH.

**Answer: B**

Adrogué, H.J. and Madias, N.E. (2000) Hyponatremia. *New England Journal of Medicine*, **342** (21), 1581–1589.
Moro, N., Katayama, Y., Igarashi, T., *et al.* (2007) Hyponatremia in patients with traumatic brain injury: incidence, mechanism, and response to sodium supplementation or retention therapy with hydrocortisone. *Surgical Neurology*, **68** (4), 387–393.

11  A 65-year-old man has been in the ICU for 2 days following a motor vehicle crash for which he sustained four rib fractures and a left femur fracture which has been repaired. He has a history of Crohn's disease and was on steroids for a recent flare-up prior to his accident. Stress-dose steroids were given shortly after arrival, and he had been doing well until today. He now is not able to tolerate his diet and he has vomited twice. Plain films of the chest and abdomen show free air. What is the most likely cause of the free air?
A *Crohn's exacerbation with subsequent perforation following stress response to injury*
B *Injury to bowel from initial crash, not identified secondary to steroid use*
C *Bowel perforation secondary to ischemia from blood loss during femur repair*
D *Beginning diet too soon after injury prior to subsequent femur operation*
E *Gastric perforation from stress ulceration*

This patient most likely had occult bowel injury on presentation. A CT of the abdomen may not show early bowel injury if there is not free air, bowel wall thickening or oral contrast (if given) extravasation at the site of perforation. Given his steroid use, he may not develop peritonitis. A much higher index of suspicion for occult injury is required for patients who have been taking steroids chronically as their *inflammatory* response will be blunted.

**Answer: B**

Martin, R.F., Rossi, R.L. (1997) The acute abdomen: an overview and algorithms. *The Surgical Clinics of North America*, **77** (6), 1227–1243.
ReMine, S.G. and McIlrath, D.C. (1980) Bowel perforation in steroid-treated patients. *Annals of Surgery*, **192** (4), 581–586.

12  A 32-year-old woman has been transferred to the ICU following a celiotomy and right hemicolectomy for a Crohn's flare-up that resulted in perforation. She had been taking 10 mg of prednisone daily prior to her presentation and was started on stress-dose steroids perioperatively. Which of the following may help improve wound healing in this patient?
A *Prolonged steroid taper to decrease the inflammatory response.*
B *Topical vitamin E*
C *Topical vitamin A*
D *Topical mitomycin C*
E *Topical hydrocortisone*

Patients who are on steroids have impaired wound healing. Vitamin A is known to reverse many of the deleterious effects of steroids in wound healing, namely the appearance of inflammatory cells, fibroblasts, deposition of ground substance, regeneration of capillaries, and epithelial migration. It should be noted that while steroids decrease wound contracture, vitamin A does not reverse this effect. While there are many animal models that demonstrate these effects of vitamin A, there is a lack of good randomized controlled trials to support the animal models. There are no studies to support topical vitamin E, mitomycin C or hydrocortisone to improve wound healing. A prolonged steroid taper will most likely worsen this patient's wound healing and should only be tailored according to her hemodynamic status and clinical picture.

**Answer: C**

Haws, M., Brown, R.E., Suchy, H., and Roth, A. (1994) Vitamin A-soaked gelfoam sponges and wound healing in steroid-treated animals. *Annals of Plastic Surgery*, **32** (4), 418–422.

Wicke, C., Halliday, B., Allen, D., *et al.* (2000) Effects of steroids and retinoids on wound healing. *Archives of Surgery*, **135** (11), 1265–1270.

**13** *A 67-year-old man is in the cardiac intensive care unit on postoperative day one following a three-vessel coronary artery bypass graft. On morning rounds it is noted that he received etomidate on induction prior to the operation. Etomidate has been shown to*

**A** *increase vasopressor needs post elective surgery but not emergent surgery*

**B** *increase mortality in patients with sepsis*

**C** *inhibit adrenal mitochondrial activity and cause reversible adrenal insufficiency*

**D** *increase hydrocortisone requirements in septic patients*

**E** *be more likely to cause hemodynamic derangement than propofol*

There have been many studies that looked at the effect of etomidate on the adrenal gland, and it is well known that there is adrenal insufficiency after etomidate administration (answer C). However, there has been controversy regarding whether or not etomidate can effect outcomes. As of late 2016, the most current studies have shown there is no change among multiple outcome indicators including ventilator days, days of hospitalization, and mortality (thus answer B is incorrect). Another recent study found no difference in vasopressor requirements with or without etomidate in patients undergoing cardiac surgery. There is no data to support an increase steroid requirement in patients that receive a single dose of etomidate. Etomidate is preferred over propofol because of its minimal effect on hemodynamics.

**Answer: C**

Gu, W.-J., Wang, F., Tang, L., and Liu, J.-C. (2015) Single-dose etomidate does not increase mortality in patients with sepsis. *Chest*, **147** (2), 335–346.

Wagner, C.E., Bick, J.S., Johnson, D., *et al.* (2014) Etomidate use and postoperative outcomes among cardiac surgery patients. *Anesthesiology. The American Society of Anesthesiologists*, **120** (3), 579–589.

**14** *A 19-year-old man is admitted to the intensive care unit following an emergent incision and drainage of a right arm abscess. He is a heroin addict and is a skin popper. On admission to the ICU his blood pressure is 143/82 mm Hg, heart rate is 143 beats/min and respiratory rate is 36 breaths/min. He complains of right arm pain and is thirsty. Postoperative labs are drawn and his blood glucose level is 832 mg/dL, bicarbonate level < 2 mmol/L, and anion gap level of > 31 mmol/L. In addition to insulin, what additional treatment is necessary?*

**A** *Sodium bicarbonate infusion*

**B** *A Foley catheter to monitor urine output*

**C** *Morphine for adequate pain control*

**D** *Fluconazole given the high incidence of fungal infections in the skin popper population.*

**E** *Intravenous hydration*

In addition to insulin, a patient with diabetic ketoacidosis require intravenous hydration. As the hyperglycemia and acidosis resolves, there will be fluid shifts from the extracellular space to the intracellular space. These patients are hypovolemic and as the fluid shifts occur, they will become hypotensive as the intravascular volume is depleted. Answer A is incorrect because as the hyperglycemia and hypovolemia are corrected the acidosis will correct as well, thus there is no indication for sodium bicarbonate. A Foley catheter is not necessary to monitor urine output. Pain control is necessary but narcotics may not be required. Last, there is no data to suggest skin poppers have a higher rate of fungal infections than the general population.

**Answer: E**

Ingelfinger, J.R., Kamel, K.S., and Halperin, M.L. (2015) Acid–base problems in diabetic ketoacidosis. *New England Journal of Medicine*, **372** (6), 546–554.

**15** *A 43-year-old man is two months status post a cadaveric renal transplant for renal failure secondary to uncontrolled hypertension is being seen in clinic for routine follow up. His laboratory data is as follows: sodium 163 mg/dL, potassium 3.2 mg/dL, chloride 108 mg/dL, bicarbonate 20 mEq/L, BUN 42 mg/dL, creatinine 1.2 mg/dL, and glucose 734 mg/dL. What is the most likely diagnosis for this patient?*

**A** *Diabetic ketoacidosis*

**B** *Tacrolimus toxicity*

**C** *Acute rejection*

**D** *Hyperglycemic hyperosmolar state*

**E** *Diabetes insipidus*

While the level of ketonemia is not known, there is lack of significant metabolic acidosis. The blood glucose level is greater than 600 mg/dL and the serum osmolality is greater than 320 mmol/kg. Similar to diabetic ketoacidosis, the treatment for hyperglycemia hyperosmolar state (HHS) is to restore circulatory volume while correcting hyperglycemia. Other electrolytes should be monitored and corrected. Typically patients who have HHS have a higher mortality and have other comorbidities upon presentation.

This is not diabetic ketoacidosis as the bicarbonate level, while low, does not meet the criteria for even mild DKA, thus answer A is incorrect. Tacrolimus toxicity manifests with neurotoxicity and nephrotoxicity. This is not acute rejection which would present with symptoms of an immune reaction to the kidney transplant (increased inflammatory markers, fever, pain, etc.). In diabetes insipidus, there would be a paradoxical increase in urine osmolarity despite a low plasma osmolarity.

**Answer: D**

Umpierrez, G. and Korytkowski, M. (2016) Diabetic emergencies – ketoacidosis, hyperglycaemic hyperosmolar state and hypoglycaemia. *Nature Reviews, Endocrinology*, **12** (4), 222–232.

16  *A 72-year-old woman arrives in the trauma bay following a ground level fall. Her Glasgow Coma Scale (GCS) is 8. Other significant exam findings include a heart rate of 42, blood pressure of 88/44 mm Hg, respiratory rate of 8 breaths/min, and a temperature of 31 °C. Imaging is negative and laboratory workup shows she is hyponatremic. She is intubated, resuscitated, and admitted to the intensive care unit. After further workup and an adequate history from her daughter, a thyroid stimulating hormone (TSH) level is checked and found to be high. Myxedema coma is suspected. What is the best course of action at this time?*

**A** *Begin intravenous levothyroxine therapy alone*
**B** *Begin intravenous levothyroxine and hydrocortisone therapy*
**C** *Slowly correct electrolyte abnormalities prior to starting any hormone therapy*
**D** *Begin broad spectrum antibiotics as there is likely occult infection*
**E** *Recheck TSH after normothermia is achieved*

Myedema coma is a rare phenomenon and one must have a high index of suspicion to make the diagnosis. Mortality rates are high given that there is usually a precipitating event that causes the myxedema coma, such as sepsis, stroke, myocardial infarction, trauma, and gastrointestinal disorders. In addition to treating the myxedema coma, a workup for inciting events should be undertaken to identify and treat the underlying cause.

When the diagnosis is made, intravenous T4 and steroid therapy should be initiated, therefore answer B is the best choice. T3 may also be initiated and patients will typically respond more quickly, however T3 is not as widely available. Once the diagnosis is made, therapy should begin immediately, so answer C is incorrect. While one may need to begin antibiotics as sepsis is the leading cause for myxedema coma, there may be other reasons for the coma so answer B is still the best choice. Hypothermia should not effect TSH level, so answer E is incorrect.

**Answer: B**

Dutta, P., Bhansali, A., Masoodi, S.R., *et al.* (2008) Predictors of outcome in myxoedema coma: a study from a tertiary care centre. *Critical Care*, **12** (1), R1.
Mathew, V., Misgar, R.A., Ghosh, S., *et al.* (2011) Myxedema coma: a new look into an old crisis. *Journal of Thyroid Research*, **2011** (12), 493462–493467.

# 16

# Hypothermia and Hyperthermia

*Raquel M. Forsythe, MD*

**1** *In a healthy 25-year-old man at rest in a neutral environment (28°C), the majority of heat exchange occurs as heat loss via*
 **A** *Convection*
 **B** *Radiation*
 **C** *Conduction*
 **D** *Transference*
 **E** *Evaporation*

Radiation exchange is the transfer of energy between objects with no direct contact. It accounts for 50% to 70% of heat lost by humans at rest in a neutral environment. Conduction involves the direct exchange of heat between the body and an object in direct contact with the body. The speed of heat exchange is related to the thermal conductivity of the object. Water has much greater thermal conductivity than the body, which accounts for the rapid heat exchange that occurs when the body is submerged in water. Convection involves the exchange of heat with the warmer or cooler air molecules passing over the skin. The amount of heat exchange by convection depends on the speed of airflow around the body. Evaporative heat loss in humans is primarily through perspiration. Unlike the other mechanisms of heat exchange, evaporation can exchange heat even in a warmer environment than the body. It is therefore the major means that the body utilizes to prevent hyperthermia in a warm thermal environment. Transference is not a mechanism by which heat is exchanged by the body.

**Answer: B**

Irwin, R. and Rippe, J. (2008) *Irwin and Rippe's Intensive Care Medicine*, 6th edn, Lippincott Wiliams & Wilkins, Philadelphia, PA.

**2** *Comparing a healthy 25-year-old and a healthy 75-year-old, which of the following is correct?*
 **A** *The younger patient has a lower basal metabolic rate*
 **B** *The younger patient has a higher heat conductance*
 **C** *The younger patient generates more heat by shivering*
 **D** *The older patient has a lower risk of hypothermia*
 **E** *The older patient has a lower sweat threshold*

Older patients have deterioration of the ability to regulate temperature, putting them at higher risk for both hypothermia and hyperthermia. Older persons require a greater change in temperature to notice ambient changes. In some cases, they may need a change in temperature of > 2°C to notice a change. The sweat volume decreases and the threshold to produce sweat increases as we age. This significantly decreases evaporative cooling. Older people have lower basal metabolic rates than do younger individuals. A decline in body mass in older patients leads to a higher heat conductance as well as less heat generated by shivering. Some elderly patients lose the ability to shiver. Older people may also experience a loss of the ability to vasoconstrict cutaneous vessels in response to cold.

**Answer: C**

Irwin, R. and Rippe, J. (2008) *Irwin and Rippe's Intensive Care Medicine*, 6th edn, Lippincott Wiliams & Wilkins, Philadelphia, PA.

**Questions 3 and 4** *A man becomes lost on a hiking trip in winter. He is found after 36 hours and brought to the emergency department. His skin is cool to the touch. He is* *lethargic with sluggish pupils. His EKG shows a heart rate of 52 beats/min with J waves (Osborn waves) noted.*

**3** *His expected core body temperature would be:*
   **A** *37°C*
   **B** *35°C*
   **C** *31°C*
   **D** *26°C*
   **E** *20°C*

This patient demonstrates signs and symptoms consistent with moderate hypothermia. Mild hypothermia is classified based on core body temperature of 35–32.2 °C. One would expect to see confusion, slurred speech, impaired judgment, and tachycardia. This patient exhibits moderate hypothermia, defined as core body temperature of <32.2–28 °C. Besides the symptoms noted above, a patient would also exhibit hypoventilation, decreased oxygen consumption and $CO_2$ production. The bradycardia that patients with moderate hypothermia exhibit is resistant to atropine. Severe hypothermia is defined as core temperature below 28 °C. At this temperature, patients may experience spontaneous ventricular fibrillation or asystole. Severe hypothermia causes a decline in blood pressure (BP) and cardiac output as well as a loss of cerebrovascular regulation. EEG activity is diminished in severe hypothermia.

**Answer: C**

Hanania, N.A. and Zimmerman, J.L. Hypothermia, in *Principles of Critical Care*, 3rd edn (eds J.B. Hall, G.A. Schmidt, and L.D.H. Wood), www.accesssurgery.com/content.aspx?aID=2282615 (accessed November 14, 2011).

**4** *After removing the man's wet clothing and confirming core body temperature with a low-reading rectal thermometer, normal saline warmed to 42°C is administered via short IV tubing. The next most appropriate step in this patient's management is:*
   **A** *Endotracheal intubation*
   **B** *Transcutaneous pacing*
   **C** *Placement of nasogastric tube with warm saline gastric lavage*
   **D** *Immersion in a 40°C water bath*
   **E** *Placement of a forced air blanket over the body*

Although some controversy exists with regard to the optimal method and rate of rewarming, with moderate hypothermia (temperature <32.2–28 °C), active rewarming is indicated. There are no controlled studies that compare rewarming protocols, so there is no level 1 evidence to guide rewarming. After removing any wet clothing or other factors that may contribute to ongoing heat loss, the patient should be placed in a controlled, warm environment. Passive external rewarming, consisting of covering the patient with an insulating material to prevent any additional heat loss can increase body temperature by 0.5–2 °C per hour. This should be performed in patients with mild or moderate hypothermia and may be sufficient treatment in patients with mild hypothermia. For patients with moderate to severe hypothermia, any cardiovascular instability, or inadequate rewarming by passive methods, more aggressive rewarming is indicated. Active external rewarming methods include forced air rewarming (Bair Hugger-type blanket), heating pads, radiant heat and submersion in a 40 °C water bath. Active external rewarming may cause vasodilatation of the extremities, facilitating transport of colder peripheral blood to the warmer core and transiently lowering core body temperature. Peripheral vasodilatation may also worsen hypotension. There are technical challenges associated with immersion in a water bath with regards to monitoring and active resuscitation. Successful use of forced air blankets, which are readily available, as the primary rewarming method has been reported, even in cases with cardiopulmonary arrest. Active core warming may be needed if active external rewarming fails. Techniques include gastric lavage with warm saline, the delivery of heated oxygen via an endotracheal tube, pleural cavity lavage through chest tubes and peritoneal lavage. Rewarming rates average 1–3 °C per hour. In cases of severe hypothermia, cardiopulmonary bypass can provide circulatory support and raise core temperatures much more quickly, up to 1–2 °C every three to five minutes, though this takes time to initiate, may require systemic anticoagulation, and may not be readily available.

**Answer: E**

Hanania, N.A. and Zimmerman, J.L. Hypothermia, in *Principles of Critical Care*, 3rd edn (eds J.B. Hall, G.A. Schmidt, and L.D.H. Wood), www.accesssurgery.com/content.aspx?aID=2282615 (accessed November 14, 2011).

Koller, R., Schnider, T.W., and Neidhart, P. (1997) Deep accidental hypothermia and cardiac arrest – rewarming with forced air. *Acta Anaesthesiologica Scandinavica*, **31**, 1359–1364.

**5** *A 22-year-old military recruit collapses at basic training. He is brought to the emergency department for treatment. Which of the following would differentiate heat exhaustion from heat stroke in this patient?*
   **A** *Lactic acidosis*
   **B** *Heart rate of 127 beats/min*

C  *Orthostatic hypotension*
D  *Temperature of 39.8 °C*
E  *Sweating*

The spectrum of heat injury encompasses heat cramps, heat exhaustion and heat stroke. Treatment of heat exhaustion does not generally require intensive care management but it is important to differentiate it from heat stroke. There are two syndromes of heat stroke: classic heat stroke typically occurs in older individuals with underlying medical problems, while exertional heat stroke predominantly occurs in younger individuals who participate in vigorous activity in a hot environment. Both syndromes can present with tachycardia and orthostatic hypotension. Sweating is present in 50% of individuals presenting with heat stroke, so this is not a useful discriminating factor between heat stroke and heat exhaustion. Heat stroke most often presents with a history of exposure to heat, severe CNS dysfunction and temperature >40 °C. However, temperature alone does not rule out heat stroke, since frequently attempts at cooling the patient have been initiated in the prehospital setting. Heat stroke involves a systemic inflammatory response that leads to organ dysfunction, predominantly encephalopathy. Lactic acidosis would not be expected in heat exhaustion but may be seen as severe in heat stroke. In classic heat stroke, it is generally the result of hypoperfusion, while in exertional heat stroke it is usually caused by anaerobic muscle metabolism.

**Answer: A**

Zimmerman, J.L. and Hanania, N.A. Hyperthermia, in *Principles of Critical Care*, 3rd edn, (eds J.B. Hall, G.A. Schmidt, and L.D.H. Wood), www.accesssurgery.com/content.aspx?aID=2282701, accessed November 14, 2011.

6  *In a patient who remains comatose after resuscitation from cardiac arrest, which of the following would be a contraindication to therapeutic hypothermia?*
   A  *Initial rhythm of asystole*
   B  *An elapsed time of six hours since the arrest*
   C  *Need for norepinephrine at 0.1 µg/kg/min*
   D  *Cardiac arrest as a result of a motor vehicle crash with a pelvic fracture*
   E  *Glasgow Coma motor score of 4 on exam*

At experienced centers, there are multiple indications for therapeutic hypothermia. The most common is cardiac arrest with coma (unable to follow commands) after return of spontaneous circulation (ROSC). Other indications include severe cerebral edema from acute liver failure (while awaiting transplantation) and refractory intracranial hypertension. In survivors of cardiac arrest, it is standard to induce therapeutic hypothermia regardless of the initial presenting rhythm. If more than 8 hours have elapsed since the return of spontaneous circulation, hypothermia may have limited value. Other contraindications include imminent cardiopulmonary collapse despite hemodynamic support or mechanical hemodynamic support, or the presence of any underlying existing terminal condition. Therapy with pressors would not, in and of itself, be a contraindication for hypothermia, unless the patient remains unstable despite aggressive support. In addition, hypothermia should be avoided in patients with life-threatening bleeding or infection. For this reason, hypothermia should not be induced in trauma patients with cardiac arrest unless bleeding can be effectively ruled out. In the case of a traumatic cardiac arrest, only if the trauma workup reveals no source of hemorrhage would hypothermia be appropriate.

**Answer: D**

Seder, D.B. and Van der Kloot, T.E. (2009) Methods of cooling: practical aspects of therapeutic temperature management. *Critical Care Medicine*, **37** (7), S211–S222.

7  *In patients undergoing operative procedures, a body temperature of 35 °C in the recovery room is associated with:*
   A  *Stimulation of the immune response to surgery*
   B  *Improved wound healing*
   C  *Increased risk of surgical site infection*
   D  *Decreased hospital length of stay*
   E  *Increased systemic vasodilation*

Perioperative hypothermia is defined as a temperature of <36 °C at any point in the perioperative period. There is significant evidence that it is associated with significant morbidity. The two main areas of increased morbidity are surgical site infection and cardiac complications. Perioperative hypothermia has a significant effect on the immune system including leukocyte migration, neutrophil phagocytosis, and cytokine antibody production. These immune changes result in a decreased resistance to surgical-site infections (SSI). Surgical-site infections have been associated with an increased risk of death, increased length of hospital stay, and an increase in hospital costs. Perioperative hypothermia can also cause an increase in circulating catecholamine levels, systemic vasoconstriction, and systemic blood pressure. These effects increase cardiac demands and lead to an increased risk of cardiac morbidity. Perioperative hypothermia, however, remains common. Recent guidelines recommend that active measures be taken to the prevention of perioperative hypothermia in an effort to reduce the risk of SSIs and morbid cardiac events. These active measures include esophageal or oral thermometry, the use of IV fluid warmers for abdominal procedures of greater than one hour duration and the use of warm forced air devices for procedures that are expected to last greater than 30 minutes.

**Answer: C**

Forbes, S.S., Eskicioglu, C., Nathens, A.B., *et al.* (2009) Evidence-based guidelines for prevention of perioperative hypothermia. *Journal of the American College of Surgeons*, **209**, 492–503.

Melling, A.C., Ali, B., Scott, E.M., *et al.* (2001) Effects of preoperative warming on the incidence of wound infection after clean surgery: a randomized controlled trial. *Lancet*, **358**, 876–880.

**8**  *The cardiovascular and hemodynamic effect of mild hypothermia (33 °C) in a healthy euvolemic patient includes:*
   A  *Increased heart rate*
   B  *Decreased myocardial contractility*
   C  *Increased cardiac output*
   D  *Increased systolic function*
   E  *No change in vascular resistance*

The effect of hypothermia on the myocardium and cardiovascular physiology are complex and depend on the patient's volume status and sedation level. It also depends on the depth of hypothermia. With mild hypothermia in an otherwise healthy, euvolemic patient, heart rate would decrease with an increase in myocardial contractility. Systolic function will improve while a mild degree of diastolic dysfunction may occur. With the decrease in heart rate, a decrease in cardiac output may be seen. Given that the metabolic rate decreases with hypothermia, the balance between oxygen supply and demand for tissues is generally stable or improved. In contrast to mild hypothermia, deep hypothermia (less than 30 °C) does decrease myocardial contractility and may also cause hypovolemia by inducing a cold diuresis and capillary leak.

**Answer: D**

Polderman, K.H. (2009) Mechanisms of action, physiological effects and complications of hypothermia. *Critical Care Medicine*, **37**, S186–S202.

**9**  *In the brain injured patient:*
   A  *Fever occurs in approximately 30% of all patients with subarachnoid hemorrhage (SAH)*
   B  *Fever in traumatic brain injury is associated with poor long-term outcomes*
   C  *Fever has no impact on the outcome after ischemic stroke*

   D  *An infectious cause for fever is rarely found after spinal cord injury*
   E  *There is no relationship between fever and cerebral vasospasm in SAH*

Fever occurs in approximately 70% of all neurologically injured patients. Only half the febrile episodes can be attributed to infection, with pneumonia the most common source of infection in these patients. Early temperature elevation after brain injury is most commonly attributed to an acute phase response. Blood within the cerebrospinal fluid spaces, particularly the intraventricular spaces, may lead to fever. Patients with subarachnoid hemorrhage (SAH) have a high rate of fever—up to 70%—and this has been implicated in the development of cerebrovascular spasm. Fever in the acute phase of SAH has been independently associated with morbidity and mortality. Fever after traumatic brain injury (TBI) is associated with increased intracranial pressure, neurologic impairment and long-term poor outcome. Spinal-cord injured patients may have difficulty maintaining normothermia. Therefore, they will most commonly have an infection causing fever, generally pneumonia or a urinary tract infection; although fever of unknown origin can also occur. In ischemic stroke patients, early fever is associated with worse stroke severity and outcomes.

**Answer: B**

Badjatia, N. (2009) Hyperthermia and fever control in brain injury. *Critical Care Medicine*, **37**, S250–S257.

**10**  *Which of the following medications does not predispose individuals to heat-related illness?*
   A  *Meclizine*
   B  *Quetiapine*
   C  *Hydroyxzine*
   D  *Aspirin*
   E  *Doxepin*

Anticholinergic medications and antihistamines may impair sweating rates and thus limit evaporative capacity. Diuretics can result in hypohydration and salt depletion – resulting in decreased plasma volume – which may predispose individuals to heat-related illness. Daily aspirin therapy in healthy middle-aged adults exercising in heat had measurable delays in skin blood flow, but a negligible effect on cardiovascular response and perception of heat. In a laboratory study of exertional heat stress, there was no difference between the rise in heart rate, internal body temperature or thermal perception between individuals taking aspirin versus placebo.

**Answer: D**

Hostler, D., Suyama, J., Guyette, FX, *et al.* (2014) A randomized controlled trial of aspirin and exertional heat stress activation of platelets in firefighters during exertion in thermal protective clothing. *Prehospital Emergency Care.* **18**(3), 359–367.

**11**   *When compared with surface cooling techniques for induced-hypothermia or targeted temperature management, intravascular cooling techniques:*
   **A** *Achieve target temperature more rapidly*
   **B** *Overcool more commonly than with surface cooling devices*
   **C** *Are more precise in the maintenance of desired temperature*
   **D** *Are associated with an increase in adverse events*
   **E** *Are associated with improved neurologic outcomes*

Data collected in the Targeted Temperature Management trial was retrospectively analyzed to determine differences between surface and intravascular cooling device effectiveness. The rate to achieve the temperature goal was similar between intravascular and surface cooling devices. Intravascular cooling devices were better at maintaining target temperature than surface devices. The incidence of adverse events was equal between the two groups. There was no difference in neurologic outcome between the two groups. While surface devices had more episodes of overcooling, there was no statistically significant difference noted.

**Answer: C**

Glover, G.W., Thomas, R.M., Vamvakas, G., *et al.* (2016) Intravascular versus surface cooling for targeted temperature management after out-of-hospital cardiac arrest – an analysis of the TTM trial data. *Critical Care,* **20**, 1–10.

**12**   *Metabolic consequences of moderate-to-severe hypothermia include all of the following, except:*
   **A** *Reduced oxygen consumption*
   **B** *Increased fat metabolism*
   **C** *Mild metabolic acidosis*
   **D** *Decreased free radical production*
   **E** *Increased insulin secretion*

Moderate-to-severe hypothermia results in a decrease in the metabolic rate, with an approximately 50–60% decrease in oxygen consumption and $CO_2$ production at 32 °C. If ventilator settings are left unchanged, hyperventilation may result with potentially deleterious consequences such as cerebral vasoconstriction. Increased fat metabolism results in increased levels of glycerol, free fatty acids, ketones, and lactate. This may result in a mild metabolic acidosis. Free radical production is reduced in hypothermia, although production is not completely prevented. Insulin secretion is reduced in hypothermia, which may result in moderate to severe insulin resistance and a need to increase insulin doses during targeted temperature management. It is important to remember that during active rewarming, endogenous insulin will increase and require attention to glucose levels and likely modification of insulin dosing.

**Answer: E**

Polderman, K.H. (2009) Mechanisms of action, physiological effects and complications of hypothermia. *Critical Care Medicine,* **37**, S186–S202.

# 17

## Acute Kidney Injury
*Remigio J. Flor, MD, Keneeshia N. Williams, MD and Terence O'Keeffe, MD*

1 *Which of the following is not part of the definition of Acute Kidney Injury (AKI)? (as per the KDIGO clinical practice guidelines – see Table 17.1).*
   A *Increase in serum creatinine by ≥ 0.3 mg/dL within 72 hours*
   B *Urine output of less than 0.5 mL/kg/hour for 6 hours*
   C *Increase in serum creatinine to ≥ 1.5 times baseline, which is known or presumed to have occurred within the prior 7 days*
   D *An increase in serum creatinine from 0.8 mg/dL to 1.3 mg/dL within 48 hours*
   E *Anuria for 12 hours*

An increase in serum creatinine by ≥0.3 mg/dL must be within 48 hours to meet the criteria for AKI, not 72 hours. A patient who has a urine output of less than 0.5 mL/kg/hour for 6 hours is one of the KDIGO criteria for defining AKI. This patient classifies as stage 1 AKI.

An increase in serum creatinine to ≥ 1.5 times baseline, which is known or presumed to have occurred within the prior 7 days is also one of the KDIGO criteria for defining AKI. This patient classifies as stage 1 AKI.

The patient in option D has an increase in serum creatinine from 0.8 mg/dL to 1.3 mg/dL within 48 hours. This meets the ≥ 0.3 mg/dL increase within 48 hours criteria for stage 1 AKI.

A patient who has a urine output of less than 0.5 mL/kg/hour for six hours meets the criteria for AKI. Furthermore, anuria for at least 12 hours meets the definition of stage 3 AKI.

The term acute renal failure (ARF) has been largely replaced by acute kidney injury (AKI). AKI is considered a more accurate description of an acute loss of kidney function that is of clinical relevance but that does not necessarily result in overt organ failure. In 2004, a consensus group of expert intensivists and nephrologists called the Acute Dialysis Quality Initiative (ADQI) group introduced the RIFLE criteria to make a uniform definition for AKI. This was later modified by the Acute Kidney Injury Network (AKIN) which provided both a staging system and diagnostic criteria for AKI. In 2012, the Kidney Disease: Improving Global Outcomes (KDIGO) Clinical Practice Guidelines for AKI revised the definition of AKI merging both the RIFLE and AKIN criteria. The KDIGO criteria only uses changes in the biomarkers of serum creatinine and urine output for adults. The only exception is in pediatric patients where GFR is used only for stage 3 AKI, otherwise GFR is not used for staging. KDIGO also accounts for the timeframe of biomarker changes. Furthermore, the criteria divides AKI into 3 stages with patients classified according to the criteria that results in the highest stage of injury.

AKI as defined by KDIGO: Increase in serum creatinine by ≥ 0.3 mg/dL (≥26.5 micromol/L) within 48 hours; or increase in serum creatinine to ≥ 1.5 times baseline, which is known or presumed to have occurred within the prior 7 days; or urine volume < 0.5 mL/kg/hour for six hours

**Answer: A**

KDIGO Clinical Practice Guideline for Acute Kidney Injury (2012) *Kidney International Supplements*, **2** (1), http://www.kdigo.org/clinical_practice_guidelines/pdf/ KDIGO%20AKI%20Guideline.pdf (accessed November 17, 2017).

Ostermann, M. and Joannidis, M. (2016) Acute kidney injury 2016: diagnosis and diagnostic workup. *Critical Care*, **20**, 1–13.

2 *Which of the following patients meet the criteria for stage 3 AKI according to the KDIGO Clinical Practice Guidelines?*
   A *6-year-old girl with an estimated GFR to 50 mL/ min/1.73 m$^2$*
   B *88-year-old man with an increase in serum creatinine to two times over baseline the past 48 hours*

**Table 17.1** The KDIGO criteria stages of AKI.

| KDIGO criteria AKI Stages | Increase in Serum Cr | Decrease in Urine Output (UOP) | Other findings |
|---|---|---|---|
| 1 | Increase ≥ 0.3 mg/dL (≥ 26.5 micromol/L) Increase to 1.5 to 1.9 times baseline | Reduction in urine output to < 0.5 mL/kg/hour for 6 to 12 hours | |
| 2 | Increase to 2.0 to 2.9 times baseline | Reduction in urine output to < 0.5 mL/kg/hour for ≥ 12 hours | |
| 3 | Increase in serum creatinine to ≥ 4.0 mg/dL (≥ 353.6 micromol/L) Increase in serum creatinine to 3.0 times baseline | Reduction in urine output to < 0.3 mL/kg/hour for ≥ 24 hours, or anuria for ≥ 12 hours | The initiation of renal replacement therapy, or, in patients < 18 years, decrease in eGFR to < 35 mL/min/1.73 m$^2$ |

**C** *45-year-old woman with an increase in baseline serum creatinine from 0.9 to 2.2 mg/dL in 48 hours*
**D** *77-year-old man who started renal replacement therapy 3 hours ago*
**E** *24-year-old man that has a urine output of 0.4 mL/kg/hour for the past 12 hours*

Estimated GFR (eGFR) is only used as part of the KDIGO criteria in pediatric patients in defining stage 3 AKI. This patient has an estimated GFR to 50 mL/min/1.73 m$^2$ which is below normal range for her age but above the eGFR <35 mL/min/1.73 m$^2$ required as criteria for stage 3 AKI.

A serum creatinine increase of 2 times over baseline the past 48 hours meets the KDIGO criteria of 2.0–2.9 times increase from baseline for stage 2 AKI.

The patient in option C had a serum creatinine increase of about 2.0 times baseline in 48 hours meeting the KDIGO criteria for stage 2 AKI.

A patient who requires the initiation of renal replacement therapy meets the criteria for stage 3 AKI.

A urine output of 0.4 mL/kg/hour for the past 12 hours meets the criteria for stage 2 AKI. Stage 3 criteria would be met if the patient had a reduction in urine output to < 0.3 mL/kg/hour for ≥ 24 hours.

The KDIGO criteria uses only changes in the biomarkers of serum creatinine and urine output for adults. An exception is made in pediatric patients where the estimated GFR (eGFR) is used only for stage 3 AKI, otherwise eGFR is not used for staging. KDIGO also accounts for the timeframe of biomarker changes. Furthermore, the criteria divides AKI into 3 stages with patients classified according to the criteria that results in the highest stage of injury.

See Table 17.1 for details on the KDIGO criteria stages of AKI.

**Answer: D**

KDIGO Clinical Practice Guideline for Acute Kidney Injury (2012) *Kidney International Supplements*, **2** (1),

http://www.kdigo.org/clinical_practice_guidelines/pdf/ KDIGO%20AKI%20Guideline.pdf (accessed November 17, 2017).
Ostermann, M. and Joannidis, M. (2016) Acute kidney injury 2016: diagnosis and diagnostic workup. *Critical Care*, **20**, 1–13.

**3** *Which of the following is not consistent with acute tubular necrosis in a patient with oliguria?*
**A** *Urine osmolality of 280 mOsm/L*
**B** *Fractional excretion of sodium (FENa) of 3%*
**C** *Urine/plasma creatinine ratio of 18*
**D** *The presence of granular casts on urine microscopy*
**E** *Urinary sodium of 12 mEq/L*

Acute tubular necrosis is one of many causes of oliguric renal failure, but can usually be distinguished from prerenal azotemia by a low urine osmolality (<350 mOsm/L), a high urinary sodium (>40 mEq/L), an elevated FENa (usually > 2%), a low urine/plasma creatinine ratio of < 20, and the presence of granular casts and renal tubular epithelial cells on microscopy.

Urinary sodium of less than 20 mEq/L is more typically found in patients with pre-renal azotemia. The FENa is the most discriminatory single test

**Answer: E**

Fauci, A., Braunwald, E., Kasper, D.L., *et al.* (2008) Acute renal failure, in *Harrison's Principles of Internal Medicine*, 17th edn, McGraw-Hill, New York, pp. 1752–1761.
Lerma, E.V. and Kelly, B. (2011) Acute tubular necrosis. eMedicine at Medscape.com, http://emedicine. medscape.com/article/238064-overview (accessed February 14, 2011).

**4** *Which of the following would not be part of an appropriate initial workup for a postoperative surgical*

patient with oliguria, a BUN of 45 mg/dL and a creatinine of 2.2 mg/dL?

A Sending urinary electrolytes and creatinine to calculate a fractional excretion of sodium (FENa)

B Assessment of intravascular volume by invasive monitoring

C Renal arteriography to assess for renal artery stenosis

D Calculation of the BUN/Cr ratio

E Placement of a Foley catheter to assess hourly urine volume

A thorough history and physical exam may provide key information regarding the likely source of the acute kidney injury (AKI). The goal is to identify whether the patient is in AKI due to a prerenal, renal or postrenal cause, as this will guide the management of the patient and help to identify what further testing may be necessary.

The initial investigation of acute kidney injury should include urinary electrolytes, a plasma chemistry panel, a complete blood count, bladder scanning and/or placement of a Foley catheter as well as an assessment of intravascular fluid volume status. Urine microscopy and urinary tract ultrasound may also form part of these initial investigations.

In the patient case presented, a renal angiogram would not be indicated as one of the first line investigations. Renal angiography is rarely indicated in the acute phase and in fact may exacerbate the situation by increasing the kidney injury due to the intravenous contrast required.

**Answer: C**

Anderson, R.J. (2007) Acute renal failure, in *Critical Care Medicine. Principles of Diagnosis and Management in the Adult*, 3rd edn (eds J.E. Parrillo and R.P. Dellinger), Mosby, Philadelphia, PA, pp. 1163–1188.

5  A 49-year-old woman is admitted to the ICU after undergoing an abdominal peritoneal resection for rectal cancer. Immediately postoperatively, the patient was noted to have decreased urine output. She responds well to a fluid bolus. She was restarted on her home medications, which included atorvastatin, aspirin 325 mg, lisinopril, and metoprolol. On postoperative day 4, she is noted to have purulent drainage from her perineal wound. Her abdomen has increased distention. Her WBC is 17 000/mm$^3$, and she is febrile to 38.9 °C. Her creatinine was 0.8 mg/dL preoperatively and is now 2.7 mg/dL. Her urine output was 10 ml in the last hour. A bladder pressure is measured and is noted to be 10 mm Hg. Which of the following is least likely to have contributed to the AKI in this patient?

A Hypovolemia

B Nephrotoxic agent

C Sepsis

D Increased abdominal pressure

E Ischemia

Hypovolemia and ischemia are not uncommon following major surgery. The patient's low urine output in the immediately postoperative period indicates hypovolemia.

ACE-inhibitors and NSAIDs are among the most common nephrotoxic drugs.

Sepsis, hypovolemia, nephrotoxic agents, ischemia, and increased abdominal pressure are all common causes of AKI. Sepsis is the most common cause of AKI and can account for up to 50% of cases.

Increased abdominal pressure is often overlooked as a cause of AKI. However, this patient's bladder pressure is not consistent with elevated intra-abdominal pressure.

**Answer: D**

Al-Mufarrej, F., Abell, L.M., and Chawla, L.S. (2012) Understanding intra-abdominal hypertensions: from bench to bedside. *Journal of Intensive Care Medicine*, **27**, 145–160.

Uchino, S., Kellum, J.A., Bellomo, R., *et al.* (2005) Acute renal failure in critically ill patients: a multinational, multicenter study. *Journal of the American Medical Association*, **294**, 813–818.

6  Which of the following patients with hyperkalemia would most benefit from dialysis?

A 58-year-old man with a potassium level of 5.2 mEq/L and a urine output of 0.4 mL/kg/hour over a 48 hour period

B 72-year-old man taking lisinopril 20 mg daily with a potassium level of 5.5 mEq/L

C 49-year-old woman with a potassium level of 5.7 mEq/L with a recent diagnosis of stage 1 AKI but decreasing levels of serum creatinine over the past 24 hours

D 56-year-old woman with a potassium level of 5.8 mEq/L which has been refractory to conservative therapy and a recent diagnosis of stage 2 AKI

E 94-year-old woman with a recent diagnosis of stage 3 AKI and a potassium level of 5.5 mEq/L, but with a good prognosis

Reversible causes of hyperkalemia such as ACE-inhibitors for hypovolemia should be addressed as they are generally responsive to medical therapy. Dialysis should be reserved for patients who are refractive to medical therapy.

A recent diagnosis of AKI may indicate the need for dialysis. However, this patient is showing evidence of an improving AKI with a decreasing serum creatinine.

A patient with hyperkalemia without easily reversible causes which has been refractory to conservative therapy is an indication for dialysis.

The patient in option E has a mild hyperkalemia with no evidence of symptoms. She would most benefit from medical therapy prior to proceeding with dialysis if needed.

**Answer: D**

Kellum, J.A., Leblanc, M., and Venkataraman, R. (2008) Acute renal failure. Clinical Evidence, ii, **2001**.

Moss, A.H. (2010) Revised dialysis clinical practice guideline promotes more informed decision-making. *Clinical Journal of the American Society of Nephrology*, **5** (12), 2380–2383.

7 *In patients with acute kidney injury from traumatic rhabdomyolysis, which of the following is true?*
   A *Serum myoglobin levels remain elevated longer than serum CK levels*
   B *Early aggressive fluid replacement with saline is the mainstay of treatment*
   C *Mannitol is strongly recommended as first line therapy in the treatment of this condition*
   D *Alkalinization of the urine using intravenous sodium bicarbonate, targeting a pH of greater than 6.0, can prevent renal failure in patients with rhabdomyolysis*
   E *Treatment should be instituted when the creatine kinase (CK) levels rise to above 3000 U/L*

Rhabdomyolysis is most commonly caused by trauma but may also be due to medications, exercise, toxins, infections, muscle enzyme deficiencies, or endocrinopathies.

The half-life of serum CK is 1.5 days, compared to 2–3 hours for serum myoglobin.

The only effective treatment seems to be aggressive intravenous fluid replacement early in the course of the disease.

Neither mannitol nor urinary alkalinization with sodium bicarbonate have been convincingly shown to reduce the need for dialysis or mortality from this condition.

Rhabdomyolysis is associated with elevated levels of creatine kinase. Levels above 5000 U/L are associated with acute kidney injury and treatment is recommended above this level.

**Answer: B**

Brown, C.V., Rhee, P., Chan, L., *et al.* (2004) Preventing renal failure in patients with rhabdomyolysis: do bicarbonate and mannitol make a difference? *Journal of Trauma*, **56** (6), 1191–1196.

Huerta-Alardín, A.L., Varon, J., and Marik, P.E. (2005) Bench-to-bedside review: Rhabdomyolysis –- an overview for clinicians. *Critical Care*, **9** (2), 158–169.

8 *Which of the following would not be considered an indication for acute dialysis?*
   A *A patient with primary hyperparathyroidism, with a serum calcium of 12 mg/dL, unresponsive to hydration and calcitonin*
   B *A pericardial friction rub in a patient with a BUN of 100 mg/dL*
   C *A patient with a prolonged international normalized ratio due to warfarin overdose*
   D *A central venous pressure of 20 cm $H_2O$ in a patient with AKI and acute pulmonary edema*
   E *A pH of 7.15, unresponsive to bicarbonate fluid therapy*

The easily remembered mnemonic of AEIOU (Acid-base, Electrolytes, Intoxications, Overload, Uremic symptoms) still provides a good working guide for the indications for dialysis in the acute setting.

Dialysis can remove electrolyte abnormalities such as hypercalcemia, hyperkalemia and hyperphosphatemia. It should be noted that hypocalcemia is more common in acute kidney injury (AKI), with hypercalcemia being much more rare, and is usually associated with the diuretic phase of rhabdomyolysis-associated AKI.

Excessive uremia can generally lead to instituting dialysis especially in patients with a BUN of greater than 100 mg/dL. Uremic symptoms are an indication for dialysis. These symptoms include pericarditis, nausea and vomiting, altered mental status, and coagulopathy.

Dialysis may be indicated for the removal of certain metabolic poisons and/or medications, however warfarin does not cross the dialysis membrane and so an overdose of this drug cannot be treated in this way. It will require reversal with vitamin K, prothrombin complex concentrate, and/or fresh frozen plasma.

Fluid overload, especially if symptomatic as demonstrated by pulmonary edema in a patient non-responsive to diuretics, is an appropriate indication for dialysis.

Patients with severe metabolic acidosis that is unresponsive to conservative therapy are also good candidates for acute dialysis.

**Answer: C**

Palevksy, P. Renal replacement therapy (dialysis) in acute kidney injury (acute renal failure): Indications, timing, and dialysis dose. Uptodate.com: http://www.uptodate.com/contents/renal-replacement-therapy-dialysis-in-acute-kidney-injury-acute-renal-failure-indications-timing-and-dialysis-dose (accessed November 12, 2016).

Sharfuddin, A., Weisbord, S.D., Palevsky, P.M., and Molitoris, B.A. (2012) Acute kidney injury, in *Brenner and Rector's The Kidney*, 9th edn (eds, M.W. Taal, G.M. Chertow, P.A. Marsden, *et al.*), W.B. Saunders, Philadelphia, PA, pp. 1044–1099.

**9** *Which of the following prevention strategies has the highest level of evidence for reducing the risk of contrast-induced nephropathy (CIN) using intravenous low-osmolar contrast media (LOCM)?*
   **A** *Ascorbic Acid plus IV saline*
   **B** *IV sodium bicarbonate alone*
   **C** *N-acetylcysteine plus IV saline*
   **D** *Intravenous saline alone*
   **E** *N-acetylcysteine plus IV sodium bicarbonate*

Ascorbic acid is an antioxidant, and as such, acts as a scavenger of reactive oxygen species which reduces oxidative stress possibly preventing CIN. There is however a low strength of evidence in randomized controlled trials that compared ascorbic acid with IV saline or N-acetylcystine.

Sodium bicarbonate acts to diminish the production of free oxygen radicals by alkalinization of tubular fluid. This is believed to be the mechanism by which CIN is prevented. An analysis of 11 randomized, controlled trials with patients who received LOCM showed no statistical difference between treatment of IV sodium bicarbonate vs. IV saline. Furthermore, an analysis of seven randomized clinical trials comparing N-acetylcysteine plus IV saline vs. sodium bicarbonate showed no clinical benefit over the use of one treatment over the other. The strength of evidence is low for the use of sodium bicarbonate over N-acetylcysteine plus IV saline.

N-acetylcysteine has both antioxidant and vasodilatory properties that is thought to protect against CIN. It acts as a direct free radical scavenger and improves blood flow via nitric oxide mediated pathways. An analysis of 40 studies showed a clinical benefit and moderate level of evidence in preventing CIN when N-acetylcysteine with IV saline was used vs. IV saline alone. Furthermore, KDIGO Clinical Practice Guidelines recommend using N-acetylcysteine with IV fluids in patents who are at an increased risk for CIN.

**Answer: C**

KDIGO Clinical Practice Guideline for Acute Kidney Injury (2012) *Kidney International Supplements*, **2** (1), http://www.kdigo.org/clinical_practice_guidelines/pdf/KDIGO%20AKI%20Guideline.pdf (accessed November 17, 2017).
Subramaniam, R.M., Suarez-Cuervo, C., Wilson, R.F., *et al.* (2016) Effectiveness of prevention strategies for contrast-induced nephropathy: a systematic review and meta-analysis. *Annals of Internal Medicine*, **164** (6), 406–416.

**10** *Which of the following signs and/or symptoms is unlikely to be observed in a patient with hyperkalemia due to stage 3 AKI?*
   **A** *Widened QRS complex in a patient with a potassium level of 5.5 mEq/L*
   **B** *Peaked T waves on the EKG*
   **C** *Left bundle branch block with a potassium level of 7.2 mEq/L.*
   **D** *Ventricular fibrillation if untreated*
   **E** *Generalized fatigue*

The EKG changes are generally related to the serum potassium level, therefore a widened QRS complex would be unlikely in a patient with a potassium level of only 5.5 mEq/L.

Early changes on the EKG consist of peaked T waves, a shortened QT interval, and ST segment depression. These are followed by bundle branch blocks and widening of the QRS complex. Without treatment the QRS morphology will eventually widen to resemble a sine wave, with ventricular fibrillation or asystole following.

Patients may be asymptomatic or can report generalized fatigue, weakness, paresthesias, palpitations, or even paralysis.

**Answer: A**

Garth, D. (2011) Hyperkalemia in emergency medicine. eMedicine at Medscape.com: http://emedicine.medscape.com/article/766479-overview (accessed February 12, 2011).
Nyirenda, M.J., Tang, J.I., Padfield, P.L., *et al.* (2009) Hyperkalaemia. *British Medical Journal*, **339**, b4114.

**11** *Which of the following laboratory findings is consistent with an intrinsic cause of acute kidney injury?*
   **A** Urine osmolality of 380 mOsm/L
   **B** BUN/Cr ratio of 18
   **C** Urine Na of 15 mEq/L
   **D** Fractional excretion of sodium (FENa) of 1%
   **E** Urine pH of 4.5

Intrinsic and prerenal causes of acute kidney injury may often be difficult to distinguish in a clinic setting.

Intrinsic causes of acute kidney injury (AKI) result in low urine osmolality (<350 mOsm/L), a low BUN/Cr ratio (<20:1), and a high urine Na (>40 mEq/L). The results shown in answers A and C are more consistent with prerenal causes of AKI.

Calculating the FENa value is considered the most discriminatory test. A FENa of < 2% suggests a prerenal cause of AKI while an elevated FENa of > 3% suggests an intrinsic cause of AKI.

Low urine pH findings are consistent with prerenal causes of AKI.

**Answer: B**

Townsend, C., Jr, Beauchamp, D., Evers, B., and Mattox, K. (2012) *Sabiston Textbook of Surgery: The Biological Basis of Modern Surgical Practice*, 19th edn, Philadelphia, PA. Elsevier Saunders, pp. 584–585

**12** *Which of the following tests is the single most discriminatory test in distinguishing the difference between a prerenal and intrinsic cause of AKI?*
  **A** *Urine Na*
  **B** *Urine osmolality*
  **C** *FENa*
  **D** *Urine specific gravity*
  **E** *BUN/Cr ratio*

Intrinsic and prerenal causes of acute kidney injury may often be difficult to distinguish in a clinic setting. Urine sodium, urine osmolality, urine specific gravity, and BUN/Cr ratio may all assist in discriminating between prerenal and intrinsic causes of AKI while not clinically apparent. However, FENa is considered the most discriminatory test.

Calculating the FENa value is considered the most discriminatory test. A FENa of < 2% suggests a prerenal cause of AKI while an elevated FENa of > 3% suggests an intrinsic cause of AKI.

**Answer: C**

Townsend, C., Jr, Beauchamp, D., Evers, B., and Mattox, K. (2012) *Sabiston Textbook of Surgery: The Biological Basis of Modern Surgical Practice*, 19th edn, Philadelphia, PA. Elsevier Saunders, pp. 584–585

**13** *In a patient with severe hyperkalemia (potassium > 6.5 mEq/dL) and widened QRS complexes, which of the following treatments should be administered first to prevent malignant ventricular arrhythmias?*
  **A** *Albuterol*
  **B** *Intravenous calcium gluconate*
  **C** *Intravenous sodium bicarbonate*
  **D** *Intravenous furosemide*
  **E** *Intravenous insulin and glucose*

Albuterol has a similar effect and onset of action as that of intravenous insulin. All the treatment choices listed can be used to treat hyperkalemia, however, calcium gluconate will have the most rapid effect by stabilizing the myocardium, thereby decreasing the risk of arrhythmias. It is usually only indicated when EKG changes are present.

Sodium bicarbonate raises pH, which results in potassium shifts into the intracellular space. Furosemide can be effective by inducing potassium loss through the kidney if the patient can still make urine, but the onset of action is slower, and large doses may be needed in AKI.

Intravenous insulin will drive potassium back into the cells and the effects occur within 30 minutes of administration. Glucose is given simultaneously to prevent hypoglycemia.

**Answer: B**

Garth, D. (2011) Hyperkalemia in emergency medicine. eMedicine at Medscape.com: http://emedicine.medscape.com/article/766479-overview (accessed Februaty 12, 2011).

Nyirenda, M.J., Tang, J.I., Padfield, P.L., and Seckl, P.L. (2009) Hyperkalaemia. *British Medical Journal*, **339**, b4114.

**14** *Which of the following statements is correct regarding the use of furosemide in acute kidney injury (AKI)?*
  **A** *Furosemide will decrease the percentage of patients with AKI who will require renal replacement therapy*
  **B** *The use of high-dose furosemide for AKI is not associated with significant side effects*
  **C** *Furosemide can convert patients from an oliguric to non-oliguric state, which is associated with a decreased hospital length of stay*
  **D** *Administration of furosemide for AKI is associated with increased mortality*
  **E** *Furosemide will induce a diuresis in some patients with acute kidney injury*

Although furosemide may produce a diuresis in some patients with acute kidney injury, it has not been conclusively shown that this has an affect on the eventual need for renal replacement therapy or the number of dialysis sessions required until the recovery of renal function. The high doses of furosemide required to induce a diuresis in this patient group carry a significant risk of ototoxicity, however, data regarding an increase in mortality due to furosemide administration is questionable. In the absence of significant benefits, the use of furosemide in acute kidney injury (AKI) is to be discouraged.

There is no conclusive evidence showing a significant effect on hospital length of stay or reduction in mortality.

**Answer: E**

Bagshaw, S.M., Delaney, A., Haase, M., *et al.* (2007) Loop diuretics in the management of acute renal failure: a systematic review and meta-analysis. *Critical Care and Resuscitation.* **9** (1), 60–68.

Ho, K.M. and Sheridan, D.J. (2006) Meta-analysis of frusemide to prevent or treat acute renal failure. *British Medical Journal*, **333** (7565), 420–423.

**15** *When used in the treatment of acute kidney injury, dopamine has all of the following effects except?*
   **A** *Tachycardia and other arrhythmias*
   **B** *An increase in the glomerular filtration rate*
   **C** *A significant rise in the urine output in the majority of patients*
   **D** *Administration of low-dose dopamine at 5 μg/kg/min is more effective than 3 μg/kg/min in preventing the need for renal replacement therapy*
   **E** *Has been shown to effectively reduce the need for renal replacement therapy*

Unwanted effects from dopamine therapy include tachycardia and arrhythmias, which can limit the use of this medication. Current recommendations preclude the use of dopamine for acute kidney injury. Therapy with low-dose dopamine will increase the glomerular filtration rate by improving renal blood flow, subsequently causing an increase in urine output in the majority of patients. This may be associated with an improvement in the serum creatinine level, and measured creatinine clearance.

There is no compelling data that doses of dopamine of 5 μg/kg/min is more effective than 3 μg/kg/min, other than increasing the risk of side effects.

Treatment with low-dose dopamine for acute kidney injury was considered beneficial in the past. However, the largest meta-analysis performed in 2005 showed no beneficial effects of low-dose dopamine on mortality, the need for real replacement therapy, or adverse events.

**Answer: E**

Friedrich, J.O., Adhikari, N., Herridge, M.S., and Beyene, J. (2005) Meta-analysis: low-dose dopamine increases urine output but does not prevent renal dysfunction or death. *Annals of Internal Medicine*, **142** (7), 510–524.

Marik, P.E. (2002) Low-dose dopamine: a systematic review. *Intensive Care Medicine*, **28** (7), 877–883.

**16** *Which of the following medications would be the least likely cause of acute kidney injury in a female patient with a new rash, white blood cells in the urine, a normal white blood cell count and eosinophilia on urine microscopy?*
   **A** *Phenytoin*
   **B** *Ketorolac*
   **C** *Heparin*
   **D** *Pantoprazole*
   **E** *Amoxicillin*

This patient presents with findings consistent with acute interstitial nephritis. This typically begins abruptly, manifesting as acute kidney injury. In most instances, the nephritis occurs within days of exposure to the offending drug. However, in some instances (particularly with non-steroidal anti-inflammatory drugs), acute interstitial nephritis begins after several months of exposure.

The most commonly associated drugs are: antibiotics (e.g., penicillins, fluoroquinolones, and sulfa drugs), rifampin, phenytoin, proton pump inhibitors, non-steroidal anti-inflammatory medications, diuretics (e.g., thiazides, furosemide), and allopurinol.

Analgesic nephropathy is 5–6 times more common in women, which is generally attributed to women taking more analgesics than men. However, a greater sensitivity to the toxic effects of analgesics or differences in analgesic metabolism in women cannot be ruled out.

Although any drug can theoretically cause acute interstitial nephritis, acute reactions to heparin are more likely to be generalized hypersensitivity or even anaphylactic. Additionally, thrombocytopenia occurs in up to 30% of patients, which can occur in a severe form as heparin-induced thrombocytopenia.

**Answer: C**

Alper, A.B. (2016) Nephritis, Interstitial. eMedicine at Medscape.com: http://emedicine.medscape.com/article/243597-overview (accessed 15 November, 2016).

Brenner, B.M., ed. (2007) Interstitial Nephritis, in *Brenner and Rector's The Kidney*, 8th edn (ed. B.M. Brenner), W.B. Saunders, Philadelphia, PA, pp. 1239–1248.

**17** *Which of the following is not an advantage of continuous renal replacement therapy over intermittent dialysis?*
   **A** *It can be used in hemodynamically abnormal patients*
   **B** *Less expensive*
   **C** *Useful to remove fluid in smaller volumes*
   **D** *More effective in lowering intracranial pressure*
   **E** *Better removal of pro-inflammatory mediators*

Although the type of renal placement therapy, as well as the dosing of the dialysis remains controversial, there are some circumstances in which continuous renal replacement therapy such as continuous venovenous hemodiafiltration offers advantages over intermittent hemodialysis. It is a much better tolerated process for the patient who is critically ill, for example in septic shock requiring vasopressor support, as there are fewer hemodynamic fluxes during dialysis. It can be available 24 hours a day, depending on the training of the nursing personnel and the equipment available in the intensive care unit. It can also remove small volumes of fluid at a time therefore allowing finer adjustments to be made regarding the amount of fluid removed. It may have benefit in septic shock by removing pro-inflammatory mediators, although this remains controversial. It also has fewer deleterious side effects on intracranial pressure, which may be important in those patients also suffering from traumatic brain injury. However, it is clear that it is not cheaper than other forms of hemodialysis, and may in fact be more expensive than other currently available therapies.

**Answer: B**

Anderson, R.J. (2007) Acute renal failure, in *Critical Care Medicine. Principles of Diagnosis and Management in the Adult*, 3rd edn. Mosby; Philadelphia, PA, pp. 1163–1188.

Pannu, N., Klarenbach, S., Wiebe, N., *et al.* (2008) Renal replacement therapy in patients with acute renal failure: a systematic review. *Journal of the American Medical Association*, **299** (7), 793–805.

18  *A 55-year-old man sustained multiple injuries in a motorcycle collision. Imaging revealed a grade 3 liver laceration with a blush. He undergoes embolization and is admitted to the ICU. On hospital day 3, the patient is noted to have decreased urinary output. His creatinine of 2.0 mg/dL, sodium is 133 mEq/L, urine creatinine 90 mg/dL, urine sodium is 10 mEq/L. What is the calculated FENa?*
   A  5.0
   B  2.0
   C  Cannot be calculated with the information given
   D  0.2
   E  1

$$FENa = ([\text{urine sodium/serum sodium}]/$$
$$[\text{urine creatinine/serum creatinine}]) \times 100$$

The FENa is this patient is consistent with a prerenal disorder. Prerenal disorders can be distinguished from renal disorders by urine sodium (<20 mEq/L), elevated urine osmolality (>500 mOsm/kg), and a FENa (<1%). Prerenal disorders account for approximately 40% of cases of AKI and usually result from hypovolemia (decreased renal blood flow). These patients require volume resuscitation. Low-output heart failure can also lead to prerenal AKI and should be within the differential.

**Answer: D**

Abnernathy, V.E. and Lieberthal, W. (2002) Acute renal failure in the critically ill patient. *Critical Care Clinics*, **18**, 203–222.

19  *All of the following are true except:*
   A  *A FENa of 0.7 is consistent with a prerenal process*
   B  *A urine sodium concentration of 12 mEq/L is consistent with a prerenal process*
   C  *Fractional excretion of urea (FEUrea) can be used in place of FENa in patients that have received diuretics*
   D  *Fractional excretion of urea (FEUrea) is < 35% in ATN*
   E  *A urine sodium concentration greater than 40 mEq/L occurs in ATN*

A FENa less than 1% is consistent with prerenal disorders. A FENa greater than 2% is consistent with renal disorders.

An elevated urine sodium (>40 mEq/L) is seen in renal disorders. The elevated sodium concentration in urine that is seen in ATN is the result of impaired sodium reabsorption. However, elevated urine sodium can be associated with prerenal conditions in patients receiving diuretics. In these patients, the FENa will be falsely elevated.

The fractional excretion of urea (FEUrea) is not influenced by diuretics and can be used to distinguish between prerenal and renal disorders. The FEUrea is < 35% in prerenal disorders and > 50% in renal disorders (ATN).

**Answer: D**

Gottfried, J., Weisen, J., Raina, R., and Nally, J.V. (2012) Finding the cause of acute kidney injury: which index of fractional excretion is better? *Cleveland Clinic Journal of Medicine*, **79**(2), 121–126.

Kasper, D.L., Fauci, A., Hauser, S., *et al.* (eds) (2015) Acute kidney injury, in *Harrison's Principles of Internal Medicine*, 19th edn, McGraw-Hill, New York.

20  *The workup for obstructive uropathy might include all of the following except?*
   A  *Rectal exam*
   B  *Ultrasonography of the urinary tract*
   C  *Placement of a Foley catheter*
   D  *Abdominal CT scan*
   E  *Renal arteriography*

The history and physical exam, in addition to additional laboratory tests, will help to guide the appropriate investigation.

A rectal exam will give information regarding the size and character of the prostate, while Foley catheterization may relieve the cause of the obstruction as well as enabling a clear quantification of the amount of urine produced.

Ultrasonography of the urogenital tract is the preferred screening modality for obstruction if suspected, as it is highly sensitive for detecting hydronephrosis, is relatively inexpensive and is safe and reproducible.

CT scanning is becoming more and more useful for evaluation of the upper urinary tract, particularly with the recent improvements in image quality from helical CT.

Renal arteriography has no place in the management of obstructive renal failure, although it may be important to investigate renal hypertension and other renovascular disorders.

**Answer: E**

Frøkiaer, J. and Zeidel, M.L. (2012) Urinary tract obstruction, in *Brenner and Rector's The Kidney*, 9th edn (eds, M.W. Taal, G.M. Chertow, P.A. Marsden, *et al.*), W.B. Saunders, Philadelphia, PA, pp. 1383–1410.

21 *Regarding nutrition for a patient with acute kidney injury requiring dialysis, which of the considerations listed below is correct?*
   A *Fat-soluble vitamin supplementation is important*
   B *Total caloric intake should be in the order of 35–40 kcal/kg/day*
   C *Enteral formulas do not need to be low in nitrogen*
   D *Caloric needs are not increased due to acute kidney injury.*
   E *Parenteral nutrition is the preferred route while the patient is on continuous renal replacement therapy.*

Nutritional management in patients with acute kidney injury requires close collaboration between physicians, nurses, and dietitians. The objective of nutrition in AKI is to provide sufficient calories and protein to preserve lean body mass, avoid starvation ketoacidosis and promote healing, while minimizing production of nitrogenous waste.

Water-soluble vitamins should be provided with the exception of vitamin C, which in high doses, promotes urinary oxalate excretion.

Total caloric intake should normally be in the range of 25–30 kcal/kg/day, and should not exceed 35 kcal/kg/day.

Patients with AKI, particularly following surgery or trauma, and patients with multiorgan failure, can frequently have protein catabolic rates above 1.5 g/kg/day. If the patient is not catabolic then protein intake should be restricted to below 0.8 g/kg/day. Catabolic patients, especially those on continuous renal replacement therapy, should receive at least 1.4 g/kg/day.

Although vigorous parenteral nutrition has been claimed to improve prognosis in AKI, the enteral route is preferred because it avoids the morbidity and costs associated with parenteral nutrition.

**Answer: C**

Brown, R.O. and Compher, C. (2010) A.S.P.E.N. clinical guidelines: nutrition support in adult acute and chronic renal failure. *Journal of Parenteral and Enteral Nutrition*, **34** (4), 366–377.

Sharfuddin, A., Weisbord, S.D., Palevsky, P.M., and Molitoris, B.A. (2012) Acute kidney injury, in *Brenner and Rector's The Kidney*, 9th edn (eds, M.W. Taal, G.M. Chertow, P.A. Marsden, *et al.*), W.B. Saunders, Philadelphia, PA, pp. 1044–1099.

22 *Which of the following is an appropriate indication for the use of sodium bicarbonate?*
   A *A patient with gram-negative sepsis undergoing CRRT, with a pH of 7.3*
   B *Post-cardiac arrest in a hospitalized patient who was cardioverted for ventricular fibrillation*
   C *A trauma patient post-splenectomy with a pH of 7.15 and a hemoglobin of 7.0 mg/dL*
   D *Severe non-gap metabolic acidosis (pH < 7.0)*
   E *Torsades de pointes*

The use of intravenous sodium bicarbonate to treat metabolic acidosis, although practiced for over 50 years, remains contentious. Patients with mild acidosis, particularly those who undergo reorientation therapy, could have this adjusted using the buffers in the dialysis solution rather than the administration of intravenous sodium bicarbonate.

The primary treatment for ventricular fibrillation is cardioversion, and if this is performed rapidly after arrest, then there is no need for the routine administration of sodium bicarbonate.

The treatment for a trauma patient who has just undergone splenectomy and remains anemic should be to transfuse with packed red blood cells and or clotting factors as necessary.

Treating this patient with sodium bicarbonate will only serve to mask the underlying hypovolemia. Sodium bicarbonate therapy has a definite role in the treatment of severe metabolic acidosis that is unresponsive to conventional fluid resuscitation, particularly in the face of acute kidney injury.

The treatment for torsade de pointes is magnesium.

**Answer: D**

Brenner, B.M., ed. (2007) Metabolic disorders, in *Brenner and Rector's The Kidney*, 8th edn (ed. B.M. Brenner), W.B. Saunders, Philadelphia, PA, pp. 943–976.

Vukmir, R.B. and Katz, L. (2006) Sodium bicarbonate improves outcome in prolonged prehospital cardiac arrest. *American Journal of Emergency Medicine*, **24** (2), 156–161.

## 18

## Liver Failure

*Muhammad Numan Khan, MD and Bellal Joseph, MD*

**1** *A 58-year-old man presents to the emergency department with an incarcerated umbilical hernia with leaking ascites. He is a known alcoholic and has been previously diagnosed with cirrhosis. Which of the following scoring systems is the most accurate predictor of increased risk for morbidity and mortality in a cirrhotic patient after an abdominal operation?*

**A** *APACHE II*
**B** *APACHE III*
**C** *Childs Class*
**D** *MELD (model for end-stage liver disease) score*
**E** *Child–Turcotte–Pugh score (CTP)*

Prognostic models are useful in estimating disease severity and survival and are used to make decisions regarding specific medical interventions. Several prognostic models are currently used in healthcare settings. Some focus on generalized health status, such as the Acute Physiology and Chronic Health Evaluation System (APACHE III). Cirrhosis of the liver is associated with increased morbidity and mortality when a patient must undergo surgery. Two models that are used commonly in the care of patients with chronic liver disease are: The Child–Turcotte–Pugh (CTP) score and the more recently described Model for End-stage Liver Disease (MELD). The CTP score was found to be better than the APACHE II and APACHE III scores in predicting short-term mortality of cirrhotic patients. The MELD is a prospectively developed and validated chronic liver disease severity scoring system that uses a patient's laboratory values for serum bilirubin, serum creatinine, and the international normalized ratio for prothrombin time (INR) to predict survival. The MELD score is the most precise tool to assess operative risk in the same patient population. The MELD score has been confirmed to be more precise in categorizing high risk cirrhotic patients for both hepatic and other abdominal operations. In patients with acute on chronic liver failure, the APACHE II scoring is a better prognostic indicator as compared to sequential organ failure assessment (SOFA), CTP, and MELD scoring system. The revised model is currently used by the United Network for Organ Sharing (UNOS) in prioritizing allocation of deceased donor organs for liver transplantation.

$$MELD = 3.78 \times \ln[\text{serum bilirubin (mg/dL)} \\ + 11.2 \times \ln[\text{INR}] + 9.57 \times \ln[\text{serum} \\ \text{creatinine (mg/dL)}] + 6.3$$

It is reported as a whole number and is rounded. The three-month mortality rates are shown in Table 18.1.

**Answer: D**

Chatzicostas, C., Roussomoustakaki, M., Notas, G., *et al.* (2003) A comparison of Child-Pugh, APACHE II and APACHE III scoring systems in predicting hospital mortality of patients with liver cirrhosis. *BMC Gastroenterology*, **3**, 7.

Duseja, A., Choudhary, N.S., Gupta, S., *et al.* (2013) APACHE II score is superior to SOFA, CTP and MELD in predicting the short-term mortality in patients with acute-on-chronic liver failure (ACLF). *Journal of Digestive Diseases*, **14** (9), 484–490.

Farnsworth, N., Fagan, S.P., Berger, D.H., *et al.* (2004) Child-Turcotte-Pugh versus MELD score as a predictor of outcome after elective and emergent surgery in cirrhotic patients. *American Journal of Surgery*, **188**, 580–583.

Wiesner, R., Edwards, E., Freeman, R., *et al.* (2003) Model for end-stage liver disease (MELD) and allocation of donor livers. *Gastroenterology*, **124** (1), 91–96

**2** *A 65-year-old woman with a history of severe alcohol abuse is brought to the emergency department after*

*Surgical Critical Care and Emergency Surgery: Clinical Questions and Answers*, Second Edition.
Edited by Forrest "Dell" Moore, Peter Rhee, and Gerard J. Fulda.
© 2018 John Wiley & Sons Ltd. Published 2018 by John Wiley & Sons Ltd.
Companion website: www.wiley.com/go/moore/surgical_criticalcare_and_emergency_surgery

**Table 18.1** Three-month mortality rates by MELD score.

| MELD Score | Mortality (%) |
|---|---|
| < 10 | 1–2 |
| 10–19 | 6.0 |
| 20–29 | 19.6 |
| 30–39 | 52.6 |
| ≥ 40 | 71.3 |

*her first episode of hematemesis. After initial resuscitation with four units of packed RBCs the patient's vital signs are stable and the bleeding has subsided. The patient undergoes upper endoscopy and esophageal varices with active bleeding are noted. Which of the following is the next best step in management of this patient:*

**A** *Transjugular intrahepatic portosystemic shunt (TIPS)*
**B** *Liver transplantation*
**C** *Check PT/INR and if deranged give activated Factor VII and vitamin K*
**D** *Oral octreotide with Vasopressin*
**E** *Band ligation of esophageal varices*

In patients with presumed cirrhosis and upper gastrointestinal bleeding, the source of the bleeding must be identified. After initial patient stabilization, upper endoscopy is indicated to search for the etiology. If varices are seen with active bleeding, ablative therapy is the appropriate next step to control local hemorrhage. Methods for ablating varices without open operation include endoscopic sclerotherapy and endoscopic band ligation. Band ligation is usually chosen because it is associated with fewer complications such as perforation and stricture. Transjugular intrahepatic portosystemic shunt (TIPS) and operative portosystemic shunting are options if endoscopic ablation is unsuccessful. Patients with cirrhosis who had acute variceal bleed, treated with TIPS had relatively low rate of mortality and a lower rate for rebleeding as compared to patients who did not undergo TIPS. Liver transplantation is never considered in the acute situation. Patients with a history of severe alcohol abuse would not meet transplant criteria. Activated factor VII is used in rare circumstances to control coagulopathic bleeding, but is never indicated in a patient for whom standard measures have been successful.

**Answer: E**

Brunicardi, F., Andersen, D., and Billiar, T. (2014) *Schwartz's Principles of Surgery*, 10th edn, McGraw-Hill, New York.

Deltenre, P., Trépo, E., Rudler, M., *et al.* (2015) Early transjugular intrahepatic portosystemic shunt in cirrhotic patients with acute variceal bleeding: a systematic review and meta-analysis of controlled trials. *European Journal of Gastroenterology and Hepatology*, **27** (9), e1–e9.

Rosemurgy, A.S. and Zervos, E.E. (2003) Management of variceal hemorrhage. *Current Problems in Surgery*, **40**, 263–343.

**3** *A 65-year-old alcoholic man with ascities undergoes emergent colectomy for a lower gastrointestinal bleed. During his postoperative recovery the urine output is consistently low. The patient has a presumed diagnosis of hepatorenal syndrome. Which of the following is most often associated with hepatorenal syndrome:*
**A** *Proteinuria of more than 3 gm/day*
**B** *Hematuria*
**C** *Low sodium concentration in the urine*
**D** *Low urine-plasma osmolality ratio (U:P < 1.0)*
**E** *BUN:CR < 10:1*

Hepatorenal syndrome (HRS) is quite common in the cirrhotic population and is found in approximately 10% of individuals admitted to the hospital with ascites. HRS is characterized by the occurrence of acute kidney injury in cirrhotic patients in the absence of other identifiable causes. It is characterized by azotemia (high levels of nitrogen such as urea, creatinine), oliguria (<500 mL per day), low urinary sodium excretion (<10 mEq/L), and increased urine-plasma osmolality ratio (U:P > 1.0) in the absence of urinary sedimentation. There are two types of HRS, Type 1 characterized by acute renal failure and rapid functional deterioration of other organs. Type 2 is characterized by slowly progressive renal failure and refractory ascites. Pathogenesis of HRS involves arterial vasodilatation of splanchnic circulation, decreased effective arterial volume, and further reduction of glomerular filtration by the renin-angiotensin-aldosterone system leading to prerenal azotemia. Hepatorenal syndrome occurs in patients with pre-existing parenchymal liver disease after a precipitating event such as surgery or a hypotensive episode (e.g., GI bleed, dialysis, sepsis). Hepatorenal syndrome progresses over days to weeks after the precipitating event. Medical management of hepatorenal syndrome includes terlipressin and albumin which is more effective than midodrine and octreotide plus albumin in improving renal function. Type 1 HRS is often resistant to medical management and requires liver transplant. Proteinuria more than 3 gm/day is associated with nephrotic syndrome. Hematuria is associated with nephritic syndrome, urothelial tumors or renal/bladder calculi.

**Answer: C**

Barbano, B., Sardo, L., Gigante, A., *et al.* (2014) Pathophysiology, diagnosis and clinical management of hepatorenal syndrome: from classic to new drugs. *Current Vascular Pharmacology*, **12** (1), 125–135.

Cavallin, M., Kamath, P.S., Merli, M., *et al.* (2015) Terlipressin plus albumin versus midodrine and octreotide plus albumin in the treatment of hepatorenal syndrome: a randomized trial. *Hepatology*, **62** (2), 567–574.

Mulholland, M.W., Lillemoe, K.D., Doherty, G. *et al.* (2011) *Greenfield's Surgery: Scientific Principles and Practice*, 5th edn, Lippincott Williams & Wilkins, Philadelphia, PA.

**4** The stent placed during transjugular intrahepatic portosystemic shunt (TIPS)

    **A** Should be followed with computed tomography scan every six months after placement

    **B** Is not covered

    **C** Is associated with postprocedure encephalopathy rates of 80%

    **D** Has a stenosis rate of greater than 50%

    **E** Is dilated until a gradient of less than 20 mm Hg is obtained

Transjugular intrahepatic portosystemic shunts (TIPS) involve creation of a low-resistance channel between the hepatic vein and the intrahepatic portion of the portal vein using angiographic techniques. The indications for TIPS include bleeding refractory to endoscopic and medical management, refractory ascities, Budd–Chiari syndrome, and hepatorenal syndromes. The stent is expanded to a diameter that reduces the portosytemic gradient to less than 12 mm Hg. TIPS is associated with postprocedure encephalopathy rates of approximately 25% and patients with renal insufficiency are at risk for worsened renal function. The long-term problem with TIPS is stenosis of the shunt, which is reported in as many as two-thirds of patients. Most centers advocate an aggressive Doppler ultrasound monitoring program with prompt balloon dilation for identified stenosis of the stent. Patients on TIPS who have recurrent stent stenosis treated with percutaneous transluminal angioplasty with paclitaxel result in prolonged secondary patency without the systemic side effects of paclitaxel.

**Answer: D**

Boyer, T.D. and Haskal, Z.J. and the American Association for the Study of Liver Diseases (2010) The role of transjugular intrahepatic portosystemp shunt (TIPS) in the management of portal hypertension: update 2009. *Hepatology*, **51**, 306.

Garcia, S.M., Langmann, M., Schnorr, B., *et al.* (2016) Use of paclitaxel-coated balloon catheter dilation to reduce in-stent restenosis in transjugular intrahepatic portosystemic shunt (TIPS). *RöFo-Fortschritte auf dem Gebiet der Röntgenstrahlen und der bildgebenden Verfahren*, **188** (4), 374–380.

Mulholland, M.W., Lillemoe, K.D., Doherty, G. *et al.* (2011) *Greenfield's Surgery: Scientific Principles and Practice*, 5th edn, Lippincott Williams & Wilkins, Philadelphia, PA.

**5** A 50-year old male was brought to ED with chief complaints of confusion, inability to concentrate, and abdominal distention. He has a history of alcoholic cirrhosis. For the past week, patient complained of constipation. He was diagnosed with hepatic encephalopathy. Which of the following is the best initial therapy to decrease blood ammonia level?

    **A** High dietary protein intake

    **B** Construction of a side-to-side portocaval shunt

    **C** Infusion of dextrose 5%

    **D** Administration of lactulose

    **E** Hemodialysis

Hepatic encephalopathy or portal-systemic encephalopathy is a reversible impairment of neuropsychiatric function associated with impaired hepatic function. Hepatic encephalopathy is a result of complex interplay of inhibitory neurotransmitters following ammonia intoxication. Precipitating factors include hypokalemia, hypovolemia, infection, sedatives, GI bleeding, and renal failure. Lactulose acts as a mild cathartic, and its breakdown products acidify the luminal contents in the colon and thereby decrease absorption of ammonia which is produced by intestinal bacteria. Neomycin and rifaximin are an alternative to Lactulose which decreases the gut bacteria and eventually reduces ammonia production. Combination of lactulose plus rifaximin is more effective than lactulose only. Hypoglycemia is also one of the precipitants of hepatic encephalopathy because hypoglycemia causes ammonia intoxication since glucose inhibits ammonia production by gut bacteria. Reversal of these factors might improve patient prognosis. Ammonia is produced when intestinal bacteria break down blood in the gastrointestinal tract. Active bleeding should be controlled and dietary protein should be limited to reduce protein load to the liver. Protein diet intake should be restricted, but prolonged restriction of protein intake should be considered with caution because of the risk of protein-calorie malnutrition in these patients. There may be benefit to administering relatively higher levels of branch-chain amino acids with minimized aromatic amino acids Portosystemic shunts interfere with ammonia metabolism in the liver. Side-to-side shunts are indicated when the patient has hepatic venous outflow obstruction.

**Answer: D**

Cameron, J, (2013) *Current Surgical Therapy*, 11th edn, Mosby, New York.

Mulholland, M.W., Lillemoe, K.D., Doherty, G. *et al.* (2011) *Greenfield's Surgery: Scientific Principles and Practice*, 5th edn, Lippincott Williams & Wilkins, Philadelphia, PA.

Sharma, B.C., Sharma, P., Lunia, M.K., *et al.* (2013) A randomized, double-blind, controlled trial comparing rifaximin plus lactulose with lactulose alone in treatment of overt hepatic encephalopathy. *The American Journal of Gastroenterology*, **108** (9), 1458–1463.

**6** Which of the following statements is the most true regarding spontaneous bacterial peritonitis?

**A** Infection is most commonly polymicrobial

**B** Diagnosis can be made clinically without paracentesis

**C** Antibiotic therapy is reserved for patients with positive ascitic fluid cultures

**D** Gram-negative enteric bacteria are often present.

**E** Diagnosis is established by elevated ascitic fluid absolute polymorphonuclear leukocyte count (PMN) > 100 cells/mm³

The diagnosis of spontaneous bacterial peritonitis is established by a positive ascitic fluid bacterial culture and an elevated ascitic fluid absolute polymorphonuclear leukocyte (PMN) count (≥250 cells/mm³). Thus paracentesis is needed. Spontaneous bacterial peritonitis is a lethal complication of ascites that affects about 10% of patients with cirrhotic ascites. Fever and abdominal pain are common manifestations. Antibiotic therapy should be instituted promptly based on elevated ascitic fluid PMN count or on symptoms even if the PMN count is lower. The infection is usually from one organism and most commonly *Escherichia coli*, or Klebsiella. Initial therapy is usually a third-generation cephalosporin. Broad spectrum antibiotic therapy is recommended after diagnosis of SBP, and shouldn't be delayed while awaiting culture results in patients with a PMN count ≥250 cells/mm³. Once culture result is available, the antibiotic coverage should be narrowed against specific bacteria. Renal failure develops in 30–40% of patients with SBP and is a major cause of death. The risk for renal failure can be reduced by infusion of albumin. Prophylaxis for SBP includes flouroquinolones and TMP-SMX. Secondary bacterial peritonitis is an infrequent complication in cirrhotic patients but the mortality is high. It is typically a polymicrobial infection that is treated with broad spectrum antibiotics such as cefotaxime and metronidazole but it rarely responds to antibiotics. An operative or radiological intervention is often necessary for definitive treatment.

**Answer: D**

Brunicardi, F., Andersen, D., and Billiar, T. (2014) *Schwartz's Principles of Surgery*, 10th edn, McGraw-Hill, New York.

Runyon, B.A., AASLD Practice Guidelines Committee (2009) Management of adult patients with ascites due to cirrhosis: an update. *Hepatology*, **49**, 2087–2107.

Runyon, B.A., (2015) Spontaneous bacterial peritonitis in adults: Treatment and prophylaxis. UpToDate.com: https://www.uptodate.com/contents/spontaneous-bacterial-peritonitis-in-adults-treatment-and-prophylaxis (accessed 16 November, 2017).

Soriano, G., Castellote, J., Álvarez, C., *et al.* (2010) Secondary bacterial peritonitis in cirrhosis: a retrospective study of clinical and analytical characteristics, diagnosis and management. *Journal of Hepatology*, **52** (1), 39–44.

**7** Which of the following is appropriate for prevention of variceal hemorrhage in a patient with varices that have never bled?

**A** Endoscopic sclerosis

**B** TIPS

**C** Surgical selective shunt

**D** Propranolol

**E** Prophylactic ligation

Of the currently available therapies most studies show some decrease in the incidence of bleeding with prophylactic propranolol. Prophylactic ligation reduces the risks of variceal bleeding. Compared with β-blockers, ligation reduces the risk for first variceal bleed but has no effect on mortality. Prophylactic ligation should be considered for patients with large esophageal varices who cannot tolerate β-blockers. Endoscopic sclerotherapy as prophylaxis has not yielded consistent benefit and may be detrimental to some patients. Surgical therapy in the form of prophylactic portacaval shunting has shown a decreased risk of bleeding in operated patients but an increased risk of hepatic failure and encephalopathy due to decreased clearance of ammonia and overall decreased survival.

**Answer: D**

Cameron, J. (2013) *Current Surgical Therapy*, 11th edn, Mosby, New York

D'Amico, G., Criscuoli, V., Fili, D., *et al.* (2002) Meta-analysis of trials for variceal bleeding. *Hepatology*, **36**, 1023–1024.

Imperiale, T.F. and Chalasani, N. (2001) A meta-analysis of endoscopic variceal ligation for primary prophylaxis of esophageal variceal bleeding. *Hepatology*, **33** (4), 802–807.

**8** *A 65-year-old man with a model for end-stage liver disease (MELD) score of 15 has intractable ascites and esophageal varices. Which of the following is the best treatment for the ascites?*

**A** *Surgical side to-side portacaval shunt*
**B** *Surgical end-to-side portacaval shunt*
**C** *Transjugular intrahepatic portosystemic shunt (TIPS)*
**D** *Peritoneovenous shunt*
**E** *Distal splenorenal shunt*

Cirrhosis is the most common cause of ascites in the United States. The goal of treatment is to decrease ascitic fluid and peripheral edema without affecting the intravascular volume. Medically intractable ascites occurs in 10% of patients with cirrhosis and ascites. The only definitive therapeutic option is liver transplantation. Other treatment options for refractory ascites include therapeutic paracentesis and TIPS. Peritoneovenous shunts and surgical portosystemic shunts have limited role. TIPS is effectively a side-to-side portacaval shunt placed through the right internal jugular vein under local anesthesia. TIPS has been shown to lead to an increase in urine output and a marked or complete reduction in ascites. A peritoneovenous shunt that drains into the internal jugular vein, reinfuses ascites into the vascular space. However, this procedure has been virtually abandoned due to an excessive rate of complications. Surgical shunts are not indicated for the treatment of ascites alone in a patient who has not had bleeding varices. Surgical shunts for ascites require a nonselective, side-to-side arrangement; therefore an end-to-side portacaval or distal splenorenal shunt are contraindicated. Shunt surgery has been associated with a high morbidity and mortality.

**Answer: C**

Boyer, T.D. and Haskal, Z.J., 2010. The role of transjugular intrahepatic portosystemic shunt (TIPS) in the management of portal hypertension: update 2009. *Hepatology*, **51**(1), pp.306–306.
Cameron, J (2013) *Current Surgical Therapy*, 11th edn, Mosby, New York.

**9** *A 60-year-old man with liver cirrhosis secondary to alcohol abuse presents to the emergency room with hematemesis and lightheadedness. The patient still drinks alcohol and appears cachectic and pale. On examination the patient has significant ascites and large collateral veins on the abdominal wall. Stool is guaiac positive. The patient has two large-bore IVs placed and aggressive hydration is started. He is also treated with IV famotidine and an IV octreotide drip. The patient continues to have hematemesis and is intubated for airway protection. Which of the following statements is most correct regarding management of this patient?*

**A** *If emergent endoscopy is not immediately available, esophageal balloon tamponade is indicated*
**B** *Immediate angiogram with possible embolization needs to be performed*
**C** *Sclerotherapy and esophageal balloon tamponade have comparable efficacy in controlling esophageal bleeding*
**D** *Transfusion of fresh frozen plasma is indicated prior to procedural interventions*
**E** *Patient should be aggressively resuscitated pending an endoscopy and anatomic diagnosis of bleeding*

The patient should be resuscitated with resuscitation and the transfusion of blood products as needed. Once this is accomplished, or if the patient has persistent bleeding, emergent endoscopy should be performed in order to establish a diagnosis and attempt hemostasis of bleeding lesion. An esophageal balloon tamponade with a Sengstaken–Blakemore or Minnesota tube is indicated in cases of confirmed esophageal variceal hemorrhage in which endoscopy therapy is unavailable, technically not feasible, or unsuccessful. Placement of an esophageal balloon should not be performed without anatomical diagnosis. Although the patient in this case is at high risk for esophageal variceal hemorrhage, severe gastrointestinal bleeding in patients with signs of chronic liver disease can result from other causes in up to 35% of cases. Endoscopic therapy with sclerotherapy or banding has been demonstrated to be more effective than an esophageal balloon tamponade in treating acute esophageal variceal hemorrhage. Without documentation of coagulopathy, there is no reason to transfuse fresh frozen plasma in this patient.

**Answer: E**

Cameron, J. (2013) *Current Surgical Therapy*, 11th edn, Mosby, New York.
D'Amico, G., Criscuoli, V., Fili, D. *et al.* (2002) Meta-analysis of trials for variceal bleeding. *Hepatology*, **36**, 1023–1024.
Villanueva, C., Colomo, A., Bosch, A., *et al.* (2013) Transfusion strategies for acute upper gastrointestinal bleeding. *New England Journal of Medicine*, **368** (1), pp.11–21.

**10** *A 25-year-old woman is brought to the hospital by family members after being found unresponsive.*

*The patient has no significant past medical history, however the family reports that she has been depressed. The patient is lethargic, and has mild diffuse abdominal tenderness, with no guarding and decreased bowel sounds. Laboratory data are significant for: alanine amino transferase 3800 U/L, aspartate aminotransferase 4300 U/L, total bilirubin 7.5 mg/dL, and INR of 2.5. Which of the following is the most likely to result in mortality in this patient?*

**A** *Uncontrolled bleeding*
**B** *Septic shock*
**C** *Brain edema*
**D** *Respiratory failure*
**E** *Acute myocardial infarction*

The patient presents with a clinical picture that is consistent with fulminant liver failure (FLF). Acute liver failure (ALF) is defined as a rapid deterioration of hepatic function, manifested by an increase in prothrombin time (PT) and a decrease of factor V, without evidence of hepatic encephalopathy. FLF involves severe, acute liver dysfunction complicated by hepatic encephalopathy in a patient with no previous liver disease. Usually one of the first findings of liver failure is jaundice. Recognition of hepatic injury may be delayed if confusion or agitation is the dominant presenting sign, particularly in hyper acute cases in which jaundice is minimal or in sub acute cases, which may be mistaken for chronic liver disease. The onset of hepatic encephalopathy is less than two weeks. Causes of ALF include viral infection, drugs, autoimmune, inherited liver diseases, and shock liver. The most common cause of ALF and FHFFLF in the United States is acetaminophen toxicity. Complications related to ALF and FLF include coagulopathy, cerebral edema and intracranial hypertension, acute portal hypertension, renal failure, infections, and multiple organ failure. The most common cause of death in patients with FLF is cerebral edema leading to increased intracranial pressure and herniation. The care for patients with FLF and ALF is supportive along with management of the underlying cause, if possible. It is important to identify patients at higher risk of death for rapid referral to transplant centers, since, in most patients, liver transplant is the only curative therapeutic modality. Post op mortality for liver transplantation is high and most occurs within 3 months of transplant, with infection being most common cause of death/graft rejection in these patients. Overt bleeding is uncommon in patients with ALF and reflects a balanced hemostatic defect. In most cases, the loss of hepatic synthesis of procoagulant factors is paralleled by the loss of hepatically derived anticoagulants. Early restoration of intravascular volume and systemic perfusion may prevent or mitigate the severity of organ failure.

This patient has no evidence of bleeding, or sepsis. Respiratory failure is common but is not the predominant cause of death. This patient is young and is not expected to have an acute myocardial infarction.

**Answer: C**

Bernal, W. and Wendon, J. (2013) Acute liver failure. *New England Journal of Medicine*, **369** (26), 2525–2534.
Germani, G., Theocharidou, E., Adam, R., *et al.* (2012) Liver transplantation for acute liver failure in Europe: outcomes over 20 years from the ELTR database. *Journal of Hepatology*, **57** (2), 288–296.

**11** Which of the following is not appropriate in regards to *acetaminophen toxicity:*

**A** *Acetaminophen toxicity leads to elevation of PT/INR within 24 hours of ingestion*
**B** *Acetaminophen is an irreversible inhibitor of cytochrome c of Electron Transport Chain(ETC)*
**C** *Acute alcohol ingestion is an additional risk factor for hepatotoxicity*
**D** *The initial manifestations of acetominophen poisoning are often mild and nonspecific*
**E** *A serum acetaminophen level must be obtained in every patient if there are signs and symptoms of liver failure*

Acute alcohol ingestion is not a risk factor for hepatotoxicity and may even be protective by competing with acetaminophen for metabolism of the cytochrome p450 enzymes, reducing the amount of toxic metabolite produced (N-acetyl-p-benzoquinoneimine (NAPQI)). Toxicity is likely to occur with single ingestions greater than 250 mg/kg or those greater than 12 g over a 24-hour period for adults. Initial manifestation of acetaminophen toxicity is often mild and non-specific. Virtually all patients who ingest doses in excess of 350 mg/kg (24.5 gms for a 70 kg person) develop severe liver toxicity (defined as peak aspartate aminotransferase (AST) or alanine aminotransferase (ALT) levels greater than 1000 IU/L) with elevation of PT/INR after 24–48 hours. Acetaminophen is rapidly and completely absorbed from the gastrointestinal tract. Serum concentrations peak between one-half and two hours after an oral therapeutic dose. In patients with severe acetaminophen poisoning, the time interval between drug ingestion and treatment with acetylcysteine is closely related to the outcome. Patients with sub-therapeutic level of acetaminophen can also cause hepatotoxicity with concomitant presence of other causes of chronic hepatic dysfunction usually chronic alcoholism or chronic acetaminophen toxicity. All patients with possible acetaminophen toxicity should have acetaminophen level after 4 hours of ingestion.

If the patient has taken it more than four hours than it should be checked immediately.

**Answer: D**

Bernal, W. and Wendon, J. (2013). Acute liver failure. *New England Journal of Medicine*, **369** (26), 2525–2534.

Lee, W.M. (2003) Drug-induced hepatotoxicity. *New England Journal of Medicine*, **349**, 1118–1127.

**12** *Which of the following is true regarding the clinical manifestations of acute acetaminophen intoxication?*

   **A** *Laboratory studies are typically elevated within 8 hours of ingestion of acetaminophen*

   **B** *Liver function abnormalities peak from 24 to 36 hours*

   **C** *Patients who develop hepatic injury usually demonstrate elevation of aminotransferase*

   **D** *Acute renal failure rarely occurs as a result of acetaminophen toxicity*

   **E** *Chronic hepatic dysfunction is a common sequel of acetaminophen poisoning*

The clinical course of acetaminophen poisoning is often divided into four sequential stages. Stage I: In the first 24 hours after overdose, patients often manifest nausea, vomiting, diaphoresis, pallor, lethargy, and malaise. Some patients remain asymptomatic. Laboratory studies are typically normal. Stage II: from 24 to 72 hours after ingestion, the clinical and laboratory evidence of hepatotoxicity and, occasionally, nephrotoxicity become evident. Of patients that develop hepatic injury, over one half will demonstrate aminotransferase elevation within 24 hours and all have elevations by 36 hours. Stage III: liver function abnormalities peak from 72 to 96 hours after ingestion. The systemic symptoms of stage I reappear in conjunction with jaundice, confusion (hepatic encephalopathy), a marked elevation in hepatic enzymes, hyperammonemia, and a bleeding diathesis. Acute renal failure occurs in 25% of patients with significant hepatotoxicity and in more than 50% of those with frank hepatic failure. Stage IV patients who survive stage III enter a recovery phase that usually begins by day 4 and is complete by 7 days after overdose. It is notable that chronic hepatic dysfunction is not typically a sequel in survivors of acetaminophen poisoning. Acute liver failure can occur after ingestion of a single large dose of acetaminophen, the risk of death is greatest with substantial drug ingestion staggered over hours or days rather than at a single time point.

Acetylcysteine is the accepted treatment for acetaminophen poisoning and is given to all patients at significant risk for hepatotoxicity. Some recommend administering acetylcysteine for all patients with fulminant hepatic failure, even if not caused by acetaminophen toxicity.

**Answer: C**

Bernal, W. and Wendon, J. (2013) Acute liver failure. *New England Journal of Medicine*, **369** (26), 2525–2534.

Blieden, M., Paramore, L.C., Shah, D., and Ben-Joseph, R. (2014) A perspective on the epidemiology of acetaminophen exposure and toxicity in the United States. *Expert Review of Clinical Pharmacology*, 7 (3), 341–348.

**13** *A 55-year-old male presents to ED with a 4-week history of shortness of breath on exertion and/or standing and was improved by lying flat. Past medical history is significant for liver cirrhosis with portal hypertension secondary to alcoholism. On physical exam, he had decreased breath sounds at the base of both lungs. ABGs showed respiratory alkalosis with $PaO_2$ of 50 mm Hg and $PaCO_2$ of 30 mm Hg. What is the most likely diagnosis?*

   **A** *Acute respiratory distress syndrome*

   **B** *Acute pulmonary edema*

   **C** *Hepatopulmonary syndrome*

   **D** *Acute exacerbation of COPD*

   **E** *Pulmonary thromboembolism*

Hepatopulmonary syndrome (HPS) is characterized by abnormal arterial oxygenation induced by pulmonary vascular dilation in the setting of liver cirrhosis or portal hypertension. It is defined by an A-a gradient of > 15 mm hg at sea level. Most patient with HPS are either asymptomatic or develop the subtle onset of dyspnea. The mechanism behind decrease $PaO_2$ is intrapulmonary vascular dilation (IPVD) due to increased level of nitric oxide. Shortness of breath is improved on lying flat due the reason that lying increased blood flow to the lungs and decreases the ventilation perfusion mismatch and hypoxemia. The best screening tool for HPS is pulse oximetry. ABGs can be used to check the A-a gradient. Contrast enhanced transthoracic echocardiography can detect intrapulmonary vascular dilation. Another method for detecting IPVD is 99 mTc macro aggregated albumin particles. Normally these particles are trapped in the microcirculation of lungs but in HPS due to dilation of vessels, it can lodge into distal capillary beds of brain, kidneys, liver or spleen. Definitive treatment for HPS is liver transplant which is indicated in severe cases. Mild to moderate cases can be managed with $O_2$ supplementation with regular monitoring with pulse oximetry. Other investigational treatment options include TIPS, embolization, and certain medication that decrease nitric oxide concentration. Acute respiratory distress syndrome commonly occurs after trauma, sepsis, or DIC. Acute pulmonary edema usually occurs after exacerbation of cardiac failure, which causes dyspnea while lying flat due to increased blood volume in lungs due to forward pump failure leading to ventilation perfusion mismatch and hypoxemia. Acute exacerbation of COPD is associated with productive cough, wheezes on auscultation and hypercapnia on ABGs. Pulmonary thromboembolism causes same ABGs changes but the dyspnea doesn't change with position and there is no change in breath sounds.

**Answer: C**

Grace, J.A. and Angus, P.W. (2013) Hepatopulmonary syndrome: update on recent advances in pathophysiology, investigation, and treatment. *Journal of Gastroenterology and Hepatology*, **28** (2), 213–219.

Raevens, S., Geerts, A., Van Steenkiste, C., *et al.* (2015) Hepatopulmonary syndrome and portopulmonary hypertension: recent knowledge in pathogenesis and overview of clinical assessment. *Liver International*, **35** (6), 1646–1660.

**14** *A 61 years old male was admitted to hospital with 2 days history of anorexia, unsteady gait, weakness, and shortness of breath. Past medical history is significant for IV drug abuse and hepatitis C. The patient also reported drinking 10 beers per day for past 30 years with increased consumption within last few months due to marital issues. On physical exam he had abdominal distension with positive fluid thrill, bilateral pedal edema and crackles as well as dullness to percussion in the left lower lobes. Which of the following electrolyte abnormality is associated with this condition?*

**A** *Hypernatremia*
**B** *Hyperkalemia*
**C** *Hypophosphatemia*
**D** *Hyponatremia*
**E** *Hypercalcemia*

Hyponatremia is a common complication of cirrhosis and ascites. The pathophysiology of hyponatremia is either due to increased anti-diuretic hormone (ADH) due to circulatory insufficiency (hypovolemic hyponatremia) or renal impairment that fails to eliminate solute free water (hypervolemic hyponatremia). Hyponatremia in cirrhosis is associated with higher morbidity and mortality, especially affecting brain functions and increased risk for hepatic encephalopathy. Sodium is the major determinant of the osmolality of ECF, hyponatremia can cause neuronal swelling leading to cerebral edema and raised ICP which can cause death if not treated. Treatment of hyponatremia depends on volume status. If patient is hypovolemic, normal saline should be used for increasing plasma volume. Hypervolemic patients can be treated with fluid restriction and/or vaptans (ADH receptor antagonist). In severe cases of hyponatremia, hypertonic saline can be used, but with caution in patients with hypervolemic status. Rapid correction of hyponatremia can cause central pontine myelinosis.

**Answer: D**

Cordoba, J., Ventura-Cots, M., Simón-Talero, M., *et al.* (2014) Characteristics, risk factors, and mortality of cirrhotic patients hospitalized for hepatic encephalopathy with and without acute-on-chronic liver failure (ACLF). *Journal of Hepatology*, **60** (2), 275–281.

Gines, P. and Guevara, M. (2008) Hyponatremia in cirrhosis: pathogenesis, clinical significance, and management. *Hepatology*, **48** (3), 1002–1010.

## 19

# Nutrition Support in Critically Ill Patients
Rifat Latifi, MD and Jorge Con, MD

1   *Which of the following is true?*
   A *The response to stress and injury has been described as the ebb phase, the catabolic flow phase, and the anabolic flow phase*
   B *The ebb phase is dominated by catabolism, typically lasts 3–10 days, but may last longer*
   C *The catabolic flow phase is dominated by circulatory changes that require resuscitation (with fluid, blood, and blood products) over a period of 8–24 hours*
   D *The ebb phase should be treated with blood and blood products*
   E *The catabolic phase emerges as the patient's metabolism shifts to synthetic activities and reparative processes*

The response to stress and injury consists of three phases: the ebb phase, the catabolic flow phase, and the anabolic flow phase. Each of these phases has distinct changes that require specific interventions in order to eliminate or minimize the consequences of illness and/or injury. The ebb phase is dominated by circulatory changes that require resuscitation (with fluid, blood, and blood products) over a period of 8–24 hours. The catabolic flow phase, dominated by catabolism, typically lasts 3–10 days, but may last longer. The anabolic flow phase emerges as the patient's metabolism shifts to synthetic activities and reparative processes. The catabolic flow phase is driven by cytokine mediators released from lymphocytes and macrophages in the cellular immune reaction, dominated by interleukin-6 (IL-6). The release of these mediators is proportional to the intensity of the injury, but the release of cytokines themselves is upregulated by hormonal and humoral events. The early nonspecific response to systemic tissue injury that is responsible for the reprioritization of protein synthesis in the liver is termed the acute phase response (APR). Depending on the magnitude and the severity of the

injury, APR is characterized by an exponential increase in positive acute phase proteins and a decrease in negative acute phase proteins. The regulation of APR, a complex process, depends on many factors. Tissue injury or infection leads to a local inflammatory response, which in turn leads to the release of many cytokines at the site of inflammation; the cytokines are eventually carried to the liver, where they act on the hepatocytes. Crystalloids, blood, and blood products may be required for the initial resuscitation based on the severity and the magnitude of the injury.

**Answer: A**

Azimuddin, K., Latifi, R., and Ivatury, R. (2003) Acute phase proteins in critically ill patients, in *The Biology and Practice of Current Nutritional Support*, 2nd edn (eds R. Latifi and S.J. Dudrick), Landes Bioscience, Austin, TX.

Hill, A.G. and Hill, G.L. (1998) Metabolic response to severe injury. *British Journal of Surgery*, **85**, 884–890.

Ingenblek, Y. and Berstein, L. (1999) The stressful condition as a nutritional adaptive dichotomy. *Nutrition*, **15** (40), 305–320.

2   *Which of the following is true?*
   A *Interleukin 1 and 6 (IL-1, IL-6) and tumor necrosis factor-alpha (TNF) are implicated in the production of acute phase proteins (APP) from the liver*
   B *Interleukin 1 and 6 affect only gastrointestinal tract and have no effect on APP*
   C *Interleukin 12 (IL-12) has no effect on Th1-mediated inflammatory responses*
   D *Interleukin 1 and 6 (IL-1, IL-6) and tumor necrosis factor-alpha (TNF) are not implicated in the production of acute phase proteins (APP) from the liver*
   E *Interleukin 1 and 6 affect APP but do not affect the gastrointestinal tract*

The catabolic flow phase is driven by cytokine mediators released by lymphocytes and macrophages in the cellular immune reaction, dominated by interleukin-6 (IL-6). The release of these mediators is proportionate to the extent of the injury. The release of cytokines is linked to upregulation of hormonal and humoral events. The hormonal events include the release of glucagon and catecholamines, thyroid hormone, growth hormone, and cortisol, and their effects – hyperglycemia, metabolic rate, release of free fatty acids and associated ketosis, insulin growth factor 1 (IGF1), and negative nitrogen balance from gluconeogenesis. A variety of cytokines have been implicated in the production of acute phase proteins from the liver, including interleukin 1 and 6 (IL-1, IL-6) and tumor necrosis factor-alpha (TNF). Interleukin-12 is a key cytokine that initiates Th1-mediated inflammatory responses. This pattern is predictable and reproducible. First, the serum concentration decreases for most of the acute phase proteins, both for positive and for negative reactants. Later, the hepatic synthesis of negative acute phase proteins decreases, and the concentration of serum albumin remains depressed for days to weeks after the injury. Albumin reaches the lowest point by postinjury day 5. Whether nutritional support in the immediate postinjury phase can alter or blunt the acute phase response has not been adequately answered.

**Answer: A**

Castell, J.V., Gomez-Lechon, M.J., David, M., *et al.* (1990) Acute-phase response of human hepatocytes: regulation of acute-phase protein synthesis by interleukin-6. *Hepatology*, **12**, 1179–1186.

Ingenbleek, Y. and Bernstein, L. (1999) The stressful condition as a nutritionally dependent adaptive dichotomy. *Nutrition*, **15**, 305–320.

Issihiki, H., Akira, S., Sugita, T., *et al.* (1991) Reciprocal expression of NF-IL6 and C/EBP in hepatocytes: possible involvement of NF-IL6 in acute phase protein gene expression. *The New Biologist*, **3** (1), 63–70.

**3** *Glutamine is an amino acid that serves as the primary fuel for small bowel enterocytes and other rapidly proliferating cells, such as cells in wounds. Which of the following is true?*
   **A** *It is an essential amino acid because it cannot be synthesized in sufficient quantities during periods of stress*
   **B** *Glutamine is involved in many immune functions, but not in the production of heat shock proteins*
   **C** *Glutamine is contraindicated in critically ill patients except TBI and perioperative SICU patients*
   **D** *Glutamine is classified as a branch-chain amino acid and should be given to patients with liver failure*
   **E** *Glutamine serves as the primary fuel for colonocytes and other slowly proliferating cells*

Glutamine is an amino acid that serves as the primary fuel for small bowel enterocytes and other rapidly proliferating cells, such as cells in wounds. Butyrate is the primary fuel source for colonocytes and slowly proliferating cells. Glutamine is classified as a non-essential amino acid because the human body can synthesize it in sufficient quantities. Yet, during periods of stress, the body's requirements may exceed its capacity to synthesize glutamine. Glutamine is involved in many immune functions, including the production of heat shock proteins. Studies have shown that supplementation with glutamine may lead to a decrease in nosocomial infections in patients with systemic inflammatory response and a decrease in pneumonia, sepsis, and bacteremia in trauma patients. Parenterally administered glutamine has been associated with a decrease in gram-negative bacteremia. Thus, the addition of glutamine to enteral nutrition has been recommended for TBI and perioperative patients in the SICU in the 2016 Society of Critical Care Medicine (SCCM)/American Society for Parenteral and Enteral Nutrition (ASPEN) nutritional guidelines.

**Answer: C**

Garrel, D., Patenaude, J., Nedelec, B., *et al.* (2003) Decreased mortality and infectious morbidity in adult burn patients given enteral glutamine supplements: a prospective, controlled, randomized clinical trial. *Critical Care Medicine*, **31** (10), 2444–2449.

McClave, S.A., Taylor, B.E., Martindale, R.G., *et al.* (2016). Guidelines for the provision and assessment of nutrition support therapy in the adult critically ill patient. *Journal of Parenteral and Enteral Nutrition*, **40** (2), 159–211.

Wischmeyer, P.E., Lynch, J., Liedel, J., *et al.* (2001) Glutamine administration reduces gram-negative bacteremia in severely burned patients: a prospective, randomized, double-blind trial versus isonitrogenous control. *Critical Care Medicine*, **29** (11), 2075–2080.

**4** *Which of the following is true regarding prealbumin, retinol-binding protein, and transferrin?*
   **A** *They are negative acute phase proteins*
   **B** *They are positive acute phase proteins*
   **C** *Neither of the above is true*
   **D** *Both of the above are true*
   **E** *Prealbumin and retinol binding protein are positive acute phase proteins, while transferrin is a negative acute phase protein*

Release of positive acute phase proteins seems to be a protective response to tissue injury. They have diverse functions as antioxidants, proteolytic inhibitors, and mediators of coagulation. The negative acute phase proteins are albumin, prealbumin, retinol-binding protein, and transferrin. Their serum concentrations fall immediately after the injury, in proportion to its severity. They are used to monitor the nutritional status of acutely ill patients. Continued and prolonged production of acute phase proteins in critically ill patients may be an indicator of ongoing sepsis and tissue damage and is associated with higher mortality rates. Perhaps some of the changes at this stage are responsible for what is defined as compensatory anti-inflammatory response syndrome (CARS).

**Answer: A**

Latifi, R. and Caushaj, P.E. (1999) Nutrition support in critically ill patients: current status and practice. *Journal of Clinical Ligand Assay*, **22**, 279–284.
Ward, N.S., Casserly, B., Ayala, A. (2008) The Compensatory Anti-inflammatory Response Syndrome (CARS) in critically ill patients. *Clinics in Chest Medicine*, **29** (4), 617–627.

5  *Severely injured and critically ill patients characteristically demonstrate significant muscle losses, negative nitrogen balance, increased nutriment requirements and:*
   A *Redistribution of amino acids from peripheral tissues to splanchnic organs when they undergo daily hemodialysis*
   B *Redistribution of amino acids from peripheral tissues to splanchnic organs*
   C *Redistribution of amino acids from peripheral tissues to splanchnic organs only after liver transplantation*
   D *Requirements and redistribution of amino acids from peripheral tissues to splanchnic organs only in severe burns*
   E *Redistribution of amino acids from peripheral tissues to splanchnic organs only in bowel ischemia*

Severely injured and critically ill patients characteristically demonstrate significant muscle losses, negative nitrogen balance, two- to three-fold increased requirements, and redistribution of amino acids from peripheral tissues to splanchnic organs. Metabolic response to injury is a striking increase in protein catabolism. Skeletal muscle and nitrogen losses following injury occur as well. The process of increased nitrogen losses is complex and correlates with increased metabolic rate, which peaks several days after injury and gradually returns toward normal over several weeks. This phenomenon

occurs consistently following major surgery, blunt injury, burns, sepsis and various other major injuries. This results in mobilization and increased utilization of nutrient substrates such as fatty acids, amino acids, and glucose. An increased muscle protein catabolism following injury has been demonstrated. Although plasma amino acid levels have been measured in critically ill and injured patients in an effort to identify specific changes related to the catabolic response, the results have been inconsistent. Nonetheless the adverse consequences for the critically ill patient are a rapid loss of muscle mass and subsequent marked debility. All amino acids are required for optimal protein synthesis; however, alanine and glutamine are the major carriers of nitrogen from muscle, constituting as much as 70% of the amino acids released from skeletal muscle following injury.

**Answer: B**

Essen, P., McNurlan, M.A., Gamrin, L., *et al.* (1998) Tissue protein synthesis rates in critically ill patients. *Critical Care Medicine*, **26**, 92–100.
Long, C.L., Schiller, W.R., Blakemore, W.S., *et al.* (1977) Muscle protein catabolism in the septic patient as measured by 3-methylhistidine excretion. *American Journal of Clinical Nutrition*, **30**, 1349–1352.

6  *Which of the following is a true statement?*
   A *Protein synthesis occurs on the surface of ribosome, or multiprotein, multi-RNA complexes that provide the enzyme, peptidyl-transferase*
   B *Protein synthesis has three steps: initiation, elongation, and termination*
   C *During elongation, the ribosome moves from the 5'-end to the 3'-end of the mRNA that is being translated*
   D *The final step of protein synthesis occurs in response to termination signals, after the final amino acid residue is placed at the carboxyl terminal of the newly synthesized protein*
   E *All of the above*

Protein synthesis occurs on the surface of ribosome, or multiprotein, multi-RNA complexes that provide the enzyme, peptidyl-transferase. Peptidyl-transferase is one of many proteins of the larger ribosomal subunit and is imbedded in the surface of the subunit. It catalyzes peptide bond formation and covalent linkage of one amino acid residue to another. The process of protein synthesis itself is called "translation," because the "language" of the nucleotide sequence on the mRNA is translated into the language of an amino acid sequence. The mRNA is translated from its 5'-end to its 3'-end producing a protein synthesized from its amino-terminal end to its carboxyl-terminal end. The direction of translation is precisely defined, with the amino terminal of the evolving protein being synthesized first and the carboxyl terminal synthesized last. The polypeptide chains produced by translation may be modified further after translation. Protein synthesis has three steps: initiation, elongation, and termination. Initiation involves assembly of the components of the translational system before the peptide bonds are formed. The termination, as the final step of protein synthesis, occurs in response to termination signals, after the final amino acid residue is placed at the carboxyl terminal of the newly synthesized protein.

**Answer: E**

Latifi, R. and Dudrick, S.J. (1993) *Amino Acids in Critically Ill and Cancer Patients*. R.G. Landes, Austin, TX.

**7** *Which of the following is true?*
  **A** *Arginine levels are increased in trauma and critical care patients*
  **B** *Arginine is part of the TPN formulas*
  **C** *Arginine and glutamine are present only in immune modulating enteral diets*
  **D** *Glutamine and arginine are present only in immune-enhancing diets*
  **E** *None of the above is true*

Arginine is a semi- or conditionally-essential amino acid, and its requirements are increased during sepsis and tissue injury. Through its role in the urea cycle, arginine takes part in the synthesis of other amino acids, urea, and nitric oxide. Arginine is important for cell-mediated immunity. It is required for the growth and function of T lymphocytes in cultures. In vivo, arginine retards thymic involution by encouraging production of thymic hormones and thymocyte proliferation. Arginine also promotes leukocyte-mediated cytotoxicity. Growth hormone receptors are widely distributed in the immune system, and by releasing growth hormone, arginine may increase the cytotoxic activity of macrophages, neutrophils, NK cells, and cytotoxic T cells. Furthermore, nitric oxide, a product of arginine metabolism, has important tumoricidal, anti-microbial, and inflammatory activities.

Glutamine is the most abundant amino acid in blood and in the body's free amino acid pool. Lymphocytes and macrophages use glutamine as a source of energy. After entering the cell, glutamine is converted to glutamate and ammonia by the action of glutaminase in the inner mitochondrial membrane. Further processing results in production of aspartate and oxidation of about 25% of glutamine to carbon dioxide. This "glutaminolysis" pathway works in conjunction with the glycolytic pathway to allow the combined use of glucose and glutamine as an

energy source for macrophages and lymphocytes. Thus, a relative deficiency of glutamine stores that occurs during critical illness is likely to lead to poor immune responses. Both arginine and glutamine are present in large quantities in immune-modulating formulas (i.e., Oxepa) and immune-enhancing formulas (i.e., Impact). Neither one of them is part of current TPN formulas. In May 2015, the Canadian Clinical Practice Guidelines Committee recommended that enteral glutamine no longer be used in critically ill patients. Two recent multicenter RCTs involving enteral glutamine have reported increased mortality rates in groups of mechanically ventilated adult patients, while demonstrating no additional benefits to other outcomes, such as nosocomial infections. Additional research is required before guideline changes to enteral glutamine are applied to other groups of patients. Recent recommendation of ASPEN is that immune-modulating formulations containing arginine be considered in patients with severe trauma.

**Answer: E**

Canadian Clinical Practice Guidelines Committee (2015) Canadian Clinical Practice Guidelines Compsition of EN: Glutamine. Critical Evaluation Research Unit (CERU): http://www.criticalcarenutrition.com/(accessed September 14, 2015).

Heyland, D., Muscedere, J., Wischmeyer, P.E., et al. (2013) A randomized trial of glutamine and antioxidants in critically ill patients. *New England Journal of Medicine*, **368**, 1489–1497.

McClave, S.A., Taylor, B.E., Martindale, R.G., et al. (2016). Guidelines for the provision and assessment of nutrition support therapy in the adult critically ill patient. *Journal of Parenteral and Enteral Nutrition*, **40** (2), 159–211.

Stroster, J.A., Uranues, S., and Latifi, R. (2015) Nutritional controversies in critical care: revisiting enteral glutamine during critical illness and injury. *Current Opinion in Critical Care*, **21**, 527–530.

**8** *TPN is indicated in which of the following clinical scenarios:*
  **A** *All trauma and critically ill patients with open abdomens admitted to an intensive critical care unit*
  **B** *Only those patients who cannot eat for more than 10 days*
  **C** *High output enterocutaneous fistulas*
  **D** *Patients with acute pancreatitis*
  **E** *First phase of management of short gut syndrome*

The general indications for the use of TPN are: 1) provision of adequate nutrition for as long as necessary intravenously when use of the gastrointestinal tract is impractical, inadequate, ill-advised, or impossible; 2) reduction of mechanical and secretory activity of the alimentary tract to basal levels in order to achieve a state of "bowel rest"; 3) provision of specially tailored formulas to improve nutritional status in patients with kidney or liver failure; and 4) reduction of the urgency for surgical intervention in patients who might eventually require operation, but in whom prolonged, progressive malnutrition will greatly increase the risk of the operation and postoperative complications. TPN efficacy has been demonstrated clearly in many pathophysiologic conditions including short-gut syndrome, fistulas, severe inflammatory bowel disease, severe acute hemorrhagic pancreatitis, chemotherapy and radiation induced enteritis, transplant patients, and severely malnourished cancer patients in their perioperative management, when provision of nutrition enterally is not possible. Other conditions in which TPN is indicated but in which its efficacy has not been clearly demonstrated in the literature include acute exacerbations of chronic pancreatitis, anorexia nervosa, cardiac cachexia, hyperemesis gravidarum, chronic protein losses, and cancer patients with mild malnutrition. In general, when the GI tract cannot be used for more than five days in patients in a catabolic state with or without evidence of malnutrition, or when patients cannot be fed for more than 4–5 days after major surgery, parenteral nutrition should be started. Areas of intense clinical investigation in which TPN may eventually be shown to be of great value are cancer patients in general, sepsis and trauma, and general perioperative support to prevent or correct malnutrition. Answer A is incorrect, as it has been clearly demonstrated that patients with an open abdomen can be fed enterally successfully. If patients who cannot eat, should not eat or cannot eat for more than 3–5 days they should be started on TPN or peripheral parenteral nutrition. One should not wait 7–10 days to start TPN. Patients with acute pancreatitis may be fed enterally. TPN should be reserved for only those patients who have severe hemorrhagic acute pancreatitis complicated with severe ileus and potentially fistulas. Short gut syndrome patients should be supported with TPN. The length of TPN depends on the patient's condition, however, most patients eventually will be able to eat. If patients cannot meet caloric requirements, then TPN is given to support oral intake, usually at night.

**Answer: C**

Dudrick, S.J. and Latifi, R. (1992) Total parenteral nutrition: current status. *Contemporary Surgery*, **41**, 41–48.

Dudrick, S.J., Latifi, R., and Fosnocht, D. (1992) Management of short bowel syndrome. *The Surgical Clinics of North America*, **71**, 625–643.

Joseph, B., Kulvatunyou, K., Tang, A., *et al.* (2011) Total parenteral nutrition in critically ill and injured patients. *European Surgery*, **43** (1), 19–23.

9 *Which of the following statements about TPN are true?*

   A *Dr. Stanley Dudrick described the growth of intravenously fed mice that experienced normal weight gain and normal growth, as compared with their orally fed counterparts*

   B *Early nutritional support via TPN has the potential to reduce disease severity, diminish complications, and decrease the intensive care unit (ICU) length of stay*

   C *TPN cannot give clinicians the ability to parenterally fulfill patients' ongoing requirement for calories, protein, electrolytes, vitamins, minerals, trace elements, and fluids*

   D *The rate of TPN use in the critical care setting has increased in recent years*

   E *TPN is imperative in all critically ill patients*

In 1967 Dudrick *et al.* described the growth of intravenously fed beagle puppies that experienced normal weight gain and normal growth, as compared with their orally fed counterparts. Early nutritional support via TPN has the potential to reduce disease severity, diminish complications, and decrease the intensive care unit (ICU) length of stay. When enteral nutrition is not possible, TPN gives clinicians the ability to parenterally fulfill patients' ongoing requirement for calories, protein, electrolytes, vitamins, minerals, trace elements, and fluids. TPN use has been studied in patients with a wide array of clinical conditions, such as trauma, cancer, inflammatory bowel disease, short gut syndrome, radiation enteritis, poor wound healing, and gastrointestinal (GI) fistula. Yet few well-designed, randomized, controlled trials of the efficacy of TPN in critically ill and injured patients have been conducted. It is well known that 20–40% of critically ill and injured patients exhibit some form of malnutrition. Of that subgroup, 85–90% can be treated with enteral nutrition. In the remaining 10–15%, enteral nutrition is contraindicated; TPN, delivered intravenously, provides the only support. Many interacting biologic and clinical factors are responsible for the development of malnutrition in critically ill and injured hospitalized patients, including a history of pre-injury or disease-specific causes, as well as the hypercatabolic states associated with trauma, sepsis, cancer, and surgical interventions.

**Answer: B**

Dudrick, S.J., Wilmore, D.W., Vars, H.M., *et al.* (1968) Long-term total parenteral nutrition with growth, development and positive nitrogen balance. *Surgery*, **64**, 134–142.

Heyland, D.K., Dhaliwal, R., Drover, J.W., *et al.* (2003) Canadian clinical practice guidelines for nutrition support in mechanically ventilated critically ill adult patients. *Journal of Parenteral and Enteral Nutrition*, **27**, 355–373.

VA TPN Cooperative Study (1991) Perioperative total parenteral nutrition in surgical patients. *New England Journal of Medicine*, **325**, 525–532.

**10** *Which of the following is true regarding lipid use in critically ill patients?*

   **A** *Lipid emulsions should be avoided in critically ill patients in the first week of ICU stay*

   **B** *Essential fatty acid deficiency occurs if patients do not receive lipids in the first seven days*

   **C** *Omega-3 and omega-6 fatty acid are currently used in TPN formulas*

   **D** *There is no biochemical test to diagnose fatty acid deficiency*

   **E** *None of the above is true*

The nature of the lipids that should be administered is currently the focus of much debate; so is the question of whether or not such innovations as structured lipids and triglycerides of varying chain lengths are of any benefit. A study by Dudrick et al. proved that the fear of essential fatty acid deficiency, if fatty emulsions are not given to critically ill and injured patients, is unfounded. In that study, designed to arrest and eliminate atherosclerotic plaque formation in patients with severe heart disease, TPN was administered, with no lipids, for 3 months. None of the patients on TPN without lipids developed fatty acid deficiency, as measured by the triene:tetraene ratio and by clinical examinations. A subsequent study found that trauma patients on TPN with no lipids had better clinical outcomes than patients on TPN with lipids. The latest guidelines of the American Society for Parenteral and Enteral Nutrition call for no fat or limited fat in the first week in the ICU. Until intravenous omega-3 fatty acids become available everywhere, we should be very cautious when using fat emulsions in critically ill and injured patients, because the effect may actually be detrimental.

**Answer: A**

Battistella, F.D., Widegren, J.T., Anderson, J.T., and Siepler, J.K. (1997) A prospective randomized trial of intravenous fat emulsion administration in trauma victims requiring TPN. *Journal of Trauma*, **43** (1), 52–58.

Gould, K.L., Martucci, J.P., Goldberg, D.I., *et al.* (1994) Short-term cholesterol lowering decreases size and

severity of perfusion abnormalities by positron emission tomography after dipyridamole in patients with coronary artery disease. A potential noninvasive marker of healing coronary endothelium. *Circulation*, **89** (4), 1530–1538.

McClave, S.A., Taylor, B.E., Martindale, R.G., *et al.* (2016). Guidelines for the provision and assessment of nutrition support therapy in the adult critically ill patient. *Journal of Parenteral and Enteral Nutrition*, **40** (2), 159–211.

**11** *Which of the following statements is true regarding use of antioxidants and micronutrients in critically ill patients?*

   **A** *Selenium supplementation does not affect the mortality of critically ill patients*

   **B** *Antioxidants are not recommended in critically ill patients*

   **C** *Antioxidants should be used only in burn patients*

   **D** *Among the antioxidants, selenium is the most effective*

   **E** *Only Vitamin C is a real antioxidant*

A meta-analysis of 21 RCTs concluded that supplementation with high dose trace elements and vitamins may improve outcomes of critically ill patients, particularly those at high risk of death.

When the results of these studies were statistically aggregated (n = 20), combined antioxidants were associated with a significant reduction in mortality (risk ratio (RR) = 0.82, 95% confidence interval (CI) 0.72–0.93, P = 0.002); a significant reduction in duration of mechanical ventilation (weighed mean difference in days = -0.67, 95% CI -1.22 to -0.13, P = 0.02); a trend towards a reduction in infections (RR = 0.88, 95% CI 0.76–1.02, P = 0.08). Overall ICU or hospital length of stay (LOS) was not affected. Furthermore, antioxidants were associated with a significant reduction in overall mortality among patients with higher risk of death (>10% mortality in control group) (RR 0.79, 95% CI 0.68–0.92, P = 0.003) whereas there was no significant effect observed for trials of patients with a lower mortality in the control group (RR = 1.14, 95% 0.72–1.82, P = 0.57). Trials using more than 500 μg per day of selenium showed a trend towards a lower mortality (RR = 0.80, 95% CI 0.63–1.02, P = 0.07) whereas trials using doses lower than 500 μg had no effect on mortality (RR 0.94, 95% CI 0.67–1.33, P = 0.75).

Among the antioxidants, selenium may be the most effective. A systematic analysis suggested that selenium supplementation, with or without other antioxidants, was associated with a reduction in mortality (RR, 0.59; 95% CI, 0.32–1.08, P = 0.09).

Another systematic and meta-analysis of nine RCTs using selenium supplementation in critically ill patients reported a reduction in 28-day mortality of borderline statistical significance (risk ratio = 0.84, 95% confidence interval 0.71–0.99, P = 0.04). The analysis of pre-defined subgroups detected no significant effects regarding the supplementation with doses of selenium ≤ 500 μg/d, administration of a load dose with a bolus and duration of treatment. Only 2 studies analyzed 6-month mortality and could not show a difference. No effects could be demonstrated on hospital length of stay, pulmonary infections, or renal failure.

The current recommendation is to provide a combination of antioxidant vitamins and trace minerals, especially including selenium, to all critically ill patients receiving specialized nutrition therapy.

**Answer: D**

Angstwurm, M.W., Engelmann, L., Zimmermann, T., *et al.* (2007) Selenium in Intensive Care (SIC): results of a prospective randomized, placebo-controlled, multiple-center study in patients with severe systemic inflammatory response syndrome, sepsis, and septic shock. *Critical Care Medicine*, **35** (1), 118–126.

Crimi, E., Liguori, A., Condorelli, M., *et al.* (2004) The beneficial effects of antioxidant supplementation in enteral feeding in critically ill patients: a prospective, randomized, double-blind, placebo-controlled trial. *Anesthesia and Analgesia*, **99** (3), 857–863.

Landucci, F., Mancinelli, P., De Gaudio, A.R., and Virgili, G. (2014) Selenium supplementation in critically ill patients: a systematic review and meta-analysis. *Journal of Critical Care*, **29** (1), 150–156.

12  *Which of the following statements about branched-chain amino acids (BCCAs) is true?*
  A  *BCCAs are contraindicated in liver failure*
  B  *BCCAs should not be used in critically ill patients*
  C  *BCCAs are contraindicated in sepsis*
  D  *BCCAs should be used in a concentration of 3%*
  E  *Although some studies have demonstrated lower mortality in sepsis, there is no recommendation to use BCAAs in sepsis*

After injury and sepsis, an energy deficit may develop in skeletal muscle and is met by increased oxidation of branched-chain amino acids (BCAAs). Evidence indicates that skeletal muscle is the major site of BCAA degradation. When critically ill patients who were unable to be fed enterally but who were given total parenteral nutrition (TPN) fortified with BCAAs at high concentration (at either 23% or 45%) they had significantly lower morbidity and mortality, as compared with patients on standard TPN (1.5 g/kg/day of protein). The decrease in mortality correlated with higher doses of BCAAs (at 0.5 g/kg/day or higher). Furthermore, BCAA-rich parenteral nutrition

formulas have been shown to correct the plasma amino acid imbalance that consistently exists in critically ill patients. Such formulas also improve plasma concentrations of prealbumin and retinol-binding protein in septic patients. In a series of trauma patients, BCAA supplementation improved nitrogen retention, transferrin levels, and lymphocyte counts. Since the concentration of BCAAs is low in septic patients, probably as a result of overuse of BCAAs, supplementation with BCAAs may be beneficial. Despite few studies showing benefit in sepsis, there is no recommendation for use of BCAA in sepsis.

**Answer: E**

Calder, P.C. (2006) Branched-chain amino acids and immunity. *Journal of Nutrition*, **136** (1 Suppl), 288S–293S.

Freund, H.R., James, J.H., and Fischer, J.E. (1981) Nitrogen-sparing mechanisms of singly administered branched-chain amino acids in the injured rat. *Surgery*, **90** (2), 237–243.

García-de-Lorenzo, A. Ortíz-Leyba, C., Planas, M., (1997) Parenteral administration of different amounts of branch-chain amino acids in septic patients: clinical and metabolic aspects. *Critical Care Medicine*, **25** (3), 418–424.

13  *Critically ill patients with ARDS:*
  A  *Should not be fed enterally for fear of aspiration and further exacerbation of pneumonias*
  B  *Should be on TPN*
  C  *Should be kept NPO as long as they are on high PEEP*
  D  *Should be given immune enhancing formulas*
  E  *Should not routinely be given immune-modulating formulas*

Immunonutrition has gained wider use in the care of critically ill and injured patients. This trend follows an increasing body of literature supporting the idea that different substrates will enhance a depressed immune system (immune-enhancing formulas) or modulate an over-reactive one (immune-modulating formulas). Although the biologic properties of immune-enhancing nutritional substrates have been well studied, their role in routine clinical care is still controversial. Multiple meta-analyses have shown that immune-modulating formulations are associated with a reduction in ventilator days, in infectious morbidity, and in hospital length of stay, as compared with standard nutritional regimens.

For example, studies have shown that nutritional formulas containing medium-chain triglycerides (MCTs) – when given in a 1:1 LCT:MCT ratio – may be beneficial to septic patients with ARDS, as evidenced by changes in the venous admixture (Qva/Qt), in the mean pulmonary artery pressure (MPAP), and in the P/F ratio. Not only does a high-fat, low- carbohydrate nutritional regimen appear to be beneficial for patients in acute respiratory failure requiring ventilatory support, but the type of fatty acids provided may also have an effect on recovery. A prospective, multicenter, double-blinded, randomized, controlled trial involving 146 patients with ARDS first showed a benefit of the eicosapentaenoic acid, gamma-linolenic acid (EPA + GLA) + antioxidants diet on pulmonary neutrophils recruitment, gas exchange, mechanical ventilation requirements, length of ICU stay, and new organ failures. In that trial, patients in the 2 randomization arms received, for at least 4–7 days, either 1) an enteral compound with EPA + GLA or 2) an isonitrogenous isocaloric standard diet. Subsequent studies by the same authors also showed a decrease in inflammatory mediators from bronchoalveolar lavage fluids (BALFs), namely, a decrease in IL-8 and in $LTB_4$, as well as an associated decrease in BALF neutrophils and protein permeability, suggesting a possible mechanism of the observed benefit. A subsequent single-center, prospective, randomized, controlled, unlabeled study expanded the criteria to include patients with ALI in addition to ARDS; oxygenation and lung compliance improved. Subsequently, another prospective, multicenter, double-blinded, randomized, controlled trial involving 165 patients showed a significant decrease in the 28-day mortality rate (absolute mortality reduction, 19.4%, $P = 0.037$) in patients with sepsis or septic shock requiring mechanical ventilation who received the EPA + GLA + antioxidants diet, as compared with the control group. Moreover, in patients on that diet vs. the control group, the number of ventilator-free days (13.4 vs. 5.8 days) and ICU-free days (10.8 vs 4.6 days) also increased, and new organ dysfunction significantly decreased.

Most recent ASPEN recommendation of 2016 do not support routine use of an enteral formulation characterized by an anti-inflammatory lipid profile (e.g., omega-3 FOs, borage oil) and antioxidants in patients with ARDS and severe ALI, due to a recent meta-analysis of 6 randomized controlled trials.

**Answer: E**

Gadek, J.E., DeMichele, S.J., Karlstad, M.D., *et al.* (1999) Effect of enteral feeding with eicosapentaenoic acid, gamma-linolenic acid, and antioxidants in patients with acute respiratory distress syndrome. *Critical Care Medicine*, **27** (8), 1409–1420.

Li, C., Bo, L., Liu, W., *et al.* (2015) Enteral immunomodulatory diet (omega-3 fatty acid, γ-linolenic acid and antioxidant supplementation) for acute lung injury and acute respiratory distress syndrome: an updated systematic review and meta-analysis. *Nutrients.* 7 (7), 5572–5585.

Pontes-Arruda, A., Aragao, A.M., Albuquerque, J.D. (2006) Effects of enteral feeding with eicosapentaenoic acid, gamma-linolenic acid, and antioxidants in mechanically ventilated patients with severe sepsis and septic shock. *Critical Care Medicine*, **34** (9), 2325–2333.

**14** *Immune-enhancing formulas:*

 **A** *Are contraindicated in trauma patients*
 **B** *Are contraindicated in sepsis*
 **C** *Are contraindicated in cancer*
 **D** *Are too expensive and should be used only in patients with insurance*
 **E** *Have been shown to reduce morbidity and complications*

Although it is difficult to isolate the precise impact of nutritional support, enteral formulas fortified with immune-enhancing substrates have been associated with a significant reduction in the risk of infectious complications and a reduction in overall hospital stay. It has been demonstrated that certain nutrients can modulate inflammatory, metabolic, and immune processes, while other can enhance the immune system. Amino acids such as arginine and glutamine improve body defenses and tumor cell metabolism; increase wound healing; and reduce nitrogen loss. RNA and omega-3 fatty acids also modulate the immune function. Immune-enhancing formulas have improved the immune response in burn, trauma, and surgical patients and have reduced infections, total complications, and length of stay. One prospective, blinded study found that an immune-enhancing enteral diet containing glutamine reduced septic complications in patients with severe trauma. Of 390 critically ill surgical and medical patients, 101 received early enteral nutrition (within 72 hours). Of those 101 patients, 50 received immune-enhancing diets and had significantly reduced requirements for mechanical ventilation and a shorter hospital stay, as compared with control patients. In a prospective, double-blind, randomized trial of patients with major burns (>50% body surface) supplemental intravenous glutamine, infused continuously over 24 hours, was significantly better than just isonitrogenous amino acid solutions.

**Answer: E**

Bower, R.H., Cerra, F.B., Bershadsky, B. *et al.* (1995) Early enteral administration of a formula (Impact) supplemented with arginine, nucleotides, and fish oil in intensive care unit patients: result of multicenter, prospective, randomized, clinical trial. *Critical Care Medicine*, **23**, 436–449.

Houdijk, A.P., Rijnsburger, E.R., Jansen, J. *et al.* (1998) Randomized trial of glutamine-enriched enteral nutrition on infectious morbidity in patients with multiple trauma. *Lancet*, **352** (9130), 772–776.

Kudsk, K., Minard, G., Groce, M., *et al.* (1996) A randomized trial of isonitrogenous enteral diets after severe trauma. An immune-enhancing diet reduces septic complications. *Annals of Surgery*, **224**, 531–543.

**15** *Which statement is true?*
  **A** *Nucleotides are not provided in TPN formulas*
  **B** *Nucleotides are not present in enteral diets and should be given intramuscularly only*
  **C** *Nucleotides are provided in TPN*
  **D** *Nucleotides should be given only in combination with glutamine*
  **E** *Nucleotides are present only in certain TPN formulas*

Nucleotides are perhaps best known for their role in the synthesis of deoxyribonucleic acid (DNA) and ribonucleic acid (RNA), hence, for their role in genetic coding. However, nucleotides also play a role in adenosine triphosphate (ATP) metabolism; they are a part of many coenzymes involved in carbohydrate, protein, and lipid synthesis. Nucleotides may be synthesized by some cells. But it is believed that rapidly dividing cells, such as epithelial cells and T lymphocytes, are unable to produce nucleotides and that, during periods of stress, a relative deficit of nucleotides develops. Nucleotides have been implicated in the modulation of immune function. Exogenous nucleotides have been found to be needed for the helper/inducer T-cell response. In the clinical setting, immune enhancing-containing nucleotides have been shown to significantly reduce infections, ventilator days, and length of hospital stay, for both critically ill and postsurgical patients. However, those studies have not addressed the isolated effects of nucleotides as a substrate, so further studies addressing them are needed. Nucleotides are not present in current TPN formulas. When TPN was used in kidney transplant patients, patients required less immunosuppressive medications.

**Answer: A**

Beale, R.J., Bryg, D.J., and Bihari, D.J. (1999) Immunonutrition in the critically ill: a systematic review of clinical outcome. *Critical Care Medicine*, **27** (12), 2799–2805.

Kulkarni, A.D., Rudolph, F.B., Van Buren, C.T. (1994) The role of dietary sources of nucleotides in immune function: a review. *Journal of Nutrition*, **124** (8 Suppl), 1442S–1446S.

Van Buren, C.T., Kulkarni, A.D., Fanslow, W.C., and Rudolph, F.B. (1985) Dietary nucleotides, a requirement for helper/inducer T lymphocytes. *Transplantation*, **40** (6), 694–697.

**16** *A meta-analysis of 24 RCTs that assessed the outcome of critically ill patients randomized to immunonutrition formulas, which included supplementation with arginine, glutamine, fish oil, and combinations of those components, showed that these formulas:*
  **A** *Had no effect in critically ill patients*
  **B** *Significantly improved the mortality of critically ill patients*
  **C** *Improved both morbidity and mortality of critically ill patients*
  **D** *Improved only morbidity but not mortality of critically ill patients*
  **E** *Improved mortality but not morbidity*

Although it is difficult to isolate the precise impact of nutritional support, enteral formulas fortified with immune-enhancing substrates, such as amino acids (arginine, glutamine), nucleotides, nucleosides, and other nutrients, have been associated with a significant reduction in the risk of infectious complications and a reduction in overall hospital stay. It has been demonstrated that certain nutrients can modulate inflammatory, metabolic, and immune processes. Amino acids such as arginine and glutamine improve body defenses and tumor cell metabolism, increase wound healing, and reduce nitrogen loss. RNA and omega-3 fatty acids also modulate the immune function. Immune-enhancing formulas have improved the immune response in burn, trauma, and surgical patients and have reduced infections, total complications, and length of stay. A meta-analysis of 24 RCTs assessed the outcome of critically ill patients randomized to an immunomodulatory diet, which included supplementation with arginine, glutamine, fish oil, and combinations of those components. The immunomodulatory diet, as compared with the control diet, had no effect on the mortality rate or the length of hospital stay. However, a subgroup analysis showed that patients with systemic inflammatory response syndrome (SIRS), sepsis, or ARDS who received fish oil alone had a significantly improved outcome in terms of the mortality rate, the rate of secondary infections, and the length of hospital stay. Immunomodulating diets supplemented with arginine, with/without additional glutamine or fish oils, did not appear to offer an advantage over standard enteral formulas in intensive care unit, trauma or burn patients.

**Answer: C**

Dogjani, A., Zatriqi, S., Uranues, S., and Latifi. R. (2011) Biology-based nutritional support of critically ill and injured patients. *European Surgery*, **43** (1): 7–12.

Marik, P.E. and Zaloga, G.P. (2008) Immunonutrition in critically ill patients: a systematic review and analysis of the literature. *Intensive Care Medicine*, **34** (11). 1980–1990.

**17** *Regarding the monitoring of tolerance and adequacy of enteral nutrition (EN) in the ICU, which of the following is correct:*

**A** *Routine monitoring of gastric residual volumes (GRV) should be part of routine care*

**B** *Gastric residual volumes correlate well to gastric emptying*

**C** *A gastric residual volume of 350 mL should always prompt cessation of feeds and further evaluation*

**D** *Elevating the head of the bed 30–45 degrees has not been shown to decrease the incidence of pneumonia*

**E** *Bundled interventions including chlorhexidine mouthwash has been shown to decrease nosocomial respiratory infections.*

Gastric residual volumes (GRV) do not correlate well with incidences of pneumonia, regurgitation, or aspiration. In a trial using a highly sensitive and specific marker for aspiration, GRVs (over a range of 150–400 mL) were shown to be a poor monitor for aspiration, with a very low sensitivity, a positive predictive value of 18.2–25%, and a negative predictive value of 77.1–77.4%. Results from 4 RCTs indicate that raising the threshold to stop feedings for GRVs from 50–150 mL to 250–500 mL did not increase the incidence of regurgitation, aspiration, or pneumonia. Current recommendations are to not checking GRVs and to use a threshold to hold tube feeds if >500 mL GRVs if compelled to check. Studies in which chlorhexidine oral care was included in bundled interventions showed significant reductions in nosocomial respiratory infections. Elevating the head of the bed 30°–45° was shown in one study to reduce the incidence of pneumonia from 23% to 5%.

**Answer: E**

McClave, S.A., Lukan, J.K., Stefater, J.A., *et al.* (2005) Poor validity of residual volumes as a marker for risk of aspiration in critically ill patients. *Critical Care Medicine*, **33** (2), 324–330.

McClave, S.A., Taylor, B.E., Martindale, R.G., *et al.* (2016). Guidelines for the provision and assessment of nutrition support therapy in the adult critically ill patient. *Journal of Parenteral and Enteral Nutrition*, **40** (2), 159–211.

**18** *Regarding delivery of enteral nutrition (EN) in the ICU, which of the following is correct:*

**A** *Post-pyloric feeding has not been shown to decrease incidence of pneumonia*

**B** *Targeting 24-hour feeding volumes is equal to targeting hourly rates.*

**C** *High-risk patients and those intolerant to bolus feeds should not receive continuous feeds.*

**D** *Prokinetics such as erythromycin should be initiated in high risk patients.*

**E** *Food coloring in enteral nutrition can be used as a marker for aspiration.*

Changing the level of infusion of EN from the stomach to the small bowel has been shown to reduce the incidence of regurgitation, aspiration, and pneumonia. Volume-based feeding protocols in which 24-hour or daily volumes are targeted instead of hourly rates have been shown to increase volume of nutrition delivered. Adding prokinetic agents such as erythromycin or metoclopramide has been shown to improve gastric emptying and tolerance of EN but has resulted in little change in clinical outcome for ICU patients. Besides food coloring being found to be associated to mitochondrial toxicity, the US Food and Drug Administration (FDA), through a Health Advisory Bulletin (September 2003), issued a mandate against the use of blue food coloring as a monitor for aspiration in patients receiving EN.

**Answer: D**

Heyland, D.K., Murch, L., Cahill, N., *et al.* (2013) Enhanced protein-energy provision via the enteral route feeding protocol in critically ill patients: results of a cluster randomized trial. *Critical Care Medicine*, **41** (12), 2743–2753.

Kortbeek, J.B., Haigh, P.I., and Doig, C. (1999) Duodenal versus gastric feeding in ventilated blunt trauma patients: a randomized controlled trial. *Journal of Trauma*. **46** (6), 992–996.

McClave, S.A., Taylor, B E., Martindale, R G., *et al.* (2016). Guidelines for the provision and assessment of nutrition support therapy in the adult critically ill patient. *Journal of Parenteral and Enteral Nutrition*, **40** (2), 159–211.

**19** *Regarding nutritional therapy in pulmonary failure, the following is correct:*

**A** *Specialty high-fat/low-carbohydrate formulations should be used*

**B** *High-fat low-carbohydrate formulations are designed to increase $CO_2$ production*

**C** *Enteral formulations with an anti-inflammatory profile typically include omega-3 fatty acids, borage oils, and antioxidants*

**D** *Serum phosphate concentrations do not affect respiratory failure*

**E** *Fluid restricted energy-dense formulations should not be used in respiratory failure*

Although an early small trial showed that high-fat/low-carbohydrate formulations reduced duration of mechanical ventilation, these findings were not reproduced in subsequent RCTs. Phosphate deficiency is associated with respiratory muscle weakness and failure to wean from mechanical ventilation. Fluid- restricted formulations may be considered for patients with fluid accumulation, pulmonary edema, and renal failure. Six RCTs have evaluated the use of additives or formulas with an anti-inflammatory lipid profile (omega-3 FO, borage oil, and antioxidants) in patients with ARDS, ALI, and sepsis. However, because studies were heterogeneous and because of conflicting data, anti-inflammatory lipid formulations are not currently recommended for routine use in ARDS/ALI as mentioned in the ASPEN 2016 guidelines.

**Answer: C**

Bech, A., Blans, M., Raaijmakers, M., *et al.* (2013) Hypophosphatemia on the intensive care unit: individualized phosphate replacement based on serum levels and distribution volume. *Journal of Critical Care*, **28** (5). 838–843.

McClave, S.A., Taylor, B E., Martindale, R G., *et al.* (2016). Guidelines for the provision and assessment of nutrition support therapy in the adult critically ill patient. *Journal of Parenteral and Enteral Nutrition*, **40** (2), 159–211.

Mesejo, A., Acosta, J.A., Ortega, C., *et al.* (2003) Comparison of a high-protein disease-specific enteral formula with a high-protein enteral formula in hyperglycemic critically ill patients. *Clinical Nutrition*, **22** (3), 295–305.

**20** *Regarding nutritional therapy in hepatic failure, the following is correct:*
   A *Actual weight is superior to dry weight or usual weight in calculating energy and protein needs in patients with cirrhosis and hepatic failure*
   B *Parenteral nutrition is contraindicated in cirrhosis*
   C *Branched-chain amino acids include lysine, isoleucine, serine, and valine*
   D *Branched-chain amino acids are of no benefit for encephalopathic patients in the ICU already receiving luminal-acting antibiotics and lactulose*
   E *Protein restriction may reduce risk from hepatic encephalopathy*

Although protein restriction was historically used to reduce risk from hepatic encephalopathy, such a strategy may worsen nutrition status, decrease lean muscle mass, and ironically lead to less ammonia removal. There is no evidence to suggest that a formulation enriched in BCAA improves patient outcomes compared with standard whole-protein formulations in critically ill patients with liver disease. In patients with hepatic encephalopathy already receiving first-line therapy (antibiotics and lactulose), there is no evidence to date that adding BCAAs

will further improve mental status or coma grade. In clinical trials, EN has been associated with decreased infection rates and fewer metabolic complications in liver disease and after liver transplant when compared with PN. Serine is not a BCAA.

**Answer: D**

Bemeur, C., Desjardins, P., and Butterworth, R.F. (2010) Role of nutrition in the management of hepatic encephalopathy in end-stage liver failure. *Journal of Nutrition and Metabolism*, **2010**, 489823.

Charlton, M. (2006) Branched-chain amino acid enriched supplements as therapy for liver disease. *Journal of Nutrition*, **136** (1), 295S–298S.

McClave, S.A., Taylor, B E., Martindale, R G., *et al.* (2016). Guidelines for the provision and assessment of nutrition support therapy in the adult critically ill patient. *Journal of Parenteral and Enteral Nutrition*, **40** (2), 159–211.

**21** *Regarding nutritional therapy in severe pancreatitis, which of the following is correct:*
   A *Jejunal feeding is superior to gastric feeding in tolerance and clinical outcome*
   B *Patients with moderate to severe acute pancreatitis benefit from parenteral nutrition over enteral nutrition*
   C *Probiotics are of no benefit to patients on enteral nutrition*
   D *Parenteral nutrition should be started when enteral nutrition has not been feasible after 72 hours from onset of pancreatitis*
   E *Strategies to improve tolerance to enteral nutrition include: early start of enteral nutrition, feeding distally, and near fat-free elemental diets*

Use of EN is preferred to PN because of decreased infectious morbidity, hospital LOS, need for surgical intervention, and mortality. Several RCTs comparing gastric with jejunal feeding in severe acute pancreatitis showed no significant differences between the two. Measures to improve tolerance to EN in patients with moderate to severe acute pancreatitis include starting EN as soon as possible within the first 48 hours of admission, feeding more distally in the GI tract, changing from a standard polymeric formula to one that contains small peptides and medium-chain triglycerides or to one that is a nearly fat-free elemental formulation, and switching from bolus to continuous infusion.

**Answer: E**

Cao, Y., Xu, Y., Lu, T., *et al.* (2008) Meta-analysis of enteral nutrition versus total parenteral nutrition in patients with severe acute pancreatitis. *Annals of Nutrition and Metabolism*, **53** (3–4), 268–275.

Chang, Y.S., Fu, H.Q., Xiao, Y.M., and Liu, J.C. (2013) Nasogastric or nasojejunal feeding in predicted severe acute pancreatitis: a meta-analysis. *Critical Care*, **17** (3), R118.

Wang, G., Wen, J., Xu, L., *et al*. Effect of enteral nutrition and ecoimmunonutrition on bacterial translocation and cytokine production in patients with severe acute pancreatitis. *Journal of Surgical Research*, **183** (2), 592–597.

**22** *Regarding nutritional therapy in burns, which of the following is correct:*

    **A** *Indirect calorimetry is almost never needed as other predictive formulas are just as accurate*

    **B** *Protein needs are increased and should be in the range of 1.5–2 g/kg/d*

    **C** *Nutrition should be held until after 48 hours, at the onset of the catabolic phase*

    **D** *Although enteral nutrition should be withheld in futile or end-of-life cases, hydration should not*

    **E** *Supplementation of enteral nutrition with parenteral nutrition is of benefit*

In an evaluation of 46 predictive equations published between 1953–2000, Dickerson et al found none of them to be precise in estimating energy expenditure measured by indirect calorimetry in 24 patients with > 20% total body surface area burns. A trial evaluating the role of supplemental PN showed that patients receiving both PN and EN had a higher incidence of infection and increased mortality compared with patients receiving EN alone. The 2001 American Burn Association guidelines, the 2013 ESPEN guidelines, and ASPEN 2016 guidelines all recommend the provision of 1.5–2 g of protein/kg/d for patients with burn injury. Based on expert consensus, very early (within 4–6 hours of injury) initiation of enteral nutrition in burn patients is recommended in ASPEN 2016 guidelines.

**Answer: B**

Dickerson, R.N., Gervasio, J.M., Riley, M.L., *et al*. (2002) Accuracy of predictive methods to estimate resting energy expenditure of thermally-injured patients. *Journal of Parenteral and Enteral Nutrition*, **26** (1). 17–29.

Herndon, D.N., Barrow, R.E., Stein, M., *et al*. (1989) Increased mortality with intravenous supplemental feeding in severely burned patients. *Journal of Burn Care and Rehabilitation*, **10** (4), 309–313.

McClave, S.A., Taylor, B E., Martindale, R G., *et al*. (2016). Guidelines for the provision and assessment of nutrition support therapy in the adult critically ill patient. *Journal of Parenteral and Enteral Nutrition*, **40** (2), 159–211.

**23** *Regarding nutritional therapy in critically ill obese patients, which of the following is correct:*

    **A** *An obese ICU patient with a history of sleeve gastrectomy should receive supplemental thiamine prior to initiating dextrose-containing IV fluids or nutrition therapy*

    **B** *In this population, high-protein/eucaloric diets are superior to high-protein/hypocaloric formulas*

    **C** *Obese patients require no additional monitoring for glucose levels compared with the non-obese population*

    **D** *Providing protein at a dose of 2 g/kg ideal body weight is sufficient for achieving a neutral nitrogen balance when BMI > 40*

    **E** *There is no evidence that patients with BMI > 40 have a higher mortality than those with BMI < 40*

Patients who have undergone procedures including sleeve gastrectomy, gastric bypass, or biliopancreatic diversion have an increased risk of micronutrient deficiency and thiamine deficiency and should be identified prior to glucose administration. Use of high-protein hypocaloric feeding in hospitalized patients with obesity is associated with possibly better outcomes than high-protein eucaloric feeding including shorter ICU stay, shorter antibiotic duration, and fewer days on mechanical ventilation. The higher incidence of diabetes mellitus and magnified insulin resistance in critical illness results in the need for increased vigilance of glucose levels. A retrospective study by Choban et al indicated that provision of protein at a dose of 2.0 g/kg ideal body weight per day was insufficient for achieving neutral nitrogen balance when BMI is > 40. Patients with a BMI > 40 clearly have worse outcomes and higher mortality than ICU patients with BMI ≤ 40.

**Answer: A**

Choban, P.S., Burge, J.C., Scales, D., and Flancbaum, L. (1997) Hypoenergetic nutrition support in hospitalized obese patients: a simplified method for clinical application. *American Journal of Clinical Nutrition*, **66** (3), 546–550.

Dickerson, R.N., Boschert, K.J., Kudsk, K.A., and Brown, R.O. (2002) Hypocaloric enteraltube feeding in critically ill obese patients. *Nutrition*, **18** (3), 241–246.

McClave, S.A., Taylor, B E., Martindale, R G., *et al*. (2016). Guidelines for the provision and assessment of nutrition support therapy in the adult critically ill patient. *Journal of Parenteral and Enteral Nutrition*, **40** (2), 159–211.

## 20

# Neurocritical Care
*Herb A. Phelan, MD*

**1** *Intracranial hypertension immediately following blunt traumatic brain injury is most commonly a result of:*
 **A** *Epidural hematoma*
 **B** *Intracellular edema*
 **C** *Diffuse axonal injury*
 **D** *Vasogenic edema*
 **E** *Both intracellular edema and vasogenic edema*

The most common cause of intracranial hypertension following blunt traumatic brain injury is intracellular brain edema. Vasogenic edema, although occasionally present in the early stages, is not a common early cause, but may result in prolonged intracranial hypertension after about 7–10 days. Epidural hematomas and diffuse axonal injury by themselves are infrequent causes.

**Answer: B**

Marmarou, A., Signoretti, S., Fatourous, P., *et al.* (2006) Predominance of cellular edema in traumatic brain swelling in patients with severe head injuries. *Journal of Neurosurgery,* **104**, 720–730.

**2** *Steroid therapy for blunt traumatic brain injury*
 **A** *Increases the chance of death from all causes*
 **B** *Reduces the mortality rate at two weeks post injury*
 **C** *Is associated with decreased infection rates*
 **D** *Must be started within 48 hours to be effective*
 **E** *Prevents late vasogenic edema if started within five days of injury*

A number of studies have consistently demonstrated no role for steroids in the management of acute traumatic brain injury. The MRC CRASH trial, published in 2004, was stopped after enrolling approximately 10 000 patients because of the clear increase in mortality from all causes in the group of patients receiving steroids. Higher infection rates were also reported. Steroids are still occasionally used to treat headaches that accompany concussion syndrome, but this is usually in the later stages of the injury and presumably reduces the mild vasogenic edema. The vasogenic edema associated with brain tumors are also treated with steroids on occasion with good symptomatic relief.

**Answer: A**

Carney, N., Totten, A.M., O'Reilly, C., *et al.* (2016) Guidelines for the management of severe traumatic brain injury, 4th edition. *Neurosurgery,* **80** (1), 6–15.
Edwards, P., Arango, M., Balica, L., *et al.* (2005) Final results of MRC CRASH, a randomized placebo-controlled trial of intravenous corticosteroid in adults with head injury-outcomes at six months. *Lancet,* **365**, 1957–1959.

**3** *The main objective of intracranial cerebral pressure monitoring following traumatic brain injury is to*
 **A** *Maintain cerebral perfusion pressure over > 70 mm Hg*
 **B** *Maintain intracranial pressures < 15 mm Hg*
 **C** *Maintain adequate cerebral perfusion and oxygenation to the non-injured brain tissue*
 **D** *Prevent secondary seizure development*
 **E** *Maintain cerebral perfusion pressure > 55 mm Hg and intracranial pressure < 10 mm Hg*

The primary objective of ICP monitoring is to maintain adequate brain tissue perfusion and oxygenation simultaneously avoiding secondary brain injury while the injured portions of the brain are allowed to heal. Generally, treatment of the intracranial pressure should be initiated when the ICP increases > 20 mm Hg. The ideal cerebral perfusion pressure currently is controversial, but lies somewhere between 50–70 mm Hg.

**Answer: C**

*Surgical Critical Care and Emergency Surgery: Clinical Questions and Answers*, Second Edition.
Edited by Forrest "Dell" Moore, Peter Rhee, and Gerard J. Fulda.
© 2018 John Wiley & Sons Ltd. Published 2018 by John Wiley & Sons Ltd.
Companion website: www.wiley.com/go/moore/surgical_criticalcare_and_emergency_surgery

Carney, N., Totten, A.M., O'Reilly, C., *et al.* (2016) Guidelines for the management of severe traumatic brain injury, 4th edition. *Neurosurgery*, **80** (1), 6–15.

**4** *A 25-year-old man is admitted to the emergency department following a motor vehicle crash. He arrives comatose and intubated with a blood pressure of 140/85 mm Hg, heart rate of 100 beats/min, $SpO_2$ of 100%, and breathing spontaneously at a rate of 14 breaths/min. A CT scan of the brain confirms a right frontal intraparenchymal cerebral hematoma. Indications for immediate operative intervention include:*

**A** *Midline shift of 3 mm on CT scan*

**B** *A Glasgow Coma Scale Score of 11 (intubated) with the intracerebral hematoma volume measurement equal to 10 $cm^3$*

**C** *A Glasgow Coma Scale Score of 7 (intubated) with a measured intracranial pressure of 8 mm Hg, a midline shift of 2 mm, and a mass lesion measuring 8 $cm^3$*

**D** *A mass lesion on CT measuring over 50 $cm^3$*

**E** *None of the above*

Patients with intraparenchymal hematomas are candidates for surgery if they develop signs of progressive neurological deterioration and the lesion is of sufficient size to warrant operative intervention. Patients with Glasgow Coma Scale Scores of 6–8 with frontal or temporal contusions greater than 20 $cm^3$ in volume with midline shift of at least 5 mm and/or cisternal compression on the CT scan, and patients with any lesion greater than 50 $cm^3$ in volume should generally be treated operatively. Patients with intraparenchymal mass lesions who do not show evidence of neurological compromise, have well controlled intracranial pressure, and no significant signs of mass effect on CT scan are generally managed nonoperatively with intensive monitoring and serial imaging.

**Answer: D**

Bullock, M.R., Chestnut, R., Ghajar, J., *et al.* (2006) Surgical management of traumatic parenchymal lesions. *Neurosurgery*, **58**, S225–S246.

**5** *A 37-year-old woman is admitted following a fall from a horse. Her initial Glasgow Coma Score prior to intubation is 8 and her vital signs are stable. A CT scan shows multiple small intraparenchymal hemorrhages in the frontal and temporal lobes with a small amount of subarachnoid hemorrhage in the right posterior parietal area. A ventriculostomy is inserted for intracranial pressure monitoring. Her initial intracranial pressure is 10 mm Hg. Approximately*

*30 hours following admission the patient's intracranial pressure increases to 25 mm Hg. There is no change in neurological examination. Initial management of the patient's change in intracranial pressure includes all of the following except:*

**A** *Drainage of cerebral spinal fluid through the ventriculostomy*

**B** *Immediate CT scan of the brain to rule out development of a mass lesion*

**C** *Osmotic diuretics*

**D** *Maintenance of normothermia*

**E** *Hyperventilation to a $PaCO_2$ of 25–30 torr*

Initial management of an elevated intracranial pressure in a patient with a ventriculostomy should be drainage of cerebral spinal fluid. Additionally, an emergency CT scan should be obtained as soon as possible to rule out development of a mass lesion that might require operative intervention. Osmotic diuretics and maintenance of body temperature within normal limits are also appropriate. Hyperventilation is not usually recommended since it may result in ischemia to normal brain tissue. Generally, hyperventilation to this level is a last resort in patients who are showing obvious signs of impending cerebral herniation.

**Answer: E**

Valadka, A.B. and Dannenbaum, M.J. (2008) Pathophysiology, clinical diagnosis, and prehospital and emergency center care. Head and central nervous system injuries, in *Current Therapy of Trauma and Surgical Critical Care* (eds J. Asensio and D. Trunkey), Mosby Elsevier, Philadelphia, PA, pp. 147–152.

**6** *Mannitol for osmotic therapy to reduce intracranial pressure*

**A** *Should never be given prior to insertion of an intracranial pressure monitor*

**B** *Is usually given at a dose of 0.1 g/kg*

**C** *Should not be given if the serum osmolality is over 295 mosm/L*

**D** *Works initially by creating osmotic gradients between blood plasma and brain cells, reducing cellular volume*

**E** *Initially reduces intracranial pressure by expanding intravascular volume, reducing blood viscosity, and increasing cerebral blood flow*

Mannitol remains a standard therapy for reducing intracranial pressure. The initial dose of mannitol is 1 g/kg and can be given emergently without intracranial pressure monitoring as long as the patient is normotensive. Mannitol is particularly useful if the patient is showing any signs or symptoms of impending herniation. Subsequent dosing to a serum osmolality up to 320 mosm/L is usually recommended as needed. Dosing to higher levels has not been shown to improve outcome and increases the risk of acute renal failure. Mannitol reduces intracranial pressure through two mechanisms. The immediate mechanism is expansion of intravascular volume, resulting in reduced blood viscosity. This results in an increase in cerebral blood flow in the areas of the brain where cerebral autoregulation remains intact and ICP falls. The second mechanism, which occurs later, involves the establishment of osmotic gradients between the serum plasma and the brain cells. This ultimately decreases intracellular volume and reduces intracranial pressure. Since mannitol also functions as a diuretic there is always a risk of reducing blood pressure and therefore cerebral perfusion pressure if the patient is not adequately volume resuscitated. For this reason, hypertonic saline has gained favor as an osmotic agent for increased ICP since it is less likely to cause hypotension.

**Answer: E**

Muizelaar, J.P., Lutz, H.A., and Becker, D.P. (1984) Effect of mannitol in ICP and CBF and correlation with pressure autoregulation in severely head-injured patients. *Journal of Neurosurgery*, **61**, 700–706.

Vialet, R., Albanese, J., Thomachot, L., *et al.* (2003) Isovolume hypertonic solutes (sodium chloride or mannitol) in the treatment of refractory posttraumatic intracranial hypertension: 2 mL/kg 7.5% saline is more effective than 2 mL/kg 20% mannitol. *Critical Care Medicine*, **31**, 1683–1687.

7  Clinical studies in both the prehospital and hospital setting following traumatic brain injury
   A  Have definitely shown that correcting hypotension and hypoxia improves mortality rate
   B  Have shown a correlation with increased mortality and systolic blood pressure < 90 mm Hg
   C  Have failed to show any relationship between avoidance of hypoxemia and improved mortality rates
   D  Are inconsistent with current recommendations for treating hypotension and hypoxemia following traumatic brain injury
   E  Suggest that systolic blood pressure is a better parameter than mean arterial pressure for monitoring patients with traumatic brain injury

There is an abundance of Level II evidence to support the dictum of avoiding hypotension and hypoxemia in patients with traumatic brain injury. Secondary brain injury may occur from episodes of hypotension and hypoxemia. Chestnut *et al.*, in reviewing data from the Traumatic Coma Data Bank, showed a correlation between a single prehospital systolic blood pressure measurement < 90 mm Hg and increased morbidity and mortality. Other studies support that repeated episodes of hypotension in the hospital setting may significantly and negatively affect mortality rates. Current Level II recommendations are that in patients with traumatic brain injury, systolic blood pressure < 90 mm Hg, and $PaO_2$ < 60 mm Hg (or $SpO_2$ < 90%) should be avoided. For obvious ethical reasons, there are no definitive Level I studies to prove this Level II evidence. There is no evidence to suggest that systolic blood pressure is a better parameter to monitor compared to mean arterial pressure. There is no consistent relationship between systolic blood pressure and mean arterial pressure. Mean arterial pressure is used to calculate cerebral perfusion pressure, so it is reasonable to maintain mean arterial pressure at levels considerably higher than those represented by a systolic blood pressure of 90 mm Hg.

**Answer: B**

Carney, N., Totten, A.M., O'Reilly, C., *et al.* (2016) Guidelines for the management of severe traumatic brain injury, 4th edition. *Neurosurgery*, **80** (1), 6–15.

Chestnut, R.M., Marshal, L.F., Clauber, M.R., *et al.* (1993) The role of secondary brain injury in determining outcome from severe head injury. *Journal of Trauma*, **34**, 216–222.

8  A 30-year-old man is admitted to the intensive care unit following a gunshot wound to the head. He is hemodynamically stable with a systolic blood pressure of 140/100 mm Hg, a heart rate of 115 beats/min, and a spontaneous respiratory rate of 22 breaths/min. The best predictor of a poor outcome is:
   A  Bihemispheric injury
   B  Bullet fragmentation
   C  Pupillary changes
   D  An admission Glasgow Coma score of < 6
   E  Presence of intraventricular blood

A number of studies in the mid-to-late 1990s showed that patients arriving post gunshot wound to the brain and a Glasgow Coma Score of 3, 4, or 5 have extremely poor outcomes in terms of mortality or survival in a chronic vegetative state. The decision to subject these patients to aggressive resuscitation remains controversial. The presence of disseminated intravascular coagulopathy (DIC) is always associated with a poor outcome. Diffuse fragmentation, bihemispheric injury, intraventricular hemorrhage, and absence of pupillary response all predict a poor outcome, but a Glasgow Coma score of < 6 is the most consistently reported negative predictor.

**Answer: D**

Levy, M.L. (2000) Outcome prediction following penetrating craniocerebral injury in a civilian population; aggressive surgical management in patients with admission Glasgow Coma Scale scores of 6 to 15. *Neurosurgery*, **8**, 1–6.

Levy, M.L., Masri, L.S., Lavine S., and Apuzzo, M.L.J. (1994) Outcome prediction after penetrating craniocerebral injury in a civilian population: Aggressive surgical management in patients with admission Glasgow Coma Scale scores of 3, 4, or 5. *Neurosurgery*, **35**, 77–85.

9  *Subarachnoid hemorrhage secondary to a ruptured cerebral artery aneurysm*
   A *Can be excluded with a normal CT scan of the brain*
   B *Usually requires a lumbar puncture to make a definitive diagnosis*
   C *Is treated in the early preoperative stages with maintenance of blood pressure < 160/90 mm Hg with intravenous anti-hypertensive medications*
   D *Does not require anticonvulsant prophylaxis*
   E *Is not associated with xanthochromia or red blood cells in the cerebral spinal fluid*

A ruptured cerebral artery aneurysm usually presents with severe headache of sudden onset, lethargy, and nuchal rigidity. Smaller bleeds may not present with severe symptoms. The initial diagnosis of subarachnoid hemorrhage is usually made by non-contrast CT scan of the brain. However, about 10% of patients presenting with early subarachnoid hemorrhage related to a ruptured cerebral artery aneurysm will have a normal CT, and the diagnosis will need to be confirmed with lumbar puncture. Lumbar puncture will typically show xanthochromia or high red blood cell counts that do not clear across serial cerebral spinal fluid samples. In addition to assuring that airway and breathing are optimized, early treatment includes maintaining blood pressure < 160/90 mm Hg. Prophylactic anticonvulsants are recommended for prevention of seizures in all cases.

**Answer: C**

Cowan, J.A., Jr., and Thompson, B.G. (2010) Neurosurgery, in *Current Diagnosis and Treatment Surgery*, 13th edn (eds G.M. Doherty and N.W. Thompson), McGraw-Hill, New York, pp. 858–859.

10  *Vasospasm following surgical or endovascular occlusion of a cerebral artery aneurysm*
    A *Is best managed with a combination of "permissive" hypertension, hemodilution, and hypervolemia*
    B *Is usually self-limited and requires no treatment*
    C *Is not typically treated with nimodipine*
    D *Is often heralded by the development of hypothermia*
    E *Is often treated with cerebral angioplasty for distal cerebral lesions*

Vasospasm following surgical or endovascular management of cerebral artery aneurysms is common and can lead to severe disability and death. Hyperthermia and mental status changes are early signs of vasospasm. Typical treatment includes "permissive" hypertension to maintain systolic blood pressure between 180–200 mm Hg (adding vasopressors if necessary), hemodilution with intravenous fluids to keep the hematocrit at approximately 30%, and hypervolemia with albumin and hypertonic saline to maintain a central venous pressure between 8–14 mm Hg. The peak time for occurrence is 4–14 days following the development of subarachnoid hemorrhage. Vasospasm should always be treated since approximately 30% of patients will develop permanent neurological deficits. Nimodipine is a commonly used drug following surgical or endovascular intervention to reduce vasospasm. Cerebral angioplasty is used for proximal vasospasm, but generally is not used for distal or diffuse vasospasm.

**Answer: A**

Cowan, J.A., Jr., and Thompson, B.G. (2010) Neurosurgery, in *Current Diagnosis and Treatment Surgery*, 13th edn (eds G.M. Doherty and N.W. Thompson), McGraw-Hill, New York, pp. 858–859.

11  *The incidence of infection from external ventriculostomy catheters for cerebral spinal fluid drainage and intracranial pressure monitoring*
    A *Increases linearly over time*
    B *Is reduced by exchanging the catheters every five days*
    C *Is reduced with the use of antibiotic-impregnated catheters*
    D *Is reduced by administering intravenous antibiotics for prophylaxis just prior to insertion*
    E *None of the above*

As with most medical devices used in the intensive care unit, ventriculostomy removal should occur as soon as possible when the perceived risk of complications outweighs the benefits of their use. Ventriculostomy catheters are used extensively for both elective and traumatic brain injury neurosurgical patients but there are very little controlled randomized data to definitively answer the question of true infection risk. Zambramski *et al.* performed a prospective randomized study on patients of all types requiring ventriculostomy. These investigators found a lower infection rate (1.3% versus 9.4%) in those patients randomized to receive a catheter impregnated with rifampin and minocycline. Park *et al.* showed a nonlinear relationship between infection risk and duration of catheter use. They found an extremely low infection rate that rose over the initial four days, but then remained constant even with prolonged catheter use for greater than 10 days. All patients in this retrospective study received antibiotics for prophylaxis, and no antibiotic impregnated catheters were used. A positive cerebral spinal fluid culture was considered an infection. Multiple other studies have failed to demonstrate a benefit in using systemic antibiotics for prophylaxis with ventriculostomy catheter insertion. There is also no evidence to support the use of routine ventriculostomy exchange at a predetermined period to prevent infection. If ventriculostomies are placed carefully, under sterile conditions, and used with closed drainage systems, minimizing manipulations and flushing, then the risk of a device-related infection is very low. Further studies are needed to arrive at a definition for ventricular device related infection versus colonization so that the true incidence can be better defined.

**Answer: C**

Park, P., Garton, H.J.L., Kocan, M.J., *et al.* (2004) Risk of infection with prolonged ventricular catheterization. *Neurosurgery*, **55**, 594–601.

Wong, G.K.C., Poon, W.S., Wai, S., *et al.* (2002) Failure of regular external ventricular drain exchange to reduce cerebrospinal fluid infection: result of a randomized controlled trial. *Journal of Neurology, Neurosurgery and Psychiatry*, **73**, 759–761.

Zambramski, J.M., Whiting, D., Darouiche, R.O., *et al.* (2003) Efficacy of antimicrobial-impregnated external ventricular drain catheters: a prospective, randomized, controlled trial. *Neurosurgery*, **98**, 725–730.

**12** *An 80-year-old man with a Glasgow Coma Scale score of 15 is admitted to the intensive care unit three hours following a fall from ground level. Bilateral proximal humerus fractures have been splinted. CT scans of the brain and cervical spine show a 1 cm left frontal lobe intracerebral contusion and chronic degenerative changes to the cervical spine without acute fracture. Neurological assessments show good motor strength and reflexes in the lower extremities. Motor strength in the upper extremities is difficult to* *fully assess due to the fractures, but the patient appears to have bilateral loss of fine motor movement in the fingers and weakness with wrist flexion and extension. These findings are most consistent with:*

**A** *Conus medullaris syndrome*
**B** *The findings on the brain CT scan*
**C** *Anterior spinal cord syndrome*
**D** *Brown–Sequard syndrome*
**E** *Central cord syndrome*

Central cord syndrome is commonly associated with falls in the elderly. The injury affects motor strength in the upper extremities more severely than the lower extremities. These patients frequently have spinal stenosis and the mechanism of injury is usually a hyperextension injury resulting in vascular compromise to the central portion of the cervical spinal cord. Since the cervical fibers controlling motor function to the upper extremities are located more medially than the lower motor fibers, the effects are more prominent in the upper extremity motor neurons. Sensory findings are variable and sphincter control may also be affected.

**Answer: E**

Cowan, J.A., Jr. and Thompson, B.G. (2010) Neurosurgery, in *Current Diagnosis and Treatment Surgery*, 13th edn (eds G.M. Doherty and N.W. Thompson), McGraw-Hill, New York, pp. 858–859.

**13** *A ventricular catheter connected to an external strain gauge transducer for intracranial pressure monitoring:*

**A** *Provides measurements that are usually lower than parenchymal ICP transducer systems*
**B** *Is more accurate than subarachnoid, subdural, and epidural monitoring systems*
**C** *Is associated with a 10% risk of significant intracerebral hematoma formation at the time of insertion*
**D** *Is the most expensive method of monitoring intracranial pressure*
**E** *Is much less accurate than parenchymal ICP transducer systems*

There are a number of devices currently used to measure intracranial pressure. The optimal device should be accurate, reliable, cost-effective, and associated with minimal patient morbidity during insertion and during the life of the device. The two most accurate systems currently available are the ventriculostomy catheter and parenchymal catheter insertion systems. Published studies show similar results in terms of measurement accuracy. Systems using subarachnoid, subdural, and epidural catheters are less accurate. In the current state of technology, ventriculostomy is considered the most accurate, reliable, and cost-effective method and remains the reference standard for comparison of all other systems. The risk of significant hematoma formation is less than 1% during insertion of a ventriculostomy. Ventriculostomy also allows therapeutic drainage of cerebral spinal fluid if the intracranial pressure is elevated, an advantage when compared to other monitoring systems.

**Answer: B**

Carney, N., Totten, A.M., O'Reilly, C., *et al.* (2016) Guidelines for the management of severe traumatic brain injury, fourth edition. *Neurosurgery*, **80** (1), 6–15.

**14** *Seizures following traumatic brain injury:*
   **A** *Are higher following blunt traumatic brain injury compared to penetrating traumatic brain injury*
   **B** *Are best prevented in the late stages of injury (after 4 weeks) with early administration of phenytoin for prophylaxis*
   **C** *Are associated with increased mortality rates if they occur early (less than 2 weeks) following traumatic brain injury*
   **D** *Are reduced in the early stages of injury (less than 2 weeks) with phenytoin*
   **E** *Are not affected by administration of anti-seizure medications for prophylaxis*

Anticonvulsants are recommended to decrease the incidence of early post-traumatic seizures. Risk factors for developing seizures following trauma include penetrating brain injury (>50% of cases), Glasgow Coma Scale scores < 10, depressed skull fractures, subdural and epidural hematomas, and intracerebral hematomas. Temkin *et al.* showed a significant reduction in early post-traumatic seizures with administration of phenytoin early after injury. No reduction in late post-traumatic seizures occurred and no difference in mortality rates was identified between those patients who developed seizures early following injury versus those without seizures. The current body of evidence indicates that anticonvulsants administered for prophylaxis prevent early post-traumatic seizures but do not significantly reduce the incidence of late post-traumatic seizures.

**Answer: D**

Temkin, N.R., Dikmen, S.S., Wilensky, A.J., *et al.* (1990) A randomized, double-blind study of phenytoin for the prevention of post-traumatic seizures. *New England Journal of Medicine*, **323**, 497–502.
Yablon, S.A. (1993) Posttraumatic seizures. *Archives of Physical Medicine and Rehabilitation*, **84**, 983–1001.

**15** *Barbiturate therapy in the management of traumatic brain injury:*
   **A** *May effectively reduce ICP in patients with intracranial hypertension refractory to other forms of therapy*
   **B** *Improves outcome when used as initial therapy in patients with diffuse brain injury*
   **C** *Has minimal effect on cardiac function and hemodynamic status*
   **D** *Is superior to standard forms of therapy for reducing ICP*
   **E** *Is best monitored for effective reduction in cerebral metabolism and cerebral blood flow by monitoring serum pentobarbital levels*

The use of barbiturates, specifically pentobarbital, to treat refractory intracranial hypertension following traumatic brain injury remains controversial. A number of randomized controlled studies were performed in the 1980s. Eisenberg *et al.* randomly allocated patients to receive pentobarbital versus continuing standard therapy in patients with Glasgow Coma Scale scores of 4–8. A large number of the control patients in this study crossed over to receive barbiturates, thus confusing the interpretation of the final results. In addition, all of these studies were performed at a time when prolonged hyperventilation, strict fluid restriction, and steroids were considered optimal conventional therapy. Therefore, the question of improving mortality and outcome with today's conventional therapy remains unanswered. This has led one group to conclude that there is no evidence that barbiturate therapy in patients with acute severe head injury improves outcome. It is well known that barbiturates can significantly reduce cardiac output and if this form of therapy is utilized, strict monitoring techniques to prevent reduction in cardiac output should be implemented. Barbiturate therapy will effectively reduce intracranial pressure. It is believed that this effect is due to a reduction in both cerebral metabolism and cerebral blood flow. Barbiturate therapy as an initial treatment is not indicated. One study actually showed increased mortality rates when barbiturates were used compared to mannitol as initial treatment. Standard forms of therapy should always be utilized initially since barbiturates have not been definitively shown to reduce ICP in the early stages following injury. If barbiturates are used in patients with intracranial hypertension refractory to standard forms of therapy, treatment is best monitored for effective reduction in cerebral metabolism and cerebral blood flow by monitoring the electroencephalogram pattern of burst suppression. Optimal reductions in cerebral metabolism and cerebral blood flow are believed to occur when burst suppression is induced. A goal of therapy remains achievement of serum pentobarbital levels in the range of 3–4 mg/dL. However, there is poor correlation among serum levels, systemic complications secondary to pentobarbital therapy, and ultimate therapeutic benefit.

**Answer: A**

Eisenberg, H.M., Frankowski, R.F., Contant, C.F., *et al.* (1988) High dose barbiturate control of elevated intracranial pressure in patients with severe head injury. *Journal of Neurosurgery*, **69**, 15–23.

Schwartz, M., Tator, C., Rowed, D., *et al.* (1984) The University of Toronto head injury treatment study: a prospective, randomized comparison of pentobarbital and mannitol. *Canadian Journal of Neurological Science*, **11**, 434–440.

16  The best order of initial management of a patient presenting with a blunt cervical spinal cord injury at the C3–C4 level is
   A  Airway management, high dose methylprednisolone, volume resuscitation, beta-agonist support, and alpha-agonist support
   B  Airway management, volume resuscitation, beta-agonist support, alpha-agonist support, high-dose methylprednisolone
   C  Volume resuscitation, vasopressor support, and high-dose methylprednisolone
   D  Airway management, volume resuscitation, and vasopressor support
   E  Airway management, volume resuscitation, beta-agonist support, alpha-agonist support, high-dose methylprednisolone

Patient with cervical spinal cord injuries are at high risk for acute respiratory failure from hypoventilation. While this may not be apparent initially, the risk may increase within the first 12–48 hours post-injury due to temporary ascending spinal cord edema. Therefore, airway concerns and close observation for signs of ventilatory failure should always be the first priority. Hypotension from neurogenic shock should be treated with prompt initiation of volume expansion. Decreased systolic blood pressure refractory to volume expansion is typically followed by a beta-agonist followed by an alpha-agonist if needed. A beta-agonist is initially preferred because of the possibility of bradycardia, which may be exacerbated by a pure alpha-agonist. High-dose methylprednisolone is still offered as an option for acute blunt spinal cord injury as a guideline by the AANS, but it is presented with the caveat that "evidence supporting harmful side effects is more consistent than any suggestion of clinical benefit." Generally, high-dose methylprednisolone is being used less and less due to the high risk of infectious complications.

**Answer: D**

Cowan, J.A. Jr. and Thompson, B.G. (2010) Neurosurgery, in *Current Diagnosis and Treatment Surgery*, 13th edn (eds G.M. Doherty and N.W. Thompson), McGraw-Hill, New York, pp. 858–859.

Matsumoto, T., Tamaki, T., Kawakami, M., *et al.* (2001) Early complications of high-dose methylprednisolone sodium succinate treatment in the follow-up of acute cervical spinal cord injury. *Spine*, **26**, 426.

17  All of the following statements concerning brain oxygenation monitoring techniques are true except:
   A  Increased mortality rates are associated with just one episode of jugular venous oxygen desaturation ($SjO_2$)
   B  $SjO_2$ levels > 5% are associated with poor neurologic outcomes
   C  $SjO_2$ levels < 60% are associated with poor neurologic outcomes
   D  Brain tissue oxygenation tension ($P_{br} O_2$) < 15 mm Hg is associated with a poor neurologic outcome.
   E  A high $SjO_2$ level is associated with cerebral infarction

A number of observational studies suggest a correlation between low brain oxygenation parameters and poor outcome following traumatic brain injury. Current thresholds to initiate therapy to improve brain tissue oxygenation, based on Level III evidence include an $SjO_2$ level < 50% and a $PbrO_2$ level < 15 mm Hg. A high $SjO_2$ (>75%) is associated with cerebral infarction as necrotic brain tissue does not extract oxygen. The question still remains whether goal directed therapy to restore $SjO_2$ and $PbrO_2$ to normal improves outcome. Technological deficiencies in $SjO_2$ monitoring and studies specifically addressing what area of the brain in which $PbrO_2$ measurements should be performed (most injured versus least injured hemisphere for example) need to be performed before these techniques in monitoring are uniformly adopted.

**Answer: C**

Carney, N., Totten, A.M., O'Reilly, C., *et al.* (2016) Guidelines for the management of severe traumatic brain injury, fourth edition. *Neurosurgery*, **80** (1), 6–15.

Cormio, M., Valadka, A.B., and Robertson, C.S. (1999) Elevated jugular venous oxygen saturation after severe head injury. *Journal of Neurosurgery*, **90**, 9–15.

Robertson, C.S., Gopinath, S.P., Goodman, J.C., *et al.* (1995) SjvO2 monitoring in head-injured patient. *Journal of Neurotrauma*, **12**, 891–896.

**18** *Progesterone for the treatment of traumatic brain injury*
 **A** *Has serious side effects that prevent its use*
 **B** *Has not been shown to reduce mortality following traumatic brain injury*
 **C** *Reduces mortality, but not morbidity following traumatic brain injury*
 **D** *Has neuroprotective effects that works primarily by mechanisms other than reducing cerebral edema*
 **E** *Has been shown to reduce both mortality and improve functional outcomes following traumatic brain injury*

Progesterone is a naturally occurring hormone and in most clinical studies has been shown to have a very high safety profile. Two Phase-II trials have been published and both have shown promising benefit in progesterone's neuroprotective effects and potential benefits in reducing both early and late mortality and improving functional outcomes following traumatic brain injury. A Phase III multicenter trial has been approved by the National Institutes of Health. A number of studies to determine the molecular mechanisms of this neuroprotective effect have been performed. These molecular effects include reduced inflammation and reduced lipid peroxidation, maintenance of blood-brain barrier, integrity and improved ionic stability. All of these molecular effects directly reduce cerebral edema following traumatic brain injury. Further studies are needed to determine whether progesterone becomes a standard therapy in the armamentarium of treatments following traumatic brain injury.

**Answer: E**

Phelan, H.A., Shafi, S., Parks, J., *et al.* (2007) Use of a pediatric cohort to examine gender differences in outcome after trauma. *Journal of Trauma*, **63**, 1127–1131.

Schumacher, M., Guennoun, R., Stein, D.G., and De Nicola, A.F. (2007) Progesterone: therapeutic opportunities for neuroprotection and myelin repair. *Pharmacology and Therapeutics*, **116**, 77–106.

Wright, D.W., Kellerman, A.L., Hertzberg, D.S., *et al.* (2007) ProTECT: a randomized clinical trial of progesterone for acute traumatic brain injury. *Annals of Emergency Medicine*, **49**, 391–402.

Xiao, G., Wei, J., Yan, W., *et al.* (2008) Improved outcomes from the administration of progesterone for patients with acute traumatic brain injury: a randomized controlled trial. *Critical Care*, **12**, 1–10.

**19** *The zone of normal cerebral autoregulation:*
 **A** *Is usually between 50 mm Hg and 150 mm Hg (cerebral perfusion pressure)*
 **B** *Is usually maintained following traumatic brain injury*
 **C** *Has no relationship to actual cerebral blood flow*
 **D** *Can be reproduced following traumatic brain injury by increasing cerebral perfusion pressure to > 70 mm Hg*
 **E** *Results in maximum cerebral vasoconstriction as cerebral perfusion pressure decreases*

Under normal conditions cerebral blood flow is maintained relatively constant between cerebral perfusion pressures of 50–150 mm Hg. Cerebral autoregulation is disrupted following traumatic brain injury. In the mid to late 1990s it became popular to push cerebral perfusion pressure to > 70 mm Hg or higher in order to enhance cerebral blood flow. This practice is generally no longer observed and in more recent years maintaining cerebral perfusion pressure to a value of approximately 60 mm Hg is recommended. The ultimate goal of managing both cerebral blood flow and the level of perfusion is to meet the metabolic demands of the brain. As cerebral perfusion pressure decreases maximal intracerebral vasodilatation occurs in order to maintain constant flow. As cerebral perfusion pressure increases the opposite occurs and cerebral vasoconstriction occurs to reduce flow and maintain normal perfusion.

**Answer: A**

Chestnut, R.M. (2006) Head trauma, in *Green-field's Surgery Scientific Principles and Practice*, (eds M.W. Mulholand, K.D. Lillemoe, G.M. Doherty, *et al.*), Lippincott Williams & Wilkins, Philadelphia, PA, pp. 374–375.

Lang, E.W. and Chestnut, R.M. (2000) A bedside method for investigating the integrity and critical thresholds of cerebral pressure autoregulation in severe traumatic brain injury patients. *British Journal of Neurosurgery*, **14**, 117–126.

**20** *Controlling elevated intracranial pressure is an important factor in pediatric patient survival following traumatic brain injury. Appropriate measures to maintain intracranial pressure < 20 mm Hg include all of the following except:*
 **A** *3% normal saline by continuous infusion*
 **B** *Prophylactic hyperventilation to maintain $PaCO_2$ < 35 mm Hg*
 **C** *Mannitol*
 **D** *Sedation and neuromuscular blockade*
 **E** *Ventriculostomy with cerebrospinal fluid drainage*

Prophylactic hyperventilation, as in adults, should be avoided in infants and children with traumatic brain injury since hyperventilation can compromise cerebral perfusion at a time when cerebral blood flow may be reduced. Aggressive hyperventilation ($PaCO_2$ < 30 mm Hg) should be considered only as a second tier option when all other forms of therapy have failed. Even in this situation, either brain tissue oxygen monitoring or jugular venous oxygen saturation should be monitored to identify ischemic changes in the brain. All of the other options given are acceptable first tier therapeutic responses for reducing intracranial pressure in infants and children.

**Answer: B**

Adelson, P.D., Bratton, S.L., Carney, N.A., *et al.* (2003) Guidelines for the acute medical management of severe traumatic brain injury in infants, children, and adolescents. *Pediatric Critical Care Medicine,* **4,** S1–S75.

Jagannathan, J., Okonkwo, D., Yeoh, H., *et al.* (2008) Long-term outcomes and prognostic factors in pediatric patients with severe traumatic brain injury and elevated intracranial pressure. *Journal of Neurosurgery Pediatrics,* **2,** 240–249.

21 *A surgical colleague consults you on a 33-year-old man on whom he performed diagnostic laparoscopy for right lower quadrant pain 12 days previously. Intra-operatively, the appendix was found to be normal and turbid fluid was found in the pelvis which later grew out* Campylobacter jejuni. *The patient had an uneventful postoperative course, but came to his clinic check yesterday complaining of weakness, malaise, and shortness of breath. He was admitted, and a subsequent chest x-ray was normal as was a chest CT. Over the ensuing 48 hours, his extremity weakness has progressed while his work of breathing has increased to the point that his surgeon now wishes to place him in the ICU. Which of the following is an incorrect statement about this patient's likeliest diagnosis?*

A *Guillain Barre Syndrome (GBS) typically presents 2–4 weeks after a relatively benign gastrointestinal or respiratory illness*

B *Campylobacter seropositivity is found in 40–70% of patients*

C *GBS has a low lethality, with an expected mortality rates of less than 3%*

D *Plasmapheresis is no longer considered a mainstay of therapy for GBS*

E *Corticosteroids are ineffective when used as monotherapy*

This patient has a fairly typical history and presenting picture for Guillain Barre Syndrome. This progressive demyelinating disorder is usually preceded by a bacterial or viral infection, with *C. jejuni* being a common etiology. Patients often initially complain of finger dysthesias and proximal lower extremity weakness which is progressive. A minority of patients will progress to needing mechanical ventilation. Both plasma exchange and intravenous immunoglobulin are effective treatments, but their concomitant use has not been shown to shorten symptoms. Steroids alone have not been shown to shorten symptoms or affect long-term neurologic function, and they do cause higher rates of insulin requirement. While a minority of patients will exhibit permanent neurologic sequelae, a large review of 5000 GBS patients showed an overall mortality rate of 2.6%.

**Answer: D**

Alshekhlee, A., Hussain, Z., Sultan, B., and Katirji, B. (2008) Guillain-Barre syndrome: incidence and mortality rates in US hospitals. *Neurology,* **70** (18), 1608–1613.

Cortese, I., Chaudhry, V., So, Y.T., *et al.* (2011) Evidence-based guideline update: plasmapheresis in neurologic disorders: report of the Therapeutics and Technology Assessment Subcommittee of the American Academy of Neurology. *Neurology,* **76** (3), 294–300.

Dalakas, M.C. (2002) Mechanisms of action of IVIg and therapeutic considerations in the treatment of acute and chronic demyelinating neuropathies. *Neurology,* **59** (12 Suppl. 6), S13–21.

Hughes, R.A., Swan, A.V., and van Doorn, P.A. (2010) Corticosteroids for Guillain-Barré syndrome. *Cochrane Database Systematic Reviews,* **2.**

22 *The management of elevated ICP's that are refractory to medical interventions is controversial. Which of the following statements about 2016's "Randomized Evaluation of Surgery with Craniectomy for Uncontrollable Elevation of Intracranial Pressure" [RESCUEicp] trial is* incorrect?

A *Surgery resulted in lower rates of death and higher rates of vegetative state at 6 months after injury than ongoing medical management.*

B *Long-term results demonstrated that cranial reconstruction is poorly tolerated.*

C *Surgery resulted in higher rates of disability and equivalent rates of good outcomes at 6 months after injury.*

D *The RESCUEicp study results stand in stark contrast to 2011's Decompressive Craniectomy [DECRA] trial*

E *The DECRA trial used decompressive craniotomy as a first-tier therapy while RESCUEicp used it as a last-tier therapy*

Critics of decompressive craniectomy have cited the concern that the procedure simply results in salvaging patients who go on to live in a persistent vegetative state. The DECRA trial in 2011 studied early decompressive craniotomy for persistently high ICPs, and found equivalent death rates at 6 months after injury for surgery vs. medical management (19% vs 18%) as well as significantly worse functional outcomes for the surgical arm. The RESCUEicp trial used decompressive craniotomy as a last-tier intervention and found better rates of survival as well as higher rates of vegetative state and disability at 6 months after injury. Tolerance of cranial reconstruction was not one of the end points studies.

**Answer: B**

Hutchinson, P.J., Kolias, A.G., Timofeev, I.S., *et al.* (2016). Trial of decompressive craniectomy for traumatic intracranial hypertension. *New England Journal of Medicine*, **375** (12), 1119–1130.

Cooper, D.J., Rosenfeld, J.V., Murray, L., *et al.* (2011) Decompressive craniectomy in diffuse traumatic brain injury. *New England Journal of Medicine*, **364**, 1493–1502.

**23** *Which of the following is NOT a new recommendation in the 2016 update of the Brain Trauma Foundation's Guidelines for the Management of Severe Traumatic Brain Injury (4th edition)?*

**A** *Early, prophylactic hypothermia is not recommended to improve outcomes for patients with diffuse axonal injury.*

**B** *Target caloric replacement should occur by 48 hours after injury to decrease mortality after TBI.*

**C** *Transgastric jejunal feeding is recommended to decrease the incidence of ventilator-associated pneumonia (VAP).*

**D** *The use of povidone-iodine for oral care is not recommended to reduce VAP and may lead to an increased risk for acute respiratory distress syndrome.*

**E** *Insufficient evidence exists to recommend levetiracetam over phenytoin for prophylaxis against early-onset seizures.*

**Answer: B**

Carney, N., Totten, A.M., O'Reilly, C., *et al.* (2016) Guidelines for the management of severe traumatic brain injury, fourth edition. *Neurosurgery*, **80** (1), 6–15.

The recent publication of the Brain Trauma Foundation's Guidelines has several new areas of recommendations. Notably, the recommendation for caloric replacement is by the 5th day at least and the 7th day at most in order to decrease mortality after TBI. The entire guidelines address 18 topics over the three major areas of TBI treatment, monitoring, and thresholds. The entire work can be perused and downloaded free of charge at www.braintrauma.org.

## 21

# Thromboembolism

*Herb A. Phelan, MD*

**1** *A 37-year-old man is admitted after suffering a grade II spleen injury in a motor vehicle collision. He is hemodynamically stable, and you undertake a course of nonoperative management. On postinjury day 3 he develops acute shortness of breath and a workup reveals a pulmonary embolism. What should be the next step in your management?*
**A** *Placement of a permanent vena cava filter*
**B** *Placement of a retrievable vena cava filter*
**C** *Immediate initiation of systemic anticoagulation*
**D** *Performance of splenectomy followed by systemic anticoagulation*
**E** *An echocardiogram to assess for signs of right heart strain followed by initiation of systemic anticoagulation at 5 days post-injury if no heart strain is found*

Prophylactic and therapeutic anticoagulation in patients with nonoperatively managed solid organ injuries is a controversial topic with a paucity of data to support any opinion. Santaniello and colleagues examined a series of 20 patients with blunt aortic injuries and concomitant Grade I or II spleen or liver injuries, which were being managed nonoperatively. These patients all underwent systemic heparinization with bypass during the repair of their blunt aortic injuries at a mean of 1.5 days post-injury, and the authors reported no failures of splenic/liver nonoperative management. Further, others have shown that low molecular weight heparin can be used as prophylaxis at 48 hours post-injury without an increase in transfusion requirement or failure rates. While extrapolation of data should always be undertaken with caution, in the setting described above systemic anticoagulation would seem to be suitable management by post-injury day 3. Because "C" is a safe option, which is the least invasive and does not involve a delay in care, it represents the best answer.

**Answer: C**

Alejandro, K.V., Acosta, J.A., Rodriguez, P.A., *et al.* (2003) Bleeding manifestations after early use of low-molecular-weight heparins in blunt splenic injuries. *American Journal of Surgery,* **69** (11), 1006–1009.

Santaniello, J.M., Miller, P.R., Croce, M.A., *et al.* (2002) Blunt aortic injury with concomitant intra-abdominal solid organ injury: treatment priorities revisited. *Journal of Trauma,* **53** (3), 442–445.

**2** *Regarding intermittent pneumatic compression devices (IPCs) and graduated compression stockings (GCSs), which of the following statements is incorrect?*
**A** *When IPCs were initially created, some systems used cuffs with large bladders and slow inflation rates, which weakens the value of older studies on the subject*
**B** *Incorrect GCS sizing or application can lead to a reverse gradient of flow which creates greater pressure proximally and increases DVT risk*
**C** *The complementary physiologic mechanisms of action for IPC and GCS account for studies that show an additive efficacy when used simultaneously*
**D** *The 2008 ACCP recommendations do not discriminate between IPCs and GCS when making recommendations about mechanical DVT prophylaxis*
**E** *If a DVT is diagnosed in a patient wearing IPCs, the device on that leg should be removed*

While many high-quality studies on the utility of IPCs are available, the various methods of application frequently make comparisons difficult, particularly in regard to older literature. Other issues with the research in the field is that studies do not specify between foot, calf, and thigh-high devices, nor do they always describe the patient and nursing compliance with the device's application (a persistent clinical problem). GCS can come in up to 12 sizes, and the limb has to be measured

*Surgical Critical Care and Emergency Surgery: Clinical Questions and Answers,* Second Edition.
Edited by Forrest "Dell" Moore, Peter Rhee, and Gerard J. Fulda.
© 2018 John Wiley & Sons Ltd. Published 2018 by John Wiley & Sons Ltd.
Companion website: www.wiley.com/go/moore/surgical_criticalcare_and_emergency_surgery

accurately to prevent incorrect pressure gradients. This incorrect gradient can occur in up to 50% of applied GCS. GCS work by reducing venous diameter and increasing venous flow, while IPCs do the same by periodically emptying the deep venous system. It is, therefore, not recommended that they be used in tandem. The ACCP guidelines do not differentiate between the two in making mechanical prophylaxis recommendations, but weak data suggest that IPCs are superior for the prevention of DVT. If a DVT is found in a patient wearing IPCs, the IPC should be removed since their action may cause embolization.

**Answer: C**

Best, A.J., Williams, S., Crozier, A., *et al.* (2000) Graded compression stockings in elective orthopaedic surgery: an assessment of the in vivo performance of commercially available stockings in patients having hip and knee arthroplasty. *Journal of Bone and Joint Surgery (British Volume,* **82**, 116–118.

Geerts, W.H., Bergqvist, D., Pineo, G.F., *et al.* (2008) Prevention of venous thromboembolism: American College of 2, chest physicians evidence-based clinical practice guidelines, 8th edn,. *Chest,* **133**, 381S–453S.

Morris, R.J. and Woodcock, J.P. (2010) Intermittent pneumatic compression or graduated compression stockings for deep vein thrombosis prophylaxis? A systematic review of direct clinical comparisons. *Annals of Surgery,* **251**, 393–396.

3 *After a 12-foot fall, a 48-year-old woman suffers a pelvic fracture and requires anterior plating on post-injury day 2. On post-injury day 5 she develops a swollen left leg and an ultrasound confirms that she has a superficial femoral DVT for which she is started on therapeutic anticoagulation. When you see her in clinic on post-injury day 32 after her discharge from a rehabilitation facility, she is complaining of a painful, swollen, heavy leg. On exam, the leg has normal skin color with no breakdown and is swollen and mildly tender to palpation. As you begin to explain her condition to her, which of the following statements about post-thrombotic syndrome (PTS) would be incorrect?*

   A *Eighty percent of symptomatic DVTs are proximal to the knee; of these, the incidence of PTS 2 years post-DVT will be 50%*

   B *Up to 10% of patients with PTS will manifest leg ulcerations*

   C *Studies have shown that the quality of life of patients suffering from PTS is poorer than patients of similar age with arthritis, chronic lung disease, or diabetes*

   D *For patients with DVT, no benefit has been shown for anticoagulation for 3 to 6 months and the use of graduated compression stockings for 2 years in reducing the incidence of PTS*

   E *The societal costs of PTS are considerable as the mean age of affected patients is 56, and more than 50% of patients are of working age.*

Thrombosis damages the deep venous valves and frequently renders them incompetent. This results in venous reflux and venous hypertension. Venous hypertension in turn can affect segments of veins and valves not involved in the original area of thrombus. This is the fundamental pathophysiology of PTS, which is characterized by pain, heaviness, and edema of the involved extremity. When it occurs in the leg, these symptoms are exacerbated by standing and ambulating. As the disease becomes more severe, it can progress to subcutaneous atrophy, hyperpigmentation, and ulceration. This condition markedly diminishes quality of life, particularly given the fact that it often affects younger patients and affects their ability to earn a livelihood. Fortunately, good data exist, which suggests that a regimen of anticoagulation and graduated compression stockings can reduce its frequency.

**Answer: D**

Kahn, S.R., Shbaklo, H., Lamping, D.L., *et al.* (2008) Determinants of health-related quality of life during the 2 years following deep vein thrombosis. *Journal of Thrombosis and Haemostasis,* **6**, 1105–1112.

Patterson, B.O., Hinchliffe, R., Loftus, I.M., *et al.* (2010) Indications for catheter-directed thrombolysis in the management of acute proximal deep venous thrombosis. *Arteriosclerosis, Thrombosis and Vascular Biology,* **30**, 669–674.

Prandoni, P., Lensing, A.W., Prins, M.H., *et al.* (2004) Below-knee elastic compression stockings to prevent the post-thrombotic syndrome: a randomized, controlled trial. *Annals of Internal Medicine,* **141**, 249–256.

4 *A 27-year-old man remains intubated in your SICU on post-injury day 6 after a motor vehicle collision in which he suffered multiple left-sided rib fractures with a large pulmonary contusion and underwent laparotomy with splenectomy. After noting that his left lower extremity is swollen, an ultrasound is obtained which shows a superficial and common femoral DVT which appears to extend above the inguinal ligament. Therapeutic anticoagulation is initiated. The following day a CT scan of the abdomen is performed to assess for an abscess. No abscess is found but the CT scan demonstrates that the DVT*

*extends proximally to just below the cava. In discussing this with his family, all of the following statements about catheter-directed thrombolytics (CDT) are correct except:*

A *While systemic thrombolysis has been shown to be effective but associated with excessively high bleeding complications, CDT uses a more localized delivery of drug to achieve lysis with lower rates of systemic complications*

B *Freshly formed thrombus responds better to CDT*

C *A filter should be placed prior to performing CDT as the lysing clot has been shown to be at high risk for embolization*

D *Venous stent placement in conjunction with thrombolysis may improve patency rates in select cases*

E *Phlegmasia caerulea dolens is a well accepted indication for CDT*

Early studies examining the question of systemic thrombolytics for DVT lysis demonstrated that the technique achieved success but with unacceptably high rates of serious bleeding complications, particularly retroperitoneal and intracranial hemorrhage. By instilling the lytic agent locally, CDT appears to markedly reduce these risks. While CDT seems to be effective in achieving lysis, the indications for the procedure remain vague. The 2008 American College of Chest Physicians (ACCP) guidelines recommend that patients with a life expectancy greater than one year, good functional status, extensive ileofemoral thrombosis, and presentation within 14 days of symptom onset be considered candidates for CDT. Ongoing studies are evaluating whether this window can be pushed to 21 days. By successfully achieving recanalization, it is hoped that post-thrombotic syndrome (PTS) can be avoided by maintaining valvular competence and avoiding venous hypertension. Filters need not be used routinely as CDT has not been shown to increase the rate of embolization. Venous stents are occasionally indicated, particularly if abnormal venous anatomy is demonstrated. In the most common of these conditions, May–Thurner syndrome, the left common iliac vein is compressed by the overlying iliac artery causing not only an extrinsic compression but chronic low-grade venous trauma from the arterial pulse as well. Given the lack of an effective alternative and the high mortality if left untreated, phlegmasia is an accepted indication for CDT.

**Answer: C**

Comerota, A.J. (2010) Hypoenergetic nutrition support in hospitalized obese patients: a simplified method for clinical application. *Perspectives in Vascular Surgery and Endovascular Therapy* January 3.

Enden, T., Sandvik, L., Klow, N., *et al.* (2007) Catheter-directed venous thrombolysis in acute iliofemoral vein thrombosis: the CaVenT study: rationale and design of a multicentre, randomized controlled, clinical trial (NCT00251771). *American Heart Journal*, **154**, 808–814.

Geerts, W.H., Bergqvist, D., Pineo, G.F., *et al.* (2008) Prevention of venous thromboembolism: American College of 2. Chest Physicians evidence-based clinical practice guidelines, 8th edn. *Chest*, **133**, 381S–453S.

Protack, C., Bakken, A., Patel, N., *et al.* (2007) Long-term outcomes of catheter directed thrombolysis for lower extremity deep venous thrombosis without prophylactic inferior vena cava filter placement. *Journal of Vascular Surgery*, **45**, 992–997.

5 *Which of the following statements about VTE in pregnancy is incorrect?*

A *Pelvic vein thromboses account for 50% of all pregnancy-related VTE*

B *Normal pregnancy is accompanied by increased levels of fibrinogen, von-Willebrand factor, and factors VII, VIII, and X*

C *The risk of VTE in pregnancy is as high during the first trimester as it is during the third trimester*

D *About 33% of pregnancy-related DVT and 50% of pregnancy-related PE occur post-partum*

E *When DVT occurs in pregnancy it is more likely to be proximal and massive*

The hypercoagulability of pregnancy is an evolutionary response to protect women from exsanguination during childbirth. Indeed, hemorrhage is still the leading cause of maternal death worldwide. In industrialized countries, however, it is VTE. Other factors that increase maternal risk for VTE are hormonally induced decreased venous capacitance, decreased venous outflow from the pelvis, and lower levels of mobility. Since the risk of VTE has been shown to be as high during the first trimester as the last, it suggests that the anatomic changes of pregnancy are less important than the hypercoagulable state that develops. Pelvic vein thromboses account for less than 1% of all DVTs, and about 10% of DVT in pregnancy. Not only are the DVTs of pregnancy more commonly proximal and massive, they are more frequently left-sided (likely due to the longer course of the left common iliac vein). Further, about one-third of pregnancy-related DVT and 50% of PE occur post-partum. Despite these risks, most women do not require anticoagulation as its complication rates are generally accepted to be higher than the risks of VTE. The exception is those women who have a history of thrombosis for whom anticoagulation can not only potentially decrease VTE risk but decrease the likelihood of spontaneous abortion as well.

**Answer: A**

Chang, J., Elam-Evans, L.D., Berg, C.J., *et al.* (2003) Pregnancy-related mortality surveillance–United States, 1991–1999. *MMWR Surveillance Summary*, **52**, 1–8.

Goldhaber, S.Z. and Tapson, V.F. (2004) A prospective registry of 5,451 patients with ultrasound-confirmed deep vein thrombosis. *American Journal of Cardiology*, **93**, 259–262.

Gordon, M. (2002) Maternal physiology in pregnancy, in *Normal and Problem Pregnancies*, 4th edn, (eds, S. Gabbe, J. Niebyl, and J. Simpson), Churchill Livingstone, New York, pp. 63–92.

James, A.H., Tapson, V.F., and Goldhaber, SZ. (2005) Thrombosis during pregnancy and the postpartum period. *American Journal of Obstetrics and Gynecology*, **193**, 216–219.

Macklon. N.S., Greer. I.A, and Bowman, A.W. (1997) An ultrasound study of gestational and postural changes in the deep venous system of the leg in pregnancy. *British Journal of Obstetrics and Gynaecology*, **104**, 191–197.

Ray, J.G. and Chan, W.S. (1999) Deep vein thrombosis during pregnancy and the puerperium: a meta-analysis of the period of risk and the leg of presentation. *Obstetrical and Gynecological Survey*, **54**, 265–271.

6 *Which of the following statements about echocardiography and its use in diagnosing PE is incorrect?*

   **A** *Transthoracic echo (TTE) is only able to visualize thrombus in right heart chambers approximately 15% of the time and thrombi in the pulmonary artery at an even lower frequency*

   **B** *A right ventricular size of 30 mm or greater in the precordial view is the most specific TTE finding for pulmonary embolism*

   **C** *Transesophageal echo (TEE) relies upon visualization of the embolus for the diagnosis of pulmonary embolism*

   **D** *The value of echocardiography is in identifying those patients with a higher mortality risk who may benefit from more aggressive management of their embolism*

   **E** *For central pulmonary embolism, TEE has a sensitivity of 95% and a specificity of 100%*

In general, TTE relies on detecting general signs of right ventricular strain as a surrogate for diagnosing pulmonary embolism, whereas TEE relies on direct visualization of thrombus to make the diagnosis. Given that another etiology of right ventricular enlargement and hypokinesis is the common condition of volume overload, it is not a very specific sign. TEE is highly sensitive and specific for central PE, but loses some of this accuracy for more peripheral emboli as the left mainstem bronchus interferes with the ultrasound beam. While TTE has much lower sensitivity for the detection of pulmonary embolism, it provides valuable information about hemodynamics, the status of the right ventricle, and the presence of pulmonary hypertension. Other TTE findings suggestive of pulmonary embolism are tricuspid regurgitation, abnormal motion of the interventricular septum, and lack of collapse of the inferior vena cava during inspiration. One of the values of echocardiography is that it can assist in risk stratification by identifying proximal emboli and giving information regarding cardiac function and compensation. Knowledge of these factors can inform decisions about thrombolytic therapy or surgical embolectomy.

**Answer: B**

Mookadam, F., Jiamsripong, P., Goel, R., *et al.* (2010) Critical appraisal on the utility of echocardiography in the management of acute pulmonary embolism. *Cardiology Review*, **18** (1), 29–37.

7 *Which of the following statements about the incidence and management of DVT and PE is incorrect?*

   **A** *Twenty to 30% of untreated calf thrombi propagate into the thigh where they pose a 40–50% chance of embolizing if they remain untreated*

   **B** *The diagnostic properties of the history and physical exam have been shown to be of very low utility in screening for DVT in critically ill patients*

   **C** *Neither antiembolic stockings nor pneumatic compression devices have been evaluated with randomized controlled trials in general medical-surgical ICU patients*

   **D** *The new anticoagulant fondaparinux holds promise as an anticoagulant in critical care due to the fact that it has an antidote which provides easy reversibility*

   **E** *Autopsy studies have shown that over 75% of PE found on post-mortem examination were clinically unsuspected prior to death*

Not only are DVT common, but they are almost universally under-recognized as multiple studies in centers that utilize aggressive screening have shown incidences of 10–30%. Further, clinical screening techniques that are of utility in ambulatory patients have been shown to be of almost no worth in ICU populations due to the infrequency of unilateral limb swelling (due to being recumbent) and the frequency of intubation, sedation, and analgesia interfering with reports of leg pain. The dearth of literature comparing mechanical prophylaxis methods in general medical-surgical patients is striking. Fondaparinux is approved for pharmacologic prophylaxis in high-risk patients, but has not been widely embraced due to its long half life, renal mode of clearance, lack of an antidote, and a lack of data on its effects in general medical-surgical units. In a 25-year longitudinal study, 9% of patients were found to have PE at autopsy, and 84% of these were clinically unsuspected.

**Answer: D**

Crowther, M.A., Cook, D.J., Griffith, L.E., *et al.* (2005) Deep vein thrombosis: clinically silent in the ICU. *Journal of Critical Care*, **20**, 334–340.

Kakkar, V.V., Howe, C.T., Flanc, C., *et al.* (1969) Natural history of postoperative deep vein thrombosis. *Lancet*, **2**, 230–232.

Karwinski, B. and Svendsen, E. (1989) Comparison of clinical and postmortem diagnosis of pulmonary embolism. *Journal of Clinical Pathology*, **42**, 135–139.

Limpus, A., Chaboyer, W., McDonald, E., *et al.* (2006) Mechanical thromboprophylaxis in critically ill patients: a systematic review and meta-analysis. *American Journal of Critical Care*, **15**, 402–410.

**8** Which of the following statements regarding the use of low-molecular-weight heparins (LMWHs) is correct?
   **A** They have been shown to have equivalent rates of heparin-induced thrombocytopenia (HIT) to unfractionated heparin (UFH)
   **B** LMWHs have a shorter half-life than UFH
   **C** LMWHs are dependent on hepatic clearance
   **D** In patients with impaired clearance, therapeutic doses of LMWHs have been shown to bioaccumulate over time while prophylactic doses do not
   **E** Due to decreased binding of LMWHs to plasma proteins as compared to UFH, hypoalbuminemic patients have less predictable dose responses with LMWH

LMWHs are glycosaminoglycans derived from UFH with a molecular weight of about 5 kDa. In comparison with UFH, they are known for having greater bioavailability, longer half-lives, more predictable dose-response curves, better safety profiles, lower rates of HIT, and no need for lab monitoring. LMWHs are also known for being renally cleared, however, and this has led to some trepidation on the part of clinicians in their use in patients with a creatinine clearance > 30 mL/min. Cook and co-workers have done a considerable amount of work in this area and have published relatively strong data that suggest that bleeding is less of a concern at prophylactic doses. In fact, in their work they have shown that for the LMWH dalteparin, bleeding complications at prophylactic doses in the setting of renal impairment are related to the concomitant use of aspirin rather than the dalteparin itself.

**Answer: D**

Cook, D., Douketis, J., Meade, M., *et al.* (2008) Venous thromboembolism and bleeding in critically ill patients with severe renal insufficiency receiving dalteparin thromboprophylaxis: prevalence, incidence and risk factors. *Critical Care*, **12**, R32.

Lim, W., Dentali, F., Eikelboom, J.W., *et al.* (2006) Meta-analysis: low-molecular-weight heparin and bleeding in patients with severe renal insufficiency. *Annals of Internal Medicine*, **144**, 673–684.

Rabbat, C.G., Cook, D.J., Crowther, M.A., *et al.* (2005) Dalteparin thromboprophylaxis for critically ill medical-surgical patients with renal insufficiency. *Journal of Critical Care*, **20**, 357–363.

**9** All of the following statements about D-dimer and its utility in the diagnosis of DVT and PE are true except:
   **A** D-dimer is primarily stored in the alpha granules of platelets and endothelial cells where, after platelet or cell activation, it translocates to the surface and is released into the plasma in soluble form
   **B** In the setting of low to intermediate risk, a negative D-dimer value can rule out PE with a sensitivity of 95% and a negative predictive value of 99% and no further testing is necessary
   **C** In prospective cohort studies, an elevated D-dimer has been shown to be associated with a threefold increased risk for future first-time DVT or PE
   **D** For patients stopping anticoagulation after DVT or PE, D-dimer has been shown to be an accurate predictor of recurrence
   **E** D-dimers accuracy in predicting risk is even higher in patients with congenital thrombophilias

D-dimer is a degradation product of cross-linked fibrin that is formed immediately after clots are degraded by plasmin. It reflects a systemic activation of clot promotion and degradation. P-selectin is a cell-adhesion molecule important in clot formation which is stored in platelets and endothelial cells in the manner described, and its use as a serum marker for DVT and PE diagnosis is currently under investigation. While the negative predictive value of a normal D-dimer is very good, its lack of specificity and elevation by general states of hypercoagulability has limited its use as a sole tool for the positive diagnosis of PE. Both observational and interventional studies have demonstrated that D-dimer is a useful predictor of recurrence of DVT and PE. To that end, a strong body of evidence suggests that if a D-dimer is still elevated after the discontinuation of anticoagulation after an event, it should be restarted.

**Answer: A**

Cushman, M., Folsom, A.R., Wang, L., *et al.* (2003) Fibrin fragment D-dimer and the risk of future venous thrombosis. *Blood*, **101**, 1243–1248.

Palareti, G., Cosmi, B., Legnani, C, *et al.* (2006) D-dimer testing to determine the duration of anticoagulation therapy. *New England Journal of Medicine*, **355**, 1780–1789.

Verhovsek, M., Douketis, J.D., Yi, Q., *et al.* (2008) Systematic review: D-dimer to predict recurrent disease after stopping anticoagulant therapy for unprovoked venous thromboembolism. *Annals of Internal Medicine*, **149**, 481–90.

**10** *Given the difficulty of using clinical diagnosis to make the diagnosis of pulmonary embolism (PE), two major, validated scoring systems have been created which stratify clinical risk for PE (the Wells score and the revised Geneva score). Which of the following is NOT a variable to be factored into the calculation of the revised Geneva score?*

**A** *Age greater than 65*
**B** *Previous surgery requiring general anesthesia within 1 month*
**C** *Hemoptysis*
**D** *Heart rate of 75 to 94 beats per minute*
**E** *Index of suspicion for PE*

While they are largely the same in many respects, the primary difference between the Wells score and the Geneva score is that the Wells score gives points for the degree of clinical suspicion for PE while the Geneva score is completely standardized. It is thought that this reliance on only objective findings as the basis for score generation makes the Geneva score of more utility for the less experienced practitioner. A criticism of the original Geneva score was that the arterial blood gas required in the scoring system had to be performed on room air, and 15% of patients were not able to tolerate this in the original study. Therefore, the revised Geneva Score dropped that component. Other variables to be taken into account besides those listed in the question are a previous history of DVT or PE, an active malignant condition, unilateral limb pain, a heart rate greater than 95 beats per minute (which gives more points than someone with a heart rate of 75 to 94 beats per minute), and pain on lower limb deep palpation. Scores are assigned based on these findings, and total scores stratify patients as being low-, moderate-, or high-risk for PE.

**Answer: E**

Le Gal, G., Righini, M., Roy, P.M., *et al.* (2006) Prediction of pulmonary embolism in emergency patients: the revised Geneva score. *Annals of Internal Medicine*, **144**, 165–171.

Wells, P.S., Anderson, D.R., Rodger, M., *et al.* (2000) Derivation of a simple clinical model to categorize patients' probability of pulmonary embolism: increasing the model's utility with the SimpliRed D-dimer. *Journal of Thrombosis and Haemostasis*, **83**, 416–420.

**11** *After admitting a 63-year-old man with a flail chest to the surgical intensive care unit, you consult the pain service to place an epidural catheter for pain control. The consultant asks for your plans regarding VTE prophylaxis, and you articulate a desire to initiate a low molecular weight heparin (LMWH) when the patient is a candidate for anticoagulation. Which of the following is not a recommendation of the 2002 Consensus Statement of the American Society of Regional Anesthesia and Pain Medicine (ASRA) on the topic of LMWHs and epidurals?*

**A** *The monitoring of anti-Xa levels is not recommended while the catheter is in place*
**B** *The presence of blood during needle and catheter placement requires that LMWH initiation be delayed for 24 hours post-procedure*
**C** *After pulling the catheter, the practitioner should wait 12 hours before initiating LMWH*
**D** *Catheter placement can be safely performed as soon as 12 hours after a prophylactic dose of LMWH*
**E** *Catheter placement can be safely performed as soon as 24 hours after discontinuing a therapeutic dose of LMWH*

The ASRA drew on the extensive European experience with LMWHs and epidural analgesia to generate their recommendations in 2002. It should be noted, however, that many of the studies that served as the basis for these recommendations were done using once-daily LMWH dosing. Anti-Xa levels are not recommended to be followed as they have not been shown to be predictive of the risk of bleeding. The ASRA also states that while LMWH initiation should be delayed for 24 hours by a "bloody tap," this does not serve as a rationale for an automatic cancellation of an elective surgery. The ASRA states that LMWH can be initiated after a 2-hour delay from the completion of catheter removal. Given the predictable nature of LMWH bioavailability, catheter placement can be safely performed 12 hours after a prophylactic dose and 24 hours after a therapeutic dose.

**Answer: C**

Horlocker, T.T., Wedel, D.J., Benzon, H., *et al.* (2003) Regional anesthesia in the anticoagulated patient: defining the risks (the second ASRA Consensus Conference on Neuraxial Anesthesia and Anticoagulation). *Regional Anesthesia and Pain Medicine*, **28** (3), 172–197.

**12** *Which of the following is a recommendation in the 2016 Clinical Practice Guidelines on VTE prevention and treatment from the American College of Chest Physicians (ACCP)?*

 **A** *Duplex ultrasound screening for DVT should be performed routinely after major trauma*

 **B** *Prophylactic vena cava filters should be placed after complete spinal cord injury*

 **C** *For trauma patients with impaired mobility who undergo inpatient rehabilitation, pharmacologic prophylaxis can be discontinued in favor of mechanical prophyalxis at the time of transfer*

 **D** *For major trauma patients in whom ongoing bleeding is not a concern, first-line pharmacologic VTE prophylaxis constitutes low-molecular-weight heparin*

 **E** *For incomplete spinal cord injury, unfractionated low dose heparin should be first-line therapy for VTE prophylaxis*

Routine screening with Duplex ultrasound has not been shown to be an effective strategy for the prevention of clinically significant VTE, and the cost is generally considered to be prohibitive. Selective screening may be of benefit in those major trauma patients in whom the initiation of early prophylaxis was delayed. The ACCP guidelines do not recommend the use of prophylactic vena cava filters under any circumstances. Major trauma patients with impaired mobility should receive prophylaxis with a low-molecular-weight heparin or a vitamin K antagonist through their inpatient stay. Strong level I evidence exists which suggests that low-molecular-weight heparin is superior to low-dose unfractionated heparin as VTE prophylaxis after major trauma. Similarly, low- molecular-weight heparin constitutes first line therapy after incomplete spinal cord as well.

**Answer: D**

Kearon, C., Akl, E.A., Ornelas, J., *et al.* (2016) Antithrombotic therapy for VTE disease: CHEST guideline and expert panel report. *Chest*, **149** (2), 315–352.

**13** *Which of the following statements about the Factor V Leiden mutation is incorrect?*

 **A** *Five percent of Caucasians are heterozygous for the mutation*

 **B** *The mutation causes resistance to activated protein C*

 **C** *Long-term anticoagulation with a vitamin K antagonist is recommended for patients who are heterozygous for the mutation*

 **D** *Venous thromboses are more common than arterial thromboses in patients with Factor V Leiden mutation*

 **E** *Venous thrombosis after general surgical or orthopedic procedures does not appear to be increased in patients heterozygous for the Factor V Leiden mutation when they are managed with well-reasoned protocols for VTE prophylaxis*

Five percent of Caucasians are heterozygous for the mutation, making it the most common inherited hypercoagulable state, as approximately 1 person in 5000 is homozygous for the disorder among the general population. Platelets carry an endogenous protein C inhibitor, which makes arterial thrombosis less common. The preponderance of the literature suggests that for patients undergoing major general surgical or orthopedic procedures, the incremental risk carried by possession of the mutation is overwhelmed by well-reasoned prophylaxis measures. Therefore, there is no basis for altering their perioperative management based on a history of Factor V Leiden. The same cannot be said for arterial thrombosis after a vascular procedure, however. Asymptomatic heterozygosity for Factor V Leiden does not constitute an indication for intervention.

**Answer: C**

Donahue, B.S. (2004) Factor V Leiden and perioperative risk. *Anesthesia and Analgesia*, **98**, 1623–1634.

Slusher, K.B. (2010) Factor V Leiden: a case study and review. *Dimensions of Critical Care Nursing*, **29** (1), 6–10.

**14** *For a patient preparing to undergo a total knee or hip replacement who is deemed to be at baseline risk for both PE and bleeding, the American Academy of Orthopedic Surgery's (AAOS) 2009 guidelines recommend that all of the following are acceptable prophylaxis regimens except:*

 **A** *Aspirin 325 mg twice a day starting on the day of surgery and continuing for six weeks*

 **B** *Low molecular weight heparin starting 12–24 hours postoperatively for 7–12 days and dosed per package insert*

 **C** *Unfractionated heparin 5000 U every 12 hours starting 24 hours postoperatively and continuing for 14 days*

 **D** *A synthetic pentasaccharide starting 12–24 hours postoperatively for 7–12 days and dosed per package insert*

 **E** *Warfarin starting the night before surgery at a dose sufficient to obtain an INR < 2.0 for 2–6 weeks*

Patients deemed to be at a baseline risk for bleeding and PE represent the majority of patients undergoing total knee and hip replacement. Further, this referral to a

**Table 21.1** The AAOS recommendations.

| PE risk | Bleeding risk | Recommendation |
|---------|---------------|----------------|
| Baseline | Baseline | Any of: |
| | | ASA 325 bid starting the day of surgery and continuing for 6 weeks |
| | | LMWH starting 12–24 h postop for 7–12 days, dosed per package insert |
| | | A synthetic pentasaccharide starting 12–24 h postop for 7–12 days, dosed per package insert. |
| | | Warfarin starting the night before surgery at a dose sufficient to obtain an INR < 2.0 for 2–6 weeks. |
| Baseline | Increased | Any of: |
| | | ASA 325 bid starting the day of surgery and continuing for 6 weeks |
| | | Warfarin starting the night before surgery at a dose sufficient to obtain an INR < 2.0 for 2–6 weeks |
| | | No prophylaxis |
| Increased | Baseline | Any of: |
| | | LMWH starting 12–24 h postop for 7–12 days, dosed per package insert. |
| | | A synthetic pentasaccharide starting 12–24 hrs postop for 7–12 days, dosed per package insert. |
| | | Warfarin starting the night before surgery at a dose sufficient to obtain an INR < 2.0 for 2–6 weeks. |
| Increased | Increased | Any of: |
| | | ASA 325 bid starting the day of surgery and continuing for 6 weeks |
| | | Warfarin starting the night before surgery at a dose sufficient to obtain an INR < 2.0 for 2–6 weeks |
| | | No prophylaxis |

"standard" PE risk is relative to other joint replacement patients and not general surgical or medical patients (who are at lower overall risk). The bleeding risk with these regimens is felt to be in the range of 3–5%. Much of the early work done in this area suggested that the timeframe for PE occurrence was six weeks, and the time frame for aspirin was created to conform to this interval. Several reports on the low molecular weight heparins suggest that the utility of their use is much shorter. Of note, unfractionated heparin is not felt by the AAOS to have a role in prophylaxis. The AAOS recommendations are summarized in table 21.1.

**Answer: C**

Johanson, N.A., Lachiewicz, P.F., Lieberman, J.R., *et al.* (2009) Prevention of symptomatic pulmonary embolism in patients undergoing total hip or knee arthroplasty. *Journal of the American Academy of Orthopedic Surgeons*, **135**, 513–520.

**15** Which of the following is NOT a new recommendation in the 2016 ACCP guideline?
  **A** *Once diagnosed with DVT, patients should not wear compression stockings for the prevention of post-thrombotic syndrome (PTS)*
  **B** *For subjects with PE and hypotension, catheter-directed thrombolytics are recommended over systemic therapy*

  **C** *For patients with acute VTE and cancer, recommended treatment is LMWH over vitamin K antagonists, dabigatran, or rivaroxaban*
  **D** *For recurrent VTE while on LMWH, the recommendation is to increase the LMWH dose*
  **E** *For patients with subsegmental PE and no known proximal DVT, simple surveillance is recommended for patients deemed to be at low-risk for recurrence (i.e., recent surgery or other transient risk factor)*

The new 2016 ACCP guidelines update twelve topics from the 9th edition and address three new topics. Among them, systemic therapy is now preferred over catheter-directed thrombolytics for PE with hypotension (Grade 2C). Compression stockings are now discouraged after DVT diagnosis (Grade 2B), and LMWH is the treatment of choice for VTE associated with cancer (Grades 2B and 2C). For recurrence of VTE while on LMWH, the recommendation is now increasing the dose rather than placement of an IVC filter (Grade 2C). Finally, for low-risk patients with subsegmental PE and no proven proximal DVT, the recommendation is for surveillance although no particular regimen is specified.

**Answer: B**

Kearon, C., Akl, E.A., Ornelas, J., *et al.* (2016) Antithrombotic therapy for VTE disease: CHEST guideline and expert panel report. *Chest*, **149** (2), 315–352.

**16** *Which of the following statements about the anti-phospholipid syndrome (APS) is incorrect?*

    **A** *Presence of the antiphospholipid antibody on a single determination constitutes a diagnosis of the syndrome*

    **B** *For patients diagnosed with APS, indefinite anti-coagulation with warfarin is recommended*

    **C** *In APS, arterial thrombosis tends to recur on the arterial side and venous thrombosis tends to recur on the venous side*

    **D** *Management of anticoagulation in APS can be complicated by artifactual elevation of the INR, requiring alternate strategies for monitoring*

    **E** *The syndrome is referred to as "primary APS" when it occurs by itself and as "secondary APS" when it occurs in conjunction with another auto-immune condition*

Antiphospholipid antibodies can occur in 5–10% of healthy donors, but these titers normally disappear over time. The diagnostic criteria for APS involves a characteristic clinical picture of thrombosis and a persistent antiphospholipid antibody titer on two separate occasions at least 12 weeks apart. Patients diagnosed with APS have high rates of recurrent thrombosis after discontinuation of anticoagulation for a period of years. Therefore, the consensus treatment is to continue anticoagulation indefinitely. Beginning an anticoagulation regimen can be difficult as the syndrome is known for occasionally interfering with standard assays. This necessitates specific inquiries with your hematology lab as to whether INR-reagents resistant to this effect are being used, and potentially following functional factor II and X assays. For reasons that are unclear, recurrences of thrombosis in APS tend to occur on the same side of the circulation as the original event.

**Answer: A**

Dentali, F. and Crowther, M. (2010) Antiphospholipid antibodies in critical illness. *Critical Care Medicine*, **38** (Suppl.), 51–56.

**17** *Which of the following statements about enoxaparin dosing and monitoring is incorrect?*

    **A** *It has been shown that hypercoagulability demonstrated on thromboelastogram (TEG) is predictive of VTE in surgical patients*

    **B** *In 2014, an underpowered RCT showed that TEG-guided enoxaparin dosing results in decreased DVT rates in SICU patients*

    **C** *Standard dosing of enoxaparin at 30 mg subcutaneously every 12 hours results in subtherapeutic anti-Xa levels in 70% of patients*

    **D** *The risk factors for subtherapeutic anti-Xa levels are male gender, obesity, and increased total body surface area*

    **E** *Trauma patients have been shown to be antithrombin-III (AT-III) deficient in multiple studies*

Despite increasing acceptance of the idea that earlier pharmacologic initiation of VTE prophylaxis should be undertaken, VTE rates in the SICU have remained persistently high and lasting decreases in VTE incidence have been difficult to demonstrate. One hypothesis for this finding is that the standard doses of enoxaparin 30 mg or unfractionated heparin 5000 U SQ every 12 hours is an inadequate dose for most patients. Indeed, using anti-XA levels as an end point, Constantini showed that the large majority of SICU patients are subtherapeutic at these doses. For a period of time, it was thought that a measure of functional coagulation such as TEG would be a better marker of efficacy, and indeed hypercoagulability on TEG has been shown to predict VTE in the SICU. Unfortunately, a recent pilot RCT did not show a decrease in VTE rates when TEG was used to drive enoxaparin dosing. Another confounder is the finding across multiple studies that trauma patients are AT-III deficient.

**Answer: B**

Costantini, T.W., Min, E., Box, K., *et al.* (2013) Dose adjusting enoxaparin is necessary to achieve adequate venous thromboembolism prophylaxis in trauma patients. *Journal of Trauma and Acute Care Surgery*, **74**, 128–135.

Louis, S.G., Van, P.Y., Riha, G.M., *et al.* (2014) Thromboelastogram-guided enoxaparin dosing does not confer protection from deep venous thrombosis: A randomized controlled pilot trial. *Journal of Trauma and Acute Care Surgery*, **76**, 937–943.

Kashuk, J.L., Moore, E.E., Sabel, A., *et al.* (2009) Rapid thrombelastography (r-TEG) identifies hypercoagulability and predicts thromboembolic events in surgical patients. *Surgery*, **146**, 764–772.

**18** *You see a 43-year-old woman in clinic who is very anxious after seeing a commercial on late-night TV for a legal firm soliciting clients who have received an IVC filter. She reports that she was told she had an IVC filter placed during an ICU admission for an MVC in 1997, and hands you a copy of her medical records which state that a Greenfield filter was placed prophylactically due to her injury burden and a perceived contraindication to pharmacologic prophylaxis. She reports no problems since her* *discharge from rehab that same year, and she had two term pregnancies in the five years after discharge. A plain film in your clinic demonstrates a strut fracture of one limb of the filter. What should be your recommendation?*

**A** *Elective operative removal*

**B** *Elective endovascular removal*

**C** *Referral to the Emergency Room for a stat CT scan of the abdomen*

**D** *Referral to the Emergency Room for a CT scan of the chest*

**E** *Expectant management*

A discussion of risk/benefit with this patient should emphasize the technical difficulties associated with attempting endovascular removal as the filter will endothelialize within a matter of months. Open removal for the sake of peace of mind should be absolutely ruled out as intraoperative exsanguination is a serious possibility. The strut fracture probably occurred during her term pregnancies as the enlarging uterus collapses the Greenfield filter, which subsequently re-expands post-partum. If a strut is broken but does not have any missing pieces, imaging of the chest is not warranted. Additionally, in the face of an asymptomatic patient, there are no indications for abdominal imaging beyond the film in clinic. She should also be made aware that the longest follow up of her type of filter is a mean of only about 9 years. On the whole, though, the most prudent course of action would seem to be reassurance. Discussions about continued follow up with imaging should be individualized to the patient since any risks associated with contemplated removal would only grow with time, prompting the question of what would be done if new information was gleaned while remaining asymptomatic.

**Answer: E**

Greenfield, L.J. and Proctor, M.C. (1995) Twenty-year clinical experience with the Greenfield filter. *Cardiovascular Surgery*, **3** (2), 199–205.

Phelan, H.A., Gonzalez, R.P., Scott, W.C., *et al.* (2009) Long-term follow-up of trauma patients with permanent prophylactic vena cava filters. *Journal of Trauma*, **67** (3), 485–489.

## 22

# Transplantation, Immunology, and Cell Biology
*Leslie Kobayashi, MD and Emily Cantrell, MD*

1 *Which of the following would be the most helpful in differentiating prerenal azotemia from the hepatorenal syndrome in a patient with liver failure?*
 A *Fractional excretion of sodium that is less than 1% (FeNa <1%)*
 B *Urine sodium of less than 10 ($U_{Na}$ <10)*
 C *Urine osmolality greater than 400 ($U_{Osm}$ >400)*
 D *Lack of response to fluid resuscitation*
 E *BUN/Creatinine ratio greater than 20*

Hepatorenal syndrome (HRS) is a severe and frequent complication of advanced cirrhosis. HRS refers to acute kidney injury within the setting of severe liver failure. It may have an insidious onset or present acutely if precipitated by a stressor, such as infection, gastro-intestinal bleeding, or dehydration. It can affect up to 40% of patients with cirrhosis. Although the underlying pathophysiology is not yet completely understood, the likely etiology is nitric oxide induced splanchnic and peripheral vasodilation secondary to portal hypertension causing a state of effective central hypovolemia resulting in activation of the renin-angiotensin-aldosterone system and subsequent renal vasoconstriction and reduction in glomerular filtration rate. HRS presents similarly to prerenal azotemia, and is, in essence, a prerenal disease with decreased renal blood flow. The FENa will be <1%, urine sodium will be low, urine osmoles will be high, and urinary sediment will generally be benign. However, because of the low serum oncotic pressure, and the high output, the low resistance state of cirrhotic patients, HRS generally will not respond to fluid challenge. This is markedly different from prerenal azotemia which will respond to volume replacement within 24–72 hours. The best treatment for hepatorenal syndrome is liver transplantation. Treatment of exacerbating conditions such as gastro-intestinal bleeding or infection is also critical. Some promising treatments include intravenous clonidine, midodrine, octreotide, norepinephrine in

patients with a low mean arterial pressure, and combination therapy with terlipressin and albumin.

**Answer: D**

Busk, T.M., Bendtsen, F., and Møller, S. (2016) Hepatorenal syndrome in cirrhosis: diagnostic, pathophysiological, and therapeutic aspects. *Expert Reviews of Gastroentrology of Hepatology*, **10** (10), 1153–1161.

Cavallin, M., Kamath, P.S., Merli, M., *et al.* (2015) Terlipressin plus albumin versus midodrine and octreotide plus albumin in the treatment of hepatorenal syndrome: a randomized trial. *Hepatology*, **62**, 567–574.

2 *A 65-year-old male develops atrial fibrillation with a rapid ventricular rate on postop day 4 following renal transplant. He is started and maintained on Diltiazem which achieves good rate control. Over the next several days, however, the patient's urine output begins to drop, and the patient's creatinine begins to rise. He also develops altered mental status, hyperkalemia, and transaminitis. He remains afebrile and hemodynamically stable. His current medications include tacrolimus, mycophenolate mofetil, prednisone, insulin, bisacodyl, and oxycodone/acetaminophen. Which of the following is the next best step in making the diagnosis?*
 A *Obtain a CT scan of the abdomen*
 B *Discontinue pain medications and follow laboratory values*
 C *Check a tacrolimus level*
 D *Obtain blood and urine cultures and begin broad spectrum antibiotics*

This patient's symptoms are likely the result of calcineurin toxicity secondary to diltiazem. Checking a tacrolimus level will confirm the diagnosis by revealing an elevated level. Drug-drug interactions with various immunosuppressants continue to be a clinically significant problem affecting many transplant recipients. Tacrolimus binds to FK-binding protein-12 and blocks proliferation of calcineurin, preventing interleukin-2 (IL-2) expression/production, thus preventing an immune response from lymphocytes. It is metabolized by cytochrome P450 3A4 (CYP3A4) in both the liver and small intestine, and clearance is primarily from biliary excretion and fecal elimination. Very little drug is cleared by the kidneys. Any medications that inhibit CYP3A4 will increase drug concentrations, and in contrast, medications that induce CYP3A4 will decrease drug concentrations (Table 22.1, Table 22.2). Diltiazem, a nondihydropyridine calcium channel blocker, as well as azole antifungals, erythromycin, clarithromycin, and amiodarone, are inhibitors of CYP3A4, will result in increased levels of tacrolimus. By contrast phenobarbital, phenytoin, rifampin, and carbamazepine are all CYP3A4 inducers and coadministration will result in decreased tacrolimus levels.

**Answer: C**

Azzi, J.R., Sayegh, M.H., and Mallat, S.G. (2013) Calcineurin inhibitors: 40 years later, can't live without. *Journal of Immunology*, **191** (12), 5785–5791.

Moini, M., Schilsky, M.L., Tichy, E.M. (2015) Review of immunosuppression in liver transplantation. *World Journal of Hepatology*, 7 (10), 1355–1368.

**Table 22.1** CYP3A4 inhibitors: increase tacrolimus levels.

| Class | Examples |
| --- | --- |
| Antifungal agents | Fluconazole, voriconazole, ketoconazole |
| Calcium channel blockers | Diltiazem, nifedipine, nicardipine, verapamil |
| Macrolide antibiotics | Erythromycin, clarithromycin |
| Promotility agents | Metoclopramide |
| Protease inhibitors | Indinavir, ritonavir, atazanavir |
| Misc. | Metronidazole, cimetidine, ciprofloxacin, amiodarone |
| Herbals | Echinacea |
| Foods | Grapefruit juice, star fruit |

**Table 22.2** CYP3A4 inducers: decrease tacrolimus levels.

| Class | Examples |
| --- | --- |
| Anticonvulsants | Carbamazepine, phenytoin, phenobarbital |
| Rifamycins | Rifampin, rifabutin |
| Misc. | Glucocorticoids, pioglitazone |
| Herbals | St. John's wort |

**3** *Regarding cyclosporine and tacrolimus and their use in liver transplant recipients, which of the following is TRUE?*
   **A** *Cyclosporine has more nephrotoxicity than tacrolimus*
   **B** *Cyclosporine has less nephrotoxicity than tacrolimus*
   **C** *Cyclosporine has a similar nephrotoxicity to tacrolimus*
   **D** *Cyclosporine is more potent than tacrolimus*
   **E** *Cyclosporine results in improved graft survival compared to tacrolimus*

Both tacrolimus and cyclosporine are classified as calcineurin inhibitors (CNI) and often used in maintenance immunosuppression following solid organ transplant. CNIs function as immunosuppressants by blocking T-cell activation by binding to specific receptors and blocking calcineurin, a calcium-dependent phosphatase within T-cells. Tacrolimus is superior to cyclosporine in increasing patient and graft survival. Fewer episodes of acute cellular rejection and steroid-resistant rejection have also been seen with tacrolimus use in the first year posttransplant compared to cyclosporine. Tacrolimus is preferred at most transplant centers because of its greater potency and improved cardiovascular side effect profile. The most common adverse side effect of CNIs is their nephrotoxic effect at high levels. Tacrolimus and cyclosporine have similar nephrotoxicity by causing vasoconstriction of the afferent glomerular arteriole and decrease glomerular filtration. Additionally they may exert direct cellular stress on renal tubular cells. When administered together tacrolimus and cyclosporine have a synergistic immunosuppressive effect and have an increased renal toxicity when compared to either agent given alone. Other common side effects of CNIs include hypertension, neurotoxicity, metabolic abnormalities, and hyperlipidemia. The diabetogenic effect of tacrolimus is greater than cyclosporine.

**Answer: C**

Moini, M., Schilsky, M.L., Tichy, E.M. (2015) Review of immunosuppression in liver transplantation. *World Journal of Hepatology*, 7 (10), 1355–1368.

Vicari-Christensen, M., Repper, S., and Basile, S., *et al.* (2009) Tacrolimus: review of pharmacokinetics, pharmacodynamics, and pharmacogenetics to facilitate practitioners' understanding and offer strategies for educating patients and promoting adherence. *Progress in Transplantation*, **19** (3), 277–248.

**4** *A patient with cirrhosis requires anticoagulation for a pulmonary embolus, heparin bolus followed by infusion fails to increase the aPTT. What is the next step in management?*

**A** *Transfuse with fresh frozen plasma*
**B** *Administer systemic tissue plasminogen activator (tPA)*
**C** *Change to an argatroban infusion*
**D** *Change to a lepirudin infusion*
**E** *Increase the dose of heparin*

Patients with cirrhosis are at higher risk for both bleeding and thrombosis-related complications. Cirrhosis results in decreased synthetic liver function which leads to decreased levels of clotting factors and elevations in prothrombin time (PT) and international normalized ratio (INR). The liver also synthesizes natural anticoagulants such as Protein C and S and antithrombin III (AT-III) which are decreased in cirrhotic patients as well. Also, patients may also suffer from microvascular consumption causing further decreases in AT-III levels. As a result, cirrhotic patients may be hypercoagulable despite having an elevated PT/INR. They may also demonstrate heparin resistance due to diminished AT-III levels, similar to the resistance seen in a patient undergoing cardiopulmonary bypass. It has been shown that decreases in AT-III levels to 70%, and 50% of normal will result in a decrease in heparin activity to 65% and 20% of baseline. Resistance is unlikely to respond to increases in heparin dose. AT-III deficiency can be reversed by transfusion with fresh frozen plasma (FFP) which contains high concentrations of Protein C and S as well as AT-III. Alternatively concentrates of AT-III are also available and may aid in avoiding volume overload associated with transfusion of large amounts of FFP.

**Answer: A**

Ha, N.B. and Regal, R.E. (2016) Anticoagulation in patients with cirrhosis: caught between a rock-liver and a hard place. *Annals of Pharmacotherapy*, **50**, 402–409.

Aggarwal, A., Puri, K., and Liangpunsakul, S. (2014) Deep vein thrombosis and pulmonary embolism in cirrhotic patients: systematic review. *World Journal of Gastroenterology*, **20**, 5737–5745.

**5** *Following renal transplantation, a patient is found to have an invasive fungal infection with Candida glabrata. Which antifungal is best suited to treat this infection?*
   **A** *Voriconazole*
   **B** *Amphotericin B*
   **C** *Fluconazole*
   **D** *Meropenem*
   **E** *Caspofungin*

The risk of invasive fungal infection (IFI) is increased in patients after a solid organ transplant and is associated with decreased survival. *Candida* and *Aspergillus* species are the most common organisms, with nonalbicans species increasing in frequency. Historically amphotericin B was the antifungal of choice, but it is associated with significant liver and renal toxicity. Newer liposomal formulations have decreased these risks. However, because of their clinical efficacy, a broad spectrum of activity, and favorable side effect profile, echinocandins are becoming the antifungal of choice in many patient populations. Echinocandins include caspofungin, micafungin, and anidulafungin. Comparisons of caspofungin to amphotericin B have shown equivalent efficacy and a more favorable side effect profile. In solid organ transplant recipients, caspofungin was found to be effective as both a first and second line treatment, with success in 87% of *Candidal* and 74% of *Aspergillus* infections. In-vitro studies have found efficacy against nonalbicans species such as *C. glabrata*, *C. krusei*, *C. Parapsilosis*, and *C. tropicalis*, as well as fluconazole resistant albicans isolates. The echinocandins also have the benefit of fewer drug-drug interactions in transplant patients. Specifically, unlike the azoles, they are not inhibitors of cytochrome P450 and are unlikely to alter pharmacodynamics of the calcineurin inhibitors used for immunosuppression. In general guidelines for fungal treatment and prophylaxis recommend posaconazole for prophylaxis in bone marrow transplant patients, caspofungin in confirmed or suspected *Candidal* IFI in neutropenic and nonneutropenic patients and for febrile neutropenia, and voriconazole in invasive *Aspergillosis*. Amphotericin B in liposomal preparation should be considered a second-line agent for IFI.

**Answer: E**

Farmakiotis, D. and Kontoyiannis, D.P. (2015) Emerging issues with diagnosis and management of fungal infections in solid organ transplant recipients. *American Journal of Transplantation*, **15**, 1141–1147.

Winkler, M., Pratschke, J., Schulz, U., *et al.* (2010) Caspofungin for post solid organ transplant invasive fungal disease: results of a retrospective observational study. *Transplant Infectious Diseases*, **12**, 230–237.

**6** *A patient with Childs C cirrhosis secondary to Hepatitis B presents with fevers, watery diarrhea, and large violaceous, bullous skin lesions on the legs after consuming raw oysters at a seafood restaurant two nights prior to presentation. What is the most appropriate antibiotic choice for this disease process?*
   **A** *Doxycycline*
   **B** *Piperacillin/Tazobactam*
   **C** *Vancomycin*
   **D** *Colistin*
   **E** *Penicillin*

This patient is infected with *Vibrio vulnificus,* an invasive, gram-negative bacillus found in warm seawater and often in raw oysters, shellfish, and other seafood. Greater than 90% of cases can be traced to ingestion of oysters within 1 to 3 days of clinical presentation. Hepatic dysfunction is the most common risk factor for *Vibrio* infection however other immunosuppressed states have also been implicated. Infection can occur as a result of ingestion or from exposure of unhealed wounds to contaminated water. Fever, malaise, and diarrhea generally precede the appearance of the typical skin lesions which present within 36–48 hours of initial symptoms. The characteristic findings are large violaceous bullae, especially on the lower extremities. Blood, stool, and wound cultures can confirm the diagnosis, but because the spread is rapid and lethal, a high index of clinical suspicion must be present, and treatment should be instituted prior to confirmatory cultures. The mortality of patients with *Vibrio* septicemia can be as high as 50% and increases to greater than 90% if septic shock occurs, or necrotizing soft tissue infection is present. Treatment is with doxycycline and ceftazidime. Alternative regimens include cefotaxime or ciprofloxacin. Additionally, there should be aggressive local wound care with drainage of any fluid collections and wide debridement of necrotic tissue.

**Answer: A**

Jones, M.K. and Oliver, J.D. (2009) Vibrio vulnificus: disease and pathogenesis. *Infection and Immunity,* 77 (5), 1723–1733.

Tsai, Y.H., Huang, T.J., Hsu, R.W., *et al.* (2009) Necrotizing soft-tissue infections and primary sepsis caused by vibrio vulnificus and vibrio cholera non-01. *Journal of Trauma,* 66, 899–905.

7   *What is the most common cause of late deaths in patients following renal transplant?*
   A *Viral infection*
   B *Bacterial infection*
   C *Chronic rejection*
   D *Cardiovascular disease*
   E *Squamous cell cancer*

The survival following renal transplantation has improved significantly over the years and now approaches 95% in one year. While the mortality of posttransplant patients is higher than the general population, it is significantly better than patients with end-stage renal disease without transplantation. The three leading causes of late death following renal transplant are cardiovascular disease, malignancy, and infections. Cardiovascular disease is the leading cause of mortality, implicated in

42–57% of deaths. Malignancy, which is increasing in frequency, is now the second most common cause, accounting for 9–27% of deaths. The increase in malignancy-related deaths is likely multifactorial, due to increased potency of immunosuppressive medications, longer posttransplant survival, and malignancy-inducing infections such as human papilloma virus and Epstein-Barr virus. Malignancy is more frequent in posttransplant patients than in the general population with the most common malignancy being squamous cell skin cancers. In contrast to malignancy, infection, which accounts for 11–22% of deaths, has been decreasing in frequency. Deaths due to infection are most prevalent in the early period.

**Answer: D**

Liefeldt, L. and Budde, K. (2010) Risk factors for cardiovascular disease in renal transplant recipients and strategies to minimize risk. *Transplant International,* **23**, 1191–1204.

Marcen, R. (2009) Immunosuppressive drugs in kidney transplantation: Impact on patient survival, and incidence of cardiovascular disease, malignancy, and infection. *Drugs,* **69**(16): 2227–2237.

8   *Which of the following statements is TRUE in regards to hyperacute rejection?*
   A *Its incidence can be decreased by the use of ABO cross-matching*
   B *It is mediated by activated T cells*
   C *It occurs within the first 3-7 days post-transplant*
   D *Biopsy reveals perivascular lymphocytic infiltrate*
   E *Treatment consists of pulsed steroids and OKT3*

With advancements in transplantation, hyperacute rejection has become a rare event and is primarily the consequence of high levels of complement-activating donor-specific antibodies at the time of transplantation. It may occur after the transplantation of an ABO incompatible organ or in the presence of preformed circulating antibodies against donor HLA when these are overlooked during the pretransplant crossmatch and antibody screening procedures. Hyperacute rejection is seen within minutes to hours of reperfusion and is most commonly seen in renal and cardiac transplants, but has also been noted following lung and liver transplants. Similar to an acute hemolytic transfusion reaction, it is caused by activation of complement by preformed antibodies to antigens present on the donor vascular endothelial cells that result in rapid agglutination, small vessel thrombosis, and graft loss. Additionally, if the graft is not removed, a severe systemic inflammatory response may occur. The graft itself will become soft, mottled, and cyanotic in appearance. A biopsy will demonstrate vascular wall edema and capillary microthrombi. Hyperacute rejection can be prevented by performing a preoperative cytotoxic cross match, and not utilizing ABO incompatible organs. The only treatment of hyperacute rejection is graft removal and emergent retransplantation.

**Answer: A**

Becker, L.E., Morath, C., and Suesal, C. (2016) Immune mechanisms of acute and chronic rejection. *Clinical Biochemistry*, **49** (4–5), 320–323.
Sureshkumar, K.K., Hussain, S.M., Carpenter, B.J., *et al.* (2007) Antibody-mediated rejection following renal transplantation. *Expert Opinion on Pharmacotherapy*, **8** (7), 913–921.

9 *Cardiac allograft vasculopathy (CAV) is an accelerated form of coronary artery disease (CAD) affecting transplanted hearts and is one of the leading causes of death following cardiac transplant patients. However, CAV differs from traditional CAD in many ways. In regards to these differences, which of the following is TRUE?*
   A *CAV affects proximal vessels whereas CAD is more prominent in distal and intramyocardial vessels*
   B *The plaque pattern of CAV is diffuse and concentric, compared to focal and eccentric in CAD*
   C *Calcium deposition is prominent in CAV but is rarely seen in CAD*
   D *Disruption of the internal elastic lamina is common in CAV, but rare in CAD*
   E *Active inflammation and progressive intimal hyperplasia and fibrosis are prominent in CAV, but not CAD*

Following cardiac transplantation, median survival is approximately 11 years and increases to 14 years for those who survive the first year. However, long-term success continues to be limited by CAV. CAV is a leading cause of long-term mortality in heart transplant, accounting for up to 1 in 8 deaths beyond a year posttransplant. CAV can be seen in 7–8% of patients at one year but increases to approximately 40% at 8 years posttransplant. In contrast to CAD which tends to affect proximal coronary arteries, CAV is diffuse and affects all cardiac vessels including intramyocardial arteries and, in some cases, coronary veins. Pathologically, smooth muscle proliferation, accumulation of inflammatory cells, and lipid deposition cause circumferential intimal thickening. Calcium deposition and disruption of the internal elastic lamina is rare. The inflammatory process involves both immune and nonimmune factors including; cytomegalovirus infection, dyslipidemia,

hyperhomocysteinemia, diabetes, hypertension, and ischemia-reperfusion injury. Additionally, CAV appears to be more prominent among patients with repeated episodes of graft rejection.

**Answer: E**

Chang, D.H. and Kobashigawa, J.A. (2015) Current diagnostic and treatment strategies for cardiac allograft vasculopathy. *Expert Review of Cardiovascular Therapy*, **13**, 1147–1154.
Chih, S., Chong, A.Y., Mielniczuk, L.M., *et al.* (2016) Allograft vasculopathy: the Achilles' heel of heart transplantation. *Journal of the American College of Cardiology*, **68**, 80–91.

10 *Of the following medications, which one has been shown to decrease CAV in heart transplant patients?*
   A *Beta blockers*
   B *Cyclosporin*
   C *Steroids*
   D *Aspirin*
   E *Statins*

CAV is a progressive inflammatory vasculopathy that is a significant cause of death after cardiac transplant. It is best diagnosed using intravascular ultrasound, as the sensitivity and specificity of angiography are much lower than with traditional CAD. However, as this is not always readily available and is invasive, the best screening test is dobutamine stress echocardiography, which has a sensitivity and specificity of 72% and 83% respectively. Prevention and treatment of CAV should be aimed at decreasing risk factors in posttransplant patients. Hyperlipidemia is common both pre- and posttransplant and can be exacerbated by the use of immunosuppressants like corticosteroids and cyclosporine. Treatment with statins, in particular, pravastatin and simvastatin, has been associated with decreased rates of CAV, decreased allograft rejection, and improved mortality. Additionally, treatment with calcium channel blockers, such as diltiazem, especially in combination with ACE inhibitors has been shown to prevent the development of CAV. Prevention and treatment of cytomegalovirus infection with ganciclovir has also been shown to reduce progression of CAV. Lastly, immunosuppressive regimens based on tacrolimus and mycophenolate mofetil appear to have less CAV compared to cyclosporine and azathioprine regimens. Newer areas of research show promise with folic acid, everolimus, and L-arginine. Antiplatelet agents, including aspirin, though commonly used in this patient population, have not been shown to prevent CAV.

**Answer: E**

Chang, D.H. and Kobashigawa, J.A. (2015) Current diagnostic and treatment strategies for cardiac allograft vasculopathy. *Expert Review of Cardiovascular Therapy*, **13**, 1147–1154.

Chih, S., Chong, A.Y., Mielniczuk, L.M., *et al.* (2016) Allograft vasculopathy: the Achilles' heel of heart transplantation. *Journal of the American College of Cardiology*, **68**, 80–91.

**11** *A patient is 36 hours postoperative from renal transplant and develops sudden onset oliguria. You are concerned for renal artery thrombosis. What is the best method to confirm this diagnosis?*
 **A** *Ultrasound*
 **B** *Operative exploration*
 **C** *Angiography*
 **D** *Renal biopsy*
 **E** *CT scan*

Although vascular complications account for only 5–10% of all posttransplant complications, they are a frequent cause of graft loss. Renal artery thrombosis is a rare but serious complication following renal transplant affecting less than 1% of patients. Thrombosis often presents with sudden onset of oliguria in the early postoperative period. Common causes include acute and hyperacute rejection, surgical trauma, kinking of the vessel, and hypercoagulable state. Ultrasound is a useful diagnostic tool and has a sensitivity and specificity in the diagnosis of renal artery thrombosis approaching 100%. It also has the benefit of being rapidly available, easily performed, noninvasive, and repeatable. Additionally, ultrasound can provide information about venous flow, flow in the renal parenchyma, and dilation of the collecting system. Lastly, while angiography is an excellent option for diagnosis and therapy, ultrasound has the benefits of avoiding contrast and radiation exposure.

**Answer: A**

Granata, A., Clementi, S., Londrino, F., *et al.* (2014) Renal transplant vascular complications: the role of Doppler ultrasound. *Journal of Ultrasound in Medicine*, **18**, 101–107.

Rodgers, S.K., Sereni, C.P., and Horrow, M.M. (2014) Ultrasonographic evaluation of the renal transplant. *Radiologic Clinics of North America*, **52**, 1307–1324.

**12** *Which of the following is a contraindication to liver transplantation?*
 **A** *Hepatitis B*
 **B** *Hepatitis C*
 **C** *Extrahepatic malignancy*
 **D** *Hepatocellular carcinoma with a single 4cm lesion*
 **E** *Hepatocellular carcinoma with three lesions, ranging in size from 1–3cm*

Indications for liver transplant include liver failure due to hepatitis B and C, cholestasis, metabolic disorders, alcohol abuse, autoimmune disorders, Budd-Chiari, polycystic liver disease, and primary biliary or hepatic malignancies. Hepatitis B currently has the highest survival rate following liver transplantation, and hepatitis C is the most common indication for liver transplant. Hepatocellular carcinoma (HCC) is now the fifth most common cancer and the third commonest cause of cancer deaths worldwide. Less than 15% of patients with HCC are candidates for resection. Also, multiple studies have shown that HCC patients have better survival and lower rates of recurrence after liver transplant compared to resection when using the Milan criteria, or UCSF extension of the Milan Criteria. The Milan criteria allow transplantation for a single HCC lesion up to 5cm, and up to three lesions each 3 cm or less. With these criteria, 4-year survival is 85%, and the recurrence rate is 8%. Extended criteria from UCSF allow a single lesion up to 6.5 cm or up to three lesions as large as 4.5 cm with a total tumor burden of 8 cm or less. Studies have revealed outcomes equivalent to the Milan criteria in experienced centers. Absolute contraindications to transplantation include extrahepatic malignancy, uncorrectable cardiac or pulmonary disease, irreversible neurologic impairment and uncontrolled sepsis.

**Answer: C**

Bhardwaj, N., Perera, M.T., and Silva, M.A. (2016) Current treatment approaches to HCC with a special consideration to transplantation. *Journal of Transplantation*, 7926264.

Busuttil, R.W. and Petrowsky, H. (2012) Liver transplantation, in *Mastery of Surgery*, 6th edn (eds J.E. Fischer and K.I. Bland), Lippincott Williams & Wilkins, Philadelphia PA, pp. 1350–1374.

**13** *What is the mechanism of action of tacrolimus and cyclosporine?*
 **A** *Prevention of activation of T-cells*
 **B** *De-activation of T-cells*
 **C** *Inhibition of antibody production*
 **D** *Prevent proliferation of T and B cells*
 **E** *Inhibit antigen recognition of T cells by binding CD3*

Both tacrolimus and cyclosporine are calcineurin inhibitors that block interleukin-2 (IL-2) mediated T-cell activation. Tacrolimus binds to FK-binding protein and cyclosporine binds to cyclophilin. The drug-protein complexes then bind to calcineurin and inhibit transcription of multiple cytokines including IL-2, IL-3, IL-4, granulocyte-macrophage colony stimulating factor (GM-CSF), interferon-gamma, and TNF-alpha. In most centers, tacrolimus is preferred over cyclosporine because of its greater potency and improved cardiovascular adverse side effect profile.

**Answer: A**

Moini, M., Schilsky, M.L., and Tichy, E.M. (2015) Review of immunosuppression in liver transplantation. *World Journal of Hepatology*, **7** (10), 1355–1368.

The U.S. Multicenter FK506 Liver Study Group. (1994) A comparison of tacrolimus (FK 506) and cyclosporine for immunosuppression in liver transplantation. *NEJM*, **331** (17), 1110–1115.

**14** *Which of the following side effects associated with calcineurin inhibitors is known to be more prominent with tacrolimus when compared to cyclosporine?*
**A** *Hypertension*
**B** *Diabetes*
**C** *Hirsutism*
**D** *Gingival hyperplasia*
**E** *Dyslipidemia*

Hypertension, neurotoxicity, metabolic abnormalities including hyperglycemia, electrolyte imbalances, hyperlipidemia, and nephrotoxicity are all common adverse side effects associated with calcineurin. Nephrotoxicity appears to be equivalent between the two drugs, while hypertension and dyslipidemia appear slightly more prominent with cyclosporine. Diabetes is significantly more common with tacrolimus, as well as gastroenterologic (nausea, diarrhea) and neurologic (headache, tremor, seizure) symptoms but to a lesser extent. In contrast hirsutism and gingival hyperplasia are more frequently associated with cyclosporine.

**Answer: B**

Moini, M., Schilsky, M.L., and Tichy, E.M. (2015) Review of immunosuppression in liver transplantation. *World Journal of Hepatology*, **7** (10), 1355–1368.

Vicari-Christensen, M., Repper, S., and Basile, S., *et al.* (2009) Tacrolimus: review of pharmacokinetics, pharmacodynamics, and pharmacogenetics to facilitate practitioners' understanding and offer strategies for educating patients and promoting adherence. *Progress in Transplantation*, **19** (3), 277–248.

**15** *14 hours following lung transplantation, a patient develops acute respiratory deterioration, with airspace disease on chest x-ray, worsening hypoxemia, and increased airway pressures. What is the most likely etiology of this patient's respiratory failure?*

**A** *Cytomegalovirus pneumonia*
**B** *Ischemia reperfusion injury*
**C** *Pseudomonas aeruginosa pneumonia*
**D** *Obliterative bronchiolitis*
**E** *Pulmonary embolism*

Early respiratory failure is a common occurrence after lung transplant, affecting between 20–55% of patients. The most common cause of early respiratory failure, accounting for greater than 50% of cases, is ischemia-reperfusion lung injury (IRLI). IRLI commonly occurs within the first 72 hours of surgery. It is characterized by rapid development of airspace disease, progressive hypoxemia with $PaO_2/FiO_2$ ratios less than 200, and increased pulmonary pressures. Risk factors for IRLI include preoperative pulmonary hypertension, right ventricular dysfunction, cardiopulmonary bypass, and prolonged cold ischemia times. IRLI along with episodes of acute rejection has been associated with increased risk of obliterative bronchiolitis (OB). OB is most prominent in the late postoperative period with a median time to diagnosis of 16–20 months. Bacterial and fungal pneumonia are also common in the early postoperative period, but generally present later than IRLI with a median time to occurrence of 34 days. Bacterial pneumonia is the earliest and most common, followed in timing and frequency by fungal and viral pneumonia. *Pseudomonas, Aspergillosis,* and CMV are the most common bacterial, fungal, and viral etiologies respectively. A pulmonary embolus may be an underdiagnosed cause of postlung transplant respiratory failure in the first month. However, it usually presents between 72 hours and 1 week and generally does not result in an infiltrate on chest x-ray.

**Answer: B**

Aguilar-Guisado, M., Givalda,.J, Ussetti, P., *et al.* (2007) Pneumonia after lung transplantation in the Resitra Cohort: A multicenter prospective study. *American Journal of Transplantation*, **7**, 1989–1996.

Campos, S., Caramori, M., and Teixeira, R., *et al.* (2008) Bacterial and fungal pneumonias after lung transplantation. *Transplantation Proceedings*, **40** (3): 822–824.

**16** *In addition to reducing pharmacologic immunosuppression, what is the treatment of choice in cases of severe or life-threatening cytomegalovirus (CMV) enteritis?*
**A** *Oral ganciclovir*
**B** *Oral valganciclovir*
**C** *IV ganciclovir*
**D** *IV valganciclovir*
**E** *Acyclovir*

Cytomegalovirus (CMV) is one of the most common viral pathogens causing clinical disease following solid organ transplant. For CMV prophylaxis oral or IV ganciclovir, or valganciclovir can be used with similar efficacy. Both are superior to acyclovir. Prophylaxis is begun in the early posttransplant period and continued for 3–6 months. However, in cases of severe CMV infection, the gold standard is IV ganciclovir. Studies have shown equivalent efficacy and similar outcomes using oral valganciclovir for nonlife-threatening infections in adult patients. IV ganciclovir, however, remains the treatment of choice for pediatric patients and in those with severe, life-threatening infections. Additionally, IV ganciclovir should be chosen for those patients in whom oral formulations would be poorly tolerated or unlikely to be absorbed, such as in enteritis. Consensus recommendations from the Infectious Diseases Section of The Transplantation Society recommend IV ganciclovir twice daily until viral eradication is seen on two consecutive titers, and for no fewer than 2 weeks.

**Answer: C**

Bruminhent, J. and Razonable, R.R. (2014) Management of cytomegalovirus infection and disease in liver transplant recipients. *World Journal of Hepatology*, **6**, 370–383.

Kotton, C.N., Kumar, D., Caliendo, A.M., *et al.* (2010) International consensus guidelines on the management of cytomegalovirus in solid organ transplantation. *Transplantation*, **89** (7): 779–795.

17 *A patient in the ICU is two weeks status postlung transplant and is diagnosed with pneumonia. Which of the following is the most likely organism involved?*
  A *Pneumocystis jiroveci*
  B *Pseudomonas aeruginosa*
  C *Staphylococcus aureus*
  D *Aspergillus fumigates*
  E *Cytomegalovirus*

Pneumonia is a common complication following lung transplant. It is the second leading cause of postoperative respiratory failure in the early (less than 1 month) period. Gram-negative rods (GNR) predominate, accounting for 83% of pneumonia, with the most common organisms being *Pseudomonas, Acinetobacter,* and *E. coli.* Gram-positive bacterial infections are most commonly due to *Staphylococcus aureus,* but are less common than GNR pneumonia and appear later in the posttransplant period. *Aspergillus* and cytomegalovirus (CMV) are less common causes of pneumonia and occur later than bacterial pneumonia, largely due to antimicrobial prophylaxis. Prophylaxis has also decreased the risk of pneumonia from atypical organisms, such as *Pneumocystis* from 10–12% to almost nil in most centers.

**Answer: B**

Aguilar-Guisado, M., Givalda, J., Ussetti, P., *et al.* (2007) Pneumonia after lung transplantation in the Resitra Cohort: A multicenter prospective study. *American Journal of Transplantation*, **7**, 1989–1996.

Campos, S., Caramori, M., Teixeira, R., *et al.* (2008) Bacterial and fungal pneumonias after lung transplantation. *Transplantation Proceedings*, **40** (3), 822–824.

Dudau, D., Camous, J., Marchand, S., *et al.* (2014) Incidence of nosocomial pneumonia and risk of recurrence after antimicrobial therapy in critically ill lung and heart-lung transplant patients. *Clinical Transplantation*, **28**, 27–36.

18 *A 55-year-old African American male with a history of scleroderma and end-stage renal disease on dialysis is admitted to the ICU following a deceased donor renal transplant. Per reports, the operation was uneventful, and induction agents included solumedrol and thymoglobulin. Postoperative, as per protocol, the patient receives a second dose of thymoglobulin after being premedicated with acetaminophen, diphenhydramine, and IV steroids. Several hours later, the patient develops severe respiratory distress (SpO$_2$=80%), tachycardia and fevers (T=104 °F). What is the next best step in the management of this patient?*
  A *Peripheral blood cultures, urine culture, and initiation of broad-spectrum antibiotics*
  B *Intubation and ventilator support with positive end-expiratory pressure*
  C *High dose steroid administration*
  D *Noninvasive ventilation and administration of diuretics*

Antithymocyte antibodies (thymoglobulin) may be administered as induction agents in higher risk patients, potentially, to reduce the chance of acute rejection. These polyclonal antibodies, derived from rabbit serum, will bind activated T-cells and induce depletion via apoptosis, antibody-mediated cytotoxicity, and complement lysis. Severe side effects include fevers, tachycardia, hypoxia, pulmonary edema, and bronchospasm secondary to cytokine release syndrome, as seen in this patient. Treatment for cytokine release syndrome is mostly supportive with early recognition, intubation for airway protection and ventilator support until the inflammatory reaction has resolved.

**Answer: B**

Deeks, E.D. and Keating, G.M. (2009) Rabbit antithymocyte globulin (thymoglobulin): a review of its use in the prevention and treatment of acute renal allograft rejection. *Drugs*, **69**, 1483–1512.

Zaza, G., Tomei, P., Granata, S., *et al.* (2014) Monoclonal antibody therapy and renal transplantation: focus on adverse effects. *Toxins,* **6** (3), 869–891.

**19** *A patient who is now 10 days out from liver transplant has become progressively septic and complains of right upper quadrant pain, labs reveal an increased white blood cell count and elevated liver function tests. CT scan reveals air in the biliary tree. What is the most likely diagnosis?*

**A** *Ascending cholangitis*
**B** *Portal vein thrombosis*
**C** *Hepatic artery thrombosis*
**D** *Hepatic abscess*
**E** *Acute rejection*

Hepatic artery thrombosis (HAT) is a rare but serious complication of a liver transplant. It occurs in 1.9–16.6% of cases and is subdivided into early and late thrombosis. Early thrombosis generally occurs in the first days to weeks and is characterized by sepsis/SIRS syndrome, elevated liver function tests, and right upper quadrant pain; it can also result in fulminant liver failure. Late thrombosis occurs a few months to a year after transplant and can present with intermittent recurrent sepsis, delayed bile leak or stricture, or asymptomatic elevation in liver function tests. Risk factors for HAT include obesity, hypercoagulable state, history of transarterial chemotherapy, surgical trauma, and technical error. Additionally, the incidence of HAT is increased among pediatric and living donor liver transplants. The gold standard for diagnosis of HAT is angiography. Imaging can also include CT scan which will show absence of opacification of the hepatic artery, liver abscess or necrosis, and stricture or necrosis of the biliary tree. Ultrasound can also be used to diagnose HAT and has the benefit of ease of use, repeatability, and independence from contrast. However, it has a lower sensitivity when compared to angiography, ranging from 50–60% compared to 80–90% in angiography. Treatment includes surgical revascularization, endovascular thrombolysis/thrombectomy, and systemic heparinization. However, urgent/emergent retransplantation is required in 50–90% of cases. Associated mortality is 50–55%, and is better with late compared to early thrombosis.

**Answer: C**

Duffy, J.P., Hong, J.C., Farmer, D.G., *et al.* (2009) Vascular complications of orthotopic liver transplantation: Experience in more than 4,200 patients. *Journal of the American College of Surgeons,* **208**: 896–905.

Piardi, T., Lhuaire, M., Bruno, O., *et al.* (2016) Vascular complications following liver transplantation: a literature review of advances in 2015. *World Journal of Hepatology,* **8**, 36–57.

**20** *Successful pancreatic transplant will result in correction of insulin dependence in up to 80% of patients at 1 year. It can also reverse or stabilize all of the following complications of diabetes **except**?*

**A** *Retinopathy*
**B** *Gastroparesis*
**C** *Nephropathy*
**D** *Macrovascular disease*
**E** *Neuropathy*

The success of pancreatic transplant has improved significantly in the last two decades. Survival is now greater than 95% at 1 year and approaches 90% at 5 years. Graft survival is 85% in combined kidney/pancreas transplants and slightly less for a solitary pancreas transplant. Insulin independence is achieved in 80% of patients at 1 year. Additionally, transplantation can stabilize diabetic retinopathy and can reverse neuropathy, gastroparesis, orthostatic hypotension, and nephropathy in the native kidneys. While there has been no evidence to suggest a benefit in macrovascular disease, there is some evidence that transplant can improve microvascular microangiopathy. Lastly, transplant recipients nearly uniformly report immunosuppression management to be easier than management of labile diabetes.

**Answer: D**

Dholakia, S., Oskrochi, Y., Easton, G., *et al.* (2016) Advances in pancreas transplantation. *Journal of the Royal Society of Medicine,* **109** (4), 141–146.

Stites, E., Kennealey, P., and Wiseman, A.C. (2016) Current status of pancreas transplantation. *Current Opinion in Nephrology and Hypertension,* **25**, 563–569.

# 23

# Obstetric Critical Care
*Gerard J. Fulda, MD and Anthony Sciscione, MD*

**1** *A 24-year-old G1, P0 woman at 21 weeks gestation is admitted to the ICU following a motor vehicle collision and minor head injury. Her GCS is 14, and a CT of the brain was unremarkable. She was intoxicated on presentation and her laboratories returned as positive for alcohol and cocaine. Her BP is 140/60 mm Hg, her heart rate is 110 beats/min, and the fetal heart rate is 160 beats/min. The mother is known to be Rh positive. The patient is now complaining of lower abdominal cramping and on examination is noted to have a moderate amount of vaginal bleeding. There is no evidence of peritonitis although there is mild abdominal tenderness over the uterus with bruising from the seat belt noted. The most appropriate next step is to*

**A** *Proceed with an emergency bedside Cesarean delivery for uterine rupture*

**B** *Perform a CT scan of the abdomen.*

**C** *Administer 300 mg RhoGAM STAT*

**D** *Perform a pelvic ultrasound of the pregnancy*

**E** *Obtain a STAT pelvic x-ray and determine the need for pelvic angiography with embolization*

This patient most likely has a placental abruption, and at this gestational age; the fetus would be nonviable. The diagnosis of abruption is usually made clinically. The focus should be on keeping the mother stable. Major trauma is associated with placental abruption and may be as high as 1–5%. The greater the energy transfers, the higher the incidence of abruption. Motor vehicle collisions are one of the leading causes of abruption; the most likely mechanism is due to mechanical shearing forces of the placenta along with uterine stretching during deceleration. The diagnosis of abruption is usually confirmed by emergency pelvic ultrasound. Early hemorrhage is typically hyperechoic or isoechoic, whereas resolving hematomas are hypoechoic within 1 week and sonolucent within 2 weeks of the abruption. Acute hemorrhage can be misinterpreted as uterine fibroids or a thickened placenta.

While an assessment of the bony pelvis is important, plain films alone would not dictate the need for embolization, especially in the face of stable vital signs. If the physical examination suggests a major pelvic fracture, then a CT of the pelvis with contrast would be indicated. Extravasation of contrast with hemodynamic or fetal instability would be an indication for angioembolization.

RhoGAM is administered to mothers with placental abruption when they are Rh negative only. As the fetus is not viable, an emergency Cesarean delivery is not warranted and exposes the mother to more risk of morbidity and mortality. In this setting the fetal and maternal risks of CT scan outweigh the potential to discover a ruptured viscous or other cause for her abdominal pain.

**Answer: D**

Harris, C.M. (2004) Trauma and pregnancy, in *Obstetric Intensive Care Manual*, 2nd edn (eds M.R. Foley, T.H. Strong Jr., and T.J. Garite), McGraw-Hill, New York, pp. 227–246.

Nyberg, D.A., Cyr, D.R., Mack, L.A., *et al.* (1987) Sonographic spectrum of placental abruption. *American Journal of Roentgenology*, **148**, 161.

Nyberg, D.A., Mack, L.A., Benedetti, T.J., *et al.* (1987) Placental abruption and placental hemorrhage: Correlation of sonographic findings with fetal outcome. *Radiology*, **358**, 357.

**2** *A woman in her 36th week of gestation presents with generalized malaise, headache right upper quadrant pain, and mild hypertension. Which clinical features favor the diagnosis of acute fatty liver of pregnancy (AFLP) versus HELLP syndrome?*

**A** *DIC is more common in HELLP than AFLP*

**B** *Both are likely to have decreased glucose levels*

**C** *Increased bilirubin levels are diagnostic for HELLP*

**D** *Fibrinogen is decreased in AFLP and normal or increased in HELLP*

**E** *CT scanning is used to distinguish the two conditions*

*Surgical Critical Care and Emergency Surgery: Clinical Questions and Answers*, Second Edition.
Edited by Forrest "Dell" Moore, Peter Rhee, and Gerard J. Fulda.
© 2018 John Wiley & Sons Ltd. Published 2018 by John Wiley & Sons Ltd.
Companion website: www.wiley.com/go/moore/surgical_criticalcare_and_emergency_surgery

Acute fatty liver of pregnancy (AFLP) is a rare condition with a very high mortality rate. The condition is thought to be due to an inherited defect in lipid metabolism. A mutation, G1528C, results in a defect in a mitochondrial protein long-chain 3-hydroxyacyl CoA dehydrogenase (LCHAD). This leads to an accumulation of hepatotoxic long chain fatty acids. It is important to distinguish AFLP from HELLP syndrome. HELLP syndrome leads to areas of hepatic necrosis while the pathology of AFLP is due to fatty infiltration of the liver. The definitive diagnosis can be made with a hepatic biopsy but is usually made clinically due to the risk and delay in performing the biopsy. Clinically, AFLP patients have a decrease in both *fibrinogen* and *glucose*, with severe hypoglycemia common. HELLP patients usually have normal levels of glucose and fibrinogen. Both conditions increase bilirubin and are associated with DIC but DIC is twice as common in AFLP (75% versus 20–40%) compared to HELLP. Diagnostic imaging with CT and ultrasound is not diagnostic but can be used to rule out other conditions leading to hepatic failure.

Treatment is directed to early delivery of the fetus. Most patients are in their third trimester when AFLP develops, and it usually resolves following delivery of the fetus. Intravenous glucose infusion and a combination of factor concentrates are usually required to correct the hypoglycemia and coagulopathy in preparation for delivery. When diagnosed and treated early there is a good chance for recovery, delays in management are often fatal.

**Answer: D**

Castro, M.A., Ouzounian, J.G., Colletti, P.M., *et al.* (1996) Radiologic studies in acute fatty liver of pregnancy. A review of the literature and 19 new cases. *Journal of Reproductive Medicine*, **41** (11), 839.

Knight, M., Nelson-Piercy, C., Kurinczuk, J.J., *et al.* (2008) A prospective national study of acute fatty liver of pregnancy in the UK. *UK Obstetric Surveillance System, Gut*, **57** (7), 951.

Rajasri, A.G., Srestha, R., and Mitchell, J. (2007) Acute fatty liver of pregnancy (AFLP)—an overview, *Journal of Obstetrics and Gynaecology*, **27** (3), 237.

3 *A 33-year-old G4, P4 Hispanic woman was diagnosed with symptomatic gallstones and had a laparoscopic cholecystectomy at 34 weeks gestation. She goes into spontaneous labor 3 days after surgery and delivers vaginally. She returns 1 week postpartum with shortness of breath, fatigue, and a nonproductive cough, worse at night, which began during the last couple of weeks of her pregnancy. Management of this patient should include:*

A *Standard heart failure care*
B *Cardiac catheterization to evaluate the LAD*
C *The administration of broad spectrum antibiotics*
D *The administration of RhoGAM*
E *A cardiac biopsy to rule out myocarditis*

This patient has developed peripartum cardiomyopathy, which should be managed in a similar way to other causes of congestive heart failure. This condition occurs late in pregnancy, within one month of delivery, and up to five months postpartum. The diagnosis is usually made clinically in a patient who develops heart failure (LV ejection fraction less than 40%) during this timeframe without a history of prior heart disease or other identifiable cause of heart failure. The etiology is unknown with immunologic and inflammatory hypothesis most often proposed. Risk factors for the development of postpartum cardiomyopathy have included older multiparous mothers, those with hypertension, drug abuse, and long-term tocolytic therapy. Since the diagnosis is made on a clinical basis, invasive diagnostic tests are not indicated unless attempting to rule out other causes of heart failure, which this patient does not have. While some authors have suggested a myocarditis as an explanation, results of a myocardial biopsy, have not been uniform and do not alter the management. There is no proven benefit to immunosuppressive therapy or the administration of immunoglobulin.

The treatment is directed to the management of heart failure. The main caveat during pregnancy is to avoid drugs such as angiotensin receptor antagonist and angiotensin converting enzyme inhibitors, which are known to be harmful to the fetus. Selective beta blockers are safe and frequently used. Diuretics should be used with caution predelivery due to the potential for volume depletion. Digoxin can be safely added as a second-line agent, hydralazine and nitroglycerin are options for vasodilators,

The prognosis is guarded with a mortality rate of 10%, and most women are left with some residual cardiac dysfunction.

**Answer: A**

Bozkurt, B., Villaneuva, F.S., Holubkov, R., *et al.* (1999) Intravenous immune globulin in the therapy of peripartum cardiomyopathy. *Journal of the American College of Cardiology*, **34** (1), 177–180.

Mason, J.W., O'Connell, J.B., Herskowitz, A., *et al.* (1995) A clinical trial of immunosuppressive therapy for myocarditis. *New England Journal of Medicine*, **333** (5), 269–275.

Sliwa, K., Fett, J., and Elkayam, U. (2006) Peripartum cardiomyopathy. *Lancet*, **368** (9536), 687–693.

**4** *A 26-year-old G1 P1 woman at 32 weeks pregnancy and a long-standing history of poorly controlled severe asthma presents to the ED with acute shortness of breath. She is intubated in the ED for respiratory distress. Considering the normal respiratory changes that occur during pregnancy, which of the following findings is not part of the normal physiologic compensation of pregnancy.*

**A** *An increase in $PaCO_2$ to 45 mm Hg*
**B** *An increased tidal volume of 40%*
**C** *An increase in oxygen consumption of 30–40 mL/min*
**D** *A decrease in functional residual capacity (FRC) by 25%*
**E** *An increase in A-a gradient by 10–15%*

The pregnant woman has an increased metabolic demand secondary to the needs of the fetus. This leads to several predictable physiologic alterations of the respiratory system. The most notable change is an increase in oxygen requirements of about 30–40 ml/min. The respiratory compensation is to increase the minute volume by increasing the tidal volume by about 40%, some of this is accomplished by a decrease in the FRC by 25%. There is a likely increase in the A-a gradient, which improves the availability of oxygen to the mother. All of these compensations lead to a decrease in $PaCO_2$. The mother can maintain a relatively normal pH due to the progressive nature of these changes which allows the kidneys time to excrete excess bicarbonate.

**Answer: A**

Zimmerman, J.L. (2007) *Fundamental Critical Care Support Manual*, 3rd edn, Society of Critical Care Medicine, Mount Prospect, Il, pp. 14.1–14.12.

**5** *A 23-year-old woman has been in active labor for several hours. The patient becomes hypoxic and is intubated in the delivery suite. By the time you arrive the patient is now hypotensive and on vasopressors. You suspect she has had an amniotic fluid embolism and anticipate all of the following **except***

**A** *Hemorrhage and accompanying disseminated intravascular coagulopathy*
**B** *Profound pulmonary vasoconstriction*
**C** *Left ventricular dysfunction*
**D** *Fetal squamous cells in the pulmonary arterial circulation*
**E** *Rapid delivery of the fetus*

The diagnosis of amniotic fluid embolism is generally made on clinical grounds and is made after other common causes of sudden shock are ruled out. Amniotic fluid embolism has an incidence of about 1 in 30,000 deliveries and is associated with protracted labor. There is a very high mortality rate if unrecognized. The underlying physiologic response to amniotic fluid embolism is vasomotor collapse due to vasodilation (not vasoconstriction) and left ventricular dysfunction. The patient presents with profound shock and hypoxia. If obtained, the chest x-ray will likely demonstrate bilateral interstitial and alveolar infiltrated. DIC can be the presenting symptom in amniotic fluid embolism and if present, increases the likelihood of the diagnosis. Fetal squamous cells have been recovered from maternal pulmonary artery blood in suspected cases.

Treatment is directed to the presenting symptoms which usually require aggressive volume resuscitation, inotropic support, mechanical ventilation, and blood component therapy. Rapid delivery of the fetus is indicated for an amniotic fluid embolism in a viable fetus.

**Answer: B**

Clark, S.L., Pavlova, Z., and Greenspoon, J. (1986) Squamous cells in the maternal pulmonary circulation. *American Journal of Obstetrics and Gynecology*, **154**, 104–106.

Gist, R.S., Stafford, I.P., Leibowitz, A.B., and Beilin, Y. (2009) Amniotic fluid embolism. *Anesthesia and Analgesia*, **108** (5), 1599–1602.

**6** *A 23-year-old G2 P1 woman is admitted to the ICU with a persistent BP of 178/112. She has 4+ proteinuria and decreased urinary output (<30 ml/hr). Which is the best initial agent for initialing controlling her hypertension?*

**A** *Sodium Nitroprusside IV*
**B** *Labetalol IV*
**C** *Enalapril*
**D** *Valsartan*
**E** *Furosemide*

Critical care pharmacotherapy in the pregnant patient involves a comprehensive understanding of the risk and benefits to both the mother and fetus. This is best accomplished in a multiprofessional model of critical care delivery including a pharmacist in the team. All antihypertensive agents can cross the placenta. Angiotensin receptor antagonist (valsartan) and angiotensin converting enzyme inhibitors (enalapril) are known to be harmful to the fetus and should not be used if possible. Nitroprusside has the potential to develop toxic metabolites over time and with high doses and should not be the primary agent selected unless treating a life-threatening malignant hypertensive crisis. Furosemide can be used for management of hypertension and is thought to be safe for the fetus. The risk in using a loop diuretic in a pregnant patient is volume depletion, and for this reason, they should be used with caution. Labetalol can be used in the pregnant patient and because it has both alpha and beta blocking properties, which may preserve placental blood flow better than other beta blockers. While not listed as a choice, calcium channel blockers such as nifedipine have also been used to manage hypertension in pregnancy.

**Answer: B**

Cooper, W.O., Hernandez-Diaz, S., Arbogast, P.G., *et al.* (2006) Major congenital malformations after first-trimester exposure to ACE inhibitors. *New England Journal of Medicine*, **354** (23), 2443.

Magee, L.A. and Duley, L. (2003) Oral beta-blockers for mild to moderate hypertension during pregnancy. *Cochrane Database Systematic Reviews*, **4**.

**7** *A woman in her first trimester is admitted to the ICU and requires mechanical ventilation. The patient has associated renal insufficiency with a Cr of 1.9 mg/dl. Which of the following is most correct?*

**A** *Lorazepam is preferred over midazolam for sedation*

**B** *Cisatracurium is preferred over vecuronium as a paralytic agent*

**C** *ACE inhibitors are preferred over digoxin in treating congestive failure*

**D** *Fosphenytoin is preferred over levetiracetam as an anticonvulsant*

**E** *Epinephrine is preferred over ephedrine for vasopressor support*

Critical care for the pregnant patient requires a broad understanding of the fetal risk of common ICU medications. Among benzodiazepines, lorazepam has been shown to be teratogenic in animal studies, for this reason, midazolam is theoretically a superior agent. Cisatracurium is classified as FDA category B in pregnancy versus C for Vecuronium. Cisatracurium has a very favorable metabolism occurring via plasma ester hydrolysis, Hoffman Degradation. Vecuronium is metabolized by the liver and not desirable in pregnant patients with hepatic dysfunction.

Digoxin is safe in pregnancy and can be used in the management of peripartum cardiomyopathy. However, digoxin is secreted into the breast milk. ACE inhibitors have shown a definitive fetal risk and should generally not be used in pregnancy.

Fosphenytoin, which is metabolized to phenytoin, is a category D agent that can cause fetal hydantoin syndrome or fetal anticonvulsant syndrome and should generally not be used in pregnancy. While there are no

controlled studies levetiracetam is listed as a pregnancy category C medication and would be preferred over fosphenytoin.

There is no preferred vasopressor in pregnancy. Ephedrine has been shown to increase both maternal blood pressure and fetal blood flow compared to epinephrine, which does not increase fetal blood flow due to vasoconstriction.

**Answer: B**

Lee, A., Ngan Kee, W.D., and Gin, T. (2002) A quantitative, systematic review of randomized controlled trials of ephedrine versus phenylephrine for the management of hypotension during spinal anesthesia for cesarean delivery. *Anesthesia and Analgesia*, **94** (4), 920–926.

**8** *A previously healthy, 31-year-old G1 P1 woman at 39 weeks gestation is admitted to the hospital when she was noted on a routine obstetrical visit to have a petechial rash and protein in her urine dipstick test. Further testing in the hospital revealed a Hb of 10.4 mg/dL with a platelet count of 40,000 and Cr = 2.6 mg/dL. The peripheral smear of the blood demonstrates schistocytes. The rest of her lab values are normal. Her BP = 160/100 mm Hg, HR = 96 beats/min, and RR 16 breaths/min. Urinary output is decreased at <30 ml/hr for the last 3 hours. The most appropriate next step is to:*

**A** *Begin induction of labor with oxytocin*

**B** *Perform a Cesarean delivery*

**C** *Assess for elevated ADAMTS13 activity*

**D** *Begin plasma expansion with colloid*

**E** *Initiate Plasmapheresis*

This patient has microangiopathic anemia, thrombocytopenia, and renal insufficiency. This triad is associated with thrombotic thrombocytopenic purpura (TTP) and hemolytic uremic syndrome (HUS). The distinction between the two is that neurologic symptoms predominate in TTP and renal failure is the hallmark of HUS. This patient's increasing Cr and decreasing urinary output suggest she has HUS. This condition has a very high maternal and fetal mortality and needs prompt action. The clinical presentation can be confused with severe sepsis and DIC, which are more common and should be ruled out as soon as possible. The placental vessels can thrombose so that a viable fetus should be delivered as soon as possible. Induction with oxytocin and a vaginal delivery would be preferable to performing a Cesarean section in this coagulopathic woman. There is some evidence that HUS can resolve with the delivery. Since there could be some confusion that this represents severe preeclampsia with or without HELLP syndrome, prompt delivery of the fetus would also be indicated. Failure to respond following delivery confirms the diagnosis of HUS over these other causes.

ADAMTS13 is protease that cleaves the von Willebrand's factor (VWF) to promote normal clotting. In the normal pregnancy VWF increases in the third trimester and ADAMTS13 activity is reduced. With acquired TTP, antibodies are produced against ADAMTS13, and the activity of ADAMTS13 is severely decreased. HUS is caused by complement activation and referred to as complement-mediated HUS

Further management of the patient who fails to improve following delivery is plasmapheresis. While consideration for plasmapheresis before delivery should be entertained induction of labor should begin as soon as the diagnosis is entertained. While the patient likely would benefit from volume expansion and invasive monitoring they are secondary considerations in the management scheme.

**Answer: A**

Ferrari, B., Maino, A., Lotta, L.A., *et al.* (2014) Pregnancy complications in acquired thrombotic thrombocytopenic purpura: a case–control study. *Orphanet Journal of Rare Diseases*, **193**, 1–8.

Fujimura, Y., Matsumoto, M., Kokame, K., *et al.* (2009) Pregnancy-induced thrombocytopenia and TTP, and the risk of fetal death, in Upshaw–Schulman syndrome: a series of 15 pregnancies in 9 genotyped patients. *British Journal of Haematology*, **144** (5), 742–754.

Natelson, E.A. and White, D. (1985) Recurrent thrombotic thrombocytopenic purpura in early pregnancy: effect of uterine evacuation. *Obstetrics and Gynecology*, **66** (3 Suppl), 54S.

Vesely, S.K., Li, X., McMinn, J.R., *et al.* (2004) Pregnancy outcomes after recovery from thrombotic thrombocytopenic purpura-hemolytic uremic syndrome. *Transfusion*, **44** (8), 1149–1158.

9   *Pregnancy increases the likelihood of venous thromboembolism (VTE). Which of the following is characteristic in pregnancy?*
    A *VTE occurs more frequently in the right leg*
    B *Antepartum VTE is most common in the third trimester*
    C *Clots general propagate up from the calf*
    D *Resistance to activated protein C occurs in the second and third trimester*
    E *D-dimer assay is frequently negative in the pregnant patient*

Venous thromboembolic disease occurs more frequently (10–50 times) in pregnant than in nonpregnant women.

The increased risk appears to occur with the onset of pregnancy and results in VTE being equally distributed throughout all trimesters. One contributing factor is increased resistance to activated protein C in the last two trimesters and increases the hypercoagulable state of pregnancy.

Of VTE in pregnancy 80% to 90% occurs on the left side, presumably due to the pelvic venous anatomy. In many cases, these VTEs originate in the pelvis and are not the result of calf DVT, which extended proximally.

D-dimer is an ELISA assay that detects the products of fibrin degradation. Routinely used in the emergency department, a negative D-dimer makes the presence of VTE unlikely. A positive result is used to evaluate the patient further. However, in the pregnant patient D-dimer levels routinely increase in the second and third trimesters, with more than half of normal pregnant women having an elevated D-dimer level. Thus D-dimer is much less valuable as a screening tool in the pregnant patient than the nonpregnant.

**Answer: D**

Bourjeily, G., Paidas, M., Khalil, H., *et al.* (2010) Pulmonary embolism in pregnancy. *Lancet*, **375** (9713), 500–512.

Heit, J.A., Kobbervig, C.E., James, A.H., *et al.* (2005) Trends in the incidence of venous thromboembolism during pregnancy or postpartum: a 30-year population-based study. *Annals of Internal Medicine*, **143** (10), 697–706.

Marik, P.E. and Plante, L.A. (2008) Venous thromboembolic disease and pregnancy. *New England Journal of Medicine*, **359** (19), 2025–2033.

Walker, M.C., Garner, P.R., Keely, E.J., *et al.* (1997) Changes in activated protein C resistance during normal pregnancy. *American Journal of Obstetrics and Gynecology*, **177** (1), 162–169.

10   A *21-year-old G1 P1 woman admitted to the ICU five days after a Cesarean delivery for arrest of descent. Her labor was complicated by prolonged rupture of the membranes. On a postoperative day 3, she was placed on clindamycin and gentamycin for a fever of 39.1. She is now on postoperative day 5, and she looks and feels well. She currently has a BP of 105/75 mm Hg, heart rate of 115 beats/min, a temperature of 38.2, a respiratory rate of 20 breaths/min, and her WBC is 13.2 × 10³/μL. Her wound appears to be healing well, and a CT of the pelvis and blood cultures are all negative. The most appropriate next step is to:*
    A *Add fluconazole to her antimicrobial regime*
    B *Perform pelvic venography*
    C *Begin systemic anticoagulation with heparin*
    D *Schedule her for a hysterectomy*
    E *Repeat the CT scan in one week*

This patient has septic pelvic thrombophlebitis. While some patients can present several weeks postpartum, most patients present 3–5 days postpartum with a persistent fever *despite* antibiotics. The clinical exam may be relatively benign and the patient not appearing severely ill. Rick factors include Cesarean section, arrested descent, and pelvic infections. Antibiotic administration along with systemic anticoagulation is the initial treatment of choice for this condition. Diagnosis can be difficult and requires a high index of suspicion. While most patients will have an elevated white blood cell count blood, cultures are frequently negative. Still, blood culture should be done because, if positive, it can assist in antibiotic selection. Without a positive culture, antibiotics should be directed towards Gram-positive cocci and enteric organisms including anaerobes.

There is no single imaging study that can reliably diagnose septic pelvic thrombophlebitis, especially septic thrombophlebitis of the deep veins. While CT and MRI have a better sensitivity than ultrasound, a negative study does not rule out the presence of a septic pelvic thrombophlebitis. Venography will not visualize the uterine veins.

There is no evidence that the patient has a systemic fungal infection and with only two days of antibiotic therapy, this is unlikely. Removal of the uterus is rarely indicated for septic pelvic thrombophlebitis, and in this patient, it is not the first choice for management.

**Answer: C**

Garcia, J., Aboujaoude, R., Apuzzio, J., and Alvare, J.R. (2006) Septic pelvic thrombophlebitis: diagnosis and management. *Infectious Diseases in Obstetrics and Gynecology*, 15614.

Pastorek, J.G. (1994) Septic pelvic-vein thrombophlebitis, in *Obstetric and Gynecologic Infectious Disease* (ed. J.G. Pastorek), Raven Press, New York, pp. 165–170.

Twickler, D.M., Setiawan, A.T., Evans, R.S., *et al.* (1997) Imaging of puerperal septic thrombophlebitis: prospective comparison of MR imaging, CT, and sonography. *American Journal of Roentgenology*, **169** (4), 1039–1043.

**11** *A 27-year-old woman at 23 weeks gestation with no prior medical problems presents to the emergency department due to the sudden onset of shortness of breath while at home. She is diaphoretic and using her accessory muscles to breathe. She has received one-liter normal saline. Her current BP = 78/50 mm Hg, HR = 142 beats/min, RR = 36 breaths/min, $SaO_2$ = 80% on a 100% nonrebreathing mask. Her chest X-ray is unremarkable.*

**A** *TPA should be administered if she remains hypotensive*

**B** *Apixaban administration in the first hour is associated with improved outcomes*

**C** *D-dimer levels can be used to determine if a spiral CT is justified*

**D** *Heparin is contraindicated without performing a confirmatory test*

**E** *Helical CT scan is associated with a significant fetal radiation exposure*

The risk of venous thromboembolic disease is significantly increased in pregnancy. A patient in her third trimester who presents with the sudden onset of hypoxia, hypotension, and a normal chest X-ray should be considered to have a pulmonary embolism until proven otherwise.

The use of thrombolytic agents in pregnancy associated pulmonary embolism has been successful. The key is to balance the risk and benefits based on the patient's condition. Compared to heparin, thrombolytics have an increased risk of causing bleeding. This patient is profoundly hypotensive and hypoxic and if uncorrected rapidly threatens both the mother and fetus. The risk of bleeding is about 6% in these patients and needs to be balanced against the risk of fetal hypoxia. In this situation, thrombolytics should be administered if she remains hypotensive.

There is no demonstrated benefit directly associated with early Apixaban administration in VTE. Due to a paucity of safety information, Apixaban is not recommended in pregnancy. While low molecular weight heparin is used during pregnancy, especially for long-term treatment, this patient is hypotensive, and heparinization via IV unfractionated heparin is effective immediately and can be reversed with protamine in the event of bleeding. Heparin should be administered when there is a strong clinical suspicion for a pulmonary embolism and before all diagnostic testing is complete.

D-dimer is an ELISA assay that detects the products of fibrin degradation. Routinely used in the emergency department, a negative D-dimer makes the presence of VTE unlikely. A positive result is used to evaluate the patient further. However, in the pregnant patient D-dimer levels routinely increase in the second and third trimesters, with more than half of normal pregnant women having an elevated D-dimer level. Thus D-dimer is much less valuable as a screening tool in the pregnant patient than the nonpregnant.

Spiral CT is the diagnostic study of choice for pulmonary embolism and should not be withheld due to a fear of radiation exposure to the fetus. While all ionizing radiation can lead to radiation damage it is generally believed that the amount of radiation from a spiral CT scan is insufficient to cause fetal deformity.

**Answer: A**

Ahearn, G.S., Hadjiliadis, D., Govert, J.A., and Tapson, V.F. (2002) Massive pulmonary embolism during pregnancy successfully treated with recombinant tissue plasminogen activator: a case report and review of treatment options. *Archives of Internal Medicines*, **162** (11), 1221–1228.

Bourjeily, G., Paidas, M., Khalil, H., *et al.* (2010) Pulmonary embolism in pregnancy. *Lancet*, **375** (9713), 500–512.

Turrentine, M.A., Braems, G., and Ramirez, M.M. (1995) Use of thrombolytics for the treatment of thromboembolic disease during pregnancy. *Obstetrical and Gynecological Survey*, **50** (7), 534–541.

Winer-Muram, H.T., Boone, J.M., Brown, H.L., *et al.* (2002) Pulmonary embolism in pregnant patients: fetal radiation dose with helical CT. *Radiology*, **224** (2), 487–492.

**12**  *A woman presents to the emergency department 1 week after an emergency Cesarean delivery complaining of lower abdominal tenderness and fever. The wound appears clean and is nontender. Her temperature is 38.6 °C, and the WBC count is $17.1 \times 10^3/\mu L$ with two bands. You are concerned she has postpartum endometritis. In this condition:*

**A**  *Early hysterectomy improves outcomes*

**B**  *The predominant organism is Streptococcus*

**C**  *The diagnosis is confirmed by visualizing gas in the uterus on CT scan*

**D**  *Gentamycin is the drug of choice*

**E**  *Can be reduced by a prophylactic dose of a first-generation cephalosporin.*

Prophylactic antibiotics, such as a first-generation cephalosporin, can reduce the incidence of endometritis by two-thirds to three-quarters in women having a Cesarean section. The majority of cases are polymicrobial and involving both aerobes and anaerobes. For this reason recommended antimicrobial coverage needs to be broad spectrum. An agent like Gentamycin has no anaerobic activity and would require an additional agent such as clindamycin.

Regimens with activity against penicillin-resistant anaerobic bacteria are better than those without. The diagnosis is usually made on the clinical basis of fever, foul lochia and uterine tenderness in a woman following Cesarean section. Imaging studies are used to rule out other diagnoses such as a pelvic abscess. Most often the CT is nonspecific and does not rely on visualizing gas in the endometrium.

Once uncomplicated endometritis has clinically improved with intravenous therapy, oral therapy is not needed. Failure to respond in 48 hours should raise the possibility of another condition and should be investigated. The differential diagnosis should include septic pelvic thrombophlebitis and pelvic abscess as well as other common postoperative infections.

**Answer: E**

French, L.M. and Smaill, F.M. (2004) Antibiotic regimens for endometritis after delivery. *Cochrane Database Systematic Reviews*, **18** (4).

Smaill, F. and Hofmeyr, G.J (2002) Antibiotic prophylaxis for cesarean section. *Cochrane Database Systematic Review*, **2**.

**13**  *A woman at 36 weeks gestation is admitted to the ICU with severe eclampsia. Antihypertensive therapy is initiated, and her blood pressure is 180/110 mm Hg. The patient complains of headaches, visual disturbances, and appears to be confused. Computed tomography (CT) demonstrates symmetric hypodensities that involve the occipitoparietal regions of the brain. An MRI of the brain demonstrates punctate and confluent hyperintense areas in the parietooccipital lobes. With respect to this condition:*

**A**  *Is generally limited to patients in their third trimester of pregnancy*

**B**  *Frequently presents with status epilepticus resistant to magnesium sulfate*

**C**  *These radiographic findings are expected to resolve in 1–2 weeks with treatment*

**D**  *Rarely necessitates delivery of the fetus*

**E**  *Is associated with a high risk of intracerebral hemorrhage when not treated*

This patient has posterior reversible encephalopathy syndrome or PRES, also referred to as reversible posterior cerebral edema syndrome or posterior leukoencephalopathy syndrome. Risk factors for PRES include hypertensive conditions, pre-eclampsia, and the immunosuppressants tacrolimus and cyclosporine. Clinically patients have headaches, mental status changes, confusion, and seizures. Diagnosis is confirmed with an MRI demonstrating vasogenic edema predominantly localized to the posterior cerebral hemispheres. With prompt treatment, the patient improves rapidly, and the MRI changes usually resolve in 1 to 2 weeks. In the pregnant patient with pre-eclampsia, magnesium sulfate is the drug of choice for PRES seizures. Prompt delivery of the fetus is usually therapeutic. PRES can occur anytime in the peripartum period as well in nonpregnant patients. There is no increased risk of intracranial hemorrhage in the patients with PRES.

**Answer: C**

Finocchi, V., Bozzao, A., Bonamini, M., *et al.* (2005) Magnetic resonance imaging in posterior reversible encephalopathy syndrome: report of three cases and review of literature. *Archives of Gynecology and Obstetrics*, **271** (1), 79–85.

Lamy, C., Oppenheim, C., Méder, J.F., and Mas, J.L. (2004) Neuroimaging in posterior reversible encephalopathy syndrome. *Journal of Neuroimaging*, **14** (2), 89–96.

**14** *A 27-year-old G1 P0 woman at 32 weeks gestation is admitted to the hospital with a diagnosis of preterm labor. Her cervix is 3 cm dilated. She is given a loading dose 4 gm IV magnesium sulfate followed by a 2 gm/h infusion. Soon after the loading dose of magnesium sulfate is infused she becomes lethargic, acutely short of breath, and her SaO$_2$ decreases to 87%. The most appropriate next step is to:*

**A** *Administer 250 ml of 3% sodium chloride solution*

**B** *Administer 5000 units heparin IV and obtain a STAT spiral CT*

**C** *Administer 10 ml of 10% Calcium chloride*

**D** *Perform an emergency Cesarean section*

**E** *Administer 20 µg/min terbutaline infusion*

This woman has tocolytic associated pulmonary edema. Volume overload is usually a contributing factor and patients present with signs and symptoms similar to other forms of pulmonary edema. The initial management consists of discontinuing the offending tocolytic, in this case, magnesium sulfate. It is important to rule out other causes of hypoxia, in this patient who had symptoms develop with the infusion of magnesium along with the accompanying lethargy suggest magnesium sulfate as the etiology. Without this association consideration to a sudden pulmonary embolism should be given and heparin and spiral CT scan would be a reasonable answer. The management tocolytic associated pulmonary edema from magnesium includes administration of 10 ml of 10% calcium chloride to counteract the effects of the magnesium. Other standard therapies such as oxygen and judicious diuresis should be given as well.

Unless there is evidence given of fetal distress Cesarean section and urgent delivery are not necessary. However, discontinuation of the tocolytic can result in a return of preterm labor. Resolution of the pulmonary edema usually occurs within 12–24 hours. Adding an additional tocolytic (terbutaline) or additional volume expansion (3% sodium chloride) will likely worsen the pulmonary edema and should not be chosen.

**Answer: C**

Samol, J.M. and Lambers, D.S. (2005) Magnesium sulfate tocolysis, and pulmonary edema: the drug or the vehicle? *American Journal of Obstetrics and Gynecology*, **192** (5), 1430–1432.

Sciscione, A.C., Ivester, T., and Largoza, M., *et al.* (2003) Acute pulmonary edema in pregnancy. *Obstetrics and Gynecology*, **101** (3), 511–515.

# 24

# Pediatric Critical Care
*Erin M. Garvey, MD and J. Craig Egan, MD*

1  *Compared to nonprotocolized care, use of a protocolized emergency department sepsis guideline is independently associated with*
   **A**  *Decreased organ dysfunction by hospital day 2*
   **B**  *Need for packed red blood cell transfusion*
   **C**  *Decrease in hospital mortality*
   **D**  *Need for vasoactive support*
   **E**  *Increased isolation of causative bacterial organism*

Protocolized emergency department sepsis guideline patients were more likely to be organ dysfunction (OD) free on hospital day 1 and hospital day 2. Protocol patients without OD were less likely to develop new OD in the first two hospital days. Protocol patients compared with usual care patients had shorter PICU and hospital LOS, and were less likely to have subsequent transfer to a higher level of care if initially admitted to the inpatient floor within 24 hours of ED arrival. There was no difference in hospital mortality between groups. Protocol patients had shorter time to initial IV antibiotics, initial IV fluid bolus, and third IV fluid bolus compared with usual care patients. Protocol patients also received a higher total volume of fluid per kg in the ED compared with usual care patients. There was no difference in need for blood transfusion, need for vasoactive support, or isolation of causative bacterial organism.

**Answer: A**

Balamuth, F., Weiss, S.L., Fitzgerald, J.C., *et al.* (2016) Protocolized treatment is associated with decreased organ dysfunction in pediatric severe sepsis. *Pediatric Critical Care Medicine*, **17**, 817–822.

2  *Early albumin infusion in children with burns greater than 15–45% total body surface area is associated with*
   **A**  *Higher 30-day mortality rate*
   **B**  *Reduced need for crystalloid fluid infusion during resuscitation with significantly fewer cases of fluid creep and shorter hospital stay*
   **C**  *Higher risk of progression to full-thickness burns and higher number of surgical procedures (debridement and grafting) performed*
   **D**  *Decreased rate of intraabdominal hypertension*
   **E**  *Higher median urine output*

There is still some controversy regarding the use of albumin in the treatment of burn patients. Fluid resuscitation of children with burn injuries is a major challenge due to greater intolerance to overresuscitation or under-resuscitation and to their diminished physiologic reserve compared with burned adults.

In a randomized controlled trial, it was hypothesized that albumin administered at 8–12 hours, rather than 24 hours after burn injury, would reduce fluid requirements, fluid creep, and length of hospital stay in children with extensive burns. The two groups received IV lactated Ringer's (LR) solution according to a modified Parkland formula (3 mL × TBSA × weight in kg) during the first 24 hours postburn. In addition to LR resuscitation, children weighing less than 30 kg also received maintenance fluids and electrolytes based on the Holliday-Segar formula in the form of isotonic saline solution (ISS) plus glucose to maintain normoglycemia while in a fasting state, which was gradually tapered down according to the rate of enteral feeding advancement. Enteral feeding was introduced as soon as possible, approximately 6 hours after arrival at the hospital. After 24 hours, the volume of LR solution was reduced to 1.5 mL × TBSA × weight in kg, associated with half of the ISS volume. Participants assigned to the intervention group received colloid in the form of 5% human albumin solution (0.5 g of albumin per kg body weight) between 8 and 12 hours after the burn accident (4-hr infusion) once daily for 3 days.

The hypothesis was confirmed as early albumin infusion allowed a reduction in fluid requirements on day 1 (−31.9%), maintenance of the reduced fluid requirements on day 2 (−19.37%), and ending resuscitation with a significantly lower fluid volume (−45.3%) on day 3 compared with delayed albumin infusion. Significantly fewer cases of fluid creep and shorter hospital stay were also observed among patients who received albumin earlier. However, there was no significant difference between groups regarding the number of surgical procedures (debridement and grafting) performed. Patients in the intervention group required less crystalloid fluid than controls over the first 3 days postburn. The median urine output was no different between groups. Duration of hospitalization was shorter for patients in the intervention group than for controls. There were no cases of intraabdominal hypertension or death in the sample studied.

**Answer: B**

Muller Dittrich, M.H., Brunow de Carvalho, W., and Lopes Lavado, E. (2016) Evaluation of the early use of albumin in children with extensive burns: A randomized controlled trial. *Pediatric Critical Care Medicine*, **17**, e280–e286.

3 *As a monitoring modality in pediatric patients, near infrared spectroscopy (NIRS) provides a continuous noninvasive assessment of tissue oxygenation and most closely correlates with which of the following?*
   A *Arterial oxygen saturation (SaO2)*
   B *Base deficit*
   C *Superior vena cava saturations (ScVO2) and mixed venous saturation (SmVO2)*
   D *Arterial partial pressure of oxygen (PaO2)*
   E *Arterial partial pressure of carbon dioxide (PaCO2)*

Multisite cerebral and somatic NIRS monitoring of patients in critical care units provides a continuous, non-invasive, real-time assessment of regional perfusion in patients at risk for multiorgan dysfunction and death. Several studies have reported the relationship between cerebral regional oxygen saturation (rSo2), somatic rSo2, and superior vena cava saturations (ScV02). Since the mixed venous saturation (SmVo2) is the flow-weighted average of regional venous saturations, attempts to show a univariate correlation between single site rSo2 and the SmVo2 should be viewed as oversimplified, just as the ScV02 shows variable agreement with SmVo2 under varying conditions. A global quasi-SmVo2 can be reasonably approximated by NIRS models that include multiple sites. The somatic-cerebral saturation difference (rSo2S−rSo2C) is characteristically 10–20% in health, but approaches 0 or negative values with the redistribution of limited systemic blood flow. In healthy neonates with normal Sao2, the at-rest average cerebral rSo2 was 78% with a somatic rSo2 of 88%, demonstrating higher oxygen extraction across the cerebral bed compared with the renal-somatic bed. In a study of healthy adults, mean

baseline cerebral rSo2 was 70% compared with 65% in adults just prior to cardiac surgery. Early work by Kurth *et al.* established baseline values for cerebral rSo2 in infants and children with and without congenital heart disease. Healthy children and those with acyanotic heart disease had baseline cerebral rSo2 values similar to the adult population with an arterial saturation (Sao2) − cerebral rSo2 difference of approximately 30%. In patients with cyanotic heart disease, cerebral rSo2 values were 46–57% with a wider Sao2–rSo2 difference of nearly 40% in patients with the hypoplastic left heart syndrome (HLHS).

In premature neonates, the quantification of somatic ischemia by the somatic-cerebral saturation relationship was more predictive of the development of necrotizing enterocolitis than the somatic rSo2 alone. Thus characterizing regional blood flow, not only by the absolute rSo2 but also by the comparative relationships between different organ beds, is useful in the interpretation of these physiologic measures. Changes in cerebral and somatic tissue oxygenation during feeding in healthy neonates were not significant, as would be expected with good physiologic reserve.

**Answer: C**

Ghanayem, N.S. and Hoffman, G.M. (2016) Near-infrared spectroscopy as a hemodynamic monitor in critical illness. *Pediatric Critical Care Medicine*, **17**, S201–S206.

4 *Regarding packed red blood cell transfusion in pediatric critically-ill patients:*
   A *Using a liberal transfusion threshold (Hb of 9.5g/ dL), does not confer any clinical benefit over a restrictive threshold (Hb of 7g/dL)*
   B *Is associated with decreased risk of death*
   C *Keeping Hb > 9.5g/dL results in lower MODS*
   D *The same transfusion threshold should be used for neonates and older children*
   E *Weaning from mechanical ventilation depends upon a Hb level > 10 g/dL*

Many risks are associated with PRBC transfusions, including infections, immunosuppression, transfusion reactions, fluid overload, and medical errors. Controlling for age and severity of illness at admission, PRBC transfusion was found to be significantly associated with increased risk of death, cardiac arrest, nosocomial infections, longer PICU stay, and longer time requiring mechanical ventilation.

The Transfusion Requirements in Pediatric Intensive Care Units study (multi-institutional, randomized, controlled trial evaluating PRBC transfusion in PICU patients) randomized to either transfusion threshold

9.5 g/dL (liberal criteria) or 7 g/dL (restrictive criteria) using leukocyte-reduced PRBC. Deaths, MODS, adverse events, ventilator days, and nosocomial infections were not significantly different in the two groups. When split into subgroups of pediatric cardiac surgery patients (125 patients) and pediatric general surgery patients (124 patients), the restrictive PRBC transfusion strategy showed no increase in MODS. Using a liberal transfusion threshold does not confer any clinical benefit over a restrictive threshold of Hb 7 g/dL. This threshold does not apply to neonatal patients or patients with active bleeding or severe hemodynamic instability. PRBC transfusions appear to be independently linked to increased risk of morbidity and mortality in critically ill pediatric patients.

**Answer: A**

Tyrrell, C.T. and Bateman, S.T. (2012) Critically ill children: to transfuse or not to transfuse packed red blood cells, that is the question. *Pediatric Critical Care Medicine*, **13**, 204–209.

5 *Definition of Pediatric Acute Respiratory Distress Syndrome (PARDS) includes chest imaging with new infiltrate(s) consistent with acute pulmonary parenchymal disease, respiratory failure not fully explained by cardiac failure or fluid overload, and*
   A *Known perinatal-related lung disease*
   B *Symptoms occur greater than 7 days after known clinical insult*

C *P/F ratio ≤ 300 on noninvasive mechanical ventilation*
D *Oxygen index (OI) < 4 on invasive mechanical ventilation*
E *Oxygen saturation index (OSI) < 5 on invasive mechanical ventilation*

Pediatric intensivists have recognized that ARDS in children (see Figure 24.1) is different from ARDS in adults.

**Answer: C**

Pediatric Acute Lung Injury Consensus Conference (PALICC) Group (2015) Pediatric acute respiratory distress syndrome: consensus recommendations from the pediatric acute lung injury consensus conference. *Pediatric Critical Care Medicine*, **16**, 428–439.

6 *Regarding conventional ventilation support for PARDS:*
   A *Only pressure control should be used*
   B *Tidal volumes should be 4-7 ml/kg*
   C *Inspiratory plateau pressure limit should be <24 cm H2O*
   D *PEEP should be kept < 10 cm H2O*
   E *Routine use of high-frequency jet ventilation is not recommended*

There are no outcome data on the influence of mode (control or assisted) during conventional mechanical ventilation. Therefore, no recommendations can be made on the ventilator mode to be used in patients with

| Age | Exclude patients with peri-natal related lung disease | | | |
|---|---|---|---|---|
| Timing | Within 7 days of known clinical insult | | | |
| Origin of Edema | Respiratory failure not fully explained by cardiac failure or fluid overload | | | |
| Chest Imaging | Chest imaging findings of new infiltrate(s) consistent with acute pulmonary parenchymal disease | | | |
| | **Non Invasive mechanical ventilation** | **Invasive mechanical ventilation** | | |
| | PARDS (No severity stratification) | Mild | Moderate | Severe |
| Oxygenation | Full face-mask bi-level ventilation or CPAP ≥ 5 cm H₂O² | 4 ≤ OI < 8 | 8 ≤ OI < 16 | OI ≥ 16 |
| | PF ratio ≤ 300 SF ratio ≤ 264¹ | 5 ≤ OSI < 7.5¹ | 7.5 ≤ OSI < 12.3¹ | OSI ≥ 12.3¹ |
| | **Special Populations** | | | |
| Cyanotic Heart Disease | Standard Criteria above for age, timing, origin of edema and chest imaging with an acute deterioration in oxygenation not explained by underlying cardiac disease.³ | | | |
| Chronic Lung Disease | Standard Criteria above for age, timing, and origin of edema with chest imaging consistent with new infiltrate and acute deterioration in oxygenation from baseline which meet oxygenation criteria above.³ | | | |
| Left Ventricular dysfunction | Standard Criteria for age, timing and origin of edema with chest imaging changes consistent with new infiltrate and acute deterioration in oxygenation which meet criteria above not explained by left ventricular dysfunction. | | | |

**Figure 24.1**

PARDS. The PALICC group recommends using patient-specific tidal volumes according to disease severity. Tidal volumes should be 3–6 mL/kg predicted body weight for patients with poor respiratory system compliance and closer to the physiologic range (5–8 mL/kg ideal body weight) for patients with better preserved respiratory system compliance.

In the absence of transpulmonary pressure measurements, an inspiratory plateau pressure limit of 28 cm $H_2O$, allowing for slightly higher plateau pressures (29–32 cm $H_2O$) for patients with increased chest wall elastance (i.e., reduced chest wall compliance) is recommended.

Moderately elevated levels of PEEP (10–15 cm $H_2O$) can be titrated to the observed oxygenation and hemodynamic response in patients with severe PARDS, and PEEP levels greater than 15 cm $H_2O$ may be needed for severe PARDS, although attention should be paid to limiting the plateau pressure as previously described. High-frequency oscillatory ventilation (HFOV) should be considered as an alternative ventilator mode in hypoxic respiratory failure in patients in whom plateau airway pressures exceed 28 cm $H_2O$ in the absence of clinical evidence of reduced chest wall compliance. Such an approach should be considered for those patients with moderate-to-severe PARDS. In HFOV the optimal lung volume can be achieved by exploration of the potential for lung recruitment by a stepwise increase and decrease of the Paw (continuous distending pressure) under continuous monitoring of the oxygenation and $CO_2$ response as well as hemodynamic variables. The routine use of high-frequency jet ventilation (HFJV) in children with PARDS is not recommended. However, in addition to the use of HFOV, HFJV might be considered in patients with severe air leak syndrome. High-frequency percussive ventilation (HFPV) is not recommended for routine ventilatory management of PARDS but can be considered in patients with PARDS and secretion-induced lung collapse that cannot be resolved with routine clinical care (e.g. inhalational injuries).

**Answer: E**

Pediatric Acute Lung Injury Consensus Conference (PALICC) Group (2015) Pediatric acute respiratory distress syndrome: consensus recommendations from the pediatric acute lung injury consensus conference. *Pediatric Critical Care Medicine*, **16**, 428–439.

**7** *Mechanical ventilatory support for PARDS should be titrated to*
   **A** *Keep SpO2 > 92%*
   **B** *Allow permissive hypercapnia in all cases*
   **C** *Maintain pH in range of 7.15–7.30*
   **D** *Keep patient comfortable*
   **E** *Keep PEEP > 10*

After optimizing PEEP, lower Spo2 levels (in the range of 88–92%) should be considered for those with PARDS with PEEP at least 10 cm $H_2O$, and permissive hypercapnia should be considered for moderate-to-severe PARDS to minimize ventilator-induced lung injury. pH should be maintained between 7.15–7.30 within lung-protective strategy guidelines and there are insufficient data to recommend a lower limit for pH. Exceptions to permissive hypercapnia should include intracranial hypertension, severe pulmonary hypertension, select congenital heart disease lesions, hemodynamic instability, and significant ventricular dysfunction.

**Answer: C**

Pediatric Acute Lung Injury Consensus Conference (PALICC) Group (2015) Pediatric acute respiratory distress syndrome: consensus recommendations from the pediatric acute lung injury consensus conference. *Pediatric Critical Care Medicine*, **16**, 428–439.

**8** *Which of the following is recommended for ancillary treatment for PARDS?*
   **A** *Prone positioning can be considered in cases of severe PARDS*
   **B** *Bicarbonate supplementation to keep pH > 7.20*
   **C** *Inhaled nitric oxide in mild cases of PARDS*
   **D** *Surfactant therapy*
   **E** *Intratracheal N-acetylcysteine*

Bicarbonate supplementation is not routinely recommended. Inhaled nitric oxide is not recommended for routine use in PARDS, however, its use may be considered in patients with documented pulmonary hypertension or severe right ventricular dysfunction. In addition, it may be considered in severe cases of PARDS as a rescue from, or bridge to, extracorporeal life support. When used, assessment of benefit must be undertaken promptly and serially to minimize toxicity and to eliminate continued use without established effect. At this time, surfactant therapy cannot be recommended as routine therapy in PARDS. Prone positioning cannot be recommended as routine therapy in PARDS; however, it should be considered an option in cases of severe PARDS. There are insufficient data to recommend chest physiotherapy as a standard of care in the patient with PARDS. At this time, corticosteroids cannot be recommended as routine therapy in PARDS. No recommendation for the use of the following ancillary treatments is supported: helium-oxygen mixture, inhaled or IV prostaglandins therapy, plasminogen activators, fibrinolytics, or other anticoagulants, inhaled β-adrenergic receptor agonists or ipratropium, IV *N*-acetylcysteine for antioxidant effects or intratracheal *N*-acetylcysteine for mobilizing secretions, dornase alpha outside of the cystic fibrosis population, and a cough-assist device.

No recommendation for the use of stem cell therapy can be supported.

**Answer: A**

Pediatric Acute Lung Injury Consensus Conference (PALICC) Group (2015) Pediatric acute respiratory distress syndrome: consensus recommendations from the pediatric acute lung injury consensus conference. *Pediatric Critical Care Medicine*, **16**, 428–439.

9  *Compared to those without a blush, pediatric blunt abdominal trauma patients with hepatic or splenic blush on computed tomography have*
   A  *Higher correlation with seatbelt signs*
   B  *Higher mortality rate*
   C  *Higher chance of needing embolization or operation*
   D  *No correlation with grade of injury*
   E  *Higher likelihood of needing blood transfusion*

Overall, blush was an uncommon event, occurring in 30 (9%) of 318 patients with hepatic or splenic injury; 18 cases of hepatic blush and 16 cases of splenic blush (four patients had injuries involving blush from both organs). Incidence of blush was found to correlate with higher grades of injury (AAST Grade IV and V). Twenty (67%) of the 30 blush patients presented with Grade IV or V hepatic or splenic injuries. Blush correlated significantly with ISS score; 80% of the blush population had overall injury severity scores greater than 15. Blush was not found to correlate significantly with age, gender, organ injured, or presence of a seatbelt sign. Of patients with a blush 50% needed a blood transfusion compared to only 12% of patients without a blush. Overall mortality was not found to be significantly different between the two populations (7% blush vs. 2% no blush). Among the blush population, two cases (7%) went to angiography, with one case (3%) of embolization; six blush cases (20%) went to the operating room. Importantly, only 17% of patients with blush (5 of the 30 patients) required definitive treatment, such as embolization, packing, or splenectomy. When blush is present, the crossover from nonoperative to operative or radiologic intervention is so small that the success rates for nonoperative management continue to be overwhelming.

**Answer: E**

Ingram, M.C., Siddharthan, R.V., Morris, A.D., *et al.* (2016) Hepatic and splenic blush on computed tomography in children following blunt abdominal trauma: Is intervention necessary? *Journal of Trauma and Acute Care Surgery*, **81**, 266–270.

10  *Comparing epinephrine to dopamine for treatment of fluid-refractory septic shock, epinephrine resulted in*
    A  *Less organ-failure free days*
    B  *Earlier resolution of shock*
    C  *More fluid boluses*
    D  *More adverse events*
    E  *More need for packed red blood cell transfusion*

The Surviving Sepsis Campaign 2012 guidelines endorse dopamine as first-line vasoactive agent in fluid-refractory septic shock. This recommendation is based more on the knowledge of pharmacologic effects of dopamine rather than strong clinical evidence. Dopamine has dose-dependent agonist effects on dopaminergic and adrenergic ($\alpha$ and $\beta$) receptors. In the general dosing range of 5–10 µg/kg/min, dopamine is inotropic via $\beta$-adrenergic stimulation; in the dosing range ~10–15 µg/kg/min, in addition to predominant inotropic effect, dopamine has a mild vasopressor effect via $\alpha 1$-adrenergic stimulation; and in the dose range of more than 15 µg/kg/min, it is predominantly a vasopressor (via $\alpha 1$-adrenergic effect) with minimal inotropic action. Epinephrine, on the other hand, has the advantage of predictable response and increasing mean arterial pressure and cardiac output, in the absence of immunosuppression. At lower infusion doses (0.05–0.2 µg/kg/min), epinephrine provides predominantly inotropic support via $\beta 1$ receptor stimulation and modest vasodilatation via $\beta 2$ receptor stimulation. At doses more than 0.2 µg/kg/min, epinephrine leads to increase in systemic vascular resistance by causing peripheral vasoconstriction due to $\alpha 1$ receptor stimulation along with $\beta 1$-mediated inotropic action. In the comparison of dopamine infusion dosage ranging from 10 to 20 µg/kg/min with epinephrine infusion dosage ranging from 0.1 to 0.3 µg/kg/min, resolution of shock in the first hour was more likely with epinephrine as compared to dopamine. Epinephrine group also had more organ failure-free days than the dopamine group, which was statistically significant. The groups were similar with respect to administration of crystalloid fluid boluses, vasopressors, and inodilator infusion, packed red cell transfusion within first 6 hours of enrollment, and renal replacement therapy. Adverse events were recorded in four children (13.8%) in the epinephrine group and five (16.1%) in the dopamine group. Between the two groups, there was no statistically significant difference in adverse events.

**Answer: B**

Ramaswamy, K.N., Singhi, S., Jayashree, M., *et al.* (2016) Double-blinded randomized clinical trial comparing dopamine and epinephrine in pediatric fluid-refractory hypotensive septic shock. *Pediatric Critical Care Medicine*, **17**, e502–e512.

**11** *In the pediatric intensive care unit population, which of the following increases the risk of ventilator-associated pneumonia?*
   **A** *Male gender*
   **B** *Body mass index*
   **C** *Nasogastric enteral nutrition*
   **D** *Younger age*
   **E** *Acid-suppressive therapy*

After adjusting for enteral nutrition (EN) days, illness severity, and site, ventilator-associated pneumonia (VAP) was significantly associated with mechanical ventilation of more than 10 days, PICU length of stay for more than 10 days, and the use of acid-suppressive medication. A significant incremental increase in the probability of VAP was detected, ranging from 1% (0–3%) when none of the factors were present, 4% (2–5%) with the use of acid-suppressive therapy, to 20% (14–28%) when all three risk factors were present. VAP was diagnosed in 6.5% of mechanically ventilated children in a large heterogeneous multicenter cohort. There was not a link between EN duration or route of delivery and VAP. No increase risk was associated with gender, BMI, enteral nutrition route, or age.

**Answer: E**

Albert, B.D., Zurakowski, D., and Bechard, L.J. (2016) Enteral nutrition and acid-suppressive therapy in the PICU: Impact on the risk of ventilator-associated pneumonia. *Pediatric Critical Care Medicine*, **17**, 924–929.

**12** *Which of the following has been associated with improved enteral nutrition tolerance in pediatric critical care unit patients?*
   **A** *Gastric residual volume measurements used to adjust feeding rate*
   **B** *Use of nutritional algorithms*
   **C** *Postpyloric feeding*
   **D** *Adjusting paralytics and vasoactive drugs*
   **E** *Metoclopramide administration*

Gastric dysmotility may be a consequence of critical illness and the therapies provided in this setting. In critically ill children, the prevalence of delayed gastric emptying (GE) has been estimated to be 50%. Gastric dysmotility may be associated with gastroesophageal reflux, which might increase the risk for aspiration of gastric contents and subsequent VAP in mechanically ventilated patients. Inadequate delivery of EN has been associated with poor clinical outcomes, such as worsening of underlying malnutrition, longer mechanical ventilation days, longer PICU stay, multiple organ dysfunction,

and increased mortality. Lack of EN may also be associated with bacterial overgrowth, altered gut integrity, and, hence, risk for bacterial translocation and systemic infection. Paralytics or vasoactive agents are often seen as barriers to EN due to their perceived effects on gastrointestinal motility. However, there is limited and equivocal evidence to support the negative effects of these drugs on gastrointestinal motility. In mechanically ventilated adults, paralytic agents were not associated with delayed GE. In critically ill children, postpyloric nutrition was associated with lower gastric residual volumes (GRV) but no difference in other markers of EN intolerance when compared with gastric nutrition. Surveys have shown that most bedside PICU providers use GRV measurements and feeding algorithms include GRV measurement as a measure of EN intolerance to guide bedside nutrition practices. The accuracy of GRV measurement to predict delayed GE or EN intolerance has not been studied in critically ill children. In critically ill children, the most common promotility agents in use are erythromycin and metoclopramide, but only erythromycin has been studied for its efficacy in preterm infants. In a study of mechanically ventilated children, postpyloric nutrition was associated with lower GRVs and improved EN delivery when compared with gastric nutrition. However, the frequency of aspiration and other markers of EN intolerance were similar between the two groups. The benefits of postpyloric nutrition have not been demonstrated in clinical trials, and postpyloric tube placement requires expertise. In circumstances when EN cannot be advanced, trophic EN (small nonnutritive amounts of EN) has been shown to provide similar benefits to early EN. The use of nutrition algorithms in PICUs has been associated with improved EN tolerance and delivery.

**Answer: B**

Martinez, E.E., Douglas, K., Nurko, S., *et al.* (2015) Gastric dysmotility in critically ill children: Pathophysiology, diagnosis and management. *Pediatric Critical Care Medicine*, **16**, 828–836.

**13** *Which of the following is true regarding venous thromboembolism (VTE) in pediatric trauma patients?*
   **A** *VTE is more common in pediatric trauma patients than in adult trauma patients*
   **B** *VTE frequency has been decreasing*
   **C** *Pelvic and femoral fractures double the risk of VTE*
   **D** *Central venous catheters do NOT increase risk of VTE*
   **E** *High Injury Severity Score ≥ 9, GCS ≤ 8, and blood transfusions increase risk for VTE*

In trauma patients 21 years and younger, the incidence of VTE is considerably lower, in the range of 0.1–0.6%. Although VTE is much less common in children compared with adults, the overall incidence of hospitalized pediatric patients diagnosed with VTE has increased by 70% in the past decade. The overall prevalence of VTE in this 2011–2012 National Trauma Data Base (NTDB) cohort was 0.41%, compared with 0.28% from the Johns Hopkins Trauma Registry. Undergoing an operation and receiving a blood transfusion were identified as risk factors for VTE. In addition, patients that were more severely injured (with an ISS $\geq$ 9 and/or Glasgow Coma Scale [GCS] $\leq$ 8) as well as those with longer hospital stays were at increased odds for developing a VTE (unadjusted odds ratios). After adjustment by multivariable logistic regression, each of these remained statistically significant independent risk factors for the development of VTE with trauma (adjusted odds ratios). In both the Johns Hopkins Trauma Registry and the 2008–2010 NTDB, increasing age, higher ISS, lower GCS, blood transfusions, and surgery were found to be independent risk factors for VTE. CVCs have been associated with VTE in several studies; however, we found that the majority of trauma patients with VTE did not have CVC-associated VTEs. It is also worth noting that although pelvic and femur fractures in adults are recognized as a risk factor for VTE, in our study we found that orthopedic injuries or blunt trauma were not independent risks for VTE in pediatric patients. Similarly, other studies in children with trauma did not demonstrate that pelvic and femoral fractures were significant risk factors for VTE. In particular, older age, higher ISS, lower GCS, surgery, and blood transfusion have been reported as VTE risk factors in children and adults. Hanson and colleagues have implemented clinical guidelines that used some of the risk factors identified in this study to classify high-risk patients; these included older age (>13-years-old) and GCS less than 9. However, their guideline incorporated other risks that were not included in this model. These other risks (such as immobility and spinal cord injury) may also be important, but these data were not captured in the NTDB. Implementation of this scoring system may prove beneficial in risk stratification and guiding VTE prophylaxis.

**Answer: E**

Yen, J., Van Arendonk, K.J., Streiff, M.B., *et al.* (2016) Risk factors for venous thromboembolism in pediatric trauma patients and validation of a novel scoring system: The risk of clots in kinds with trauma score. *Pediatric Critical Care Medicine*, **17**, 391–399.

**14** *Which of these is the single greatest risk factor of in-ICU acute kidney injury (AKI) for pediatric ICU patients?*
   **A** *Unplanned ICU admission*
   **B** *Circulatory or respiratory disorder*
   **C** *Use of nephrotoxic medications*
   **D** *Use of ECMO*
   **E** *Use of IV radiologic contrast*

Studies have estimated the incidence of AKI in hospitalized children ranges from 9% to 64%. Critically ill patients are at increased risk of developing AKI. Seven risk factors associated with the development of AKI were pre-existing at the time of ICU admission whereas five occurred during the patient's ICU care. The single greatest risk factor for AKI was the administration of nephrotoxic medications during the ICU stay. Unadjusted analyses revealed the development of AKI was associated with younger age; unplanned ICU admissions; cardiac surgical or medical ICU admissions; ICD admission diagnosis codes of circulatory disorders, infectious disease, and respiratory disorders; and receiving one or more nephrotoxic medications prior to ICU admission. During their ICU care, patients who experienced sepsis, shock, septic shock or organ dysfunction or received IV radiologic contrast, mechanical ventilation, ECMO, or one or more nephrotoxic medications, were significantly more likely to develop AKI. Increasing age, unplanned admission to the ICU, admission diagnoses of circulatory or respiratory system, increasing Pediatric Risk of Mortality Score (PRISM), in-ICU respiratory dysfunction, use of ECMO, and administration of nephrotoxic medication(s) both prior to and during the ICU admission increased the odds of developing AKI. Noncardiac surgical admissions, use of IV radiologic contrast, and in-ICU neurologic dysfunction were associated with a reduced occurrence of AKI. A recent meta-analysis of observational studies revealed that the risk of AKI, death, and dialysis in patients receiving contrast medium was similar to those who did not. The single greatest risk factor of in-ICU AKI was the administration of nephrotoxic medications. Twenty-nine medications were considered to have important nephrotoxic effects: acyclovir, amikacin, amphotericin, captopril, carboplatin, cidofovir, cisplatin, cyclophosphamide, cyclosporine, enalapril, enalaprilat, ethacrynic acid, flucytosine, foscarnet, furosemide, ganciclovir, gentamicin, hydrochlorothiazide, ibuprofen, ifosfamide, indomethacin, ketorolac, methotrexate, penicillin, ramipril, sirolimus, tacrolimus, tobramycin, and vancomycin.

**Answer: C**

Slater, M.B., Gruneir, A., Rochon, P.A., *et al.* (2016) Risk factors of acute kidney injury in critically ill children. *Pediatric Critical Care Medicine*, **17**, e391–e398.

**15** *Pediatric patients who sustain blunt trauma to the liver or spleen*

    **A** *Must be observed in the hospital on bedrest for the number of days equal to injury grade plus one*

    **B** *Require hemoglobin checks every 6 hours for a minimum of 48 hours*

    **C** *Have a high likelihood of needing surgery for liver/ spleen bleeding*

    **D** *Should be transfused to keep hemoglobin > 10.0 g/dL*

    **E** *Are more likely to need surgery if ≥ 40 mg/kg of blood products are required in the first 24 hours*

The incidence of pediatric blunt abdominal injury is approximately 9 per 100,000 children. In the United States alone, an estimated 8200 children per year are hospitalized for liver or spleen injury. Recent publications suggest that the initial guidelines required excessive periods of hospitalization, and management based on hemodynamic status rather than grade is safe and cost effective. Hemodynamic-based management allows for an abbreviated period of bed rest with markedly shorter periods of hospitalization. Utilization of the ICU is reserved for patients with recent or ongoing bleeding. Nonoperative management of solid organ injury in children has become standard in the decades following the initial American Pediatric Surgical Association (APSA) guidelines, with more than 96% of isolated injuries managed without surgery. Scheduled hemoglobin rechecks are no longer required once stability has been established. A transfusion threshold of 7.0 g/dl has also been demonstrated as safe in a randomized controlled trial of critically ill children, as well as in prospective trauma studies. Very few, if any, patients who stop bleeding start bleed again during the period of hospitalization as suggested by the APSA guidelines. With the significant influx of information supporting changes in management, new guidelines have been published (see Figure 24.2). Failure of nonoperative management of liver and spleen injuries in children occurs early. In a study by Holmes and colleagues looking at children who

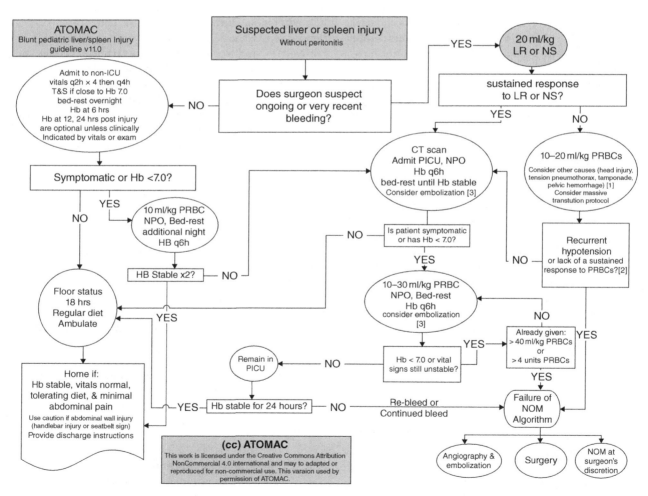

**Figure 24.2**

fail nonoperative management, the median time from admission to laparotomy was 3 hours with 38% failing by 2 hours of admission, 59% by 4 hours, 72% by 9 h, 76% by 12 hours, 87% by 24hours, and 94% by 48 hours. Reasons for failure include shock or persistent hemorrhage (49%), peritonitis or bowel injury (42%), pancreatic injury (8%), and ruptured diaphragm (1%). Consensus evidence suggests 40 ml/kg of blood products during the first 24 hours may suggest a breakpoint at which nonoperative management is less likely to be successful. Recurrent hypotension in a pediatric trauma patient occurs late and may be an ominous sign. The majority of children with contrast extravasation do not need angioembolization, and the current role appears to be limited to children who are otherwise failing non-operative management.

**Answer: E**

Notrica, D.M. (2015) Pediatric blunt abdominal trauma: current management. *Current Opinion in Critical Care,* **21**, 531–537.

**16** *Regarding pediatric blunt kidney trauma:*
   A *Low-grade injuries rarely require operative intervention*
   B *Collecting system hematoma is not a risk for non-operative failure*
   C *Urinomas under 2 cm require surgical drainage*
   D *Angioembolization, internal drainage, and percutaneous drainage should not be utilized in children*
   E *Late hypertension is common*

Renal injuries occur less frequently than liver or spleen injury. Failure of nonoperative management occurs in approximately 3% of cases, predominately in high-grade injuries. Risk factors for failure may include collecting system hematomas, urinomas greater than 4 cm, presence of dissociated renal fragments, and interpolar extravasation. Angioembolization, internal drainage, and percutaneous drainage are adjuncts to renal salvage in selective cases. Late hypertension is uncommon.

**Answer: A**

Notrica, D.M. (2015) Pediatric blunt abdominal trauma: current management. *Current Opinion in Critical Care,* **21**, 531–537.

**17** *Which of the following applies to blunt abdominal trauma in pediatric patients?*
   A *Pancreatic injuries are best managed non-operatively, regardless of location and grade*
   B *Delay in diagnosis and repair of bowel injuries dramatically increases morbidity and mortality*
   C *Blunt duodenal injuries in young children are strongly associated with non-accidental trauma*
   D *Lap belt bruising indicates that the child was protected from other injuries*
   E *Endovascular management of blunt abdominal aortic trauma has been well-studied and has consistently good long-term outcomes*

Grade 1 and 2 pancreatic injuries (contusion, minor laceration) are best managed nonoperatively. Those injuries with a transected main pancreatic duct of the body (grade 3) have fewer complications with distal pancreatectomy, and appear to further benefit from a laparoscopic approach. Roux-en-Y drainage of the distal pancreas is an option for more proximal injuries (grade 4). Fewer complications, fewer pseudocysts, a shorter time to return to enteral feeds, fewer procedures, and shorter hospitalization are seen with an operative approach. Successful endoscopic management has also been reported, and may have advantages in injury to the pancreatic head. Motorized vehicles and handlebar injuries are the most common mechanisms of blunt abdominal trauma. Of non-operative management of solid organ injury failures 15% are because of concurrent intestinal injury. Delay in diagnosis, even beyond 24 hours, was not uncommon. The delay, however, did not negatively impact outcome. With more than 20% of the patients having severe traumatic brain injury and a GCS less than six, such delays in diagnosis would be expected. In a series of destructive bowel injuries, there was no difference in complications between immediate and delayed repair in patients with open abdomens because of trauma. In those with less devastating mechanisms, laparoscopy has been utilized to evaluate and repair bowel injury. Blunt duodenal injuries in young children are another significant source of bowel injuries. Many are delayed presentations and these injuries in young children are strongly associated with nonaccidental trauma.

Blunt abdominal aortic injury is rare. When it occurs, it is often associated with severe deceleration forces. Concurrent injuries include lap belt injuries, Chance fractures, bowel injury, disruption of the cauda equina, and abdominal fascia disruption. Endovascular management of children with blunt abdominal aortic trauma has been reported. Advantages include avoiding operation or contamination in patients with concurrent bowel injury. Long-term studies in children are not available.

**Answer: C**

Notrica, D.M. (2015) Pediatric blunt abdominal trauma: current management. *Current Opinion in Critical Care,* **21**, 531–537.

**18** *In neonates and infants, the most common cause of abdominal compartment syndrome (ACS) is*
   **A** *Small bowel obstruction*
   **B** *Non-accidental trauma*
   **C** *Intussusception*
   **D** *Hirschsprungs disease*
   **E** *Necrotizing enterocolitis*

Mortality from ACS in pediatric patients is currently reported between 25% and 85%, and without treatment approaches 100%. Many conditions are associated with ACS. Primary ACS results from intraabdominal pathology such as infectious enterocolitis, bowel obstruction, or bowel perforation, and frequently requires surgical or interventional radiological treatment. Secondary ACS results from conditions originating outside the abdominopelvic compartment such as sepsis, trauma, or burns, resulting in shock states and may be related to fluid resuscitation and edema of the abdominal compartment. ACS occurs from the development of sustained intraabdominal hypertension (IAH) that ultimately leads to cardiovascular and respiratory compromise. Mortality was significantly higher in the ACS group both overall (64%) and at 28 days (52%) compared to the non-ACS group (0% and 2%, respectively). Achievement of primary fascial closure was significantly higher in the non-ACS group. In the neonatal group, the most common diagnostic category in the ACS group was necrotizing enterocolitis (NEC). In the infant group, patients with ACS also most commonly had NEC. In the children group, patients in the ACS group most commonly fell in the "Other" category. Both the 28-day mortality and overall hospital mortality were significantly higher in the ACS group. The highest mortality was seen in infants who were likely premature, as evidenced by lower birth weights and diagnoses of NEC. Approximately 30% of patients who had urgent laparotomies had ACS. Multiple nonoperative management strategies to reduce elevated IAH have been outlined in the literature and demonstrated to improve patient survival: 1) evacuation of intraluminal contents of the intestines by gastric suctioning, use of rectal tubes or enemas, and gastro- and coloprokinetics; 2) evacuation of intraabdominal space occupying lesions such as ascites, hemo- or pneumoperitoneum, which may require paracentesis; 3) optimization of fluid administration by goal-directed therapies and controlling capillary leak syndrome with diuretics, continuous renal replacement therapy, or dialysis; 4) improving abdominal wall compliance with adequate analgesia, sedation, and neuromuscular blockade. Independent risk factors associated with IAH were the presence of abdominal distension and a plateau pressure of more than 30 cm $H_2O$. The presence of IAH was associated with higher mortality and prolonged ICU stay.

In the ICU 18.8% patients died, and IAH was an independent risk factor for mortality.

**Answer: E**

Thabet, F.C., Bougmiza, I.M., Chehab, M.S., *et al.* (2016) Incidence, risk factors, and prognosis of intra-abdominal hypertension in critically ill children: A prospective epidemiology study. *Journal of Intensive Care Medicine*, **31**, 403–408.

Thomas, S., Kriplani, D, Crane, C., *et al.* (2016) Outcomes in pediatric patients with abdominal compartment syndrome following urgent exploratory laparotomy. *Journal of Pediatric Surgery*, **52** (7), 1144–1147.

**19** A massive hemothorax occurs in a patient who receiving heparin anticoagulation on extracorporeal membrane oxygenation (ECMO). Recommendations for management include:
   **A** Continue full anticoagulation regardless of type of intervention planned
   **B** Chest tube placement, then clamping the chest tube to tamponade the bleeding
   **C** Discontinue anticoagulation, chest tube drainage, administer tranexamic acid IV, and surgical evacuation if necessary
   **D** Halt any attempts at weaning off of ECMO
   **E** Tissue plasminogen activator (tPA) irrigation through the chest tube

**Answer: C**

Hemorrhage is an important complication of ECMO with a reported incidence of 12.2%. Hemothorax is associated with an 80–100% risk of mortality when conventionally treated, such as by adjusting the heparin dosage or with drainage of the pleural hemorrhage. The patients with ECMO-related massive hemothorax were initially managed by simultaneous replacement of blood volume and drainage of hemothorax by chest tube thoracostomy. Low-dose heparin infusion as part of the ECMO circuit (100 U/kg heparin) was discontinued and all subjects were prescribed 500 mg q8h tranexamic acid via intravascular injection to control bleeding (Figure 24.3). Pleural epinephrine irrigation through the chest tube at a rate of 5 mg epinephrine/1000 mL normal saline was also used. Each time 200 mL was infused and retained for 15 min and then released, and the procedure was repeated no more than five times. In addition, the surgical indications included continuous blood loss > 300 mL/hour over a period of 4 hours, persistent blood transfusion requirements, continued bleeding for 24 hours, or, more often, the accumulation of blood clots in one-third or more of the chest cavity that resulted in compromised cardiopulmonary status. The surgical strategies included

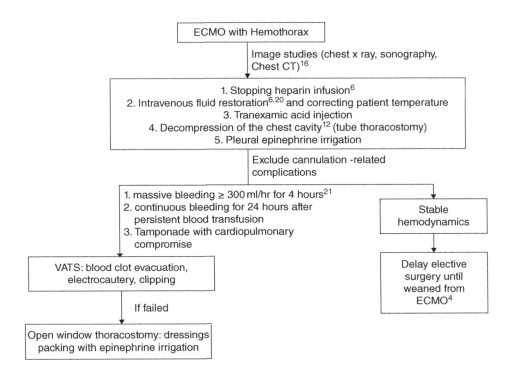

**Figure 24.3**

video-assisted thoracoscopic surgery (VATS) for detecting the source of the bleeding and evacuating the blood clots. Hemostasis was achieved by clip ligation and electrocautery. VATS was converted to open-window thoracostomy with dressing and packing if control of the refractory bleeding failed. The wet dressings were frequently changed for postoperative hemostasis, and continuous pleural epinephrine irrigation was administered through a chest tube. For treating patients with hemothorax-complicated ECMO, we propose a therapeutic algorithm for the treatment of these critically ill patients. Treatment of the underlying disease and adjusting the anticoagulant therapy are mandatory when hemothorax occurs. Major surgical intervention must be postponed, if possible, until near the termination of ECMO therapy or until the patient can be rapidly weaned off ECMO because bleeding tendency contributes to postoperatively persistent hemothorax. For the treatment of retained hemothorax, VATS is the favored alternative to thoracotomy for evacuation and adequate hemothorax drainage. However, to avoid prolonged surgery and to control intractable hemothorax, conversion to open window thoracostomy due to soaked dressings is another alternative method for treating critically ill patients.

Huang, P.M., Ko, W.J., Tsai, P.R., *et al.* (2012) Aggressive management of massive hemothorax in patients on extracorporeal membrane oxygenation. *Asian Journal of Surgery*, **35**, 16–22.

**20** *When placing a veno-venous cannula in the internal jugular vein for extracorporeal membrane oxygenation (ECMO) for respiratory failure, correct cannula position should be verified by*

**A** *Measuring the distance from the neck to the xiphoid before insertion*

**B** *Plain CXR alone after insertion*

**C** *Transthoracic echocardiography after insertion*

**D** *Real-time fluoroscopy during insertion*

**E** *Flow characteristics of the ECMO circuit during insertion*

Reports of vascular or cardiac perforation while on ECMO or during cannulation are sporadic and have included injury to the SVC, RA and RV. The historical rate of hemorrhagic pericardial tamponade for respiratory neonatal ECMO in the ELSO registry was 0.53% (~1985–2010). The reported rate of hemorrhagic pericardial tamponade on cardiac ECMO is historically higher at 1.8%. There were 11 reports of cannula-related perforation for a rate of 0.74%. When rates of perforation were distinguished by brand/design, the incidence of perforation was much higher for the wire-reinforced bicaval design 3.6% (10/279). In contrast, we observed a perforation rate of 0.1% (1/1203) in catheters that were designed to be positioned in the atrium. When cardiac perforation did occur, it generally happened in the right atrium (10/11 or 91%); all survey atrial perforations were associated with a wire-reinforced design and all but one involved the bicaval design (Figure 24.4).

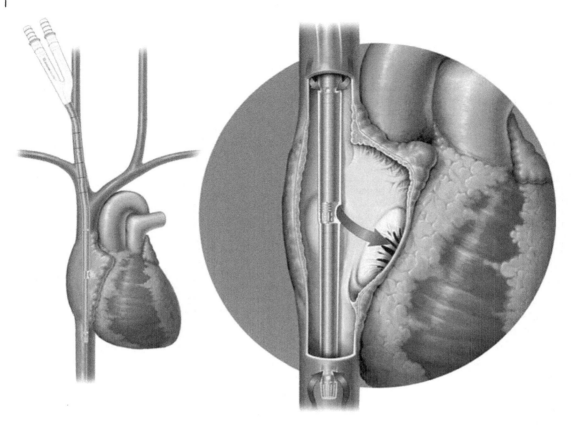

**Figure 24.4**

One-half (5/10) of the atrial perforations resulted in death, all five with the bicaval design. There was also one perforation in the IVC with the bicaval catheter. With the bicaval cannula, there were four cases of tamponade in which a perforation was not confirmed. One patient underwent sternotomy for tamponade, but a perforation was not found, two were managed with drains only, and in one patient with confirmed tamponade the patient expired prior to intervention.

The bicaval design often requires placement with wire and/or ECHO guidance in addition to standard chest radiographs. In our experience, we have noted excellent flow through the bicaval cannula even when the cannula becomes dislodged or malpositioned, thus flow characteristics may not be indicative of malposition. Correct positioning of bicaval dual-lumen catheters is therefore a

major challenge. The current standard of care for catheter placement is to use fluoroscopy and/or transesophageal echocardiography. Finally, it is very important to tightly secure the cannula to the skin in order to prevent longitudinal displacement and/or axial rotation.

**Answer: D**

Johnson, S.M., Itoga, N., Garnett, G.M., *et al.* (2014) Increased risk of cardiovascular perforation during ECMO with bicaval, wire-reinforced cannula. *Journal of Pediatric Surgery*, **49**, 46–50.

Langer, T., Vecchi, V., Belenkiy, S.M., *et al.* (2013) Pressure-guided positioning of bicaval dual-lumen catheters for venovenous extracorporeal gas exchange. *Intensive Care Medicine*, **39**,151–154.

# 25

# Envenomations, Poisonings, and Toxicology

*Michelle Strong, MD*

1 *Whole-bowel irrigation (WBI) is a technique to prevent absorption of drugs. Large volumes of polyethylene glycol electrolyte (PEG) solution are administered until the rectal effluent is clear. Which of the following statements about WBI are incorrect?*

  A *A nasogastric tube may be necessary to administer the electrolyte solution*

  B *This technique has been suggested for enhancing elimination of substances not well absorbed by activated charcoal*

  C *It is contraindicated for patients with ileus, GI obstruction, or hemodynamic instability*

  D *It should not be used for sustained-release or enteric-coated medications*

  E *The head of the bed should be elevated to 45*

Whole-bowel irrigation is a technique to prevent absorption of drugs by administering large volumes of polyethylene glycol solution until the rectal effluent is clear or toxin elimination is confirmed. A nasogastric tube is often necessary to effectively administer the electrolyte solution. The airway must be protected in patients with a depressed level of consciousness or respiratory depression. The head of the bed should be elevated to 45° to decrease the likelihood of aspiration. Whole-bowel irrigation is contraindicated in patients with ileus, GI obstruction or perforation, hemodynamic instability or intractable vomiting. This technique has been suggested to enhance elimination of substances that are not absorbed well by activated charcoal such as iron or lithium, potentially toxic ingestions of sustained-release or enteric coated medications, or in the situation of packaged illicit drug ingestion (body packing/stuffing). Currently, whole-bowel irrigation has no other indications than those mentioned above.

**Answer: D**

Mokhlesi, B., Leiken, J.B., Murray, P., *et al.* (2003) Adult toxicology in critical care: Part I: general approach to the intoxicated patient. *Chest*, **123**, 577–592.

Zimmerman, J.L. (2003) Poisonings and overdoses in the intensive care unit: General and specific management issues. *Critical Care Medicine*, **31**, 2794–2801.

Zimmerman, J.L. and Rudis, M. (2001) Poisonings, in *Critical Care Medicine*, 2nd edn. (eds J.E. Parrillo and R.P. Dellinger), Mosby, St. Louis, MO, pp. 1501–1524.

2 *Antidepressant overdose is a significant source of patient mortality with the majority due to tricyclic antidepressants (TCA). The clinical presentation of TCA toxicity can be categorized as anticholinergic effects, cardiovascular effects, and seizures. Which agent used in the management of the cardiovascular toxicity of TCA overdose is correct:*

  A *Bretylium*

  B *Sodium bicarbonate*

  C *Physostigmine*

  D *Procainamide*

  E *Dobutamine*

The cardiovascular toxicity of tricyclic antidepressants (TCA) poisoning consists of sinus tachycardia with the prolongation of the QRS, QTC, and PR intervals. Serum alkalinization remains the mainstay of therapy. Patients should receive sodium bicarbonate immediately when there is widening of the QRS interval and it should be continued until the QRS interval narrows or the pH >7.55. Therapy is based on studies that show that sodium bicarbonate narrows the QRS complex, improves systolic blood pressure, and controls ventricular arrhythmias in TCA overdose. Lidocaine is the drug of choice in cyclic antidepressant overdose complicated by refractory ventricular arrhythmias. Bretylium can exacerbate

*Surgical Critical Care and Emergency Surgery: Clinical Questions and Answers*, Second Edition.
Edited by Forrest "Dell" Moore, Peter Rhee, and Gerard J. Fulda.
© 2018 John Wiley & Sons Ltd. Published 2018 by John Wiley & Sons Ltd.
Companion website: www.wiley.com/go/moore/surgical_criticalcare_and_emergency_surgery

hypotension. Procainamide and other class 1a antiarrhythmics can add to cardiac toxicity and should be avoided. Hypotension tends to be refractory to fluid resuscitation and many patients will require vasopressors. Direct acting alpha-adrenergic agonists (norepineprine, phenylephrine) are preferred because they counteract the alpha-adrenergic antagonist effects of TCAs. Dobutamine is not used because it will likely worsen hypotension and not counteract the alpha-adrenergic antagonistic effects. Although TCAs possess some anticholinergic effects, cardiotoxicity is prominent. Physostigmine may worsen cardiac function and is associated with cardiac arrest in the setting of TCA overdose.

**Answer: B**

Blackman, K., Brown, S.G., and Wilkes, G.J. (2001) Plasma alkalinization for tricyclic antidepressant toxicity: a systematic review. *Emergency Medicine (Fremantle)*, **13**, 204–210.

Mokhlesi, B., Leiken, J.B., Murray, P., *et al.* (2003) Adult toxicology in critical care: part I: general approach to the intoxicated patient. *Chest*, **123**, 577–592.

Pentel, P. and Peterson, C.D. (1980) Asystole complicating physostigmine treatment of tricyclic antidepressant overdose. *Annals of Emergency Medicine*, **9**, 588–590.

Zimmerman, J.L. (2003) Poisonings and overdoses in the intensive care unit: General and specific management issues. *Critical Care Medicine*, **31**, 2794–2801.

3 *Analgesics are the most common agents that result in toxicity necessitating hospitalization throughout the world. Acetaminophen accounts for the majority of toxicity. Which of the following statements about acetaminophen toxicity is incorrect?*

A *Acetaminophen accounts for the highest number of deaths from poisonings in the United States*

B *The Rumack–Matthew nomogram uses acetaminophen levels to determine the need for N-acetylcysteine administration in patients with repeated ingestions or extended release formulations of acetaminophen*

C *N-acetylcysteine therapy is most effective when initiated in the first eight hours of ingestion*

D *Concomitant use of activated charcoal and N-acetylcysteine therapy improves patient outcomes*

E *King's College criteria for prognosis in acetaminophen-induced hepatotoxicity indicate that if serum creatinine is >3.4 mg/dL, INR >6.5, and grade III or worse encephalopathy occur within a 24-hour period the patient should be listed for transplantation*

Acetaminophen accounts for the majority of deaths from poisoning in the United States. N-acetylcysteine (NAC) is an antidote used in preventing acetaminophen-induced hepatotoxicity. The Rumack–Matthew nomogram uses acetaminophen levels to determine the need for NAC administration. The nomogram is useful *only* for single acute ingestions. N-acetylcysteine therapy is most effective when initiated in the first 8 hours following ingestion but may be initiated as late as 24 hours after significant ingestion. The Rumack–Matthew nomogram should *not* be used for chronic ingestions and is inaccurate in sustained-release products. Activated charcoal adsorbs acetaminophen and many coingestants and should be administered to patients with concern for acetaminophen or multiple drug overdoses. The concomitant use of activated charcoal and NAC therapy improves patient outcomes. No NAC dose adjustment is necessary. Acetaminophen-induced hepatitis may progress to fulminant hepatic failure, and appropriate referral to liver transplantation may be necessary. King's College criteria for prognosis of acetaminophen-induced hepatotoxicity are often used and the patient should be listed for transplantation if the arterial pH <7.3 after adequate fluid or resuscitation or if all three of the following occur within a 24-hour period: serum creatinine is >3.4 mg/dL, INR > 6.5, and grade III or worse encephalopathy.

**Answer: B**

Alapat, P.M. and Zimmerman, J.L. (2008) Toxicology in the critical care unit. *Chest*, **133**, 1006–1013.

Rumack, B.H. and Matthew, H. (1975) Acetaminophen poisoning and toxicity. *Pediatrics* 55 (6), 871–876.

Spiller, H.A. and Sawyer, T.S. (2007) Impact of activated charcoal after acute acetaminophen overdoses treated with N-acetylcysteine. *Journal of Emergency Medicine* **33**, 141–144.

4 *Toxidromes are combinations of specific signs and symptoms that reflect effects of a drug class on particular neuroreceptors. Which signs, drug/toxin and drug treatments (listed in order of signs: drug/toxin:treatment) are incorrect:*

A *Mydriasis, blurred vision, dry skin, ileus, urinary retention: atropine: benztropine*

B *Salivation, lacrimation, urination, diarrhea, GI cramps, emesis: organophosphates: pralidoxime*

C *Hypertension, tachycardia, mydriasis, diaphoresis: cocaine: benzodiazepines*

D *Confusion, stupor, slurred speech, apnea: benzodiazepines: flumazenil*

E *Altered mental status, slow shallow breaths, miosis: opiates: naloxone*

Management strategies are often geared toward the syndrome and not a specific agent. The anticholinergic toxidrome is manifested by mydriasis, blurred vision, tachycardia, dry skin, hypoactive bowel sounds, and urinary retention. It is caused by antihistamines, atropine, tricyclic antidepressants (TCA), benztropine, and phenothiazines. It is treated by physostigmine, except in life threatening TCA overdose because of worsening of conduction disturbances. Benztropine causes this syndrome; it does *not* treat it. Cholinergic toxidrome includes salivation, lacrimation, urination, diarrhea, GI cramps, emesis (SLUDGE). It is caused by organophosphates and is treated by pralidoxime. Signs of sympathomimetic toxidrome are hypertension, tachycardia, mydriasis, and diaphoresis. It is caused by cocaine, amphetamines, and phencyclidine (PCP) and treated by benzodiazepines. Sedative/hypnotic toxidrome is reflected by confusion, stupor, slurred speech, and apnea. It is caused by anticonvulsants, antipsychotics, benzodiazepines, and ethanol. Flumazenil is an antidote for benzodiazepine overdose. The narcotic toxidrome consists of altered mental status, slow shallow breaths, and miosis. It is caused by opiates and treated by the antidote naloxone.

**Answer: A**

Mokhlesi, B., Leiken, J.B., Murray, P., *et al.* (2003) Adult toxicology in critical care: Part I: general approach to the intoxicated patient. *Chest*, **123**, 577–592.

Weier, A. and Kleinschmidt, K. (2010) How are patients who are admitted to the intensive care unit after common poisonings diagnosed and managed?, in *Evidence-based Practice of Critical Care* (eds C.S. Deutschman and P.J. Neligan), Saunders, Philadelphia, PA, pp. 632–636.

5   *A 25-year-old woman ingested 10 tablets of carisoprodol 350 mg, 30 tablets of ibuprofen 200 mg and 10 tablets of cephalexin 500 mg 2 hours ago. On presentation to the emergency department (ED), she is lethargic but arouses to voice. Which of the following is the most appropriate method of gastric decontamination?*

   A  *Syrup of Ipecac*
   B  *Whole-bowel irrigation*
   C  *Sorbitol cathartic*
   D  *Activated charcoal*
   E  *Gastric lavage*

There is little evidence that any method of gastric decontamination is of benefit in overdose patients, however, activated charcoal is the best response. Activated charcoal adsorbs most ingested drugs and is generally effective and well tolerated. It is especially effective if given early. Ipecac syrup should not be used routinely in the management of poisoned patients. There is no evidence that ipecac improves outcomes and insufficient data to support administration soon after ingestion. Whole-bowel irrigation may be used in intoxications where activated charcoal is ineffective. It is considered for drugs such iron, lithium, sustained-release agents, and illicit drug packets. Cathartics have been used to decrease the transit time through the GI tract and thus, decrease absorption. No evidence exists to support this theory and, thus, they generally are not recommended. Gastric lavage should not be used in the management of poisoned patients because of complications including hypoxia, laryngospasm, gastrointestinal perforation, and aspiration pneumonia. There is also no clear benefit to its clinical outcome.

**Answer: D**

Chyka, P.A., Seger, D., Krenzelok, E.P., *et al.* (2005) Position paper: single-dose activated charcoal. *Clinical Toxicology*, **43**, 61–87.

Krenzelok, E.P., McGuigan, M., Lheureux, P., *et al.* (2004) Position paper: Ipecac syrup. *Journal of Toxicology and Clinical Toxicology*, **42**, 133–143.

Tenenbein, M. and Lheureux, P. (2004) Position paper: whole-bowel irrigation. *Journal of Toxicology and Clinical Toxicology*, **42**, 843–854.

6   *Salicylate poisoning is very common and sometimes fatal. Which one of the following features of salicylate toxicity or treatment of salicylate toxicity is incorrect:*

   A  *The toxidrome for salicylates includes nausea, vomiting, dyspnea, diaphoresis, dizziness, and tinnitus*
   B  *Significant ingestions of salicylates result in respiratory acidosis or mixed metabolic alkalosis and respiratory acidosis*
   C  *Administration of sodium bicarbonate to raise the plasma pH to 7.45 to 7.50 induces urinary alkalinization that in turn increases renal clearance of salicylates*
   D  *Hemodialysis is indicated for salicylate levels >100 mg/dL, significant metabolic derangements that do not rapidly clear with resuscitation, or renal insufficiency*
   E  *Activated charcoal is useful for acute salicylate ingestions, but not in cases of toxicity from chronic exposure*

The salicylate toxidrome includes nausea, vomiting, dyspnea, diaphoresis, dizziness, and hearing changes. Poisoned patients suffer from respiratory alkalosis or mixed anion-gap metabolic acidosis and respiratory alkalosis. At toxic levels, salicylates are metabolic poisons that affect multiple organ systems by uncoupling oxidative phosphorylation. This leads to accumulation of organic acids, such as lactic acid and ketoacids, and metabolic acidosis with an elevated anion gap. Respiratory alkalosis occurs through direct central stimulation. Sodium bicarbonate is administered to raise the plasma pH to between 7.45 and 7.5 to induce renal clearance. Raising the urinary pH from 6.1 to 8.1 results in a >18-fold increase in renal clearance by trapping the salicylate ion in the renal tubules. Hemodialysis is indicated for salicylate levels >100 mg/dL, significant metabolic derangements that do not rapidly clear with resuscitation, or renal insufficiency. Activated charcoal is only useful in acute salicylate ingestions. Multidose activated charcoal to enhance elimination is controversial.

**Answer: B**

Mokhlesi, B., Leiken, J.B., Murray, P., *et al.* (2003) Adult toxicology in critical care: Part I: general approach to the intoxicated patient. *Chest*, **123**, 577–592.

O'Malley, G.F. (2007) Emergency department management of the salicylate-poisoned patient (abstract). *Emergency Medicine Clinics of North America*, **25**, 333–346.

Prescott, L.F., Balali-Mood, M., Critchley, J.A., *et al.* (1982) Diuresis or urinary alkalinisation for salicylate poisoning? *British Medical Journal (Clinical Research Edition)*, **285**, 1383–1386.

**7** *Carbon monoxide (CO) is a nonirritating, colorless, odorless gas that is a common cause of morbidity and mortality. Which statement about CO poisoning is correct?*

   **A** *CO gas is formed by the complete combustion (oxidation) of carbon-containing materials*

   **B** *Pulse oximetry accurately reflects oxygen saturation because it can distinguish carboxyhemoglobin from oxyhemoglobin*

   **C** *CO binds to hemoglobin more readily than oxygen and decreases oxyhemoglobin and blood oxygen-carrying capacity*

   **D** *The severity of CO poisoning is independent of concentration and duration of exposure*

   **E** *Delayed neuropsychiatric sequelae from CO poisoning are directly correlated to the clinical severity of the toxin*

CO is an insidious gas that is formed by the *incomplete* combustion of carbon-containing materials. Complete oxidation of these materials produces carbon dioxide. CO poisoning occurs from smoke inhalation, automobile exhaust, and poorly ventilated charcoal or gas stoves. CO binds to hemoglobin with an affinity 240 times greater than oxygen and decreases oxyhemoglobin saturation and oxygen-carrying capacity. CO toxicity results in impaired transport and release of oxygen causing cellular hypoxia and cyctochrome oxidase blockade causing direct inhibition of cellular respiration. The severity of CO poisoning is dependent on the concentration of CO, duration of exposure, and the minute ventilation. Mild exposure (carboxyhemoglobin 5–10%) may result in headache and mild dyspnea. Higher carboxyhemoglobin concentrations (10–30%) cause headache, dizziness, dyspnea, irritability, nausea, and vomiting. Concentrations >50% lead to coma, seizures, cardiovascular collapse, and death. However, the delayed neuropsychiatric sequelae (DNS) *do not* correlate with the clinical severity of CO poisoning. Delayed neuropsychiatric sequelae may occur over a long period of time (3 to 240 days) and there is no accurate way of predicting which patients will acquire DNS. At 1 year, 50–75% of patients with DNS will have a full recovery. Administration of 100% supplemental oxygen decreases the half-life of carboxyhemoglobin from 5–6 hours to 45–90 min. Hyperbaric oxygen decreases the half-life to 15–30 min. Hyperbaric oxygen treatment at 6–12 hour intervals within a 24-hour period of exposure has been shown to decrease significantly DNS at both 6 weeks and 12 months.

**Answer: C**

Mokhlesi, B., Leiken, J.B., Murray, P., *et al.* (2003) Adult toxicology in critical care: Part I: General approach to the intoxicated patient. *Chest*, **123**, 577–592.

Weaver, L.K., Hopkins, R.O., Chan, K.J., *et al.* (2002) Hyperbaric oxygen for acute carbon monoxide poisoning. *New England Journal of Medicine*, **347**, 1057–1067.

Zimmerman, J.L. (2003) Poisonings and overdoses in the intensive care unit: general and specific management issues. *Critical Care Medicine*, **31**, 2794–2801.

**8** *An obtunded, hemodynamically stable patient with bipolar disorder is admitted to the ICU. She is chronically treated with lithium but had an ingestion of a large number of sustained-release lithium approximately 4 hours prior to admission. The patient's lithium level upon admission is 3.7 mEq/L (therapeutic range 0.5 to 1.25 mEq/L). Which one of the following is the most appropriate intervention at this time?*

   **A** *Normal saline solution diuresis*

   **B** *Hemodialysis*

   **C** *Administer activated charcoal*

   **D** *Close observation and repeat lithium level in 6–8 hours*

   **E** *Administer sodium polystyrene sulphonate (Kayexalate®)*

Lithium is a monovalent cation used for the treatment of bipolar disorders. It is rapidly absorbed via the GI tract and eliminated by glomerular filtration with 80% being reabsorbed in the renal tubules. The greatest risk of lithium ingestion is central nervous system toxicity including delirium, tremor, ataxia, hyperreflexia, seizures, and coma. Toxicity is more likely to occur in individuals who chronically ingest lithium. In this patient, hemodialysis should be instituted. Lithium is a prototypical dialyzable agent because of its low molecular weight, lack of protein binding, and prolonged half-life (18 hours). Hemodialysis is indicated for serum levels >3.5 mEq/L in acute indigestion, 2.5 mEq/L in chronic ingestion, symptomatic patients, or patients with renal insufficiency. The level will be decreased effectively by hemodialysis; however, repeat levels must be obtained after dialysis to assess for rebound increase as lithium shifts from the intracellular to extracellular space. Close observation and repeat levels are necessary after initial hemodialysis. Saline diuresis is not effective in enhancing the elimination of lithium. Volume replacement is appropriate in these patients because lithium causes a nephrogenic diabetes insipidus. Sodium polystyrene sulfonate (Kayexalate®) does bind lithium and may decrease absorption, it will also cause hypokalemia and is thus, not recommended. Activated charcoal is ineffective since lithium is not adsorbed to it.

**Answer: B**

Markowitz, G.S., Radhakrishnan, J., Kiambham, N., *et al.* (2000) Lithium nephrotoxicity: a progressive combined glomerular and tubulointerstitial nephropathy. *Journal of the American Society of Nephrology*, **11**, 1439–1448.

Mokhlesi, B., Leiken, J.B., Murray, P., *et al.* (2003) Adult toxicology in critical care: part II: specific poisonings. *Chest*, **123**, 897–922.

Timmer, R.T. and Sands, J.M. (1999) Lithium intoxication. *Journal of the American Society of Nephrology*, **10** (3), 666–674.

**9** *Toxicity due to nonethanol alcohols is encountered in the ICU. Which of the following statements about nonethanol alcohols is correct?*

**A** *Ethylene glycol is metabolized by alcohol dehydrogenase to formaldehyde and then to formic acid*

**B** *Accumulation and precipitation of oxalic acid to calcium oxalate in the renal tubules produces crystals and contributes to the development of renal tubular necrosis after methanol ingestion*

**C** *Propylene glycol toxicity in the ICU is usually associated with prolonged, high dose infusions of midazolam*

**D** *The treatment of choice for ethylene glycol and methanol poisoning is to enhance elimination of metabolites by administering fomepizole or ethanol which induces the alcohol dehydrogenase enzyme*

**E** *The classic characterization of ethylene glycol and methanol ingestions is an anion gap metabolic acidosis and/or an osmolar gap*

Toxicity due to nonethanol alcohols is encountered in the ICU. These ingestions are infrequent but can result in significant morbidity and mortality. Ethylene glycol is metabolized by alcohol dehydrogenase to glycoaldehyde and glycolic acid and then eventually to glyoxylic acid and oxalic acid. Methanol is metabolized by alcohol dehydrogenase to formaldehyde, which is then converted to formic acid. Accumulation and precipitation of calcium oxalate crystals in the renal tubules that leads to the development of acute tubular necrosis occurs after *ethylene glycol* ingestion. Fomepizole and ethanol are *inhibitors* of alcohol dehydrogenase (not inducers) and thus, inhibit the formation of toxic metabolites of both substances. Fomepizole is the preferred agent because it does not exacerbate the inebriated state. Metabolic acidosis with an elevated anion gap and an elevated osmolar gap are classic features of nonethanol intoxication. Late presentations may not manifest an osmolar gap if the alcohol has already been metabolized to acid metabolites, but an anion gap acidosis will be obvious.

**Answer: E**

Ammar, K.A. and Heckerling, P.S. (1996) Ethylene glycol poisoning with a normal anion gap caused by concurrent ethanol ingestion: Importance of the osmolar gap. *American Journal of Kidney Disorders*, **27**, 130–3.

Kruse, J.A. (1992) Methanol poisoning. *Intensive Care Medicine* **18**, 391–7.

Mokhlesi, B., Leiken, J.B., Murray, P., *et al.* (2003) Adult toxicology in critical care: part II: specific poisonings. *Chest*, **123**, 897–922.

Zimmerman, J.L. (2003) Poisonings and overdoses in the intensive care unit: General and specific management issues. *Critical Care Medicine*, **31**, 2794–2801.

**10** *The American Academy of Clinical toxicology and the European Associations of Poison Centres and Clinical Toxicologists (AACT/EAPCCT) have published position papers on the management of poisoned patients. Which one of the following statements from these guidelines is incorrect?*

**A** *Gastric lavage should not be used routinely in the management of poisoned patients because of complications including hypoxia, laryngospasm, gastrointestinal perforation, and aspiration pneumonia*

**B** *Ipecac syrup should not be used routinely in the management of poisoned patients due to insufficient evidence that it improves outcomes*

**C** *Single dose activated charcoal should not be used routinely in the management of poisoned patients. It should be considered if the toxin is known to be adsorbed by charcoal and has been ingested within 1 hour*

**D** *Urine alkalinization is not considered a first line treatment for patients with severe salicylate poisoning who do not meet criteria for hemodialysis*

**E** *Administration of multidose activated charcoal should be considered for patients that have ingested life-threatening amounts of carbamazepine, dapsone, phenobarbital, quinine, or theophylline*

The American Academy of Clinical Toxicology and the European Associations of Poison Centres and Clinical Toxicologists (AACT/EAPCCT) have published position papers on the management of poisoned patients. These papers function as clinical practice guidelines for elimination strategies for poisoned patients. Gastric lavage should not be used routinely in the management of poisoned patients because of complications including hypoxia, laryngospasm, gastrointestinal perforation, and aspiration pneumonia. In addition, there is no clear benefit to clinical outcome. Ipecac syrup should not be used routinely in the management of poisoned patients. There is no evidence that ipecac improves outcomes and insufficient data to support administration soon after ingestion. Single-dose activated charcoal should not be used routinely in the management of poisoned patients. However, it should be considered if the toxin is known to be adsorbed by charcoal and has been ingested within 1 hour. Studies reveal the effectiveness decreases after the first hour. Administration of multidose activated charcoal should be considered for patients that have ingested life-threatening amounts of carbamazepine, dapsone, phenobarbital, quinine, or theophylline. Studies have shown enhanced elimination of these drugs. None have demonstrated clinical benefit. Urine alkalinization is a *recommended* first-line treatment for patients with severe salicylate poisoning who do not meet criteria for hemodialysis.

**Answer: D**

Chyka, P.A., Seger, D., Krenzelok, E.P., *et al.* (2005) Position paper: single-dose activated charcoal. *Clinical Toxicology*, **43**, 61–87.

Krenzelok, E.P., McGuigan, M., Lheureux, P., *et al.* (2004) Position paper: Ipecac syrup. *Journal of Toxicology and Clinical Toxicology*, **42**, 133–143.

Proudfoot, A.T., Krenzelok, E.P., and Vale, J.A. (2004) Position paper on urine alkalinization. *Journal of Toxicology and Clinical Toxicology*, **42**, 1–26.

Vale, J.A., Krenzelok, E.P., and Barceloux, G.D. (1999) Position statement and practice guidelines on the use of multidose activated charcoal in the treatment of acute poisoning. *Clinical Toxicology*, **37**, 731–751.

Vale, J.A. and Kulig, K. (2004) Position paper: gastric lavage. *Journal of Toxicology and Clinical Toxicology*, **42**, 933–943.

**11** A 66-year-old obese man who was recently discharged from the inpatient medical service is found down by his wife with a small hematoma on his scalp. His finger stick glucose by paramedics was 24 mg/dL. He is given 1 ampule of 50% dextrose and arouses. He is brought in as trauma activation to the ED. He is initially alert and answering questions with the following vital signs: BP 150/88 mm Hg, HR 84 beats/min, RR 13 breaths/min, temperature 37.1 °C. His physical exam is unremarkable except for the small cephalohematoma and his trauma workup is negative. The patient's wife states that he is a diabetic and takes an oral medication. During a recent admission he had renal failure that resolved. During this evaluation, the patient becomes confused, lethargic and diaphoretic. His repeat finger stick glucose is 33 mg/dL. He again responds to 50% dextrose, but becomes unresponsive 30 minutes later. The patient is intubated for airway protection and admitted to the ICU. He is started on an IV infusion of 10% dextrose, but still requires several boluses of 50% dextrose for hypoglycemia. Which one of the following treatments is most likely to benefit this patient?

**A** *Administration of 50% dextrose via nasogastric tube*

**B** *Administration of subcutaneous octreotide*

**C** *Administration of intravenous thiamine 100 mg*

**D** *Administration of intramuscular glucagon*

**E** *Administration of 20% dextrose via peripheral IV*

This patient's presentation is suggestive of possible overdose with a hypoglycemic agent. Severe, prolonged hypoglycemia is characteristic of ingestion of large doses of sulfonylureas. Sulfonylurea agents stimulate insulin release from the pancreas, resulting in hypoglycemia. Risk factors for hypoglycemia from therapeutic use include: age > 65 years, multiple medications, frequent hospitalizations, use of agents with longer durations of action (e.g. chlorpropamide and glyburide), and impaired drug clearance; renal insufficiency can increase the risk of hypoglycemia four-fold. Patients with a sulfonylurea overdose and symptomatic hypoglycemia are immediately treated with IV dextrose. However, IV dextrose should not be used as monotherapy because it may cause hyperglycemia that triggers increased insulin release, leading to recurrent episodes of hypoglycemia. Octreotide is a somatostatin analogue that inhibits release of insulin from the pancreas and has been found to be effective in treating hypoglycemia and shortening the period of hypoglycemia. The most important mechanism of action is G-protein-mediated decrease in calcium influx through voltage-gated channels in pancreatic beta islet cells, which diminishes calcium-mediated insulin release. The dose of octreotide is 50 to 150 µg administered by intramuscular, or subcutaneous, injection every 6 hours. If thiamine deficiency (from alcoholism or other forms of malnutrition) is suspected, IV thiamine 100 mg is given in conjunction with glucose, but will not treat symptomatic hypoglycemia. Glucagon given IM stimulates hepatic glycogenolysis and raises serum glucose levels slightly. The efficacy of glucagon is dependent upon hepatic glycogen stores, which may be depleted in the setting of prolonged hypoglycemia. The short duration of action of glucagon further limits its effectiveness. Central venous access is required for administering concentrated glucose solutions due to hyperosmolarity that can cause endothelial damage. Oral administration of dextrose in a severely ill patient is unreliable.

**Answer: B**

Carr, R. and Zed, P.J. (2002) Octreotide for sulfonylurea-induced hypoglycemia following overdose. *Annals of Pharmacotherapy*, **36**, 1727–1732.

Fasano, C.J., O'Malley, G., Dominici, P., *et al.* (2008) Comparison of octreotide and standard therapy versus standard therapy alone for the treatment of sulfonylurea-induced hypoglycemia. *Annals of Emergency Medicine*, **51**, 400–406.

Green, R.S. and Palatnik, W. (2003) Effectiveness of octreotide in a case of refractory sulfonylurea-induced hypoglycemia. *Journal of Emergency Medicine*, **25**, 283–287.

Shorr, R.I., Ray, W.A., Daugherty, J.R., *et al.* (1997) Incidence and risk factors for serious hypoglycemia in older persons using insulin or sulfonylureas. *Archives of Internal Medicine*, **157**, 1681–1686.

**12** *A lethargic 35-year-old man is admitted to the ICU. The patient had been brought to the emergency department for evaluation by some friends after hiking. Upon admission, his vitals are BP 105/62 mm Hg, HR 125 beat/min, RR 28 breaths/min, temperature 36.5 °C. His physical examination is remarkable for bleeding gums and an ecchymotic, edematous left lower extremity from foot to knee with a small wound near the ankle. A surgical consult was obtained and compartment pressures are 21 mm Hg. He has a Foley catheter in place with brownish red urine. His laboratory studies are remarkable for platelets $92 \times 10^3/\mu L$, PTT 43 and INR 1.8; BUN 35 mg/dL, serum creatinine 1.6 mg/dL and CK 5416 U/L. Which one of the following interventions would be most beneficial to this patient?*

**A** *Placement of tourniquet to the thigh of the left lower extremity*
**B** *Administration of piperacillin/tazobactam 3.375 gm IV every 6 hours*
**C** *Transfusion of platelets and fresh frozen plasma*
**D** *Administration of Crotalinae (pit viper) antivenom (Polyvalent Crotalidae ovine immune Fab)*
**E** *Fasciotomy of the left lower extremity*

The physical findings in this patient are concerning for compartment syndrome. However, the wound on the lower leg and history are concerning for a snakebite. FabAV consists of the purified Fab fragments of sheep immunoglobulin (IgG) raised against the antivenom of four snakes. These Fab fragments bind venom in the intravascular space and are renally excreted. The half-life of FabAV is shorter than Crotalinae venom substances. Thus, recurrent toxicity is possible despite initial control of local and systemic effects and may necessitate repeated FabAV administration. FabAV appears most effective when given within 6 hours of envenomation. Methods, such as tourniquets, incision and oral suction, mechanical suction devices, cryotherapy, surgery, and electric shock therapy, have been advocated in the past, but are *no longer recommended*. Tourniquets can damage nerves, tendons, and blood vessels, and oral suction can lead to infection. Although snake bites may result in the inoculation of bacteria, infections are rare. Antibiotics should *not* be administered unless there is established infection or heavily contaminated wounds. Transfused platelets and coagulation factors in fresh frozen plasma are inactivated by Crotalinae venom and should be avoided in patients with Crotalinae-induced coagulopathy unless the patient has significant bleeding that is uncontrolled by high-dose antivenom administration. Increased compartment pressures result from this extrinsic pressure and can be reduced with the administration of adequate amounts of antivenom and elevation. Elevation, which is usually avoided in true compartment syndrome, results in the drainage of subcutaneous edema and contributes to the reduction of the source of increased tissue pressure. If there is a concern for clinically significant, increased tissue, or compartment pressures, direct measurement with an appropriate device should be performed to guide additional management with antivenom and elevation. The indications for fasciotomy in this context are unclear. An animal model of direct compartmental injection of venom demonstrated improved outcomes with antivenom alone versus antivenom plus fasciotomy. However, in this model, fasciotomy was performed immediately after venom injection. Thus, surgical intervention for elevated compartment pressures following Crotalinae snake bite is controversial and should be guided by a medical toxicologist and surgeon with extensive experience caring for victims with snake bite. In this patient, compartment pressures are still below the recommended value for performing extremity fasciotomy (30 mm Hg).

**Answer: D**

Gold, B.S., Barish, R.A., and Dart, R.C. (2004) North American snake envenomation: diagnosis, treatment and management. *Emergency Medical Clinics of North America*, **22**, 423–443.

Gold, B.S., Dart, R.C., and Barish, R.A., *et al.* (2003) Resolution of compartment syndrome after rattlesnake envenomation utilizing non-invasive measures. *Journal of Emergency Medicine*, **24**, 285–288.

Gold, B.S., Dart, R.C., and Barish R.A. (2002) Bites of venomous snakes. *New England Journal of Medicine*, **347**, 347–356.

Seifert, S.A., Boyer, L.V., Benson B.E., *et al.* (2009) AAPCC database characterization of native US venomous snake exposures, 2001–2005. *Clinical Toxicology*, **47**, 327–335.

**13** *All of the following statements are true regarding valproic acid overdose except:*

**A** *Hypernatremia has been associated with high drug levels*

**B** *Administration of L-carnitine is recommended for patients with hyperammonemia, lethargy, coma, and hepatic dysfunction*

**C** *Cerebral edema may occur 24–72 hours after ingestion*

**D** *There is no concern for toxicity if there are therapeutic drug levels and no CNS depression 2 hours after ingestion*

**E** *Hemodialysis or combined hemodialysis and hemoperfusion methods have been effective in severe toxicity*

Increased use of valproic acid (VPA) for bipolar disorder, seizures, migraine headaches, and neuropathic pain has led to increased overdose. Central nervous system depression is the most common symptom of acute overdose or toxicity ranging in severity from mild drowsiness to coma or fatal cerebral edema. The onset and progression of CNS depression is usually rapid but may be delayed as long as 72 hours with ingestion of delayed

release preparations. Valporic acid serum levels often peak several hours after ingestion. Thus, levels should be assessed every 2 to 4 hours until a decline in level is noted indicating that a peak level has been reached. If peak levels have not yet been achieved, there is concern for rebound levels that could lead to increased CNS depression. Supportive care is the principal treatment for VPA intoxication and results in good outcomes in the vast majority of patients. Because VPA-induced hyperammonemia and hepatotoxicity may be mediated in part by carnitine deficiency, the administration of L-carnitine (50 mg/kg/day) is recommended for patients with hyperammonemia, lethargy, coma, and hepatic dysfunction. Although experience is limited, hemodialysis and hemodialysis-hemoperfusion modalities have been reported be to be effective in severe toxicity. Recent reports show that early intervention may correlate with rapid clinical improvement.

**Answer: D**

Licari, E., Calzavacc, P., Warrillow, S.J., *et al.* (2009) Life-threatening sodium valproate overdose: A comparison of two approaches to treatment. *Critical Care Medicine*, **37**, 3161–3164.

Ohtani, Y., Endo F., and Matsuda I. (1982) Carnitine deficiency and hyperammonemia associated with valproic acid therapy. *Journal of Pediatrics*, **101**, 782–785.

Szthankrycer, M.D, (2002) Valproic acid toxicity. *Journal of Toxicology and Clinical Toxicology*, **40**, 789–801.

**14** *A 25-year-old man with known drug abuse history is brought to the ED for evaluation after fleeing police and then collapsing clutching his chest. On arrival to the hospital, EMS reports that he had a witnessed generalized tonic-clonic seizure en route. His current vitals are BP 180/93 mm Hg, HR 125 beats/min, RR 20 breaths/min, temperature 38.7 °C. He is agitated, diaphoretic, and mumbling. Which one of the following should NOT be administered to this patient?*

**A** *Nitroglycerin*

**B** *Metoprolol*

**C** *Lorazepam*

**D** *Oxygen*

**E** *Phentolamine*

This patient presents with sympathomimetic syndrome consistent with cocaine or amphetamine intoxication. Clinical symptoms include tachycardia, hypertension, hyperthermia, agitation, mydriasis, and psychosis. Cocaine-associated chest pain (CACP) accounts for approximately 40% of all cocaine-related visits to the emergency department and evaluation of these patients includes an ECG, chest radiograph, and biochemical markers to exclude myocardial infarction. Early management of patients with CACP includes administration of oxygen and reduction of sympathetic outflow using benzodiazepines given intravenously. Benzodiazepines should be given to patients who are anxious, agitated, hypertensive, or tachycardic; nitroglycerin should be given in addition to patients with hypertension. Beta-blockers are **contraindicated** in patients who have recently used cocaine (<24 hours), and in patients with CACP. Beta-blockers may lead to unopposed alpha-adrenergic stimulation which can cause coronary arterial vasoconstriction, ischemia, and infarction. Phentolamine, an alpha-adrenergic antagonist, can be used to reduce cocaine-induced coronary artery vasoconstriction when managing CACP or hypertension that is unresponsive to benzodiazepines.

**Answer: B**

Hollander, J.E. (1995) The management of cocaine-associated myocardial ischemia. *New England Journal of Medicine*, **333**, 1267–1272.

Lange, R.A., Cigarroa, R.G., Yancy C.W. Jr., *et al.* (1989) Cocaine-induced coronary-artery vasoconstriction. *New England Journal of Medicine*, **321**, 1557–1562.

Lange, R.A., Hillis, L.D. (2001) Cardiovascular complications of cocaine use. *New England Journal of Medicine*, **345**, 351–358.

**15** *A 20-year-old woman is brought to the hospital after being found down next to a bottle of sustained-release metoprolol. By history from family, the patient was last seen awake three hours prior to arrival. Initial vital signs revealed a temperature pf 37.0 °C, BP 102/40 mm Hg, HR 122 beats/min, respirations 20 breaths/min. The patient was given activated charcoal. Approximately 90 minutes later, the patient has decreased mental status, BP 73/30 mm Hg and HR 55 beats/min. Which one of the following would be the appropriate sequence of interventions most appropriate to stabilize this patient assuming the preceding intervention is unsuccessful?*

**A** *Calcium chloride IV, transcutaneous pacing, then transvenous pacing*

**B** *Atropine 1 mg IV, then transcutaneous pacing*

**C** *Glucagon IV, calcium chloride IV, then transcutaneous pacing*

**D** *Transcutaneous pacing then transvenous pacing*

**E** *Calcium chloride IV, glucagon IV, then transvenous pacing*

β-Adenergic blockers produce adverse effects primarily through bradycardia and hypotension. Central nervous system depression may occur with lipid-soluble agents such as propranolol, timolol, metoprolol, and acebutolol. Hypotension often results from negative inotropic effects rather than bradycardia. Glucagon is considered the *initial drug of choice*, because it produces chronotropic and inotropic effects and does not require β-receptors for activity. The goal of treatment is improvement in blood pressure and perfusion rather than increase in heart rate. Calcium chloride 10% may be effective in reversing hypotension. Transcutaneous pacing and transvenous pacing may be considered in refractory cases. Additional drugs that had variable efficacy include atropine, epinephrine, isoproterenol, and dopamine. Milrinone (phosphodiesterase inhibitors), intra-aortic balloon pump, or cardiopulmonary bypass may be considered if there is no response to other interventions.

**Answer: C**

Alapat, P.M. and Zimmerman, J.L. (2008) Toxicology in the critical care unit. *Chest*, **133**, 1006–1013.

Bailey, B. (2003) Glucagon in β-blocker and calcium channel blocker overdoses: a systemic review. *Journal of Toxicology and Clinical Toxicology*, **41**, 595–602.

Mokhlesi, B., Leiken, J.B., Murray, P., *et al.* (2003) Adult toxicology in critical care: part II: specific poisonings. *Chest*, **123**, 897–922.

**16** *A 56-year-old woman with chronic renal failure is status post a left carotid endarterectomy. She is admitted to the ICU with severe hypertension. The surgeon would like the systolic blood pressure <140 mm Hg. After 24 hours of treatment with nitroprusside, the patient develops confusion and metabolic acidosis. Her symptoms are best prevented/treated with administration of which one of the following agents?*

**A** *Cyanocobalamin*

**B** *Thiosulfate*

**C** *Glucagon*

**D** *Sodium bicarbonate*

**E** *Calcium chloride*

This patient is developing signs and symptoms consistent with cyanide toxicity from nitroprusside. Nitroprusside has been shown to cause toxicity through the release of cyanide and accumulation of thiocyanate. Cyanide toxicity presents with unexplained cardiac arrest and changes in mental status, including convulsions, encephalopathy, and coma. Metabolic acidosis may also be present as a late finding. Risk of cyanide toxicity can be decreased by utilizing recommended doses of nitroprusside for short periods of time. An infusion of thiocynate is used to prevent and treat the symptoms of cyanide toxicity.

Hydroxocobalamin is safe and effective in preventing and treating cyanide toxicity associated with the use of nitroprusside. However, cyanocobalamin is not effective as an antidote or able to prevent cyanide toxicity. Glucagon and calcium chloride are used to counteract the effects of β-blockers and calcium channel blockers, respectively. Sodium bicarbonate is used to treat tricyclic antidepressant toxicity.

**Answer: B**

Curry, S.C. (2005) Sodium nitroprusside, in *Critical Care Toxicology* (eds J. Brent, K. Wallace, K. Burkhart, *et al.*) Mosby, Philadelphia, PA, pp. 843–850.

Schulz, V., Gross, R., Pasch, T., *et al.* (1982) Cyanide toxicity of sodium nitroprusside in therapeutic use with and without sodium thiosulfate. *Klinische Wochenschrift*, **60**, 1393–1400.

Varon, J. and, Marik, P.E. (2000) The diagnosis and management of hypertensive crises. *Chest*, **118**, 214–227.

**17**  *A 25-year-old woman presented to the emergency department with a week of pain, swelling, and ulceration to her lower extremities (see Figure 25.1a and Figure 25.1b). She uses heroin daily, however due to a recent job loss, she was forced to obtain cheaper homemade heroin substitutes. She initially developed blistering of the area, which had progressed*

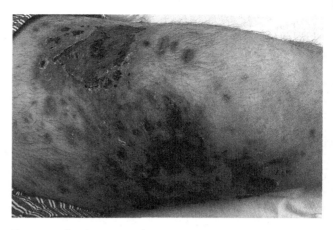

**Figure 25.1b** Ulceration to lower extremities.

*to painful necrotic ulcers. On exam, her temperature was 101 °F, heart rate 125 beats/min, blood pressure 115/60 mm Hg. Her right anterior thigh was swollen, with erythema and several large necrotic ulcerations. She was admitted to the hospital and treated with intravenous antibiotics and wound care.*

*Which of the following drugs is likely the cause of this patient's presentation?*

A  *Cocaine*
B  *Methamphetamine*
C  *Ecstasy (MDMA)*
D  *Krokodil*
E  *Phencyclidine (PCP)*

There has been a dramatic increase in the observed number of reports on the use of Krokodil (also known as Crocodile, Krok, or Croc) in the last few years. Krokodil use was first reported in Siberia in 2002 and has mostly been described in European countries. This deadly mixture however has made its way into the United States with a few cases reported. It is known as the "drug that eats junkies," and "Russia's deadly designer drug." It is characterized as the "flesh eating" or "flesh rotting" drug. The main active ingredient of Krokodil is desomorphine, a synthetic derivative of morphine. It can be manufactured at home from codeine, along with several other easily available additives, and is significantly cheaper than heroin. Its regular use results in severe damage to the vasculature, muscles, and bones, and in multiorgan failure with a mean survival time of 2 years after its first use. Krokodil refers both to chlorocodide, a codeine derivate, and to the excessive gross desquamation from gangrenous inflammation at the injection site that resembles scales of a crocodile. The use of desomorphine is prohibited internationally. It is a scheduled I drug under the United States Code Controlled Substance Act. Desomorphine first emerged in the Russian drug scene around 2002–2003 under the term

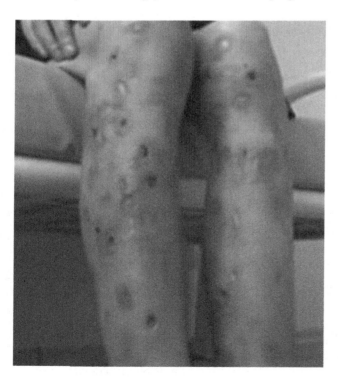

**Figure 25.1a** Ulceration to lower extremities.

Krokodil. At that time, there was a decreased import of Afghan heroin into local drug markets and a tendency back to the production of homemade drugs. A dramatic increase in the number of addicted individuals was then observed, which is thought to be a result of the easy availability of Krokodil from a simple production process that can be accomplished at home with little cost. Most Krokodil users claim to be former heroin users who switched. Due to the high dependence potential and the toxicity of Krokodil, the mean survival time after first use is reported to be 2 years. The victims of Krokodil are usually young people between ages 18 and 25, who turn to this drug for economic reasons. Desomorphine is an opioid analgesic that was first synthesized in the United States in 1932. It was originally synthesized with the intention of creating an alternative to morphine with an improved side-effect profile. However desomorphine showed increased dependence potential compared to morphine. It is almost entirely free from the emetic effects that morphine has. Its chemical structure renders desomorphine more lipophilic than morphine favoring penetration in the brain leading to a higher analgesic potency. It has eight to ten times higher analgesic potency, faster onset of action, and shorter half-life compared with morphine, which accounts for its increased addictive potential. Due to this short elimination half-life, patients with desomorphine dependence inject more frequently than those with heroin dependence.

Repeated administration of desomorphine can cause physical and psychological dependency, tolerance, and a withdrawal syndrome if the substance is no longer used, similar to heroin. Other effects are similar to those of opiates such as miosis, flushing, constipation, urinary retention, nausea, vomiting, sedation, and respiratory depression. Specifically with Krokodil, due to the high degree of contamination with various toxic byproducts, injection of Krokodil causes immediate tissue damage to blood vessels, muscle, and bone. Multisystem organ dysfunction can occur including thyroid (due to iodine) and cartilage (due to phosphorus). Heavy metal poisoning can also occur with chronic use. Abscess formation, thrombophlebitis, gangrene, necrosis, and autoamputation are common occurrences. Skin sloughs off at the injection site, often exposing the bone below. The ill effects of Krokodil are not limited to localized injuries and include pneumonia, sepsis, meningitis, osteomyelitis and osteonecrosis, neurologic injury (such motor and memory impairment), ulceration and tissue damage at sites distant from the injection site, liver injury, renal impairment, and death. These complications occur shortly after Krokodil is injected. Present accounts often involve young individuals presenting to emergency departments with severe complications. Additionally, practices common to homemade drug production are known to potentiate blood-borne virus transmission such as HIV and hepatitis C. The short duration of action (about 1.5 hours) and less than an hour time required for the home preparation of Krokodil leads its addicts to be trapped in a 24-hour daily cycle of cooking and injecting to avoid withdrawal. High concentrations of iodine in the injected solution disrupt the endocrine system, causing thyroid disorders, while high concentrations of heavy metals cause central nervous system effects such as speech and motor impairment, poor memory, and concentration. Jaw osteonecrosis, which is resistant to medical treatment, can develop in the maxillofacial region in users due to red phosphorus contamination.

Because of the high degree of contamination with different toxic chemicals, which vary among users, scientific analysis of the chemical composition is not available. Desomorphine can be detected in blood samples within a couple of hours and in urine samples within 2–3 days after Krokodil administration. Routine testing in the acute clinical setting is not typically available. Diagnosis is therefore based on the history provided by the patient as well as the clinical presentation. Soon after use, patients will present with a physical exam consistent with other opioids ingestions/injection. Although extensive tissue damage is typically described, this can also be seen in patients who develop skin and soft-tissue infections from heroin use. In chronic Krokodil users, it may be worthwhile screening for heavy metal poisoning given the contamination during the manufacture process.

In regions where Krokodil use is problematic, poor access to proper health care may exacerbate the described complications. Medical help is reportedly only sought during the late stages of tissue injury and may end with severe mutilation, amputation, and death. If someone seeks care, extensive wound care and IV antibiotics is typically indicated. In many cases, amputation is the only solution. Existing reports have emphasized the high potency of desomorphine and the need for frequent redosing, resulting in binge patterns that can last over days. During these binges, sleep deprivation, poor hygiene, and malnutrition places users at risk for further complications. Variations in the potency of desomorphine place users at increased risk of overdose. Treatment must consider not only the local tissue destruction that occurs, but also the distant tissue injury and multisystem organ damage that can occur. In the setting of respiratory depression, naloxone (0.4–2 mg IV; repeat every 2–3 min until desired effect is achieved) can be administered.

**Answer: D**

Azbel, L., Dvoryak, S., and Altice, F.L. (2013) "Krokodil" and what a long strange trip it's been. *International Journal of Drug Policy*, **24**, 275–280.

Thekkemuriyi, D.V., John, S.G., and Pillai, U. (2014) "Krokodil"—a designer drug from across the Atlantic, with serious consequences. *American Journal of Medicine*, **127**, e1–e2.

**18** *Match the correct mechanism of action with the correct drug of abuse.*

   **A** *MDMA (Ecstasy/Bath salts)*
   **B** *Cocaine*
   **C** *Synthetic Marijuana (Spice/K2)*
   **D** *Caffeine*
   **E** *PCP*

1) *Increased affinity of the NDMA receptor*
2) *Affinity for and efficacy at the CB1CB2 receptors (receptor agonists)*
3) *Adenosine receptor blockade resulting in increased glutamate activity*
4) *Increased serotonin, norepinephrine and less so dopamine reuptake*
5) *Increased dopamine reuptake*

**Answers: A–4, B–5, C–2, D–3, E–1**

**MDMA** and the other ring-substituted amphetamine derivatives act by increasing the net release of the monoamine neurotransmitters (serotonin, noradrenaline and, to a smaller extent, dopamine) from their respective axon terminals. MDMA does not act by directly releasing serotonin but, rather, by binding to, and thus blocking, the transporter involved in its reuptake. It is clear that the increase in the net release of serotonin (and possibly dopamine) is the major mechanism of action underlying the distinctive mental effects of MDMA, whereas the increased release of noradrenaline is mainly responsible for the physical effects that it shares with amphetamine.

The psychostimulant effects of **cocaine** appear to be mediated by its ability to enhance dopaminergic activity within the mesocorticolimbic circuit. Additionally, it is the intensity with which cocaine produces alterations in dopaminergic circuitry that have enabled this drug to prevail as one of the most addictive substances known to man. Specifically, the D1 dopamine receptor and intracellular signaling mediated by this receptor subtype.

**Synthetic cannabinoids** are receptor agonists that bind to the same endogenous cannabinoid receptors as THC, Cannabinoid 1, and Cannabinoid 2 (CB1/CB2). JWH-018 is one of the earliest and best characterized compounds. JWH compounds are named after John W. Huffman, a chemist from Clemson University who synthesized many SC compounds to research CB1/CB2 receptors. CB1 receptors are found throughout the body but are densely concentrated in the brain, spinal cord, and peripheral nervous system affecting pain. This receptor is responsible for most of the psychoactive effects of cannabinoids such as elevating a person's mood. Other effects mediated by this receptor include inducing analgesia, memory impairment, and altering one's sense of time. CB2 receptors are found primarily in tissues of the immune system and have a role in pain as well. Activating these receptors modulate the immune system and are anti-inflammatory. CB2 receptors have been the focus of research due to the possibility that they could decrease pain caused by inflammation without the psychoactive effects of CB1 receptors. The chemical structures of SCs are very different than THC. They are also far more potent than traditional marijuana. For example, JWH-018 has four times the affinity for the CB1 receptor and ten times the affinity for the CB2 receptor. Also, THC is a partial agonist at the CB1 receptor and many of the SCs are full agonists. In addition to the JWH compounds, there are multiple other groups of SCs including CP compounds, HU compounds (developed at Hebrew University) and the benzoylindoles. All are far more potent agonists at the CB receptors compared to THC.

**Caffeine** belongs to a class of compounds called methylxanthines, which act as CNS stimulants. The stimulating effects of caffeine are due to its ability to block the receptors for the inhibitory neurotransmitter adenosine. Caffeine blocks both the Al and A2 adenosine receptor subtypes, having its more potent effect on the A1 receptor. Adenosine inhibits the release of various neurotransmitters, in particular the excitatory amino acid glutamate. Therefore, caffeine blockade of adenosine receptors results in increased glutamate activity.

**PCP** antagonizes the actions of the excitatory amino acid neurotransmitter glutamate at the N-methyl-D-aspartate (NMDA) receptor, one of the receptor subtypes for glutamate. Glutamate is found throughout the brain and increases the flow of calcium ions into cells to cause excitatory actions. The NMDA receptor controls the calcium ion channel acted on by glutamate and binding of PCP to the receptor blocks calcium entry into the cell. It is likely that the diverse behavioral effects of PCP are due to the fact that glutamate is widely distributed in the brain and regulates the activity of a number of other neurotransmitter systems.

Carrel, M.E. (1990) PCP and hallucinogens. *Advances in Alcohol and Substance Abuse*, **9**, 167–190.

Hollister, L.E. (1986) Health aspects of cannabis. *Pharma Review*, **38**, 1–20.

Kalant, H. (2001) The pharmacology and toxicology of "ecstasy" (MDMA) and related drugs. *Canadian Medical Association Journal*, **165**, 917–928.

Nehlig, A., Daval, J.L., and Derby, G. (1992) Caffeine and the central nervous system: Mechanisms of action, biochemical, metabolic and psychostimulant effects. *Brain Research Reviews*, **17**, 139–170.

Woolverton, W.L. and Johnson, K.M. (1992) Neurobiology of cocaine abuse. *Trends in Pharmacological Sciences*, **13**,193–200.

# 26

## Common Procedures in the ICU
*Joanelle A. Bailey, MD and Adam D. Fox, DO*

**1** When preparing to place a central venous catheter (CVC) in a hemodynamically normal patient, which of the following have been shown to help reduce the risk of central line-associated bloodstream infection (CLABSI):
A Antisepsis of the skin with chlorhexadine rather than povidone-iodine solution
B Aseptic technique without the use of maximal sterile barrier precautions
C Use of catheters that are not antibiotic-impregnated
D Placement of the CVC in the femoral vein
E Preprocedural hand hygiene is unnecessary if aseptic technique is utilized

Catheter-related blood stream infections remain a significant problem in the intensive care unit (ICU). Prevention of these infections begins with the appropriate preparation. Standard hand hygiene prior to and following insertion should apply in all cases. Current recommendations call for antiseptic cleansing of the skin insertion site with >0.5% chlorhexadine preparation with alcohol solution. Studies have shown a significantly reduced infection rate with this preparation as compared to povidone-iodine or alcohol. When deciding on location for the CVC, placement in the subclavian vein has been shown to have the lowest rate of infection as compared to the internal jugular and femoral approaches; the subclavian site should be avoided in patients with advanced kidney disease in order to avoid venous stenosis. The choice of catheter may also play a role in reducing infection. Using an antimicrobial-impregnated CVC is recommended for patients in whom it is expected that the catheter will remain in place for an extended period of time. Once the site and catheter has been selected, it is imperative that full barrier precautions and personal protective equipment be utilized, this includes cap, mask, sterile gown, sterile gloves, and a large sterile drape. Additional methods that have been recommended include limiting the number of ports/lumens to those

essential the management of the patient, daily review of line necessity, and using a sterile, transparent dressing with an antimicrobial foam disc.

**Answer: A**

Momoz, O., Lucet, J.C. and Kerforne, T., *et al.* (2015) Skin antisepsis with chlorhexidine-alcohol versus povidone iodine-alcohol, with and without skin scrubbing, for prevention of intravascular-catheter-related infection (CLEAN): an open-label, multicenter, randomized, controlled, two-by-two factorial trial. *Lancet*, **386** (10008), 2069–2077.
O'Grady, N.P., Alexander, M., Burns, L.A., *et al.* (2001) Healthcare Infection Control Practices Advisory Committee (HICPAC). Guidelines for the Prevention of intravascular catheter-related infections. *Clinical Infectious Diseases*, **52** (9):e162–e193.

**2** Regarding the use of ultrasound guidance versus the landmark technique for the routine placement of a CVC:
A The landmark technique has a lower incidence of carotid puncture
B The landmark technique increases the chance of success at the first attempt to cannulate the internal jugular as compared to ultrasound
C The landmark technique results in faster venous cannulation times
D The benefits of ultrasonic localization can be generalized for all access sites (internal jugular, subclavian, femoral)
E The landmark technique reduces the chance of hematoma formation as compared to ultrasound use

Anatomic landmarks have traditionally been used to guide central venous catheter placement, but with increasing use of portable ultrasound (US) in the ICU, there have been multiple studies evaluating its use in the

*Surgical Critical Care and Emergency Surgery: Clinical Questions and Answers*, Second Edition.
Edited by Forrest "Dell" Moore, Peter Rhee, and Gerard J. Fulda.
© 2018 John Wiley & Sons Ltd. Published 2018 by John Wiley & Sons Ltd.
Companion website: www.wiley.com/go/moore/surgical_criticalcare_and_emergency_surgery

placement of CVCs. In general, these studies have supported the use of two-dimensional US for placement of CVCs. Findings include: reduction in the number of passes to cannulation, lower incidence of artery puncture/hematoma complications, and higher overall success rate. There are several caveats to these findings. Data on insertion based on experience level of providers is lacking, as are data on patients at high risk for complications. In addition, no study has compared the efficacy of US-guided vs. landmark technique in patients needing emergent central venous access. However, given the overall data, the Agency for Healthcare Research and Quality recommends that real-time ultrasound guidance be utilized for CVC insertion as a way to improve patient care.

**Answer: D**

Brass, P., Hellmich, M., Kolodziej, L., *et al.* (2015) Ultrasound guidance versus anatomical landmarks for internal jugular vein catheterization. *Cochrane Database Systematic Reviews*, **1**.

Fragou, M., Gravvanis, A., Dimitriou, V., *et al.* (2011) Real-time ultrasound-guided subclavian vein cannulation versus the landmark method in critical care patients: A prospective randomized study. *Critical Care Medicine*, **39** (7), 1607–1612.

**3** All the following are true regarding arterial catheterization except:
   A The need for frequent arterial blood gases (three or more in a 24-hour time period) is an indication for arterial catheterization
   B Carpal tunnel syndrome is a relative contraindication
   C The Allen test should be performed prior to radial artery catheterization to ensure adequate ulnar collateral flow
   D End-arteries such as the brachial artery should be avoided except when more preferable sites are not available
   E The risk of permanent ischemic complications in radial artery cannulation is rare.

As with any procedure, understanding the indications for and complications of arterial catheterization is crucial. Indications for indwelling arterial catheter placement include hemodynamic monitoring, frequent arterial blood gas sampling (three or more per 24 hours), and arterial administration of medications. Complications include bleeding, infection, arteriovenous fistula formation, and distal ischemia secondary to thrombosis or embolization. Radial artery cannulation is a relatively safe procedure that has an incidence of permanent ischemic complications of 0.09%. Multiple sites can be

utilized for cannulation, but to minimize complications, sites with limited collateral circulation (such as the brachial artery) should be avoided. The Allen test attempts to assess ulnar arterial flow to the hand prior to radial arterial line placement. While theoretically pleasing, the clinical utility of this test is dubious. As such, many practitioners have abandoned this as a precursor to radial artery cannulation. Relative contraindications to arterial cannulation include trauma or burns to the ipsilateral extremity, carpal tunnel syndrome, damaged or infected skin at the access site, coagulopathy, and Raynaud's disease.

**Answer: C**

Brzezinski, M., Luisetti, T., and London, M.J. (2009) Radial artery cannulation: A comprehensive review of recent anatomic and physiologic investigations. *Anesthesia and Analgesia*, **109** (6), 1763–81.

Gabrielli, A., Layon, A.J., and Yu, M. (eds) (2009) *Civetta, Taylor, and Kirby's Critical Care*, Lippincott Williams & Wilkins. Philadelphia, PA, pp. 409–428.

Irwin, R.S. and Ripe, J.M. (eds) (2008) *Intensive Care Medicine*. Lippincott Williams & Wilkins, Philadelphia, PA, Table 3.1, pp. 38–47.

Shiloh, A.L., Savel, R.H., Paulin, L.M., and Eisen, L.A. (2011) Ultrasound-guided catheterization of the radial artery: a systematic review and meta-analysis of randomized controlled trials. *Chest*, **139** (3), 524–529.

**4** A 76-year-old man with significant cardiac and pulmonary history is being treated for septic shock secondary to pneumonia. He has just been placed on his second vasopressor despite aggressive fluid resuscitation. To rule out a cardiogenic component to his shock, you decide to place a pulmonary artery catheter (PAC). Which of the following is true regarding PAC:
   A Pulmonary artery occlusion pressures correlate poorly with volume responsiveness
   B Placement is contraindicated in patients with tricuspid regurgitation
   C The catheter should never be pulled back without first inflating the balloon
   D Ventricular arrhythmias caused by PAC placement are usually permanent
   E The PA catheter cannot be placed through the femoral vein

Use of pulmonary artery catheters (PAC) has declined in the recent years as contemporary studies have questioned the utility of the procedure. The correlation between pulmonary artery occlusion pressures ("wedge" pressures) and response to volume administration is poor. However, if a PAC is to be used it is important to understand the information it can provide. Indications for which the PAC may be beneficial include assessment and management of: complicated cardiovascular illnesses, cardiogenic shock and mixed shock states, and complications of myocardial infarction.

Absolute contraindications to placement include right-heart thrombus or tumor, and tricuspid/pulmonary valve endocarditis; severe coagulopathy is a relative contraindication. Caution should be used in the patient with new left bundle branch block as it may precipitate complete heart block. In patients with right-sided valve disease, such as tricuspid regurgitation, caution should be used due to increased difficulty of catheter passage. The process of insertion should start with vascular access and can be done from multiple different sites, including the femoral vein. The right internal jugular and left subclavian vein approaches facilitate passage of the catheter into the pulmonary artery due to the curvature of the catheter. It is important to recognize that while the balloon needs to be inflated to advance the catheter, it should always be deflated prior to withdrawal. Many complications are possible and include balloon rupture, knotting of the catheter, pulmonary infarction, thrombosis, embolism, arrhythmias, and perforation.

Early complications include ventricular arrhythmias and are usually self-limited. Air embolism may occur if the ports were not properly flushed prior to the procedure; symptoms include chest pain, dyspnea, tachycardia, and hypotension.

**Answer: A**

Kelly, C.R. and Rabbani, L.E. (2013) Pulmonary-artery catheterization. *New England Journal of Medicine*, **369**, e35.1–e35.7.

Kumar, A., Anel, R., Bunnell, E., *et al.* (2004) Pulmonary artery occlusion pressure and central venous pressure fail to predict ventricular filling volume, cardiac performance, or the response to volume infusion in normal subjects. *Critical Care Medicine*, **32** (3), 691–699.

5  *An 80-year-old man with symptomatic bradycardia requires temporary cardiac pacing. What should be considered when placing a temporary transvenous cardiac pacemaker?*

   **A** *Both bradyarrhythmias and tachyarrhythmias may be treated by this method*

   **B** *These can be used in patients with a prosthetic tricuspid valve*

   **C** *Femoral venous access is the preferred placement route*

   **D** *Most common positioning is in the right atrium*

   **E** *There is no role for ultrasound guidance in the placement or capture of a transvenous pacemaker*

The purpose of temporary cardiac pacing is to treat an arrhythmia until it resolves, or until long-term therapy can be initiated. Temporary transvenous cardiac pacemakers are most often placed for symptomatic bradycardia but can also be used for overdrive pacing in patients with tachyarrhythmias. Contraindications include intermittent, mild symptoms where the arrhythmia is well tolerated and a prosthetic tricuspid valve, which may be damaged by the pacemaker lead.

Although the preferred access approach is through the right internal jugular or left subclavian vein, transvenous pacemaker may also be placed via the femoral or brachial veins. The most common cardiac chamber to place the device is the right ventricle. With the increasing portability of bedside ultrasound, there is a role for its use in the placement of the pacemaker, as well as assessment of functionality and complications.

**Answer: A**

Harrigan, R.A., Chan, T.C., and Moonblatt, S. (2007) Temporary transvenous pacemaker placement in the emergency department. *Journal of Emergency Medicine*, **32** (1), pp. 105–111.

Laboviz, A.J., Noble, V.E., Bierig, M. (2010) Focused cardiac ultrasound in the emergent setting: a consensus statement of the American Society of Echocardiography and American College of Emergency Physicians. *Journal of the American Society of Echocardiography*, **23** (12), 1225–1230.

6  *A patient diagnosed with recurrent pulmonary embolism (PE) is to undergo inferior vena cava (IVC) filter placement. When advising the patient on potential complications of the procedure, what should be mentioned?*

   **A** *They are not to undergo MRI after IVC filter placement*

   **B** *Following IVC filter placement, the risk of recurrent PE is eliminated*

   **C** *The presence of the filter increases the risk of caval thrombosis*

   **D** *Renal complications are unlikely, independent of filter placement position*

   **E** *Migration, perforation, and poor retrieval rates are uncommon*

The use of the IVC filter has increased significantly in recent years, likely due to newer technology, which allows for removal once the indication for the filter has passed. Indications for inferior vena cava filters vary amongst professional groups, but include: recurrent pulmonary embolism (PE) despite anticoagulation, known deep venous thrombosis (DVT), or PE with contraindication to anticoagulation, and known deep venous thrombosis DVT/PE with complications of anticoagulation. Controversy exists as to which trauma patients may benefit (if at all) from a filter. Many filters exist and there seems to be a trend toward placement of retrievable filters despite poor retrieval rates. The majority of IVC filters currently used in the United States are MRI compatible, but individual product information should be sought. They can be placed via transabdominal ultrasound, endovascular ultrasound, or fluoroscopically. It is important to understand that the placement of the IVC filter actually carries with it a risk of both deep femoral vein and inferior vena cava thrombosis. For this reason, the standard placement of filter should be below the renal veins to reduce the risk of renal vein thrombosis and subsequent kidney loss should caval thrombosis occur. No therapy is perfect, and IVC filters are not an exception to this rule; there is a 0.5–6% risk of recurrent pulmonary embolism with the filter in place, and 0.4% rate of clinically significant penetration of the IVC.

**Answer: C**

American College of Radiology (2016) *ACR-SIR-SPR Practice Parameter for the Performance of Inferior Vena Cava (IVC) Filter Placement for the Prevention of Pulmonary Embolism*. The American College of Radiology, Reston, VA.

Sarosiek, S., Crowther, M., and Sloan, M. (2013) Indications, complications, and management of inferior vena cava filters. *Journal of the American Medical Association: Internal Medicine*, **173** (7), 513–517.

**7** *For an ICU patient requiring endotracheal intubation, which of the following statements is correct?*

   **A** *Rapid sequence intubation is the best technique for intubation*

   **B** *Ensuring that the ear and sternal notch are in the same plane greatly facilitates visualization during orotracheal intubation*

   **C** *In a patient who is able to be ventilated, repeated attempts at direct laryngoscopy are not associated with worse outcomes*

   **D** *If using videolaryngoscopy or fiberoptic technique, rescue airway such as laryngeal mask airway (LMA) is unnecessary*

   **E** *There is no difference in success rate between direct laryngoscopy and videolaryngoscopy*

Rapid sequence intubation (RSI) is a method of intubating patients in which a sedative agent and short-term paralytic agent are administered prior to intubation. While useful in many situations, eliminating a patient's ability to breathe spontaneously may not always be

beneficial. For instance, a patient who is hypoxic but maintaining stable oxygen saturation through spontaneous respiration may be converted to a patient who is progressively hypoxic. If unable to be intubated, adverse events may follow. Whatever method of intubation is selected, preprocedural preparation is imperative. Correct positioning of the patient (accomplished by aligning the ear and sternal notch in a parallel plane, the "sniffing" position) ensures the best visualization possible and increases the chances of success. Although you may "take your time" securing the airway if the patient is oxygenating and hemodynamically normal, there is some evidence that repetitive laryngoscopy, either direct or by videolaryngoscopy, may place the patient at high risk for potentially life-threatening airway and nonairway related complications. Videolaryngoscopy has become the latest technique for the difficult and failed intubation. These devices present a magnified image from the tip of the blade onto a video screen. It has been demonstrated that this technique frequently improves intubation success in patients with difficult airways.

**Answer: B**

Collins, J.S., Lemmens, H.F., Brodsky, J.B., *et al.* (2004) Laryngoscopy and morbid obesity: a comparison of the "sniff" and "ramped" positions. *Obesity Surgery*, **14** (9), 1171.

American Society of Anesthesiologists (2013) Practice guidelines for management of the difficult airway: an updated report by the American Society of Anesthesiologists Task Force on Management of the Difficult Airway. *Anesthesiology*, **118** (2), 1–20.

**8** *An ICU patient requires a tracheostomy. When deciding between surgical tracheostomy (ST) or percutaneous dilatational tracheostomy (PDT), which of the following is correct?*

   **A** *Both techniques can be easily performed in the ICU setting*

   **B** *PDT is preferred in patients with difficult anatomy*

   **C** *Overall complications rates are similar for ST and PDT*

   **D** *Tracheostomy is contraindicated in patients with severe thrombocytopenia*

   **E** *ST is the preferred procedure in patients with high positive end-expiratory pressure (PEEP)*

PDT was first introduced in the mid-1980s and has since become a standard technique in the ICU due to multiple reports of its safety, cost savings, and ease of performance. There are no outcome benefits that have been found in comparing these two techniques; overall complication rates are similar, as well as similar rates of bleeding. There is, however, a lower incidence of wound infection with PDT, but a higher incidence of injury to the posterior wall of the trachea. Because PDT can be performed at the bedside, surgeons and nonsurgeons alike have adopted the procedure. Previous tracheostomy is not a contraindication to either technique. Previously, body habitus including morbid obesity and short neck along with recent cervical spine surgery, high PEEP, and coagulopathy were thought to be absolute contraindications to PDT. These contraindications have become relative, as more experience has been gained with the procedure. An experienced operator is the key to performing the procedure in this cohort of patients.

**Answer: C**

Batuwitage, B., Webber, S., and Glossop, A. (2014) Percutaneous tracheostomy. *Continuing Education in Anesthesia, Critical Care & Pain*, **14** (6), 268–272.

Beiderlinden, M., Groeben, H., and Peters, J. (2003) Safety of percutaneous dilational tracheostomy in patients ventilated with high positive end-expiratory pressure (PEEP). *Intensive Care Medicine*, **29** (6), 944–948.

Kluge, S., Meyer, A., Kuhnell, P., *et al.* (2004) Percutaneous tracheostomy is safe in patients with severe thrombocytopenia. *Chest*, **126**, 547–551.

**9** *After a successful PDT performed at the patient's bedside, a discussion ensues with the resident staff about potential complications of tracheostomy. All the following are considered early complications except:*
   **A** *Tracheostomy tube dislodgement*
   **B** *Pneumothorax*
   **C** *Hemorrhage*
   **D** *Tracheo-innominate fistula*
   **E** *Subcutaneous emphysema*

When considering complications of tracheostomy, it may be useful to divide these into early (≤7 days) and late complications (>7 days). Tracheostomy tube dislodgement can occur at any time but is most hazardous in the days after initial placement; the most devastating sequelae of tracheostomy tube dislodgement is death secondary to loss of airway. Because the tract between the trachea and skin is not well developed early after tracheostomy, attempting to replace the tracheostomy tube may lead to creation of a false passage without restoration of the airway. For this reason, oral endotracheal intubation is the procedure of choice should the tracheostomy tube be lost in the early postoperative period. Early dislodgement is usually due to a technical problem. There are multiple ways to help prevent this including proper placement of the stoma, avoidance of excessive neck hyperextension, and suturing the tube to the skin

along with using tracheostomy tape. Subcutaneous emphysema can occur secondary to positive pressure itself, or a forceful cough against a tightly sutured or packed wound. Subcutaneous emphysema should resolve without intervention over the following days. A pneumothorax can also be a consideration and can be evaluated with a chest x-ray. Due to the anatomic position of the apices of the lung in the neck, there is a 0–5% risk of pneumothorax with tracheostomy and a postprocedural chest radiograph is widely considered to be standard of care. Hemorrhage can occur in 5.7% of patients. Most minor bleeding can be controlled with simple packing, but can become life threatening if it causes airway obstruction. Major hemorrhage occurs in a smaller percentage of patients and may require exploration and hemorrhage control in the operating room.

A rare but devastating late complication of tracheostomy is tracheoinnominate (TI) fistula. In general, it will occur in the first month after the procedure but can happen as late as a year due to elevated tracheostomy tube cuff pressures or contact between the distal end of the tracheostomy tube and the innominate artery. Pulsation of the tracheostomy tube may be clue. A TI fistula will frequently present with a "herald bleed"; bright red blood from around the tracheostomy site, which abates spontaneously, only to be followed by exanguinating hemorrhage. Should late bleeding occur in a patient with a tracheostomy, it should prompt further diagnostic workup. If bleeding occurs in a patient with a high index of suspicion for a TI fistula, the first step should be overinflation of the tracheostomy tube balloon. Should this control the bleeding initially, the patient should be brought to the operating room for definitive repair. If the bleeding continues, the tracheostomy tube should be removed and a finger placed in the tracheal stoma for direct anterior compression of the fistula (the Utley maneuver). A small orotracheal tube should then be passed with its inflated cuff beyond the level of the fistula. Finally, the patient should be transported to the operating room for repair.

**Answer: D**

Fernandez-Bussy, S., Mahajan, B., Folch, E., *et al.* (2015) Tracheostomy tube placement: early and late complications. *Journal of Bronchology & Interventional Pulmonology*, **22** (4), 357–364.

Ridley, R.W. and Zwischenberger, J.B. (2006) Tracheoinnominate fistula: surgical management of an iatrogenic disaster. *Journal of Laryngology and Otology*, **120**, 676–680.

**10** *A 24-year-old man who presented after a high-speed motor vehicle collision with a traumatic brain injury and bilateral pulmonary contusions is now requiring* *pressure control ventilation with an inverse I:E ratio and inspired oxygen fraction 90%. Nursing staff describes a large volume of thick secretions and the patient is now febrile. In regards to fiber-optic bronchoscopy, all the following statements are correct except:*

**A** *Hypoxia is a relative contraindication*

**B** *Intracranial pressure may spike during the procedure*

**C** *Pneumothorax may occur in over 30% of patients*

**D** *Can safely be done in unstable cardiac patients*

**E** *The FiO$_2$ should be dialed up to 100% regardless of the patients' saturations*

Flexible bronchoscopy is generally a well-tolerated procedure with multiple potential diagnostic and therapeutic indications. As with other interventions, the practitioner must be aware of the possible complications and contraindications. Mortality in experienced hands should not exceed 0.1%. Careful patient selection is the key to keeping the incidence of complications low. Hypoxia should prompt caution given multiple studies that demonstrate a decline in oxygenation that can persist for some time postprocedure. If bronchoscopy is still deemed necessary in a hypoxic patient, minimizing procedure time, withdrawing the bronchoscope frequently, and providing maximal oxygen support will help prevent persistent hypoxia. Bronchoscopy has been noted to raise intracranial pressure but there may not be permanent sequelae. Known complications of flexible bronchoscopy include cardiac arrhythmias, bronchospasm, pneumothorax, and vasovagal reactions. Unless biopsies are being taken, pneumothorax is a rare complication of fiber-optic bronchoscopy (<2%).

**Answer: C**

Gorman, S.R. and Beamis, J.F., Jr. (2005) Complications of flexible bronchoscopy. *Clinical Pulmonary Medicine*, **12** (3), 177–183.

Kerwin, A.J., Croce, M.A., and Timmons, S.D. (2000) Effects of bronchoscopy on intracranial pressure in patients with brain injury: a prospective clinical study. *Journal of Trauma*, **48**, 878–883.

**11** *A 58-year-old man has been on the ventilator for eight days after complicated aortic aneurysm repair. He is now febrile and is noted to have a new infiltrate on chest x-ray. Regarding the use of bronchoscopy for the diagnosis of pneumonia, which of the following statements is correct?*

**A** *Quantitative protected brush specimens represent the gold standard in ventilator-associated pneumonia diagnosis*

**B** *To ensure accurate diagnostic testing, a BAL specimen must be obtained from each lobe of the lung*

**C** *To ensure accurate diagnostic testing, at least 100 ml saline should be instilled*

**D** *Bronchoscopy should be performed for diagnostic purposes even in patients with severe hypoxia on maximal ventilator settings*

**E** *The bronchoscope need only be advanced into the orifice of the desired lobe for appropriate sampling*

Bronchoscopy can be a useful tool in making the diagnosis of pneumonia and in identifying the causative organism(s). Bronchoscopy allows for the performance of either a bronchoalveolar lavage (BAL) or protected brush specimen (PBS) but neither has been definitively accepted as the standard of care for diagnosis of ventilator-associated pneumonia. When performing BAL, one need not sample from every lobe but instead attention should be directed to the location of suspected infection. If the disease process is diffuse, there is some controversy as to the location for the best sample but in general, should be taken from the most affected segment. Once chosen, the bronchoscope should be advanced until wedged into a subsegmental bronchus. Saline is then instilled and suctioned into a trap. At least 100–120 ml should be instilled and most advocate discarding the first 35–50 ml as this is likely contaminated from the more proximal airways. One must also be cognizant of the need to retrieve as much as possible as this will increase the yield of the specimen. The risks and benefits must be considered prior to performance of bronchoscopy; caution should be used in patients who may not tolerate further hypoxia as a result of this procedure.

**Answer: C**

Chastre, J. and Fagon, J.Y. (2002) Ventilator-associated pneumonia. *American Journal of Respiratory Critical Care Medicine*, **165**, 867–903.

Combes, A., Luyt, C.E., Trouillet, J.L., and Chastre, J. (2010). Controversies in ventilator-associated pneumonia. *Seminars in Respiratory and Critical Care Medicine*, **31** (1), 47–54.

Irwin, R.S. and Rippe, J.M. (eds) (2008) *Intensive Care Medicine*, Lippincott Williams & Wilkins, Philadelphia, PA.

**12** *With regard to performing endoscopy in the intensive care unit, which of the following statements is correct?*

**A** *Orotracheal intubation should be performed prior to upper endoscopy*

**B** *Lower gastrointestinal endoscopy for bleeding should not be performed without first ensuring that there is not an upper gastrointestinal source*

**C** *Endoscopy is absolutely contraindicated in the presence of coagulopathy*

**D** *Lower GI endoscopic decompression is the first line procedure in acute colonic pseudoobstruction (Ogilvie's Syndrome)*

**E** *There is no role for endoscopic retrograde cholangiopancreatography (ERCP) in the ICU*

Both upper and lower endoscopies can be carried out safely in the ICU environment. Adequate sedation is needed prior to these procedures but there is no need for orotracheal intubation in many patients unless it is warranted for airway protection or other concerning circumstances. While the majority of bleeding per rectum is from a lower gastrointestinal source (distal to the ligament of Treitz), upwards of 11% of cases will actually have an upper gastrointestinal origin. Coagulopathy is a relative contraindication to performance of endoscopy and the decision to proceed or not must be based on a thorough assessment of the potential risks and benefits of the procedure. After ruling out mechanical causes of obstruction in patients suspected to have acute colonic pseudo-obstruction, neostigmine administration is the initial treatment of choice. Many scenarios exist in which ICU patients are too ill for transport. Multiple procedures, including bedside laparoscopy, ERCP, and abdominal explorations have been shown to be safe in the ICU setting when performed by experienced personnel.

**Answer: B**

Chudzinski, A.P., Thompson, E.V., and Ayscue, J.M. (2015) Acute colonic pseudoobstruction. *Clinics in Colon and Rectal Surgery*, **28** (2), 112–117.

Saleem, A., Gostout, C.J., and Peterson, B.T. (2011) Outcome of emergency ERCP in the intensive care unit. *Endoscopy*, **43** (6), 549–551.

**13** *When placing a percutaneous endoscopic gastrostomy (PEG), all the following have been utilized to reduce complications EXCEPT:*

**A** *Preprocedural antibiotic*

**B** *Transillumination*

**C** *1:1 ballottement*

**D** *Placing the patient in the reverse Trendelenburg position*

**E** *Visualizing simultaneous air return while aspirating a syringe at the same time as endoscopic visualization of an intragastric needle*

PEG tube placement has become the preferred method for enteral access in the patient who will require long-term feeding access. It is less invasive than an open gastrostomy tube and can be performed in a variety of locations, including the ICU. Considerations prior to placement should include previous abdominal surgery and known anatomic variation of the gastrointestinal tract. PEG tubes are associated with ~1% mortality rate, ~3% major complication rate, and a 13% minor complication rate. Prior to beginning the procedure, prophylactic antibiotics (i.e. a first-generation cephalosporin) should be given to reduce infection rate. Because PEG placement requires the blind passage of a needle, wire, and ultimately gastrostomy tube between the skin and gastric lumen, techniques have been developed to minimize the risk of injuring intervening structures (e.g. colon). After adequate endoscopic insufflation of the stomach, digital indentation of the skin should be visualized as directly translated to the gastric wall (a phenomenon known as 1:1 ballottement). In addition, light from the endoscope should be visualized passing through the abdominal wall (transillumination). Lastly, there are several papers that describe using a "finder" needle and fluid-filled syringe to appropriately locate the stomach. Advancing the needle while simultaneously aspirating should show air return when in the lumen. If this air return is noted prior to gastric visualization of the needle, the assumption is that there is an interposed loop of bowel between the stomach and abdominal wall. There is no evidence that positioning the patient in reverse Trendelenburg position can help reduce complication rates.

**Answer: D**

Rahnemai-Azar, A.A., Rahnemaiazar, A.A., Naghshizadian, R., *et al.* (2014) Percutaneous endoscopic gastrostomy: Indications, technique, complications and management. *World Journal of Gastroenterology*, **20** (24), 7739–7751.

**14** *A patient in the ICU requires abdominal paracentesis for respiratory compromise secondary to ascites. With regard to paracentesis in the ICU, which of the following statements is correct?*

**A** *Coagulopathy is a contraindication to paracentesis*

**B** *Ultrasound-guided paracentesis has success rates equivalent to landmark-guided paracentesis*

**C** *The urinary bladder should be decompressed prior to paracentesis*

**D** *Paracentesis-induced circulatory dysfunction (PICD) may occur after the removal of even small volumes of fluid*

**E** *Paracentesis should not be performed in the pregnant woman*

Paracentesis has been used in the ICU for both diagnostic and therapeutic purposes. Correction of coagulopathy is not absolutely mandatory but should be considered.

The preferred site of access for paracentesis is the anterior abdominal wall, lateral to the bladder and epigastric vessels. Because a distended bladder may be at higher risk for inadvertent puncture, decompression of the bladder is recommended prior to paracentesis. Use of ultrasound may increase the success rate of paracentesis relative to the traditional landmark technique (95% versus 61% in one prospective randomized trial). Paracentesis-induced circulatory dysfunction (PCID) is a condition characterized by hyponatremia, azotemia, and increase in plasma rennin activity and typically only occurs after large- volume paracentesis. Infusion of albumin has been shown to diminish the chances of this occurring. Caution should be used when performing paracentesis in the pregnant patient. It should only be attempted with an imaging technique such as ultrasound.

**Answer: C**

Grabau, C.M., Crago, S.F., Hoff, L.K., *et al.* (2004) Performance standards for therapeutic abdominal paracentesis. *Hepatology*, **40**, 484–488.

Nazeer, S.R., Dewbre, H., and Miller, A.H. (2005) Ultrasound-assisted paracentesis performed by emergency physicians vs. the traditional technique: a prospective, randomized study. *American Journal of Emergency Medicine*, **23** (3), 363–367.

Ruiz-Del-Arbol, L., Monescillo, A., Jimenez, W., *et al.* (1997) Paracentesis-induced circulatory dysfunction: Mechanism and effect on hepatic hemodynamics in cirrhosis. *Gastroenterology*, **113** (2), 579–586.

**15** With regard to the use of lumbar puncture in the ICU, which of the following statements is correct?
   A To reduce the risk of adverse events, lumbar puncture must be performed under fluoroscopy
   B CSF pressure measurement is accurate no matter the position of the patient when sampling takes place
   C Lumbar puncture can safely be performed in most patients without first obtaining a CT scan of the brain
   D Irreversible hearing loss is a rare but potentially devastating complication of lumbar puncture
   E Utilization of ultrasound to identify landmarks is superior to the palpation technique

Lumbar puncture can be utilized in the ICU to sample cerebrospinal fluid (CSF) for a variety of reasons. In adults, CSF aspiration can usually be done under local anesthetic. Patients with previous lumbar surgery or congenital abnormal anatomy may require fluoroscopically guided needle placement but, in general, anatomic landmarks can be used. Prior to performing a lumbar puncture, a CT scan of the brain has been recommended in the following patients: immunocompromised states (e.g. HIV, posttransplant), history of central nervous system disease, new onset seizures, papilledema, abnormal level of consciousness, and focal neurologic deficits. The accuracy of CSF pressure measurement is limited by the patient's position. Cerebrospinal fluid pressure measurements are not accurate if performed when the patient is in a seated position; this can be rectified by reclining the patient into a lateral position. Several complications of lumbar puncture exist. These include spinal headache, hemorrhage, and hearing loss. Hearing loss after lumbar puncture is thought to be due to changes in intracranial pressure. While it is generally reversible, rare cases of long-term hearing loss have been reported. There is mixed literature (mostly in non-ICU patients) regarding the superiority of ultrasound-guided LP. Some suggestion exists that it may be beneficial in the morbidly obese patient.

**Answer: D**

Doherty, C.M. and Forbes, R.B. (2014) Diagnostic lumbar puncture. *Ulster Medical Journal*, **83** (2), 93–102.

Michel, O. and Brusis, T. (1992) Hearing loss as a sequel of lumbar puncture. *Annals of Otology Rhinology and Laryngology*, **101**, 390–394.

Nomura, J.T., Leech, S.J., Shenbagamurthi, S., *et al.* (2007) A randomized controlled trial of ultrasound-assisted lumbar puncture. *Journal of Ultrasound Medicine*, **26**, 1341–1348.

Tunkel, A.R., Hartman, B.J., Kaplan, S.L., *et al.* (2004) Practice guidelines for the management of bacterial meningitis. *Clinical Infectious Disorders*, **39**, 1267–1284.

# 27

## Diagnostic Imaging, Ultrasound, and Interventional Radiology

*Keneeshia N. Williams, MD, Remigio J. flor, MD and Terence O'Keeffe, MD*

1   Which of the following is **false** regarding the assessment of a pericardial effusion?
   A  *Pericardial effusions are always present in dependent segments*
   B  *Diastolic collapse of both atriums in a significant pericardial effusion occurs in ventricular systole*
   C  *Peritoneal free fluid can be confused with a pericardial effusion on the anterior view of the heart in a subcostal 4-chamber view*
   D  *Several views of a pericardial effusion via a transthoracic echocardiography (TTE) may be needed to identify its presence and amount*
   E  *A pleural effusion typically shows a complex echotexture on ultrasound*

Pericardial effusion is often found in critically ill patients and can be life-threatening. It is characterized as a diastolic fluid-filled space located within the two layers of the pericardium via a TTE. If a pericardial effusion is erroneously diagnosed in an unstable patient, an unwarranted pericardiocentesis may be performed with the strong possibility of cardiac chamber perforation, pericardial tamponade, and death.

A pericardial effusion is always located along the posterior wall, lateral, and inferior wall. These are all dependent segments of the heart.

A significant pericardial effusion will cause diagnostic collapse of both atriums. The right atrium and right ventricular outflow tracts are the first to collapse. Once the effusion has become very severe, the left atrium and left ventricle will become collapsed as well. On TTE, the collapse of both atriums can be seen in atrial diastole or ventricular systole when a pericardial effusion is present.

Peritoneal free fluid, or ascites, always appears in the subcostal views, anterior to the right cardiac chambers, but may mimic a pericardial effusion. Viewing the falciform ligament within the fluid confirms the diagnosis. Additionally, examination of the rest of the abdomen will further assist in diagnosing ascites.

Pericardial effusions may be regional or circumferential, and may be irregularly distributed. Therefore, several views via transthoracic echocardiography TTE may be needed to identify its presence and amount.

The image of a pericardial fluid on ultrasound is typically anechoic. However, when the effusion contains purulence or clots, it can sometimes show a complex echotexture.

**Answer: E**

Blanco, P. and Volpicelli, G. (2016) Common pitfalls in point-of-care ultrasound: a practical guide for emergency and critical care physicians. *Critical Ultrasound Journal*, **8**, 1–12.

2   Which one of the following views is **not** part of a goal-directed echocardiography (GDE) examination?
   A  Parasternal long-axis
   B  Color Doppler analysis of the mitral
   C  Apical four-chamber view
   D  6th intercostal space in B-mode
   E  Inferior vena cava (IVC) view

The goal directed echocardiography (GDE) gives the provider the ability to rapidly assess cardiac anatomy and function in a patient with hemodynamic failure.

In accordance to the American College of Chest Physicians/La Societe de Reanimation de Langue Francaise (ACCP/SRLF) competence standards, the GDE has five standard views that include the parasternal long-axis, parasternal short-axis, apical four-chamber, substernal, and inferior vena cava (IVC) views. These main views allow for the rapid identification of potentially life-threatening causes of hemodynamic failure that may lead to a life-saving procedure.

Both the mitral and aortic valves may be analyzed via color Doppler in conjunction with the standard five views of GDE to further assist the provider in the ultrasonic assessment.

*Surgical Critical Care and Emergency Surgery: Clinical Questions and Answers*, Second Edition.
Edited by Forrest "Dell" Moore, Peter Rhee, and Gerard J. Fulda.
© 2018 John Wiley & Sons Ltd. Published 2018 by John Wiley & Sons Ltd.
Companion website: www.wiley.com/go/moore/surgical_criticalcare_and_emergency_surgery

B-mode is a setting used in eFAST or thoracic ultrasound to detect abnormalities between the parietal and visceral pleura. This is not part of the standard GDE.

**Answer: D**

Walley, P.E., Walley, K.R., Goodgame, B., *et al.* (2014) A practical approach to goal-directed echocardiography in the critical care setting. *Critical Care*, **18** (6), 1–11.

Whitson, M.R. and Mayo, P.H. (2016) Ultrasonography in the emergency department. *Critical Care*, **20**, 227.

Shokoohi, H., Boniface, K.S., Pourmand, A., *et al.* (2015) Bedside ultrasound reduces diagnostic uncertainty and guides resuscitation in patients with undifferentiated hypotension. *Critical Care Medicine*, **43** (12), 2562–2569.

3   Which of the following is **NOT** true regarding the use of ultrasound in the evaluation of a trauma patient?

   A Ultrasound assessment of penetrating abdominal trauma has a high sensitivity for detecting the need for operative intervention.

   B Ultrasound assessment of penetrating abdominal trauma has a high specificity for detecting the need for operative intervention.

   C The sensitivity of using the standard probe during an abdominal ultrasound to assess for fascial penetration is low.

   D An eFAST exam allows for the evaluation of intraperitoneal fluid in addition to pneumothorax and hemothorax.

   E It is a noninvasive and inexpensive imaging modality that has become the standard of care for the evaluation of blunt abdominal trauma.

The use of ultrasonography for the initial assessment of trauma patients at the bedside has become standard of care across the United States.

The use of abdominal ultrasound for detecting the need for operative intervention in a patient who has sustained a penetrating trauma to the abdomen carries a **low** sensitivity and a **high** specificity. The sensitivity ranges from 28–48% likely due to the fact that in the absence of hemoperitoneum does not rule out the presence of intraabdominal injury. The best management for a patient with a penetrating abdominal wound and a negative FAST exam is serial abdominal examinations, local wound exploration, or diagnostic peritoneal lavage.

The use of abdominal ultrasound for detecting the need for operative intervention in a patient who has sustained a penetrating trauma to the abdomen carries a **low** sensitivity and a **high** specificity. The specificity ranges from 94–100%. The mere presence of hemoperitoneum does not necessarily correlate with the presence of a significant injury that requires laparotomy. The decision for operative exploration is often taken after enough evidence has been gathered via clinical and anatomical assessments. The ultrasound information does not alter the management plan.

The use of a high frequency linear probe (8-10 mHz) allows for better resolution of superficial structures including the fascia. This probe should be used in place of the standard probe for the evaluation of possible fascia penetration.

The FAST (focused assessment sonography for trauma) exam is widely used as a modality to assess intraperitoneal hemorrhage. The eFAST (extended focused assessment sonography for trauma) includes the assessments made in a FAST plus evaluation of the thoracic cavity for the presence of pneumo- or hemothorax.

It has become standard of care to use an abdominal ultrasound for the evaluation of a patient who has sustained blunt trauma via the FAST or eFAST exams. Ultrasonography has the advantages of being able to be performed rapidly at the patient's bedside and is noninvasive, inexpensive, portable, and may be easily repeated.

**Answer: A**

Biffl, W.L., Kaups, K.L., Cothren, C.C., *et al.* (2009) Management of patients with anterior abdominal stab wounds: A Western Trauma Association multicenter trial. *Journal of Trauma*, **66** (5), 1294–1301.

Hamada, S.R., Delhaye, N., Kerever, S., *et al.* (2016) Integrating eFAST in the initial management of stable trauma patients: the end of plain film radiography. *Annals of Intensive Care*, **6** (1), 62.

Murphy, J.T., Hall, J., and Provost, D. (2005) Fascial ultrasound for evaluation of anterior abdominal stab wound injury. *Journal of Trauma*, **59** (4), 843–846.

Soffer, D., McKenney, M.G., Cohn, S., *et al.* (2004) A prospective evaluation of ultrasonography for the diagnosis of penetrating torso injury. *Journal of Trauma*, **56** (5), 953–959.

4   The eFAST (extended focused assessment sonography for trauma exam) will readily give the provider the ability to detect all of the following **except**?

   A Hemopericardium

   B Sternal fracture

   C Retroperitoneal injuries

   D Diaphragm injury

   E Pneumothorax

The extended focused assessment sonography for trauma (eFAST) exam is a widely used bedside technique for evaluating intraperitoneal and injury thoracic injury.

Pericardial ultrasound can readily detect hemopericardium. In patients who have sustained precordial or transthoracic wounds, the sensitivity of ultrasound evaluation shows 100% sensitivity and 99.3% specificity.

Sternal fracture is another diagnosis that can be made using ultrasound, and some reports suggest that ultrasound is more sensitive and specific for this injury than plain radiology. The eFAST does not readily detect retroperitoneal or intraparenchymal injuries.

A gross injury with organs migrating from the abdomen into the chest is highly indicative of a diaphragmatic rupture. Although a rare occurrence, it can be detected using thoracic ultrasound in the hands of a skilled and experienced operator.

A normal ultrasound examination of the thoracic cavity demonstrates the rib, the sliding of the pleura, and the presence of a comet tail artifact. The presence of air between the visceral and parietal pleura, as seen in a pneumothorax, does not allow for the transmission of ultrasound waves. Therefore, the normal findings of pleural sliding and a comet tail are absent and a diagnosis of pneumothorax can readily be made.

**Answer: C**

Gentry Wilkerson, R., and Stone, M.B. (2010) Sensitivity of bedside ultrasound and supine anteroposterior chest radiographs for the identification of pneumothorax after blunt trauma. *Academic Emergency Medicine*, **17** (1), 11–17.

Kirkpatrick, A.W., Ball, C.G., Nicolaou, S., *et al.* (2006) Ultrasound detection of right-sided diaphragmatic injury; the "liver sliding" sign. *American Journal of Emergency Medicine*, **24** (2), 251–252.

You, J.S., Chung, Y.E., Kim, D., *et al.* (2010) Role of sonography in the emergency room to diagnose sternal fractures. *Journal of Clinical Ultrasound*, **38** (3), 135–137.

5 Which of the following is true regarding CT scan evaluation of patients who have suffered blunt abdominal trauma?
   A Oral contrast extravasation is an indirect finding of blunt bowel injury on CT imaging.
   B The absence of free intraperitoneal fluid on CT imaging has a high positive predictive value.
   C Mesenteric hematoma is a direct finding of blunt bowel injury seen on CT imaging.
   D The presence of vessel beading and abrupt vessel termination are highly specific for surgically important blunt bowel injury.
   E Small bowel wall thickening has a high sensitivity in detecting surgically important blunt bowel injury on CT imaging.

There are two basic types of findings bowel injury on CT imaging: direct and indirect. Oral contrast extravasation is a direct finding of blunt bowel injury on CT imaging. Mesenteric hematoma is an indirect finding of blunt bowel injury seen on CT imaging. In the absence of free intraperitoneal fluid, CT imaging has a high negative predictive value. The presence of vessel beading and abrupt vessel termination are highly specific for surgically important blunt bowel injury, both over 90% specific. Small bowel wall thickening has been shown to have a low sensitivity and specificity of detecting surgically important blunt bowel injury on CT imaging.

**Answer: D**

Butela, S.T., Federle, M.P., Chang, P.J., *et al.* (2001) Performance of CT in detection of bowel injury. *American Journal of Roentgenology*, **176**, 129–135.

Scott, D., Steenburg, S.D., Petersen, M.J., Shen, C., and Lin, H. (2015) Multi-detector CT of blunt mesenteric injuries: usefulness of imaging findings for predicting surgically significant bowel injuries. *Abdominal Imaging*, **40** (5) 1026–1033.

6 Which of the following statements is correct regarding splenic artery embolization following blunt trauma?
   A The success rate of nonoperative management of the spleen is improved from 50% to 75% with embolization techniques.
   B The need for further intervention occurs in up to 25% of patients after the first 24 hours of nonoperative management.
   C Although angiography has been shown to be safe in children, contrast blush in the pediatric population does not warrant the routine use of angiography.
   D Angiography has been shown to be safe in adults but should be used with caution in the pediatric population.
   E Splenic abscess is a common complication following splenic artery embolization.

A. The success rate of non-operative management of the spleen has been reported to be over 95% with embolization.

The need for further intervention is rare after 24 hours of nonoperative management of splenic injuries. Patients with grade 1 splenic injuries may be discharged after 24 hours, with no further intervention. Although further intervention is also rare after 24 hours of nonoperative management in patients with Grade II to V injuries, these patients require close monitoring for up to two weeks in an inpatient or outpatient setting.

Contrast blush on CT scan has been cited as a risk factor for failure of nonoperative management in adult patients. There have been few studies that have addressed the significance of contrast blush in the pediatric population. Recent studies have shown that pediatric patients with a hepatic or splenic blush on CT scan can be managed without angiography or embolization.

Angiography with embolization has been shown to be safe in both the adult and pediatric population.

Splenic abscess is a rare complication of splenic artery embolization. A CT scan of the abdomen should be considered in any patient with signs of infection with no obvious source.

**Answer: C**

Bansal, S., Karrer, M., Hansen, K., and Partrick, D. (2015) Contrast blush in pediatric blunt splenic trauma does not warrant the routine use of angiography. *American Journal of Surgery*, **210** (3), 345–350.

Kiankhooy, A., Sartorelli, K.H., Vane, D.W., and Bhave, A.D. (2010) Angiographic embolization is safe and effective therapy for blunt abdominal solid organ injury in children. *Journal of Trauma*, **68** (3), 526–531.

Zarzaur, B.L., Kozar, R., Meyers, J.G., *et al.* (2015). The splenic injury outcome trail: An American Association for the Surgery of Trauma multi-institutional study. *Journal of Trauma and Acute Care Surgery*, **79** (3), 335–342.

7  Regarding the need for pelvic angiography in a patient with a significant pelvic fracture, all of the following are true **except**?
   A Patients with ongoing or recurrent bleeding after angiography should undergo repeat angiography.
   B Indications for pelvic angiography are hemodynamic instability, with a significant pelvic fracture, and no identifiable thoraco-abdominal source of hemorrhage.
   C Patients with hemodynamic instability after preperitoneal packing should undergo angiography.
   D Fracture pattern on pelvic x-ray alone predicts mortality and need for angiography.
   E Large pelvic hematomas may signify arterial injury and need for angiography.

A. Patients with ongoing or recurrent bleeding after angiography should undergo repeat angiography.The generally accepted indications for pelvic angiography are hemodynamic unstable patients with a significant pelvic fracture, and no thoracic, abdominal, or other sources of hemorrhage. Patients who undergo pre-peritoneal packing should undergo angiography. Prior studies have shown that the type of fracture, particularly those involv-

ing ligamentous disruption of the sacroiliac joint, have an increased risk of bleeding and will more likely require angio-embolization, which impacts mortality. There is an increased rate of need for angiography in patients with pelvic hematomas larger than $500\,cm^3$ in size. However, neither the presence or absence of a pelvic hematoma, nor the size of the pelvic hematoma will reliably exclude the presence of active arterial hemorrhage and should not guide the decision for angiography.

**Answer: D**

Brown, C.V., Kasotakis, G., Wilcox, A., *et al.* (2005) Does pelvic hematoma on admission computed tomography predict active bleeding at angiography for pelvic fracture? *American Surgeon*, **71** (9), 759–762.

Cullinane, D.C., Schiller, H.L., Zielinski, M.D., *et al.* (2011) Eastern Association for the Surgery of Trauma practice management guidelines for hemorrhage in pelvic fracture—update and systemic review. *Journal of Trauma*, **71** (6), 1850–1868.

8  All of the following are possible complications of pelvic angiography **except**?
   A Gluteal muscle necrosis
   B Impotence
   C Poor fracture healing
   D Groin hematoma
   E Recurrent hemorrhage

Gluteal muscle necrosis is the most feared complication following pelvic angio-embolization. However, the incidence is usually extremely low in most patient groups. This complication has been especially reported in patients who have hemodynamic instability, prolonged immobilization, and primary gluteal trauma. Although controversial, bilateral internal iliac artery embolization has been associated with an increased risk of erectile dysfunction due to compromise of the blood supply. To date, there has been no suggestion that embolization of vessels for hemorrhage and severe pelvic trauma has a significant impact on the healing of the fracture site. Surgical wound breakdown, however, is a known complication of embolization. Groin hematoma is a complication of any angiographic procedure caused by hemorrhage from the arterial puncture site. Thrombosis is also a risk associated with this procedure. There is a significant rate of recurrent hemorrhage in patients with the most severe pelvic fractures, and this should be taken into account at the time of the original procedure; an arterial sheath may be left in place for ease of access for repeat angiography if this becomes necessary.

**Answer: C**

Cullinane, D.C., Schiller, H.L., Zielinski, M.D., *et al.* (2011) Eastern Association for the Surgery of Trauma practice management guidelines for hemorrhage in pelvic fracture—update and systemic review. *Journal of Trauma*, **71** (6), 1850–1868.

Matityahu, A., Marmor, M., Elson, J.K., *et al.* (2013) Acute complications of patients with pelvic fractures after pelvic angiographic embolization. *Clinical Orthopedics and Related Research*, **471**, 2906–2911.

Travis, T., Monsky, W.L., London, J., *et al.* (2008) Evaluation of short-term and long-term complications after emergent internal iliac artery embolization in patients with pelvic trauma. *Journal of Vascular and Interventional Radiology*, **19** (6), 840–847.

**9** In patients with penetrating trauma to zone II of the neck, which of the following would be true regarding the use of CT angiography for diagnostic evaluation?

**A** Use of CT angiography does not reduce the negative operation exploration rate

**B** Violation of the platysma is still an indication for mandatory operation

**C** Most patients with hard signs should undergo CT scan if hemodynamically stable

**D** CT scanning should only be performed in hemodynamically stable patients

**E** Diagnosis of an injury by CTA always requires an operative intervention

The use of CT angiography as an initial screening modality in penetrating neck trauma has been well established. More than one study has shown that the negative exploration rate can be reduced by using this modality as an initial screening tool for the presence of injury. Violation of the platsyma is no longer regarded as a mandatory indication for exploration, as significant injuries can be effectively ruled out by CT angiography of the neck. CT scanning has greater than 90% sensitivity for injuries, including the aero-digestive tract. Although there have been recent studies that have shown a reduced negative exploration rate when CT angiography is performed, even in the presence of hard signs, this remains controversial. The current recommendation is that patients with hard signs on physical examination should be explored in the operating room. It is imperative to protect the airway in these patients. Additionally, it is important to avoid bedside exploration in the emergency department as tamponaded bleeding may be disrupted. CT Angiography of the neck is not appropriate in patients who are hemodynamically unstable. Not all injuries that are seen on CTA will require an intervention. Nonoperative management of internal jugular vein injuries for example, has been safely performed in patients who were otherwise stable.

**Answer: D**

Osborn, T.M., Bell, R.B., Qaisi, W., *et al.* (2008) Computed tomographic angiography as an aid to clinical decision making in the selective management of penetrating injuries to the neck: a reduction in the need for operative exploration. *Journal of Trauma*, **64** (6), 1466–1471.

Schroll, R., Fontenot, T., Lipesey, M., *et al.* (2015) Role of computed tomography angiography in the management of zone II penetrating neck traumas in patients with clinical hard signs. *Journal of Trauma and Acute Care Surgery*, **79** (6), 943–950.

Sperry, J.L., Moore, E.E., Coimbra, R., *et al.* (2013) Western Trauma Association Critical Decisions in Trauma: penetrating neck trauma. *Journal of Trauma and Acute Care Surgery*, **75** (6), 936–940.

**10** Which of the following is true regarding the use of CT arteriography in penetrating peripheral vascular trauma?

**A** Sensitivity for the presence of an arterial injury is less than 75%.

**B** Use of 64-slice multidetector CT scanning allows for the integration of extremity CT angiography into routine thoraco-abdominal trauma imaging protocols

**C** If artifact exists due to bullets or bullet fragments, it will render the study unevaluable

**D** Poor timing of contrast material bolus is rarely an issue in CTA

**E** Approximately 15% of extremity CTA studies are nondiagnostic and will require further evaluation by formal angiography

Most reports evaluating CT angiography in vascular trauma quote sensitivity and specificity of greater than 90% and it has become the first-line investigation in many trauma centers for suspected arterial injury. If correctly performed, extremity angiography can be performed using the same contrast bolus that is given for the evaluation of the chest and abdomen that is routinely performed for trauma. In the study by Inaba *et al.*, 19% of studies had streak artifact but only one study was nondiagnostic (1.9%). Good diagnostic quality CT angiographic extremity examinations require careful patient preparation, to give images that will provide the necessary information. The extremity to be studied should be immobilized and careful attention to IV contrast bolus timing is necessary to make sure that the arteries are sufficiently opacified or that the CT table does not "overrun" the exam. This has been one of the barriers to the wider implementation of this technology as well as the significant postprocessing power that is required to analyze the images. Most studies only report a 1–2% nondiagnostic exam rate most usually due to streak artifact from metallic foreign bodies, although the presence of foreign bodies by no means is a guarantee that the study will be unreadable.

**Answer: B**

Inaba, K., Potzman, J., Munera, F., *et al.* (2009) Multi-slice CT angiography for arterial evaluation in the injured lower extremity. *Journal of Trauma and Acute Care Surgery*, **60**, 502–507.

Peng, P.D., Spain, D.A., Tataria, M., *et al.* (2008) CT angiography effectively evaluates extremity vascular trauma. *American Surgeon*, (**2**), 103–107.

Pieroni S., Foster B.R., Anderson S.W., *et al.* (2009) Use of 64-row multidetector CT angiography in blunt and penetrating trauma of the upper and lower extremities. *Radiographics*, **29** (3), 863–876.

11 With regards to penetrating peripheral vascular trauma, all of the following are true **except**:
   A Patients with flow-limiting intimal flap on CT angiography should undergo exploration.
   B Patients with posterior knee dislocations should undergo CT arteriography.
   C CT angiography can be considered in a hemodynamically stable patient with obvious vascular injury in the absence of hard signs.
   D The injured extremity should be compared to the noninjured extremity when determining the ankle-brachial index.
   E Duplex ultrasonography has a specificity of 50% and should be avoided.

**Answer: E**

An intimal defect documented on an imaging study is expected to heal approximately 90% of the time without operation. Patients who maintain flow to the hand or foot and have no clinical findings suggestive of a developing pseudoaneurysm or arteriovenous fistula, may be discharged home with no further intervention. However, patients with flow-limiting intimal defects should be explored. Posterior knee dislocation is associated with popliteal arterial injuries. These patients should undergo diagnostic imaging to rule out popliteal artery injury. Imaging can often provide additional information in operative planning. This can be particularly valuable in patients with multiple fracture sites or shot gun injuries with multiple levels of injury. If the location of the injury makes it necessary, and hard signs are present, a surgeon-performed arteriogram or duplex ultrasonography study can be rapidly performed. It is important to compare the injured extremity to the noninjured extremity. A low ankle-brachial index may represent peripheral vascular disease versus an acute arterial injury. Duplex

ultrasonography has a sensitivity of 50% to 100%, and specificity of greater than 95%. The main disadvantage of duplex ultrasonography is that it is operator-dependent and requires a trained vascular technician or surgeon.

Feliciano, D.V., Moore, F.A., Moore, E.E., *et al.* (2011) Evaluation and management of peripheral vascular injury. Part 1. Western Trauma Association/critical decisions in trauma. *Journal of Trauma*, **70**, 1551–1556.

Fox, N., Rajani, R.R., Bokhari, F., *et al.* (2012) Evaluation and management of penetrating lower extremity arterial trauma: an Eastern Association for the Surgery of Trauma practice management guideline. *Journal of Trauma and Acute Care Surgery*, **73**, S315.

Wallin, D., Yaghoubian, A., Rosing, D., *et al.* (2011) Computed tomographic angiography as the primary diagnostic modality in penetrating lower extremity vascular injuries: a level I trauma experience. *Annals of Vascular Surgery*, **25**, 620.

12 Regarding the use of preoperative MRCP to detect common bile duct stones, which of the following is true?
   A MRCP is less sensitive than endoscopic ultrasound for the detection of common duct stones
   B A negative MRCP is sufficient to avoid performing an ERCP
   C Routine MRCP should be considered for all patients with gallstones
   D Performing an MRCP in patients with suspected choledocholithiasis increases hospital length of stay
   E The ability of an ERCP to perform a therapeutic procedure and stone removal as well as diagnosing common duct stones makes this the procedure of choice

With the improvement in technology and easy availability of MRI in most centers, the use of magnetic resonance cholangiopancreatography has exploded in the last decade. This provides a noninvasive technique, to image the bile ducts, that does not carry the risks of general anesthesia and postoperative pancreatitis that are two of the disadvantages of an endoscopic cholangiopancreatogram. However, this is purely a diagnostic test, and is unable to therapeutically address any stones present.

Most literature shows an equivalent accuracy rate of 95% between endoscopic ultrasound and MRCP for detecting common bile duct stones. A negative MRCP is generally felt to be of sufficient accuracy that the risks of a subsequent ERCP are not warranted, with the caveat that the laboratory and clinical exam should also be concordant. Although some authorities have argued that

MRCP should be considered in ALL patients, the additional expense and inconvenience are not necessary in the vast majority of routine cholelithiasis cases. The issue of length of stay depends on the access to MRI that is present in the hospital and may or may not present an issue. Given the scarcity of advanced endoscopists available to perform ERCP, this may in fact be more of a rate-limiting step than MRI. While it is correct that an ERCP has the ability to be both a therapeutic as well as diagnostic procedure, the requirement for general anesthesia, special endoscopic equipment, scarcity of trained endoscopists, and risk of post-procedure pancreatitis mean that MRCP can often be a sensible first step in evaluating for common duct stones.

**Answer: B**

Giljaca, V., Gurusamy, K.S., and Takwoingi, Y., *et al.* (2015) Endoscopic ultrasound versus magnetic resonance cholangiopancreatography for common bile duct stones. *Cochrane Database Systematic Reviews*, **26** (2).

Taylor, A.C., Little, A.F., Hennessy, O.F., *et al.* (2002) Prospective assessment of magnetic resonance cholangiopancreatography for noninvasive imaging of the biliary tree. *Gastrointestinal Endoscopy*, **55** (1), 17–22.

Eshgi, F. and Abdi, R. (2008) Routine magnetic resonance cholangiography compared to intra-operative cholangiography in patients with suspected common bile duct stones. *Hepatobiliary and Pancreatic Diseases International*, **7** (5), 525–528.

13 In a trauma patient who is pregnant in her first trimester who presents after a rollover MVC with abdominal pain, which is the following is TRUE regarding imaging of this patient?
    A The patient should only undergo a FAST exam due to risk to the fetus
    B Ionizing radiation should be avoided at all costs
    C MRI imaging is the modality of choice to evaluate for intra-abdominal injuries
    D CT scan of the abdomen should only be done in the last trimester
    E It is acceptable to perform CT in patients with a high index of suspicion

While trauma in pregnancy is rare, it can be a complication in up to 5–7% of all pregnancies. Concern for fetal development and dosing of ionizing radiation has led to a major reluctance to perform necessary imaging on these patients. Although there are theoretical risks to the fetus from x-rays and CT scans, these are mostly less than the risk of misdiagnosis and delay in identifying significant injuries that could threaten the health of both the mother and the child.

While the FAST exam should certainly be the initial modality of choice to evaluate patients with blunt abdominal trauma, it carries all the usual problems with sensitivity and in fact may be less accurate in the pregnant trauma patient. It should certainly not be relied upon as the sole imaging study. Given the choice of imaging that is potentially harmful but has the possibility of direct benefit to the mother and/or the fetus, any direct benefit should outweigh the potential risks of problems in the future, so it is NOT accurate to say that ionizing radiation should be completely avoided. We should image gently and appropriately but not hesitate where it is necessary (see EAST guidelines). Many trauma centers currently have relatively easy access to MRI scanners, which makes it an attractive choice. While it is certainly an option, the length of time taken, lack of ability to provide direct care for the patient during the scan, and the need usually to transport the patient away from the trauma area makes this less than ideal, and only suitable for the completely stable patient. Additionally, MRI is not currently recommended for pregnant patients in the first trimester, as it is unclear whether the magnetic field of MRI can affect the delicate developmental process of cell migration in the first trimester. If necessary, a CT scan can be done in ANY trimester. Clearly the risks to the fetus are lower in the last trimester, but again, a fetus in the first trimester will not be viable if the mother does not survive, and the focus should, as always in pregnant trauma patients, be on care of the mother's injuries. CT scans can and should be performed in pregnant trauma patients if the index of suspicion is high enough to warrant imaging. Intravenous contrast should be used as in a regular CT scan for trauma due to the need for evaluation of the perfused organs, as per the usual case in trauma, and there does not seem to be excessive risks to the fetus.

**Answer: E**

Barraco, R.D., Chiu, W.C., Clancy, T.V., *et al.* (2010) Practice management guidelines for the diagnosis and management of injury in the pregnant patient: the EAST Practice Management Guidelines Work Group. *Journal of Trauma*, **69** (1), 211–214.

Raptis, C.A., Mellnick, V.M., Raptis, D.A., *et al.* (2014) Imaging of trauma in the pregnant patient. *Radiographics*, **34** (3), 748–763.

Tirada, N., Dreizin, D., Khati, N.J., *et al.* (2015) Imaging pregnant and lactating patients. *Radiographics*, **35** (6), 1751–1765.

14 Which of the following is TRUE regarding the use of so-called "triple-contrast" CT scans, that is, PO, IV, and rectal contrast for penetrating torso trauma?

**A** These studies are best used for the evaluation of patients with penetrating flank or back wounds

**B** They are poorly tolerated by patients

**C** The addition of rectal contrast does not increase the sensitivity for the presence of bowel injuries.

**D** These scans can still be performed in patients who have other clinical indications for surgery

**E** The use of oral contrast in patients with penetrating trauma is not safe

The use of triple contrast CT scans to evaluate for penetrating torso trauma was described many years ago as a way to evaluate the retroperitoneal organs and increase the sensitivity of this study in this population of trauma patients. The purported advantages are in helping to identify subtle injuries, trajectory of the wound, as well as helping to select patients who might be candidates for nonoperative management. The "added" benefit of rectal contrast is most effective in the diagnosis of extraperitoneal colonic injuries, where patients have sustained penetrating wounds to the flanks or back. These types of injuries are notoriously difficult to diagnose.

The added benefit of rectal contrast is only really worthwhile for those retroperitoneal structures such as the ascending and descending colon. The pancreas, stomach, and solid organs can also be better imaged with the contrasting media in place. We would recommend the addition of rectal contrast only in this group of patients. Although the use of rectal contrast in the trauma patient is by no means ideal, it is usually fairly well-tolerated in the stable patient, without other distracting injuries. Concern for patient tolerance should not be a consideration in ordering this study, although local protocols may have to be developed to provide clarity over who is responsible for the installation of the rectal contrast for example, physician, CT tech, nurse.

The addition of rectal contrast does seem to confer a small advantage to the accuracy of the CT exam. Most studies have concluded that a negative triple-contrast helical CT scan has a negative predictive value of 98–100%. There have been no direct randomized trials comparing triple contrast versus IV contrast alone in trauma patients so it is difficult to quantify the additional advantage, which is why we would specifically recommend it for those patients with penetrating back and flank injuries.

In patients who have clear indications for surgery for example, evisceration, peritonitis, CT scans should not be performed, and especially not a CT scan with PO contrast. These patients should proceed directly to the operating room. Multiple studies have shown that the use of PO contrast in an awake and hemodynamically stable trauma patient is safe. Intoxicated patients, those with traumatic injuries, or with indications for the OR

should not be given PO contrast. In those cases, a CT scan with IV contrast alone may have to suffice. Theoretical concerns over aspiration of oral contrast media due to gastric distention or ileus have not been borne out in clinical practice.

**Answer: A**

Chiu, W.C., Shanmuganathan, K., Mirvis, S.E., *et al.* (2001) Determining the need for laparotomy in penetrating torso trauma: a prospective study using triple-contrast enhanced abdominopelvic computed tomography. *Journal of Trauma*, **51** (5), 860–869.

Como, J.J., Bokhari, F., Chiu, W.C., *et al.* (2010) Practice management guidelines for selective nonoperative management of penetrating abdominal trauma. *Journal of Trauma*, **68** (3), 721–733.

Lozano, J.D., Munera, F., Anderson, S.W., *et al.* (2013) Penetrating wounds to the torso: evaluation with triple-contrast multidetector CT. *Radiographics*, **33** (2), 341–359.

15 Which of the following is TRUE regarding the use of imaging in the evaluation of blunt cerebrovascular injuries (BCVI)

**A** CTA is the most accurate test for the evaluation of BCVI

**B** MRA has been shown to be as accurate as CTA for the evaluation of BCVI

**C** Injury patterns that place patients at relatively high risk for BCVI include: C1/C2 fractures, basal skull fractures, cervical spine fractures with involvement of the transverse foramen, LeFort II or III fractures.

**D** The incidence of injuries in most screening series is 5–10%

**E** If an injury is identified on imaging, anticoagulation with aspirin for 6 months is adequate therapy.

Although blunt cerebrovascular injury is rare, it can have devastating consequences, and so there has been an increased focus over the last decade in identifying patients at risk for these injuries, and also investigating which imaging modality is the most efficacious for diagnosis. While there is still some controversy regarding the use of formal angiography as opposed to CT angiography, most trauma centers have adopted an approach of liberal use of CTA as an initial screening tool.

The question of the most accurate test for diagnosing BCVI still remains controversial with some authorities questioning the true accuracy of CTA, with angiography remaining the gold standard. While CTA is probably the most **effective** initial screening test for the injuries, the most **accurate** test remains formal digital subtraction angiography

While MRA has been effective in diagnosing BCVI, there is little data to compare its effectiveness with either CTA or formal angiography. The extra length of time involved, the need for transportation from the immediate trauma area, as well as the need to assess patients for the presence of metallic foreign objects have limited its adoption. It remains more costly, more inconvenient, and no more accurate and so has not been routinely adopted.

Screening for BCVI should in fact only occur in patients at high risk, such as those mentioned in this question. Additional risk factors include high-energy mechanisms with TBI and a low GCS, "clothesline" type injuries, near hanging or a neck seatbelt sign with significant hematoma.

Although the consequences of these injuries can be devastating, the actual incidence in most studies screening high-risk patients is only 1–2%. This is one of the rare circumstances where active screening is warranted despite such a low probability of discovering a lesion.

The data regarding the optimal therapeutic regime is still of low quality, but the current recommendations for treatment of BCVI is for full anticoagulation with intravenous heparin, unless there is a contra-indication to this therapy. Some more recent studies have suggested that aspirin alone may be sufficient in low grade injuries for example, grade I or II, but there is no prospective validation of this at the moment.

**Answer: C**

Biffl, W.L., Cothren, C.C., Moore, E.E., *et al.* (2009) Western Trauma Association critical decisions in trauma: screening for and treatment of blunt cerebrovascular injuries. *Journal of Trauma*, **67** (6), 1150–1153.

Bromberg, W.J., Collier, B.C., Vogel, T.R., *et al.* (2010) Blunt cerebrovascular injury practice management guidelines: the Eastern Association for the Surgery of Trauma. *Journal of Trauma*, **68** (2), 471–477.

Paulus, E.M., Fabian, T.C., Savage, S.A., *et al.* (2014) Blunt cerebrovascular injury screening with 64-channel multidetector computed tomography: more slices finally cut it. *Journal of Trauma and Acute Care Surgery*, **76** (2), 279–285.

16   All of the following decrease the sensitivity and specificity of the FAST exam (Focused Assessment with Sonography for Trauma) except:
   A  Abdominal tenderness on exam
   B  Lumbar spine fracture
   C  Traumatic aortic rupture
   D  Pelvic fracture
   E  Ecchymosis/abrasion of the anterior abdominal wall (seatbelt sign)

The utility of ultrasound as a tool for the evaluation of the trauma patient was pioneered in Europe and Japan. In the early 1990s its use became popularized in the United States after a series of studies reported sensitivity ranging from 79–93% and a specificity ranging from 95–100% for the evaluation of hemoperitoneum after blunt mechanism. These studies also reported that ultrasound techniques can be learned in an expeditious fashion and that ultrasound provides a rapid assessment for hemoperitoneum as a point of care tool. However, there are several important situations where there are potential pitfalls in the accuracy of the FAST exam (Figure 27.1).

Abdominal tenderness can prevent the operator creating a sufficient probe/patient interface and can interfere with the accuracy of the FAST exam, increasing the likelihood of both false negative and false positive studies. Intrathoracic injuries have never been shown to interfere with the accuracy of the abdominal exam. Additionally pelvic fractures, thoracolumbar spine fractures, seatbelt sign on the anterior abdominal wall, abdominal tenderness on exam, lower rib fractures, and hematuria. In fact, the sensitivity of the FAST exam was reported to be as low as 26% in patients with pelvic fracture. A suggested algorithm for the use of FAST in pelvic fracture is shown in Figure 27.1.

**Answer: C**

Ballard, R.B., Rozycki, G.S., Newman, P.G., *et al.* (1999) An algorithm to reduce the incidence of false-negative FAST examinations in patients at high risk for occult injury. *Journal of the American College of Surgeons*, **189** (2), 145–150.

Bode, P.J., Niezen, A., van Vugt, A.B., and Schipper, J. Abdominal ultrasound as a reliable indicator for conclusive laparotomy in blunt abdominal trauma. *Journal of Trauma*, **34** (1), 27–31.

Friese, R.S., Malekzadeh, S., Shafi, S., *et al.* (2007) Abdominal ultrasound is an unreliable modality for the detection of hemoperitoneum in patients with pelvic fracture. *Journal of Trauma*, **63** (1), 97–102.

McKenney, M., Lentz, K., Nunez, D., *et al.* (1994) Can ultrasound replace diagnostic peritoneal lavage in the assessment of blunt trauma? *Journal of Trauma*, **37** (3), 439–441.

Rozycki, G.S., Ochsner, M.G., Jaffin, J.H., and Champion, H.R. (1993) Prospective evaluation of surgeons' use of ultrasound in the evaluation of trauma patients. *Journal of Trauma*, **34** (4), 516–526.

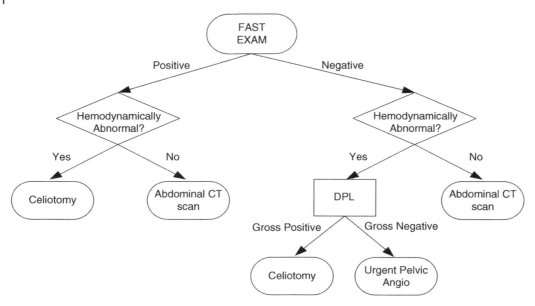

**Figure 27.1** The FAST exam.

17 Regarding the use of ultrasound for central venous catheter (CVC) placement, which of the following is FALSE?

A Duplex ultrasound is necessary to be able to tell the difference between arteries and veins

B Ultrasound identification of the vessel, followed by CVC placement, is more effective than landmark placement alone

C There is an operator learning curve with the dynamic or "real-time" ultrasound technique for CVC placement

D For internal jugular CVCs, ultrasound increases the "first-stick" success rate

E Ultrasound has no role to play in the placement of subclavian CVCs

The use of ultrasound has become standard of care for the placement of internal jugular vein central lines, and has now become part of the routine accomplishments of practitioners in the ICU. Its rapid adoption was fueled by many studies showing the superiority of this approach.

Duplex ultrasound combines both pulse echo imaging and Doppler waves, which improves the resolution of vessel images and enables accurate measures of velocity. It is these features that help distinguish the blood flow in arteries as opposed to veins, as this depends on the frequency of the ultrasound as well as the velocity of the blood flow. It is also important to remember that this is dependent on the angle of insonation, and this can be a cause of confusion if the probe was held incorrectly. Although useful, the collapsibility of the vein as opposed to the artery is the usual method of distinguishing between the two, and this obviously does not require duplex mode.

Ultrasound used as a "static" technique is not associated with increased success rates compared to the standard landmark technique. This refers to the use of ultrasound to merely map the vessels and then the ultrasound probe is not used when the vein is actually being accessed. The disadvantage of the dynamic or real-time technique is that there is a significant operator learning curve, related to using the ultrasound and the needle for access at the same time. This is fairly easily overcome, and this learning curve is not steep. It has been shown in multiple studies, particularly for the internal jugular route, that ultrasound can increase the "first-stick" success rate as well as the overall success rate. Although ultrasound has a limited role to play in the placement of subclavian central lines in patients with the appropriate anatomy of sound may still prove useful in imaging the subclavian artery and vein.

**Answer: B**

Brass, P., Hellmich, M., Kolodziej, L., *et al.* (2015) Ultrasound guidance versus anatomical landmarks for subclavian or femoral vein catheterization. *Cochrane Database System Reviews*, **9**, 1.

Denys, B.G., Uretsky, B.F., and Reddy, S. (1993) Ultrasound-assisted cannulation of the internal jugular vein. A prospective comparison to the external landmark-guided technique. *Circulation*, **87**, 1557–1562.

Hind, D., Calvert, N., McWilliams, R., *et al.* (2003) Ultrasonic locating devices for central venous cannulation: meta-analysis. *British Medical Journal*, **327**, 361–364.

Karakitsos, D., Labropoulos, N., DeGroot, E., *et al.* (1994) Real-time ultrasound-guided catheterization of the internal jugular vein: a prospective comparison with the landmark technique in critical care patients. *Critical Care*, **10** (6), R162.

Mansfield, P.F., Hohn, D.C., Fornage, B.D., *et al.* (1995) Complications and failures of subclavian-vein catheterization. *New England Journal of Medicine*, **331**, 1735–1738.

**18** In which of the following patients could a pelvic X-ray be safely omitted?

**A** 23-year-old man following a motorcycle crash at high speed, hemodynamically stable but complaining of pain in the left hip

**B** 78-year-old woman following a ground level fall

**C** 47-year-old man who was ambulatory after a rear-end collision at 45mph

**D** 32-year-old woman, with a BP of 90/60 mm Hg and severe pain over the sacrum

**E** 16-year-old man following a bicycle crash, with blood at the urinary meatus

Pelvic x-rays are notoriously inaccurate for the diagnosis of pelvic fractures, with a false negative rate somewhere between 20–30%. However there are a certain group of patients in which they provide useful information as a screening tool, particularly if those patients are not undergoing abdominal and/or pelvic CT scanning. More and more, pelvic x-rays are being omitted in neurologically normal, hemodynamically stable patients who are undergoing abdomen and pelvis CT scans as part of their workup.

The patient in choice A is at risk of either a femur fracture or pubic rami fractures and should therefore be imaged. The patient in choice B requires imaging due to the increased fracture risk in the elderly because of osteoporosis. The 47-year-old man described here, who was ambulatory at the scene, is unlikely to have a clinically significant pelvic fracture and as long as a clinical exam is reliable (i.e. the patient is not intoxicated or has other distracting injuries) the x-ray could safely be emitted with a low risk for missed injury. Any patient with significant mechanism for pelvic trauma that is hemodynamically unstable should have a pelvic x-ray performed to help assess whether the patient should go directly to the angiography suite for embolization. Any signs or symptoms of possible urethral trauma mandate a pelvic x-ray as part of the workup prior to placement of Foley catheter as a retrograde urethrogram may be necessary.

**Answer: C**

Guillamondegui, O.D., Pryor, J.P., Gracias, V.H., *et al.* (2002) Pelvic radiography in blunt trauma resuscitation:

a diminishing role. *Journal of Trauma*, **53** (6), 1043–1047.

Kessel, B., Sevi, R., Jeroukhimov, I., *et al.* (2007) Is routine portable pelvic X-ray in stable multiple trauma patients always justified in a high technology era? *Injury*, **38** (5), 559–563.

Obaid, A.K., Barleben, A., Porral, D., *et al.* (2006) Utility of plain film pelvic radiographs in blunt trauma patients in the emergency department. *American Surgeon*, **72** (10), 951–954.

Soto, J.R., Zhou, C., Hu, D., *et al.* (2015) Skip and save: utility of pelvic x-rays in the initial evaluation of blunt trauma patients. *American Journal of Surgery*, **210** (6), 1076–1079, 1079–1081.

**19** Surgeon-performed cardiac ultrasound in the ICU can be shown to accurately assess all of the following EXCEPT?

**A** Filling status

**B** Cardiac output

**C** Pericardial effusion

**D** Presence of pulmonary hypertension

**E** Right ventricular function

There has been increasing interest in echocardiography performed by surgeons and/or intensivists at the bedside in recent years, partly due to the increasingly sophisticated ultrasound machinery that is now available, which is also much more portable. Multiple studies have shown that subjective measurements can be taken of global cardiac function as well as accurate assessments of the filling status of the IVC and the heart.

Filling status of both the cardiac chambers as well of the IVC has been shown to be feasible in the majority of patients, even in the trauma bay. Cardiac output can be measured by a number of techniques, but these are limited by the need to obtain adequate images during the examination, which is not always possible in the trauma patient, particularly those with subcutaneous emphysema or other chest trauma. The presence of absence of pericardial effusions has long been part of the FAST exam, and can be easily extended into the ICU. Pulmonary hypertension usually requires more sophisticated machinery and time and is usually not part of the intensivist-performed focused echocardiographic exam. Subjective measures of ventricular function (either right or left) can be made using various different echocardiographic views, although quantification is not usually attempted with limited exam cardiac ultrasound.

**Answer: D**

Ferrada, P., Anand, R.J., Whelan, J., *et al.* (2011) Limited transthoracic echocardiogram: so easy any trauma attending can do it. *Journal of Trauma*, **71** (5), 1327–1331; discussion 1331-2.

Ferrada, P., Murthi, S., Anand, R.J., *et al.* (2011) Transthoracic focused rapid echocardiographic examination: real-time evaluation of fluid status in critically ill trauma patients. *Journal of Trauma*, **70** (1), 56–62, 62–64.

Gunst, M., Sperry, J., Ghaemmaghami, V., *et al.* (2008) Bedside echocardiographic assessment for trauma/critical care: the BEAT exam. *Journal of American College Surgeons*, **207** (3), e1–e3.

Levitov, A., Frankel, H.L., Blaivas, M., *et al.* (2016) Guidelines for the appropriate use of bedside general and cardiac ultrasonography in the evaluation of critically ill patients. Part II: cardiac ultrasonography. *Critical Care Medicine*, **44** (6), 1206–1227.

**20** Which of the following is NOT a concerning finding for aortic injury on the CXR of a 27-year-old motorcyclist who drove into a tree at highway speed?

**A** Widened mediastinum

**B** Depression of the left main bronchus

**C** Apical (pleural cap)

**D** Multiple posterior rib fractures at the costovertebral junction

**E** Large left hemothorax

With the use of whole body CT scanning for trauma becoming more and more prevalent, the relevance of the humble initial CXR has somewhat fallen by the wayside. However, this simple tool can not only diagnose pneumo- or hemothoraces, as well as confirm ETT after intubation, but can also help provide data to help screen for more major injuries in high-risk patients.

Widened mediastinum is the classic finding for a contained aortic rupture, with blood spilling into the superior mediastinum and causing this increase in the mediastinal contents, which appears as an enlargement on the CXR. Normal mediastinal width is approximately 8 cm when supine, or 6 cm when upright. The sensitivity of a mediastinal hematoma for aortic injury is low, only about 12.5%; conversely a normal good-quality CXR has about a 97% negative predictive value for aortic injury.

This is caused by the hematoma expanding in the superior mediastinum and pushing the left bronchus down. An apical cap may be present when the rupture is contained and the blood tracks in the extrapleural space, between the parietal pleura and the chest wall, causing the appearance of a hematoma. It is preferentially forced upwards by the high pressure of aortic blood. Although rib fractures per se are indicative of chest trauma, which de facto increases the risk of thoracic aortic rupture, there is no evidence of **posterior** rib fractures being pathognomic of an increased of aortic rupture

So called "free" rupture of the thoracic aorta into the pleural cavity can be a cause of large left-sided hemothoraces, and this injury should always be considered in these cases, especially if the patient has a large volume collected after tube thoracostomy, or if the output remains high and appears to be arterial. These patients will require emergent transport to the operating room, and surgical intervention.

**Answer: D**

Langdorf, M.I., Medak, A.J., Hendey, G.W., *et al.* (2015) Prevalence and clinical import of thoracic injury identified by chest computed tomography but not chest radiography in blunt trauma: multicenter prospective cohort study. *Annals of Emergency Medicine*, **66** (6), 589–600.

Mokrane, F.Z., Revel-Mouroz, P., Saint Lebes, B., *et al.* (2015) Traumatic injuries of the thoracic aorta: The role of imaging in diagnosis and treatment. *Diagnostic and Interval Imaging*, **96** (7–8), 693–706.

O'Conor, C.E. (2004) Diagnosing traumatic rupture of the thoracic aorta in the emergency department. *Emergency Medicine Journal*, **21** (4), 414–419.

# Contents

Contributors   *ix*
About the Companion Website   *xv*

**Part One     Surgical Critical Care**   *1*

1   **Respiratory and Cardiovascular Physiology**   *3*
    *Marcin Jankowski, DO and Frederick Giberson, MD*

2   **Cardiopulmonary Resuscitation, Oxygen Delivery, and Shock**   *15*
    *Filip Moshkovsky, DO, Luis Cardenas, DO and Mark Cipolle, MD*

3   **ECMO**   *23*
    *Andy Michaels, MD*

4   **Arrhythmias, Acute Coronary Syndromes, and Hypertensive Emergencies**   *33*
    *Rondi Gelbard, MD and Omar K. Danner, MD*

5   **Sepsis and the Inflammatory Response to Injury**   *51*
    *Juan C. Duchesne, MD and Marquinn D. Duke, MD*

6   **Hemodynamic and Respiratory Monitoring**   *59*
    *Stephen M. Welch, DO, Christopher S. Nelson, MD and Stephen L. Barnes, MD*

7   **Airway and Perioperative Management**   *69*
    *Stephen M. Welch, DO, Jeffrey P. Coughenour, MD and Stephen L. Barnes, MD*

8   **Acute Respiratory Failure and Mechanical Ventilation**   *79*
    *Adrian A. Maung, MD and Lewis J. Kaplan, MD*

9   **Infectious Disease**   *89*
    *Yousef Abuhakmeh, DO, John Watt, MD and Courtney McKinney, PharmD*

10   **Pharmacology and Antibiotics**   *97*
    *Michelle Strong, MD and CPT Clay M. Merritt, DO*

11   **Transfusion, Hemostasis, and Coagulation**   *109*
    *Erin Palm, MD and Kenji Inaba, MD*

12   **Analgesia and Anesthesia**   *121*
    *Marquinn D. Duke, MD and Juan C. Duchesne, MD*

**13** **Delirium, Alcohol Withdrawal, and Psychiatric Disorders** *129*
*Peter Bendix, MD and Ali Salim, MD*

**14** **Acid-Base, Fluid, and Electrolytes** *135*
*Joshua Dilday, DO, Asser Youssef, MD and Nicholas Thiessen, MD*

**15** **Metabolic Illness and Endocrinopathies** *145*
*Andrew J. Young, MD and Therese M. Duane, MD*

**16** **Hypothermia and Hyperthermia** *153*
*Raquel M. Forsythe, MD*

**17** **Acute Kidney Injury** *159*
*Remigio J. Flor, MD, Keneeshia N. Williams, MD and Terence O'Keeffe, MD*

**18** **Liver Failure** *169*
*Muhammad Numan Khan, MD and Bellal Joseph, MD*

**19** **Nutrition Support in Critically Ill Patients** *177*
*Rifat Latifi, MD and Jorge Con, MD*

**20** **Neurocritical Care** *189*
*Herb A. Phelan, MD*

**21** **Thromboembolism** *199*
*Herb A. Phelan, MD*

**22** **Transplantation, Immunology, and Cell Biology** *209*
*Leslie Kobayashi, MD and Emily Cantrell, MD*

**23** **Obstetric Critical Care** *219*
*Gerard J. Fulda, MD and Anthony Sciscione, MD*

**24** **Pediatric Critical Care** *227*
*Erin M. Garvey, MD and J. Craig Egan, MD*

**25** **Envenomations, Poisonings, and Toxicology** *239*
*Michelle Strong, MD*

**26** **Common Procedures in the ICU** *253*
*Joanelle A. Bailey, MD and Adam D. Fox, DO*

**27** **Diagnostic Imaging, Ultrasound, and Interventional Radiology** *261*
*Keneeshia N. Williams, MD, Remigio J. flor, MD and Terence O'Keeffe, MD*


**Part Two** **Emergency Surgery** *273*

**28** **Neurotrauma** *275*
*Faisal Shah Jehan, MD and Bellal Joseph, MD*

**29** **Blunt and Penetrating Neck Trauma** *287*
*Leslie Kobayashi, MD and Barret Halgas, MD*

**30  Cardiothoracic and Thoracic Vascular Injury**  *299*
*Leslie Kobayashi, MD and Amelia Simpson, MD*

**31  Abdominal and Abdominal Vascular Injury**  *307*
*Leslie Kobayashi, MD and Michelle G. Hamel, MD*

**32  Orthopedic and Hand Trauma**  *317*
*Brett D. Crist, MD and Gregory J. Della Rocca, MD*

**33  Peripheral Vascular Trauma**  *327*
*Amy V. Gore, MD and Adam D. Fox, DO*

**34  Urologic Trauma and Disorders**  *337*
*Jeremy Juern, MD and Daniel Roubik, MD*

**35  Care of the Pregnant Trauma Patient**  *345*
*Ashley McCusker, MD and Terence O'Keeffe, MD*

**36  Esophagus, Stomach, and Duodenum**  *359*
*Matthew B. Singer, MD and Andrew Tang, MD*

**37  Small Intestine, Appendix, and Colorectal**  *371*
*Vishal Bansal, MD and Jay J. Doucet, MD*

**38  Gallbladder and Pancreas**  *385*
*Matthew B. Singer, MD and Andrew Tang, MD*

**39  Liver and Spleen**  *393*
*Cathy Ho, MD and Narong Kulvatunyou, MD*

**40  Incarcerated Hernias**  *403*
*Cathy Ho, MD and Narong Kulvatunyou, MD*

**41  Necrotizing Soft Tissue Infections and Other Soft Tissue Infections**  *409*
*Jacob Swann, MD and LTC Joseph J. DuBose, MD*

**42  Obesity and Bariatric Surgery**  *415*
*Gregory Peirce, MD and LTC Eric Ahnfeldt, DO*

**43  Thermal Burns, Electrical Burns, Chemical Burns, Inhalational Injury, and Lightning Injuries**  *423*
*Joseph J. DuBose, MD and Jacob Swann, MD*

**44  Gynecologic Surgery**  *431*
*K. Aviva Bashan-Gilzenrat, MD*

**45  Cardiovascular and Thoracic Surgery**  *439*
*Jonathan Nguyen, DO and Bryan C. Morse, MS, MD*

**46  Pediatric Surgery**  *453*
*Matthew Martin, MD, Aaron Cunningham, MD and Mubeen Jafri, MD*

**47  Geriatrics**  *465*
*K. Aviva Bashan-Gilzenrat, MD and Bryan Morse, MS, MD*

**48** **Telemedicine and Telepresence for Surgery and Trauma** *477*
*Kalterina Latifi, MS and Rifat Latifi, MD*

**49** **Statistics** *483*
*Alan Cook, MD*

**50** **Ethics, End-of-Life, and Organ Retrieval** *491*
*Allyson Cook, MD and Lewis J. Kaplan, MD*

**Index** *501*

# Contributors

*Yousef Abuhakmeh, DO*
CPT MC, US Army
General Surgery Resident
William Beaumont Army Medical Center
El Paso, TX, USA

*LTC Eric Ahnfeldt, DO*
Chairman, Military Committee for American Society of
Metabolic and Bariatric Surgery Director
Metabolic and Bariatric Surgery Program Director
General Surgery Residency
William Beaumont Army Medical Center
El Paso, TX, USA

*Joanelle A. Bailey, MD*
Resident In Surgery
Rutgers New Jersey Medical School
Newark, NJ, USA

*Vishal Bansal, MD*
Trauma Medical Director
Scripps Mercy Hospital
San Diego, CA, USA

*Stephen L. Barnes, MD*
Professor of Surgery & Anesthesia
Division Chief of Acute Care Surgery
University of Missouri School of Medicine
MU Health
Columbia, MO, USA

*K. Aviva Bashan-Gilzenrat, MD*
Assistant Professor of Surgery
Division of Acute Care Surgery
Morehouse School of Medicine
Grady Health
Atlanta, GA, USA

*Peter Bendix, MD*
Department of Surgery
Section of Trauma and Acute Care Surgery
University of Chicago Medicine
Chicago, IL, USA

*Emily Cantrell, MD*
Trauma and Acute Care Surgery Fellow
Division of Trauma, Surgical Critical Care
Burns and Acute Care Surgery
UCSD Medical Center
San Diego, CA, USA

*Luis Cardenas, DO*
Medical Director, Surgical Critical Care
Program Director, Surgical Critical Care Fellowship
Christiana Care Health System
Newark, DE, USA

*Mark Cipolle, MD*
Director of Outcomes Research, Surgical Service Line
Christiana Care Health System
Newark, DE, USA

*Jorge Con, MD*
Director Trauma, eHealth and International Research
Fellowship
Westchester Medical Center
Valhalla, NY, USA

*Alan Cook, MD*
Clinical Assistant Professor
Department of Surgery
University of Arizona Phoenix Campus
Chandler Regional Medical Center
Chandler, AZ, USA

*Allyson Cook, MD*
Surgical Critical Care Fellow
Stanford University
Stanford, CA, USA

*Jeffrey P. Coughenour, MD*
Associate Professor of Surgery &
Emergency Medicine
Division of Acute Care Surgery
University of Missouri School of Medicine
MU Health
Columbia, MO, USA

*Brett D. Crist, MD*
Associate Professor
Department of Orthopaedic Surgery
Vice Chairman of Business Development
Director Orthopaedic Trauma Service
Director Orthopaedic Trauma Fellowship
University of Missouri
Columbia, MO, USA

*Aaron Cunningham, MD*
General Surgery Resident
Oregon Health Sciences University
Portland, OR, USA

*Omar K. Danner, MD*
Chief of Surgery for MSM
Grady Memorial Hospital
Associate Professor of Surgery
Director of Trauma
Department of Surgery
Morehouse School of Medicine
Atlanta, GA, USA

*Gregory J. Della Rocca, MD*
Associate Professor
Department of Orthopaedic Surgery
University of Missouri
Columbia, MO, USA

*Joshua Dilday, DO*
CPT MC, US Army
General Surgery Resident
William Beaumont Army Medical Center
El Paso, TX, USA

*Jay J. Doucet, MD*
Professor of Surgery
Head, Division of Trauma, Surgical Critical Care
Burns & Acute Care Surgery
University of California San Diego Health, San Diego
CA, USA

*Therese M. Duane, MD*
Professor of Surgery, University of North Texas, Chief
of Surgery and Surgical Specialties, John Peter Smith
Health Network, Fort Worth, TX, USA

*LTC Joseph J. DuBose, MD*
Associate Professor of Surgery, Uniformed Services
University of the Health Sciences
Associate Professor of Surgery, University of Maryland
R Adams Cowley Shock Trauma Center
University of Maryland Medical System
Baltimore, MD, USA

*Juan C. Duchesne, MD*
Professor of Surgery
Section Chief Trauma
Department of Tulane Surgery
TICU Medical Director
Norman McSwain Level I Trauma Center
New Orleans, LA, USA

*Marquinn D. Duke, MD*
Trauma Medical Director
North Oaks Medical Center
Clinical Instructor of Surgery, Tulane University
Clinical Assistant Professor of Surgery
Louisiana State University
New Orleans, LA, USA

*J. Craig Egan, MD*
Chief, Division of Pediatric Surgery
Director, Pediatric Surgical Critical Care
Phoenix Children's Hospital
Phoenix, AZ, USA

*Remigio J. Flor, MD*
CPT MC, USARMY
General Surgery Residency
William Beaumont Army Medical Center
El Paso, TX, USA

*Raquel M. Forsythe, MD*
Assistant Professor of Surgery and
Critical Care Medicine
University of Pittsburgh Medical Center
Presbyterian Hospital
Pittsburgh, PA, USA

*Adam D. Fox, DO*
Assistant Professor of Surgery
Section Chief, Trauma
Division of Trauma Surgery and Critical Care
Rutgers NJMS
Associate Trauma Medical Director NJ Trauma Center
University Hospital, Newark, NJ, USA

*Gerard J. Fulda, MD*
Associate Professor, Department of Surgery
Jefferson Medical College, Philadelphia, PA, US
Chairman Department of Surgery
Physician Leader Surgical Service Line
Christiana Care Health Systems, Newark, DE, USA

*Erin M. Garvey, MD*
Pediatric Surgery Fellow
Phoenix Children's Hospital
Phoenix, AZ, USA

Rondi Gelbard, MD
Assistant Professor of Surgery
Associate Medical Director, Surgical ICU
Associate Program Director
Surgical Critical Care Fellowship
Emory University School of Medicine
Atlanta, GA, USA

Frederick Giberson, MD
Clinical Assistant Professor of Surgery
Jefferson Health System
Philadelphia, PA, USA
Program Director, General Surgery Residency
Vice Chair of Surgical Education
Christiana Care Health System
Newark, DE, USA

Amy V. Gore, MD
Resident In Surgery
Rutgers New Jersey Medical School
Newark, NJ, USA

Barret Halgas, MD
CPT MC, US Army
General Surgery Resident
William Beaumont Army Medical Center
El Paso, TX, USA

Michelle G. Hamel, MD
Trauma and Acute Care Surgery Fellow
Division of Trauma, Surgical Critical Care
Burns and Acute Care Surgery
UCSD Medical Center
San Diego, CA, USA

Cathy Ho, MD
Acute Care Surgery Fellow
Banner University Medical Center
Tucson, AZ, USA

Kenji Inaba, MD
Associate Professor of Surgery
Emergency Medicine and Anesthesia
Division of Trauma and Critical Care
LAC + USC Medical Center
University of Southern California
Los Angeles, CA, USA

Mubeen Jafri, MD
Assistant Professor of Surgery
Oregon Health Sciences University
Portland, OR, USA

Marcin Jankowski, DO
Department of Surgery
Division of Trauma and Surgical Critical Care
Hahnemann University Hospital
Drexel University College of Medicine
Philadelphia, PA, USA

Faisal Shah Jehan, MD
Research Fellow
Division of Trauma, Critical Care
Emergency General Surgery, and Burns
Department of Surgery
University of Arizona
Tucson, AZ, USA

Bellal Joseph, MD
Professor of Surgery
Vice Chair of Research
Division of Trauma, Critical Care
Emergency General Surgery, and Burns
Department of Surgery
University of Arizona
Tucson, AZ, USA

Jeremy Juern, MD
Associate Professor of Surgery
Medical College of Wisconsin
Milwaukee, WI, USA

Lewis J. Kaplan, MD
Associate Professor of Surgery
Perelman School of Medicine, University of
Pennsylvania Department of Surgery
Division of Trauma, Surgical Critical Care and
Emergency Surgery
Section Chief, Surgical Critical Care
Philadelphia VA Medical Center
Philadelphia, PA, USA

Leslie Kobayashi, MD
Associate Professor of Clinical Surgery
Division of Trauma, Surgical Critical Care
Burns and Acute Care Surgery
UCSD Medical Center
San Diego, CA, USA

Narong Kulvatunyou, MD
Associate Professor
Program Director Surgical Critical Fellowship/
Acute Care Surgery Fellowship
University of Arizona Health Science Center
Department of Surgery, Section of Trauma, Critical
Care & Emergency Surgery
Tucson, AZ, USA

*Kalterina Latifi, MS*
Director, eHealth Center
Westchester Medical Center Health Network
Valhalla, NY, USA

*Rifat Latifi, MD*
Professor of Surgery, New York Medical College
Director, Department of Surgery
Chief, Divisions of Trauma and General Surgery
Westchester Medical Center
Professor of Surgery, NYMC
Valhalla, NY, USA

*Matthew Martin, MD*
Clinical Professor of Surgery
University of Washington School of Medicine
Seattle, WA
Professor of Surgery
Uniformed Services University for the Health Sciences
Bethesda, MD, USA

*Adrian A. Maung, MD*
Associate Professor of Surgery
Section of General Surgery
Trauma and Surgical Critical Care
Department of Surgery
Yale School of Medicine
Adult Trauma Medical Director Yale
New Haven Hospital
New Haven, CT, USA

*Ashley McCusker, MD*
Acute Care Surgery Fellow
Banner University Medical Center
Tucson, AZ, USA

*Courtney McKinney, PharmD*
Clinical Pharmacist, Chandler Regional Medical Center
Clinical Instructor, Department of
Pharmacy Practice and Science
University of Arizona College of Pharmacy Tucson
AZ, USA

*CPT Clay M. Merritt, DO*
General Surgery Resident
William Beaumont Army Medical Center
El Paso, TX, USA

*Andy Michaels, MD*
Clinical Associate Professor of Surgery
Oregon Health and Science University
Surgeon
Tacoma Trauma Trust
Medecins Sans Frontieres/Doctors Without Borders
International Committee of the Red Cross, Portland
OR, USA

*Bryan C. Morse, MS, MD*
Assistant Professor of Surgery
Emory University SOM-Department of Surgery
Grady Memorial Hospital, Atlanta, GA, USA

*Filip Moshkovsky, DO*
Assistant Professor of Clinical Surgery
University of Perelman School of Medicine
Traumatology, Surgical Critical Care
and Emergency Surgery
Reading Health System
Reading, PA, USA

*Christopher S. Nelson, MD*
Assistant Professor of Surgery
Division of Acute Care Surgery
University of Missouri School of Medicine
MU Health
Columbia, MO, USA

*Jonathan Nguyen, DO*
Assistant Professor of Surgery
Division of Acute Care Surgery
Morehouse School of Medicine
Grady Health
Atlanta, GA, USA

*Muhammad Numan Khan, MD*
Research Fellow
Division of Trauma, Critical Care
Emergency General Surgery, and Burns
Department of Surgery
University of Arizona,
Tucson, AZ, USA

*Terence O'Keeffe, MB, ChB, MSPH*
Professor, Surgery Division Chief
Trauma, Critical Care
Burn and Emergency Surgery Chief of Staff
Banner University Medical Center
Tucson, AZ, USA

*Erin Palm, MD*
Division of Trauma and Critical Care
LAC + USC Medical Center
University of Southern California
Los Angeles, CA, USA

*Gregory Peirce, MD*
MAJ MC, US Army
Chief of General Surgery
Weed Army Community Hospital
Fort Irwin, CA, USA

**Herb A. Phelan, MD**
Professor of Surgery
University of Texas Southwestern Medical Center
Department of Surgery
Division of Burns/Trauma/Critical Care
Dallas, TX, USA

**Daniel Roubik, MD**
CPT MC, US Army
General Surgery Resident, William Beaumont Army
Medical Center, El Paso, TX, USA

**Ali Salim, MD**
Professor of Surgery
Harvard Medical School
Division Chief of Trauma
Burns and Surgical Critical Care
Brigham and Women's Hospital
Boston, MA, USA

**Anthony Sciscione, MD**
Director of Obstetrics and Gynecology Residency
Program and Maternal Fetal Medicine
Christiana Care Healthcare System
Newark, Delaware
Professor of Obstetrics and Gynecology
Jefferson Medical College
Philadelphia, PA, USA

**Amelia Simpson, MD**
Trauma and Acute Care Surgery Fellow
Division of Trauma, Surgical Critical Care
Burns and Acute Care Surgery
UCSD Medical Center
San Diego, CA, USA

**Matthew B. Singer, MD**
Acute Care Surgery
The Institute of Trauma and Acute Care, Inc. Pomona
CA, USA

**Michelle Strong, MD**
Medical Director of Shock Trauma ICU
St. David's South Austin Medical Center
Austin, TX, USA

**Jacob Swann, MD**
MAJ MC, US Army
General Surgery Resident
William Beaumont Army Medical Center
El Paso, TX, USA

**Nicholas Thiessen, MD**
Acute Care Surgeon
Chandler Regional Medical Center
Chandler, AZ, USA

**Andrew Tang, MD**
Associate professor of surgery
Banner University Medical Center-Tucson
Tucson, AZ, USA

**John Watt, MD**
Associate Program Director
General Surgery Residency
William Beaumont Army Medical Center
Acute Care Surgeon
Chandler Regional Medical Center
Chandler, AZ, USA

**Stephen M. Welch, DO**
Department of Surgery
Division of Acute Care Surgery
University of Missouri Health Care
Columbia, MO, USA

**Keneeshia N. Williams, MD**
Assistant Professor of Surgery
Emory University SOM-Department of Surgery
Grady Memorial Hospital
Atlanta, GA, USA

**Andrew J. Young, MD**
Staff Surgeon
Naval Hospital
Bremerton, WA, USA

**Asser Youssef, MD**
Clinical Associate Professor of Surgery
University of Arizona College of Medicine - Phoenix
Phoenix, AZ, USA

# About the Companion Website

This book is accompanied by a companion website:

**www.wiley.com/go/moore/surgical_criticalcare_and_emergency_surgery**

The website features:

- MCQs

**Part Two**

**Emergency Surgery**

# 28

# Neurotrauma

*Faisal Shah Jehan, MD and Bellal Joseph, MD*

**1** *A 40-year-old man presents two weeks after being discharged from the hospital after an all-terrain-vehicle (ATV) accident in which he suffered a frontal bone fracture and mild traumatic brain injury. He now complains of a "whooshing" sound in his left ear, diplopia, left-eye proptosis, headaches, and fevers. Physical exam revealed conjunctival injection and pulsatile exopthalmos. A computed tomography (CT) scan of the brain showed a known displaced frontal bone fracture. The angiogram is depicted in Figure 28.1 and Figure 28.2. What is the most likely diagnosis?*

**A** *Cavernous sinus thrombosis*
**B** *Occlusion of the internal carotid artery proximal to the ophthalmic artery origin*
**C** *Carotid cavernous fistula*
**D** *Retrobulbar hematoma*
**E** *Unrecognized intraorbital foreign body, with possible cellulitis*

**Answer: C**

**2** *What should be the initial treatment of choice for the patient?*
**A** *Anticoagulation*
**B** *Two weeks of antibiotics followed by repeat angiography*
**C** *Carotid artery ligation*
**D** *Transarterial detachable balloon embolization*
**E** *Glue embolization of major arterial feeders followed by resection*

Carotid-cavernous fistula (CCF) is an abnormal communication between the carotid artery and the venous plexus of the cavernous sinus. According to Barrow classification, CCFs are divided into four types based on their etiology, rate of flow, and source of feeder vessels. Type A CCFs are direct, high-flow lesions connecting the carotid artery and cavernous sinus, and they often

result from a single, endothelialized tear in the carotid wall. Types B, C, and D fistulas are low-flow, indirect lesions that vary by anatomy. Signs and symptoms usually appear a few weeks after the injury and result from increased venous pressure transmitted through the valveless ophthalmic veins. Symptoms and signs include headache, orbital bruit, pulsating exophthalmos, chemosis, diplopia, proptosis, dilation of retinal veins, optic disc swelling, and vision loss. Although CT or MRI may reveal enlarged extraocular muscles, dilated ophthalmic veins, and enlarged affected cavernous sinus, the gold standard is cerebral angiography, which reveals direct opacification of an enlarged cavernous sinus, early filling of ophthalmic veins and diminished opacification of the distal arterial system.

The management of patients with CCF includes monitoring of ophthalmologic status, treatment of ophthalmologic complications, and closure of the CCF. The main treatment goal is to occlude the fistula without compromising carotid patency. The treatments of choice are endovascular procedures, which are associated with low morbidity and mortality. Endovascular occlusion using detachable balloons has a success rate of 90–100% with low complication rates (2 to 5%). The overall recurrence rate is 1–3.9%, and recurrence often responds to second embolization.

**Answer: D**

Fabian, T.S., Woody, J.D., Ciraulo, D.L., *et al.* (1999) Post-traumatic carotid cavernous fistula: frequency analysis of signs, symptoms, and disability outcomes after angiographic embolization. *Journal of Trauma*, **47** (2), 275–281.

Xu X.Q., Liu S., Zu Q.Q., *et al.* (2013) Follow-up of 58 traumatic carotid-cavernous fistulas after endovascular detachable-balloon embolization at a single center. *Journal of Clinical Neurology*, **9** (2), 83–90.

*Surgical Critical Care and Emergency Surgery: Clinical Questions and Answers*, Second Edition.
Edited by Forrest "Dell" Moore, Peter Rhee, and Gerard J. Fulda.
© 2018 John Wiley & Sons Ltd. Published 2018 by John Wiley & Sons Ltd.
Companion website: www.wiley.com/go/moore/surgical_criticalcare_and_emergency_surgery

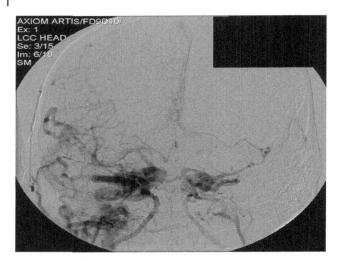

**Figure 28.1**

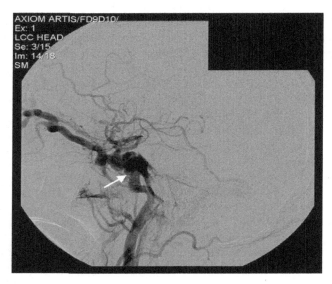

**Figure 28.2**

**3** *Basilar skull fractures are associated with ecchymosis of the mastoid process, periorbital ecchymosis, cranial nerve palsy, hemotympanum, and rhinorrhea. The presence of cerebral spinal fluid (CSF) rhinorrhea can be confirmed by which of the following assays?*

**A** *Hypoglycorrhachia*

**B** $\beta_2$ *-transferrin*

**C** *α-fetoprotein*

**D** *Sodium level*

**E** *WBC count*

Beta-2 transferrin is a protein found only in CSF and perilymph. It was first described in 1979 for its use in the detection of CSF leakage. With a sensitivity of 94—100%, and specificity of 98—100%, this assay has become the gold standard in detection of CSF leakage. The only other source is the vitreous humor of the eye. Currently fluorescein-soaked cotton pledgets have also been used for the perioperative diagnosing of CSF rhinorrhea, which has an accuracy of 100% as compared to $\beta_2$-transferrin testing. Other commonly employed tests include measuring the glucose level of the fluid (CSF glucose >30 mg%, whereas lacrimal and mucous secretions are <5 mg%) or placing the fluid on a piece of linen and seeing whether a ring of blood surrounded by a larger concentric ring of clear fluid develops ("halo" sign).

**Answer: B**

Haft, G., Mendoza, S.A., Weinstein, S.L., *et al.* (2004) Use of beta-2-transferrin to diagnose CSF leakage following spinal surgery. *Iowa Orthopedic Journal*, **24**, 115–118.

Saafan, M.E., Ragab, S.M., and Albirmawy, O.A. (2006) Topical intranasal fluorescein: the missing partner in algorithms of cerebrospinal fluid fistula detection. *The Laryngoscope*, **116** (7), 1158–1161.

**4** *A 20-year-old man presents to the trauma bay after a motor vehicle accident. He has spontaneous eye opening, is confused and localizes only to pain. His Glasgow Coma Score is*

**A** *5*

**B** *7*

**C** *9*

**D** *13*

**E** *15*

The Glasgow Coma Scale (GCS) should be determined for all injured patients (see Table 28.1). It is calculated by adding the scores of the best motor response, best verbal response, and eye opening. Scores range from 3 (the lowest) to 15 (normal). Scores of 13 to 15 indicate mild head injury, 9 to 12 moderate injury and less than 9 severe injury. The GCS is useful for both triage and prognosis. The GCS score has been shown to have a significant correlation with outcome following severe TBI, both as the sum score or as just the motor component. Recent studies have shown that pupil reactivity together with the GCS motor component correlates best with mortality. In patients with different motor response between the left and right side, the best movement is used.

**Answer: D**

Brain Trauma Foundation (2000) *Early Indicators of Prognosis in Traumatic Brain Injury*, Brain Trauma Foundation, New York, p. 163.

Brunicardi, F.C. (2010) *Schwartz's Principles of Surgery*, 9th edn, McGraw-Hill, New York, pp. 145, 1524.

**Table 28.1** Glasgow Coma Scale.

| | 1 | 2 | 3 | 4 | 5 | 6 |
|---|---|---|---|---|---|---|
| **Eyes** | Does not open eyes | Opens eyes to painful stimuli | Opens eyes to response to voice | Opens eyes spontaneously | N/A | N/A |
| **Verbal** | Makes no sounds | Incomprehensible sounds | Inappropriate words | Confused, disoriented | Oriented, converses normally | N/A |
| **Motor** | Makes no movements | Extension to painful stimuli (decerebrate response) | Abnormal flexion to painful stimuli (decorticate response) | Flexion/ Withdrawal to painful stimuli | Localizes painful stimuli | Obeys commmands |

Teasdale, G. and Jennett, B. (1974) Assessment of coma and impaired consciousness. A practical scale. *Lancet* **2**, 81–84.

Hoffmann, M., Lefering, R., Rueger, J.M., *et al.* (2012) Pupil evaluation in addition to Glasgow Coma Scale components in prediction of traumatic brain injury and mortality. *British Journal of Surgery*, **99** (S1), 122–130.

5  *A 30-year-old man experienced a high-speed motorcycle collision and experienced transient right upper extremity sensory changes. A computed tomography (CT) scan of the head was negative; however, the CT scan of the cervical spine revealed a fracture into the foramen transversarium of the fifth cervical vertebrae. CT angiography of the cervical spine revealed a pseudoaneurysm of the vertebral artery. No other injuries were identified. What would be the most appropriate next step in the management of this patient?*

   A *Antiplatelet agents*
   B *Anticoagulation*
   C *Endovascular treatment*
   D *Surgical intervention*
   E *Repeat angiography*

Blunt vertebral artery injury is associated with complex cervical spine fractures involving subluxation, extension into the foramen transversarium, or upper C1 to C3 fractures. CT angiography should be obtained after trauma in patients with neurologic signs and symptoms that are not explained by the CT-scan or in blunt trauma patients presenting with epistaxis from a suspected arterial source. Routine screening should incorporate these findings to maximize yield while limiting the use of invasive procedures. The gold standard for the diagnosis of blunt cerebrovascular injury is cerebral digital subtraction arteriography, and should be only performed if the suspicion remains high and the findings of other imaging are equivocal. The incidence of vertebral artery injury among total blunt trauma admissions ranged from 0.20% to 0.77%. The most appropriate initial treatment of this injury is systemic anticoagulation initially with heparin and subsequent conversion to warfarin. Endovascular treatment is an option when the lesion does not resolve with systemic anticoagulation; however, it should not be the initial treatment choice. Acute pseudoaneurysms are unstable lesions and the walls of these structures are weak, making the stent deployment more dangerous in the acute setting. Repeat angiography should be performed. Antiplatelet agents should be reserved for patients who have undergone endovascular stent placement or those in whom systemic anticoagulation is contraindicated. Figure 28.3 presents an algorithm for the diagnosis and management of blunt cerebrovascular injuries in adults.

**Answer: B**

Biffl, W.L., Cothren, C.C., Moore, E.E., *et al.* (2009) Western Trauma Association critical decisions in trauma: screening for and treatment of blunt cerebrovascular injuries. *Journal of Trauma and Acute Care Surgery*, **67** (6), pp. 1150–1153.

Cothren, C.C., Moore, E.E., Biffl, W.L., *et al.* (2003) Cervical spine fracture patterns predictive of blunt vertebral artery injury. *Journal of Trauma*, **55** (5), 811–813.

Feliciano, D., Mattox, K., and Moore, E. (2005) *Trauma*, 6th edn, McGraw-Hill, New York.

Inamasu, J. and Guiot, B.H. (2006) Vertebral artery injury after blunt cervical trauma: an update. *Surgical Neurology*, **65** (3), 238–245.

6  *A 19-year-old man falls 20 feet from a building and arrives at the Trauma Bay with a Glasgow Coma Scale (GCS) score of 5, a dilated and nonreactive left pupil and a blood pressure of 90/45 mm Hg. After definitive airway management and fluid resuscitation, the patient is also found to have an unstable pelvic fracture and a femur fracture. His GCS improves to 8 however his left pupil remains nonreactive. The initial management of this patient is:*

   A *Administer pentobarbital immediately*
   B *Administer high doses of mannitol immediately*

**Signs/Symptoms of BCVI**

Arterial hemorrhage from
  neck/nose/mouth (?OR)
Expanding cervical hemusoma
Cervical bruit in pt < 50 yrs old
Focal neurologic defect: TIA,
  hemispheres, vertebrobasilar
  symptoms, Horner's Syndrome
Stroke on CT or MRI
Neurologic deficit inconsistent
  with head CT

**Risk Factors for BCVI**

High energy transfer mechanism
  associated with:
Displaced mid-face fracture
  (LeFort II or III)
Basilar skull fracture with
  carotid canal involvement
CHI consistent with DAI and
  GCS < 6
Cervical Vertebral body or
  transverse foremen fracture,
  subtraction, or ligamentous
  injury at any level: any
  fracture at C1-C3
Near hanging with anoxia
Clothesline type injury or seat
  belt abrasion with significant
  swelling, pain, or altered MS.

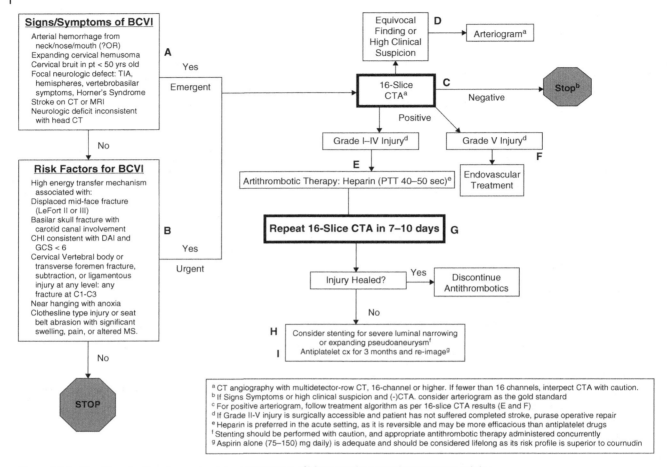

a CT angiography with multidetector-row CT, 16-channel or higher. If fewer than 16 channels, interpect CTA with caution.
b If Signs Symptoms or high clinical suspicion and (-)CTA. consider arteriogram as the gold standard
c For positive arteriogram, follow treatment algorithm as per 16-slice CTA results (E and F)
d If Grade II-V injury is surgically accessible and patient has not suffered completed stroke, purase operative repair
e Heparin is preferred in the acute setting, as it is reversible and may be more efficacious than antiplatelet drugs
f Stenting should be performed with caution, and appropriate antithrombotic therapy administered concurrently
g Aspirin alone (75–150) mg daily) is adequate and should be considered lifelong as its risk profile is superior to cournudin

**Figure 28.3** Algorithm for the diagnosis and management of blunt cerebrovascular injuries in adults.

**C** *Complete the primary survey, resuscitate the patient with blood products and if the patient is stable then obtain a computed tomography (CT) scan*

**D** *Complete the primary survey and insert an intracranial monitor and obtain a CT scan*

**E** *Take the patient directly to the operating room with no further workup*

Mannitol and hyperventilation are recommended for those patients with acute head injury as a temporary measure to control elevated intracranial pressure. Hyperventilation may be commenced immediately and it is recommended as a temporizing measure for the reduction of elevated ICP, but mannitol should be withheld until the primary survey is complete and adequate intravascular volume and urine outputs are achieved. Mannitol is effective for control of raised ICP but arterial hypotension (systolic blood pressure 90 mm Hg) should be avoided. As this patient is hypotensive which is most likely from the pelvic and femur fracture and not the head injury, mannitol would not be the first-line therapy.

Mannitol also causes diuresis and hypovolemia. Urine output is a method to help determine fluid status and this clinical variable would be lost. The mechanism of action of mannitol is still debated however there are some beneficial effects. First it acts to immediately expand the plasma by reducing hematocrit and blood viscosity (improved rheology). The improved rheology improves cerebral blood flow and $O_2$ delivery, reducing intracranial pressure quickly. Second, it draws edema from adjacent cerebral parenchyma into the intravascular compartment. Finally, it may act as a free radical scavenger. Mannitol should only be considered after sources of bleeding are ruled out and if the patient does not have hypovolemia. High-dose barbiturate is recommended to control elevated ICP refractory to maximum standard medical and surgical treatment and the patient should be hemodynamically stable. The use of barbiturates as prophylaxis against the development of intracranial hypertension is not recommended. Placement of intracranial monitor is not done blindly without first obtaining a CT scan of the head. Taking the patient directly to the operating room without CT scan is rarely done unless in the austere environment. Another alternative is 5% hypertonic saline, which will resuscitate and decrease intracranial pressure.

**Answer: C**

Brain Trauma Foundation (2016) *Guidelines for the Management of Severe Traumatic Brain Injury*, 4th edn, Brain Trauma Foundation, New York, S-50, S-63.

Feliciano, D., Mattox, K., and Moore, E. (2005) *Trauma*, 6th edn, McGraw-Hill, New York.

Joseph, B., Aziz, H., Snell, M., *et al.* (2014) The physiological effects of hyperosmolar resuscitation: 5% vs 3% hypertonic saline. *American Journal of Surgery*, **208** (5), 697–702.

7 Which of the following statements regarding intracranial pressure (ICP) monitoring is true?
   A Intraparenchymal monitor measurements have better accuracy than ventricular catheters
   B ICP monitoring is appropriate in all patients with an abnormal head CT scan and GCS < 12
   C ICP monitors carry a 1% risk of hemorrhage and 5% infection risk
   D ICP monitoring is indicated in all patients with a GCS 3 to 8 and a normal CT scan of the head
   E Risk factors for elevated intracranial pressure after traumatic brain injury are an age over 40 and systolic blood pressure greater than 90 mm Hg

Management of severe TBI patients using information from ICP monitoring is recommended to reduce in-hospital and 2-week postinjury mortality. Intracranial pressure (ICP) should be monitored in all salvageable patients with a severe traumatic brain injury (TBI; GCS score of 3 to 8 after resuscitation) and an abnormal CT scan. An abnormal CT scan of the head is one that reveals hematomas, contusions, swelling, herniation, or compressed basal cisterns. ICP monitoring is also indicated in patients with severe TBI with a normal CT scan if two or more of the following features are noted at admission: age over 40 years, unilateral or bilateral motor posturing, or systolic blood pressure (BP) < 90 mm Hg. Ventricular catheter ICP measurements are accurate but carry a higher risk of complications than do intraparenchymal monitors. There is a 1% risk of hemorrhage and 5% infection risk with ICP monitoring.

**Answer: C**

Alali, A.S., Fowler, R.A., Mainprize, T.G., *et al.* (2013) Intracranial pressure monitoring in severe traumatic brain injury: results from the American College of Surgeons Trauma Quality Improvement Program. *Journal of Neurotrauma*, **30** (20), 1737–1746.

Brain Trauma Foundation (2016) *Guidelines for the Management of Severe Traumatic Brain Injury*, 4th edn, Brain Trauma Foundation, New York, S-133, S-134.

Lane, P.L., Skoretz, T.G., Doig, G. and Girotti, M.J., (2000) Intracranial pressure monitoring and outcomes after traumatic brain injury. *Canadian Journal of Surgery*, **43** (6), 442.

8 A 24-year-old woman was the front seat passenger in a rollover motor vehicle collision. On primary survey the patient was unable to move her lower extremities and had abduction and pronation of the upper extremities. Workup revealed complete transection of the spinal cord at the C7 level. This injury most likely spares which of the following function:
   A Respiratory effort
   B Deep tendon reflexes below the level of the lesion
   C Pain and temperature sensations below the level of the lesion
   D Sympathetic vascular tone
   E Position and vibratory sensations from the lower limbs

**Answer: A**

9 The use of high-dose steroids after spinal cord injury:
   A Is not routinely recommended
   B Has little risk
   C Is indicated in all patients excluding those who are pregnant or < 14 years of age
   D Is indicated in all patients
   E May have improved outcome if steroids are given within 24 hours of injury

Injuries to the spinal cord, particularly complete injuries, remain essentially untreatable. The phrenic nerves, which are the motor nerves to the diaphragm, arise from the third, fourth, and fifth cervical roots; therefore, diaphragmatic respiration would not be disturbed by a cord transaction at C7. Anesthesia, areflexia, and flaccidity below this level would be anticipated. Hypotension results from any transaction above T5 because of the loss of sympathetic vascular tone.

The use of steroid in the treatment of acute spinal cord injury is not proven as a standard of care, nor can it be considered a recommended treatment. Evidence of the drug's efficacy and impact is weak and may only represent random events. A prospective randomized study comparing methlprednisolone with placebo demonstrated a significant improvement in outcome (usually one or two spinal levels) for those who received corticosteroids within 8 hours of injury. The National Acute Spinal Cord Injury Study (NASCIS) I and II papers provided a basis for the common practice of administering high-dose steroids to patients with acute spinal cord injury. The papers indicate greater motor and sensory recovery at 6 weeks, 6 months, and 1 year after acute spinal cord injury in patients who received steroids. However, the NASCIS trial data have been extensively criticized; as many argue that the selection criteria and study design were flawed, making the results ambiguous. Significant risks of high-dose steroids, particularly infectious complications, have been identified. Currently consensus recommendations do not endorse the administration of steroids. Of note, patients with gunshot injuries, or cauda equina injury, as well as those on chronic steroid therapy, who were pregnant, or who were less than 14 years of age were excluded from the trials. The benefit of steroid use in treatment of acute spinal cord injury is controversial as supporting literature is insufficient.

**Answer: A**

Bracken, M.B., Shepard, M.J., Collins, W.F., *et al.* (1990) A randomized controlled trial of methylprednisolone or naloxone in the treatment of acute spinal cord injury. *New England Journal of Medicine*, **322**, 1405.

Hurlbert, R.J. (2001) The role of steroids in acute spinal cord injury: an evidence-based analysis. *Spine*, **26**(24S), S39–S46.

Schroeder, G.D., Kwon, B.K., Eck, J.C., *et al.* (2014) Survey of cervical spine research society members on the use of high-dose steroids for acute spinal cord injuries. *Spine*, **39** (12), 971–977.

Short, D.J., El Masry, W.S. and Jones, P.W. (2000) High dose methylprednisolone in the management of acute spinal cord injury–a systematic review from a clinical perspective. *Spinal Cord*, **38** (5), 273–286.

**10** *A 22-year-old man has a motor vehicle accident and presents with a Glasgow Coma Scale (GCS) of 6. After primary survey and initial resuscitation the patient is found to have a left-side subarachnoid hemorrhage. Appropriate initial treatment of this patient with a severe traumatic brain injury (GCS < 8) injury includes?*
**A** *Lasix to decrease cerebral swelling*
**B** *Placement of ventriculostomy*
**C** *Hyperventilation to a $PCO_2 < 30\,mm\,Hg$*
**D** *Repeat CT scan within 1 hour*
**E** *Barbiturate coma*

**Answer: B**

**11** *The recommended target cerebral perfusion pressure in a patient with traumatic brain injury is*
**A** *100–110 mm Hg*
**B** *90–100 mm Hg*
**C** *80–90 mm Hg*
**D** *70–80 mm Hg*
**E** *60–70 mm Hg*

**Answer: E**

**12** *Therapy for increased intracranial pressure (ICP) in a patient with a traumatic brain injury is instituted when the ICP is greater than*
**A** *12 mm Hg*
**B** *22 mm Hg*
**C** *32 mm Hg*
**D** *42 mm Hg*
**E** *52 mm Hg*

Attention to the management of severe traumatic brain injuries is now focused on maintaining or enhancing cerebral perfusion rather than merely lowering intracranial pressure (ICP). It has been found that hyperventilation to a $PaCO_2 < 30\,mm\,Hg$ to induce cerebral vasoconstriction actually exacerbates cerebral ischemia in spite of decreasing ICP. These secondary iatrogenic cerebral injuries cause more harm than previously appreciated. Treatment must avoid the effects of decreased cardiac output due to the excessive use of osmotic diuretics, sedatives, or barbiturates, and hypoxia. Nevertheless, the measurement of ICP is important and is efficiently accomplished with a ventriculostomy catheter. The catheter also allows withdrawal of cerebral spinal fluid, which is the safest method for lowering ICP.

Intracranial pressure is normally less ≤ 15 mm Hg in adults, however, therapy is not usually initiated until the ICP reaches 22 mm Hg. ICP levels above 22 mm Hg are associated with high mortality and it is currently the standard to manage these patients aggressively even though there is a lack of supporting scientific evidence. Information from an ICP monitor should be used in addition to clinical and radiologic findings to improve outcomes following severe TBI. Cerebral perfusion pressure (CPP) is an important measurement for assuring adequate cerebral perfusion. CPP is the difference between mean arterial pressure (MAP) and the ICP. The recommended target cerebral perfusion pressure (CPP) value for improved survival and favorable outcomes is between 60 and 70 mm Hg. CPP can be improved by either lowering ICP or raising MAP. Maintaining ICP of 70–80 mm Hg has not improved outcome but has increased the incidence rate of adult respiratory distress syndrome (ARDS). Recent studies have shown that management based on CPP monitoring in combination with ICP monitoring reduces both mortality and morbidity when compared to previous methods of management based on ICP monitoring alone. The goal of fluid therapy is to achieve a euvolemic state. Arbitrary fluid restriction is not indicated as it may increase likelihood for hypotension. Iatrogenic hypotension from hypovolemia can worsen secondary brain injury. Whether boosting MAP with pressors or intropes in patients with an elevated ICP resistant to treatment improves outcome is unclear, although recent data suggest it does. Alternative to mannitol which can lower ICP but can also cause hypotension, is the use of hyperosmolar therapy with hypertonic saline which is commercially available in concentrations of 3%, 5%, and 23%.

**Answer: B**

Aries, M.J., Czosnyka, M., Budohoski, K.P., *et al.* (2012) Continuous determination of optimal cerebral perfusion pressure in traumatic brain injury. *Critical Care Medicine*, **40** (8), 2456–2463.

Brain Trauma Foundation (2016) *Guidelines for the Management of Severe Traumatic Brain Injury*, 4th edn, Brain Trauma Foundation, New York, S-172 and S-181.

Huang, S.J., Hong, W.C., Han, Y.Y., *et al.* (2006) Clinical outcome of severe head injury using three different ICP and CPP protocol-driven therapies. *Journal of Clinical Neuroscience*, **13** (8), 818–822.

Mangat, H.S., Chiu, Y.L., Gerber, L.M., *et al.* (2015) Hypertonic saline reduces cumulative and daily intracranial pressure burdens after severe traumatic brain injury. *Journal of Neurosurgery*, **122** (1), 202–210.

Shackford, S.R., Bourguignon, P.R., Wald, S.L., *et al.* (1998) Hypertonic saline resuscitation of patients with head injury: a prospective, randomized clinical trial. *Journal of Trauma and Acute Care Surgery*, **44** (1), 50–58.

**13** *A 75-year-old woman is brought to the trauma unit after a motor vehicle crash. She presents with a Glasgow Coma Score of 14. She has a large laceration to the right parietal region of her head and is currently alert but confused. Her primary and secondary exam is normal. While a chest and pelvic x-ray are being obtained she is noted to become much more lethargic and is responsive only to pain. Which of the following findings is most likely the cause for her condition?*
  **A** *Diffuse axonal injury*
  **B** *Cerebral contusion*
  **C** *Subdural hematoma*
  **D** *Epidural hematoma*
  **E** *Subarachnoid hemorrhage*

**Answer: D**

**14** *A CT-scan was performed in the above patient who showed a biconvex-lens shaped hematoma. She now has lateralizing signs and her mental status deteriorated to a Glasgow Coma Scale of 5. Her pupil on her right side is dilated compared to the left and she is not moving her left side. Which of the following is the next best step in the management of this patient?*
  **A** *Steroids to reduce inflammation*
  **B** *Lasix to decrease brain edema*
  **C** *Emergency craniotomy with evacuation of hematoma*
  **D** *Repeat the head CT in 24 hours*
  **E** *Admit to the ICU with neurological exam every 4 hours*

Epidural hematoma often presents with a lucid interval followed by sudden neurologic deterioration. After intubation, immediate CT scanning of the head is indicated to identify the site of the lesion and assess the degree of mass effect. If focal signs are present, suggesting a mass effect, empiric therapy with hyperventilation and osmolar therapy (mannitol or hypertonic saline) may be indicated as a temporizing attempt while the patient is being taken to surgery for emergent decompression. Unchecked hematoma expansion leads to elevated intracranial pressure and clinical signs, such as an ipsilateral dilated pupil (due to uncal herniation with compression of the oculomotor nerve), or the Cushing reflex (i.e. hypertension, bradycardia, and respiratory depression/irregularity). The pupils will be dilated on the side of the injury and hematoma whereas the motor deficit will be on the opposite side of the injury. Increase in the ICP from the hematoma will culminate in brain herniation and death unless immediate decompression is undertaken. Acute epidural hematoma is associated with arterial bleeding from the middle meningeal artery, a branch of maxillary artery. Surgical evacuation is recommended for all patients with acute epidural hematoma with a hematoma volume greater than 30 ml, clot thickness of >15 mm on CT, midline shift >5 mm, or GCS score <9 with pupillary abnormalities (anisocoria). Nonoperative management for small epidurals includes close observation and serial brain imaging. Glucocorticoid therapy is not indicated following head injury, and may be associated with increased mortality.

**Answer: C**

Bullock, M.R., Chesnut, R., Ghajar, J., *et al.* (2006) Surgical management of acute epidural hematomas. *Neurosurgery*, **58** (3), S2–S7.

Greenberg, M. (2016) *Handbook of Neurosurgery*, 7th edn, Thieme Medical Publishers, New York.

Khaled, C.N., Raihan, M.Z., Chowdhury, F.H., *et al.* (2008) Surgical management of traumatic extradural haematoma: Experiences with 610 patients and prospective analysis. *The Indian Journal of Neurotrauma*, **5** (2), 75–79.

**15** *A 55-year-old man is brought to a level I trauma center after a motor bike crash. His head hit the light* *pole and was found unconscious by the paramedics. After initial evaluation he was found to have an intact airway, and his vital signs were normal and GCS was 8. Secondary survey showed a scalp laceration on the left, and a left wrist deformity. A noncontrast head CT scan was obtained which showed a small left sided crescent shaped hematoma with no midline shift. Which of the following is the best step in the management of this patient?*

A *Emergency craniotomy with evacuation of hematoma*

B *Steroids to reduce inflammation*

C *Lasix to decrease brain edema*

D *Observe the patient in an intensive care unit with intracranial pressure monitoring and serial head CT scans*

E *Discharge the patient home from the emergency department*

**Answer: D**

16 *Which of the following statements regarding subdural hematoma is correct?*

A *Is the least common traumatic extra-axial mass lesion of the brain, occurring in approximately 20–40% of severe injuries*

B *Is generally a diagnosis of exclusion*

C *Most commonly occur in the subfrontal and anterior temporal regions of the brain*

D *Is usually due to shearing of venous sinuses and occurs between the dura and arachnoid layers*

E *May present with a lucid interval similar to an epidural hematoma*

Subdural hematoma is the most common traumatic mass lesion of the head, occurring in approximately 20–40 % of severe head injuries. It usually results from shearing of the bridging cortical veins that drain from the surface of the brain to the dural sinuses. Rupture of these vessels causes bleeding into the space between the dura and arachnoid layer of the meninges. The incidence of acute traumatic subdural hematoma is highest among middle-aged men. However, patients with significant cerebral atrophy (the elderly, those with a history of chronic alcohol abuse, and those with previous traumatic brain injury) are also at high risk as the brain can travel further tearing the veins. Patients with acute subdural hematoma are primarily managed conservatively. Those with diminished consciousness should be observed in an intensive care unit with intracranial pressure monitoring and serial head CT scans. Surgical evacuation is recommended for patients who have clot thickness >10 mm or midline shift >5 mm. Intracerebral hematomas most commonly occur in the subfrontal and anterior temporal

regions of the brain not subdural hematomas. The brain on the side of the impact collides with the skull and the energy is directly transferred to the brain tissues causing hematoma. However, intracerebral hematomas on the opposite side of the direct injury are often due to the initial pulling and tearing of the veins as the brain is pushed towards the site of impact. Contre-coup injury is not due to the brain bouncing inside the skull as the contre-coup injury is often a larger injury than the site of the primary injury. Diffuse axonal injury is generally a diagnosis of exclusion. Patients with severe head injury whose CT scan does not reveal significant lesions or those who remain in vegetative or severely disabled despite evacuation of mass lesions are given the diagnosis of diffuse axonal injury.

**Answer: D**

Brunicardi, F.C. (2010) *Schwartz's Principles of Surgery*, 9th edn, McGraw-Hill, New York, pp. 145, 1524.

Bullock, M.R., Chesnut, R., Ghajar, J., *et al.* (2006) Surgical management of acute epidural hematomas. *Neurosurgery*, **58** (3), S216.

Victor, M. and Ropper, A. (2001) Craniocerebral trauma, in *Adams and Victor's Principles of Neurology*, 7th ed, (ed. V.M. Ropper), McGraw-Hill, New York, pp. 925–953.

17 *Which of the statements regarding subarachnoid hemorrhage following trauma is correct?*

A *Mass effect from the subarachnoid blood is a major concern*

B *They have a characteristic crescent shape on CT of the head*

C *Usually produces meningismus (stiff neck and headache)*

D *Subarachnoid hemorrhage is the most common indication for operative intervention after traumatic brain injury*

E *May produce noncommunicating hydrocephalus as a complication*

Subarachnoid hemorrhage (SAH) refers to extravasation of blood into the subarachnoid space between the pial and arachnoid membranes. It usually causes headache, dizzinesss, and changes in the patient's mental status; neck stiffness (meningismus) may occur. The hemorrhage is small and rapidly diluted by the CSF, no localized mass effect occurs. This type of hemorrhage after trauma has little surgical significance. Radiologic clues of a traumatic subarachnoid hemorrhage include localized bleeding in the superficial sulci or basal cisterns, adjacent skull fracture, and cerebral contusion. Isolated subarachnoid hemorrhage in the setting of mild traumatic brain injury (GCS ≥ 13) is associated with a benign neurological outcome. Rarely does subarachnoid hemorrhage leads to progressive communicating hydrocephalus that requires shunting.

**Answer: C**

Brunicardi, F.C. (2010) *Schwartz's Principles of Surgery*, 9th edn, McGraw-Hill, New York, pp. 145, 1524.

Moore, A.J. (2005) *Neurosurgery Principles and Practice*, Springer, London.

van Gijn, J. and Rinkel, G.J.E. (2001) Subarachnoid haemorrhage: diagnosis, causes and management. *Brain*, **124** (2), 249–278.

**18** *A 58-year old man presented to a level I trauma center after a motor vehicle crash. Primary survey was intact, on secondary survey he had a 2 cm laceration on the right side of his forehead and fracture of his right tibia and left ankle. Patient was neurologically intact. Initial CT scan of the head revealed subdural hemorrhage 6 mm in size. Which of the following statements is true regarding venous thromboembolism (VTE) prophylaxis in this patient?*

**A** *It is safe to initiate chemical VTE prophylaxis in patients with intracranial hemorrhage who have neurologically intact examination.*

**B** *Chemical VTE prophylaxis can be safely initiated at 24 hours if head bleed is <8 mm and there is no progression on repeat CT scan.*

**C** *Chemical VTE prophylaxis is not safe in patients with intracranial hemorrhage.*

**D** *Chemical VTE prophylaxis can be safely initiated at 72 hours if head bleed is <8 mm and there is no progression on repeat CT scan.*

**E** *Prophylactic placement of IVC filter is recommended*

Traumatic brain injury (TBI) patients are at high risk for developing venous thromboembolism (VTE), the rate can be as high as 30%. Patients who are at low risk for progression of intracranial bleeding and have a stable repeat head CT scan at 24 hours, pharmacologic prophylaxis can be safely initiated. Patients with moderate risk, subdural or epidural hematoma >8 mm, contusion or interventricular hemorrhage >2 cm, multiple contusions per lobe or evidence of progression at 24 hours, pharmacologic prophylaxis can be initiated at 72 hours if CT scan is stable. Prophylactic placement of IVC filter should be considered only in patients at high risk for progression of intracranial hemorrhage with ICP monitor placement craniotomy evidence of progression at 72 hours. Delay in initiation of prophylaxis for greater than 4 days significantly increases the risk of venous thromboembolism.

**Answer: B**

Farooqui, A., Hiser, B., Barnes, S.L., and Litofsky, N.S. (2013) Safety and efficacy of early thromboembolism chemoprophylaxis after intracranial hemorrhage from traumatic brain injury: Clinical article. *Journal of Neurosurgery*, **119** (6), 1576–1582.

Ekeh, A.P., Dominguez, K.M., Markert, R.J., and McCarthy, M.C. (2010) Incidence and risk factors for deep venous thrombosis after moderate and severe brain injury. *Journal of Trauma and Acute Care Surgery*, **68** (4), 912–915.

Kwiatt, M.E., Patel, M.S., Ross, S.E., *et al.* (2012) Is low-molecular-weight heparin safe for venous thromboembolism prophylaxis in patients with traumatic brain injury? A Western Trauma Association multicenter study. *Journal of Trauma and Acute Care Surgery*, **73** (3), 625–628.

**19** *A 37-year-old man presents to ED after being involved in a motorcycle accident and was not wearing a helmet. At scene he had a GCS of 7 and was intubated by EMS. On arrival to ED patient was hypotensive and tachycardic while the secondary survey was positive for scalp laceration with depressed skull fracture, abnormal pupillary size, and bruises on the rest of the body. CT scan showed depressed parietal bone fracture with multiple intracranial hemorrhages, diffuse neuronal injury, and cerebral edema. His ICP was noted to be 26 mm Hg. Which of the following treatment for decreasing ICP is associated with improved neurological outcomes?*

**A** *IV Mannitol 0.7 g/kg bodyweight*

**B** *Hyperventilation*

**C** *Frontotemporoparietel decompressive craniectomy*

**D** *Bifrontal decompressive craniectomy*

**E** *Intermittent CSF drainage*

The critical care management for severe TBI is aimed at optimizing ICP and cerebral perfusion pressure (CPP) as well as maintaining adequate oxygenation and blood pressure to prevent secondary brain injury. ICP should be monitored in patients with GCS of 3–8 and abnormal head CT (hematomas, contusions, swelling, herniation, or compressed basal cisterns). Multiple treatment options are available for optimizing ICP which includes hyperventilation, mannitol, decompressive craniectomy (DC), and CSF drainage. A large frontotemporoparietel DC (≥12 cm×15 cm) has a better prognosis as compared to small frontotemporoparietel DC in terms of mortality and neurological outcomes. Bifrontal craniectomy is effective in reducing ICP but has not shown any mortality benefit. Mannitol is effective in reducing the ICP, but should be avoided in patients with BP less than 90 mm Hg. Hyperventilation is considered as a temporary option for reducing ICP and should not be used for a long-term therapy as it causes more brain ischemia. CSF drainage is also an alternative therapy to DC for lowering ICP.

**Answer: C**

Brain Trauma Foundation (2016) *Guidelines for the Management of Severe Traumatic Brain Injury*, 4th edn, Brain Trauma Foundation, New York, S-26, S-27.

Bor-Seng-Shu, E., Figueiredo, E.G., Amorim, R.L., *et al.* (2012) Decompressive craniectomy: a meta-analysis of influences on intracranial pressure and cerebral perfusion pressure in the treatment of traumatic brain injury: a review. *Journal of Neurosurgery*, **117** (3), 589–596.

Eberle, B.M., Schnüriger, B., Inaba, K., *et al.* (2010). Decompressive craniectomy: surgical control of traumatic intracranial hypertension may improve outcome. *Injury*, **41** (9), 894–898.

Bratton, S.L., Chestnut, R.M., Ghajar, J., *et al.* (2007) VI. Indications for intracranial pressure monitoring. *Journal of Neurotrauma*, **24** (Supplement 1), S-37.

Maas, A.I., Stocchetti, N., and Bullock, R. (2008) Moderate and severe traumatic brain injury in adults. *The Lancet Neurology*, 7 (8), 728–741.

**20** *A 23-year-old man involved in a motor vehicle collision arrived at the ED with a Glasgow Coma Scale (GCS) score of 8, and a dilated and nonreactive left pupil. His blood pressure was 85/45 mm Hg and heart rate 105 beats/min. The patient was intubated at the scene. There is an obvious deformity of the right femur and the right tibia. The initial use of which one of the following will decrease this patient's ICP without compromising the BP:*

**A** *Normal (0.9%) saline*
**B** *Hypertonic saline*
**C** *Mannitol*
**D** *Barbiturates*
**E** *Dextrose(5%) water*

Hypertonic saline refers to any saline solution with a concentration of sodium chloride (NaCl) higher than physiologic (0.9%). Commonly used preparations include 2%, 3%, 5%, 7%, and 23% NaCl. Hypertonic saline has an important role in preventing and treating the effects of secondary brain injury. It works primarily as an osmotic agent preventing and limiting brain edema and the subsequent increase in ICP. Mannitol can also be used to lower ICP but because of its diuretic effects its use is limited by the accompanying hypotension in TBI patients. Current therapies used for ICP control (mannitol, barbiturates) risk further reducing perfusion to the brain either by lowering blood pressure and cerebral perfusion

pressure (CPP) or by causing cerebral vasoconstriction (hyperventilation). Ideally, a therapeutic intervention should effectively reduce ICP while preserving or improving CPP. On the other hand, hypertonic saline may benefit patients with TBI while preserving or even improving hemodynamic parameters. This makes hypertonic saline a suitable choice in TBI patients with ICP elevation and concurrent hypovolemia. Normal saline and dextrose water can further increase the ICP and aggravate the situation.

**Answer: B**

Brain, T.F. (2007) Guidelines for the management of severe traumatic brain injury. II. Hyperosmolar therapy. *Journal of Neurotrauma*, **24**, S14.

Doyle, J.A., Davis, D.P., and Hoyt, D.B. (2001) The use of hypertonic saline in the treatment of traumatic brain injury. *Journal of Trauma and Acute Care Surgery*, **50** (2), 367–383.

Joseph, B., Aziz, H., Snell, M., *et al.* (2014) The physiological effects of hyperosmolar resuscitation: 5% vs 3% hypertonic saline. *American Journal of Surgery*, **208** (5), 697–702.

Rickard, A.C., Smith, J.E., Newell, P., *et al.* (2014) Salt or sugar for your injured brain? A meta-analysis of randomised controlled trials of mannitol versus hypertonic sodium solutions to manage raised intracranial pressure in traumatic brain injury. *Emergency Medicine Journal*, **31** (8), 679–683.

Wade, C.E., Grady, J.J., Kramer, G.C., *et al.* (1997) Individual patient cohort analysis of the efficacy of hypertonic saline/dextran in patients with traumatic brain injury and hypotension. *Journal of Trauma and Acute Care Surgery*, **42**(5S), 61S–65S.

**21** *A 45-year-old man presented to the ED with a history of loss of consciousness after a fall from a ladder. His primary and secondary exam is intact with a normal neurologic exam and Glasgow Coma Scale (GCS) score of 15. His vital signs are stable. A CT scan of the head was obtained which shows a minor epidural hematoma of 3 mm and no skull fracture. His past medical history is significant for occasional heartburn for which he sometimes uses over the counter antacids. He is not currently using medications. According to the Brain Injury Guidelines (BIG) what is the next best step in the management of this patient?*

**A** *Observation for 6 hours with neurologic exams*
**B** *Discharge home with family*
**C** *Admission to the ICU*
**D** *Hospitalization with a neurosurgical consult*
**E** *Neurosurgical consult with RHCT in 6 hours*

**Table 28.2** Brain injury guidelines.

| Variables | BIG 1 | BIG 2 | BIG 3 |
|---|---|---|---|
| LOC | Yes/No | Yes/No | Yes/No |
| Neurologic examination | Normal | Normal | Abnormal |
| Intoxication | No | No/Yes | No/Yes |
| CAMP | No | No | Yes |
| Skull Fracture | No | Non-displaced | Displaced |
| SDH | ≤4mm | 5–7 mm | ≥8 mm |
| EDH | ≤4mm | 5–7 mm | ≥8 mm |
| IPH | ≤4mm, 1 location | 3–7 mm, 2 locations | ≥8 mm, multiple locations |
| SAH | Trace | Localized | Scattered |
| IVH | No | No | Yes |
| **THERAPEUTIC PLAN** | | | |
| Hospitalization | No Observation (6hrs) | Yes | Yes |
| RHCT | No | No | Yes |
| NSC | No | No | Yes |

BIG, brain injury guidelines; CAMP, Coumadin, Aspirin, Plavix; EDH, epidural hemorrhage; IVH, intraventricular hemorrhage; IPH, intraparenchymal hemorrhage; LOC, loss of consciousness; NSC, neurosurgical consultation; RHCT, repeat head computed tomography; SAH, subarachnoid hemorrhage; SDH, subdural hemorrhage

This patient presented to the ED after a fall with a normal neurologic exam and a minor epidural hematoma on head CT scan. According to the Brain Injury Guidelines (BIG), any patient with a traumatic brain injury with a normal neurologic exam, no skull fracture, who is not using any anticoagulants with EDH size < 4 mm on the initial CT scan, is classified as BIG-1, and doesn't require hospitalization, repeat head CT scan, or a neurosurgical consult. The recommended management for BIG 1 patients is observation in the ED for 6 hours with repeat neurologic examinations. Patients with ICH size between 5–7 mm and a nondisplaced skull fracture on the initial CT scan are classified as BIG 2 and they need hospitalization without a neurosurgical consult or the need for a repeat heat CT scan, if the neurologic examination of the patient remains stable. While patients who are on antiplatelet or anticoagulation medications, or an abnormal neurologic examination finding, and concerning CT scan findings (displaced skull fractures, and diffused ICH size > 8 mm), are classified as BIG 3. The recommended therapeutic plan for these patients is hospitalization, a neurosurgical consult, and a follow-up head CT scan. Management of TBI patients according to the BIG guidelines (see Table 28.2) has decreased the number of unnecessary repeat head CT scans and neurological consults, resulting in conservation of health care resources.

**Answer: A**

Joseph, B., Friese, R.S., Sadoun, M., *et al.* (2014) The BIG (Brain Injury Guidelines) project: defining the management of traumatic brain injury by acute care surgeons. *Journal of Trauma and Acute Care Surgery*, **76** (4), 965–969.

Joseph, B., Aziz, H., Pandit, V., *et al.* (2014) Prospective validation of the brain injury guidelines: Managing traumatic brain injury without neurosurgical consultation. *Journal of Trauma and Acute Care Surgery*, **77** (6), 984–988.

Joseph, B., Haider, A.A., Pandit, V., *et al.* (2015) Changing paradigms in the management of 2184 patients with traumatic brain injury. *Annals of Surgery*, **262** (3), 440–448.

Velmahos, G.C. (2015) Brain injury guidelines for small head injuries. *Journal of the American Medical Association Surgery*, **150** (9), 872–873.

**22** *A 55-year-old man presented to the ED after being hit by a car. Primary survey is intact; on secondary survey the patient has a scalp laceration and bruises on the shoulder and bilateral lower extremities. He has a Glasgow Coma Scale (GCS) score of 12. His vitals are stable. The patient is on an unknown antiplatelet/anticoagulant medication. An initial head CT scan was obtained which showed a subdural hematoma (SDH). Which of the following medication is not associated with increased risk of progression of his intracranial bleed?*

**A** *Low-dose (81 mg) aspirin*
**B** *Dabigatran*
**C** *Warfarin*
**D** *Clopidogrel*
**E** *Rivaroxaban*

Patients with intracranial hemorrhage who are on preinjury antiplatelet/anticoagulant medications have a risk of progression of the bleed on repeat head CT scan (RHCT). However, the use of low dose (81 mg) aspirin, commonly referred to as "baby aspirin" in the general population, is not associated with progression of the initial injury on RHCT or clinical deterioration. Therefore, prehospital low-dose aspirin therapy shouldn't be used as a sole criterion to recommend a routine repeat head CT in traumatic brain injury. On the other hand, a number of studies have consistently shown that preinjury warfarin and clopidogrel use in TBI patients results in the progression of intracranial hemorrhage. Although the literature regarding the newer anticoagulants is insufficient, a few studies have shown that these newer agents (Factor Xa and direct thrombin inhibitors) are associated with increased risk of progression of intracranial hemorrhage following traumatic brain injury.

**Answer: A**

Beynon, C., Potzy, A., Sakowitz, O.W., and Unterberg, A.W. (2015) Rivaroxaban and intracranial haemorrhage after mild traumatic brain injury: A dangerous combination? *Clinical Neurology and Neurosurgery*, **136**, 73–78.

Joseph, B., Aziz, H., Pandit, V., *et al.* (2014) Low-dose aspirin therapy is not a reason for repeating head computed tomographic scans in traumatic brain injury: a prospective study. *Journal of Surgical Research*, **186** (1), 287–291.

Joseph, B., Pandit, V., Aziz, H., *et al.* (2014) Clinical outcomes in traumatic brain injury patients on preinjury clopidogrel: a prospective analysis. *Journal of Trauma and Acute Care Surgery*, **76** (3), 817–820.

Joseph, B., Sadoun, M., Aziz, H., *et al.* (2014) Repeat head computed tomography in anticoagulated traumatic brain injury patients: still warranted. *The American Surgeon*, **80** (1), 43–47.

Nishijima, D.K., Offerman, S.R., Ballard, D.W., *et al.* (2013) Risk of traumatic intracranial hemorrhage in patients with head injury and preinjury warfarin or clopidogrel use. *Academic Emergency Medicine*, **20** (2), 140–145.

## 29

# Blunt and Penetrating Neck Trauma
*Leslie Kobayashi, MD and Barret Halgas, MD*

**1** *Regarding zones of the neck, which of the following statements is true?*
   **A** *Zone II is bounded by the clavicle and cricoid cartilage*
   **B** *Zone II injuries require angiography*
   **C** *Zone I and III injuries require mandatory surgical exploration*
   **D** *Clinical presentation rather than zone of injury is the primary determinant of operative versus non-operative management*
   **E** *Zone II is the least surgically accessible*

Zone I is bounded by the clavicles and cricoid cartilage (see Figure 29.1). Zone II lies between the cricoid cartilage and the angle of the mandible and is the most easily accessible surgically. Zone III extends from the angle of the mandible to the base of the skull, and is the most difficult area to explore, sometimes requiring transection of the mandible, dislocation of the jaw, or drilling into the skull base to expose vital structures. Zone I and III injuries are typically investigated with CTA, endoscopy, or conventional angiography. Traditionally, all Zone II injuries underwent mandatory operative exploration, however this resulted in an unacceptably high rate of negative explorations. The primary determinant of operative versus nonoperative management is clinical presentation. Patients with hard signs of vascular or aerodigestive injury require surgical exploration regardless of location of the injury. Those with soft signs undergo further evaluation via imaging. Hard signs of vascular injury include arterial bleeding, pulsatile or expanding hematoma, absence of pulse distal to the injury, bruit or thrill at the injury site, unexplained shock or anemia. Hard signs of aerodigestive injury include bubbling from the injury site, large volume hemoptysis or hematemasis, stridor, or massive subcutaneous emphysema. Soft signs of vascular injury include nonexpanding and nonpulsatile hematomas or minor bleeding from the site of injury.

Soft signs of aerodigestive injury include odynophagia, small hemoptysis or hematemasis, hoarseness, or minor subcutaneous emphysema.

**Answer: D**

Ball, C.G. (2015) Penetrating nontorso trauma: the head and the neck. *Canadian Journal of Surgery*, **58** (4), 284–285.

Sperry, J.L., Moore, E.E., Coimbra, R., *et al.* (2013) Western Trauma Association critical decisions in trauma: penetrating neck trauma. *Journal of Trauma and Acute Care Surgery*, **75** (6), 936–940.

Shiroff, A., Gale, S.C., Martin, N.D., *et al.* (2013) Penetrating neck trauma: a review of management strategies and discussion of the "No Zone" approach. *American Surgeon*, **79** (1), 23–29.

**2** *A man was stabbed in the neck just above the cricoid. He is hemodynamically stable, however there is a large pulsatile hematoma. What is the next step in management?*
   **A** *Rapid sequence intubation in the ER followed by surgical exploration*
   **B** *Emergent cricothyroidotomy in the ER followed by surgical exploration*
   **C** *Intubation in the operating room followed by surgical exploration of the neck*
   **D** *Observation in the intensive care unit*
   **E** *Placement of laryngeal mask airway (LMA) followed by surgical exploration*

This patient has a penetrating injury to Zone II with hard signs of vascular injury that requires surgical exploration. Because the patient is stable the best course of action is to proceed immediately to the operating room for airway control. The operating room has several advantages over the ER. It is a controlled environment,

*Surgical Critical Care and Emergency Surgery: Clinical Questions and Answers*, Second Edition.
Edited by Forrest "Dell" Moore, Peter Rhee, and Gerard J. Fulda.
© 2018 John Wiley & Sons Ltd. Published 2018 by John Wiley & Sons Ltd.
Companion website: www.wiley.com/go/moore/surgical_criticalcare_and_emergency_surgery

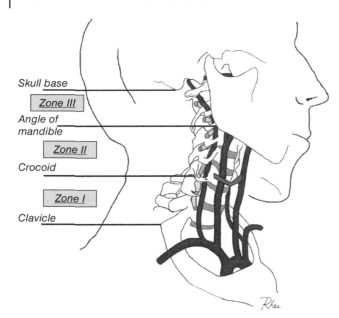

**Figure 29.1** The vascular anatomy and zones of the neck. Figure courtesy of Peter Rhee. A full color version of this figure appears in the plate section of this book.

and conversion to a surgical airway can occur with the aid of extra personnel, specialized surgical equipment, better positioning, improved lighting, and sterile technique. This is likely to be a difficult intubation due to distortion of the airway from the hematoma and the need for a surgical airway is high. Direct laryngoscopy (DL) is not tolerated well in the awake patient and medications used in rapid sequence intubation (RSI) may convert an urgent airway into an emergent airway. Because of this a good alternative to DL is fiberoptic awake intubation, which provides the ability to intubate without RSI medications, visualization of the airway and airway injuries, and potentially prevent further disruption of existing tracheal injuries during blind intubation. Cricothyroidotomy is a good option for the unstable patient, but should only be used if endotracheal intubation fails in the stable patient. Additionally, preservation of as much intact airway as possible is important if there is a tracheal injury.

**Answer: C**

Gale, S.C. and Mattox, K.L. (2009) Trauma to the head, face, and neck, in *Acute Care Surgery: A Guide for General Surgeons* (eds V.H. Gracias, P.M. Reilly, M.G. McKenney, and G.C. Velmahos), McGraw-Hill, New York, pp. 99–108.

Koletsis, E., Prokakis, C., Baltayiannis, N., *et al.* (2012) Surgical decision making in tracheobronchial injuries on the basis of clinical evidence and the injury's anatomical

setting: a retrospective analysis. *Injury*, **43** (9), 1437–1441.

Prokakis, C., Koletsis, E.N., Dedeilias, P., *et al.* (2014) Airway trauma: a review on epidemiology, mechanisms of injury, diagnosis and treatment. *Journal of Cardiothoracic Surgery*, **9**, 117–124.

3 *In a patient with cervical spinal cord injury, which pulmonary function test best predicts deteriorating lung function?*
   A *Decrease functional residual capacity*
   B *Decreased minute ventilation*
   C *Decreased vital capacity*
   D *Decreased negative inspiratory force*
   E *Decreased diffusion capacity*

Changes in pulmonary physiology after spinal cord injury (SCI) include decreased vital capacity, total lung capacity, end respiratory volume, inspiratory capacity, and $FEV_1$. Residual volume is increased and no change is noted in functional residual capacity. Respiratory complications occur in 36–83% of patients, and a large proportion will require mechanical ventilation. Injury above C3–C5 will result in loss of phrenic nerve function; below C5 loss of accessory muscles inhibit pulmonary function. Because these patients are challenging airways, many advocate early elective intubation. However, mechanical ventilation is not inevitable, and select patients can be observed if carefully monitored. Strong consideration should be given to serial assessment of vital capacity in these patients as decreased vital capacity may precede clinical evidence of respiratory compromise. Vital capacity below 10 mL/kg of ideal body weight is an indication for urgent intubation. Vital capacity is the maximum amount of air expelled after a maximum inspiration. It is equal to the inspiratory reserve volume plus the tidal volume plus the expiratory reserve volume.

**Answer: C**

Berly, M. and Shem, K. (2007) Respiratory management during the first five days after spinal cord injury. *Journal of Spinal Cord Medicine*, **30**, 309–318.

Schilero, G.J., Spungen, A.M., Bauman, W.A., *et al.* (2009) Pulmonary function and spinal cord injury. *Respiratory Physiology*, **166**, 129–141.

4 *Following a motor vehicle collision, the patient in Figure 29.2 initially presents with a GCS of 15. CT scan of the head and noncontrast CT of the cervical spine are normal. The patient acutely decompensates to a GCS of 13 and develops weakness in the left arm and leg. What is the next step in diagnosis?*

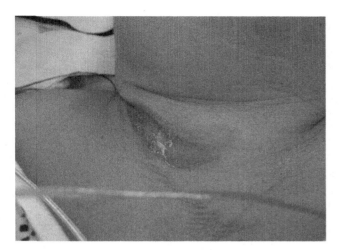

**Figure 29.2** A seat belt sign over the neck in Zone I. A full color version of this figure appears in the plate section of this book.

A *CT scan of the cervical spine*
B *Repeat CT scan of the head*
C *MRI*
D *CT Angiogram*
E *Ultrasound*

An acute neurological decompensation with lateralizing signs is concerning for a cerebrovascular event. CT imaging is not sensitive in the hyperacute phase (0–6 hours) to assess for ischemic damage in the brain. The patient has a seat belt sign above the level of the clavicle suggesting blunt cerebrovascular injury (BCVI). The Denver screening criteria is a useful tool intended to reduce the rate of CT angiography (see Table 29.1). Four vessel angiography remains the gold standard for diagnosis of BCVI, however advanced CT angiography with multichannel (16–64) detectors has become an almost equivalent screening modality. CTA has the benefit of being quick, widely available, and easy to perform, and does not require the presence of a specially trained angiography team. It also avoids the morbidity associated with an arterial puncture and uses a lower contrast dose than traditional angiography. Studies have shown detection rates similar to historical controls with four vessel angiography. Sensitivity ranges from 83–100% with negative predictive values of 92–98%. Duplex sonography, MRI/MRA, and four-slice CT angiography are not recommended.

**Answer: D**

Biffl, W.J., Cothren, C., Moore, E.E., *et al.* (2009) Western Trauma Association Critical decision in Trauma: Screening for and treatment of blunt cerebrovascular injuries. *Journal of Trauma*, **67** (6), 1150–1153.
Morales-Uribe, C., Ramírez, A., Suarez-Poveda, T., *et al.* (2016). Diagnostic performance of CT angiography in

**Table 29.1** Denver screening criteria.

| Signs/Symptoms of BCVI |
| --- |
| Arterial hemorrhage |
| Cervical bruit in patient < 50 years of age |
| Expanding cervical hematoma |
| Focal neurologic deficit |
| Neurologic exam incongruous with head CT scan findings |
| Stroke on secondary CT scan |
| **Risk Factors for BCVI** |
| High-energy transfer mechanism with: LeForte II or III fracture |
| Cervical-spine fracture patterns: subluxation, fractures extending into the transverse foramen, fractures of C1-C3 |
| Basilar skull fracture with carotid canal involvement |
| Diffuse axonal injury with a Glasgow Coma Scale (GCS) score < 6 |
| Near hanging with anoxic brain injury |

neck vessel trauma: systematic review and meta-analysis. *Emergency Radiology*, **23** (5), 421–431.

5 *A 24-year-old woman presents with an anterior Zone II stab wound. Upon exploration, a laceration to the anterior trachea is noted across the first and second tracheal rings. The next step in her evaluation would include:*
A *Exploration of the innominate artery*
B *Exposure of the brachiocephalic vein*
C *Inspection of the bilateral recurrent laryngeal nerves*
D *Examination of the superior laryngeal nerve*
E *Examination of the posterior tracheal wall*

The trachea is relatively protected from injury by the chin, sternum, and spinal column posteriorly. Tracheal injury is present in only 5% of all cervical neck trauma and only 1% of thoracic trauma. Neck exploration is typically performed via a longitudinal incision along the medial border of the sternocleidomastoid. A cervical collar incision can be used for bilateral exploration. Lateral retraction of the SCM and carotid sheath will allow of optimal visualization of the trachea and esophagus. The presence of an anterior tracheal injury makes evaluation of the posterior wall of the trachea and the esophagus of paramount importance as concomitant injuries are present in 10–15% of cases. Peritracheal dissection should be minimized to only what is required to identify and repair associated injuries because aggressive dissection can devascularize the trachea. Absorbable sutures with extraluminal knots are recommended for primary repair. Exploration of the ipsilateral carotid sheath and contents should be performed as well. Exploration of the innominate artery or brachio-cephalic vein is not indicated unless there is suspicion for injury. Positively identifying the superior or recurrent laryngeal nerves is not recommended, as dissection can actually increase the incidence of injury.

**Answer: E**

Britt, L.D. (2007) Penetrating neck trauma, in *Mastery of Surgery*, 5th edn (eds J.E. Fischer and K.I. Bland), Lippincott Williams & Wilkins, Philadelphia PA, pp. 381–386.

Lyons, J. D., Feliciano, D. V., Wyrzykowski, A. D., and Rozycki, G. S. (2013). Modern management of penetrating tracheal injuries. *The American Surgeon*, **79** (2), 188–193.

Prokakis, C., Koletsis, E.N., Dedeilias, P., *et al.* (2014) Airway trauma: a review on epidemiology, mechanisms of injury, diagnosis and treatment. *Journal of Cardiothoracic Surgery*, **9**, 117–124.

6   *Screening for blunt cerebrovascular injury (BCVI) is most indicated in which of the following situations?*
    A  *Basilar skull fracture*
    B  *Seat belt sign on the chest*
    C  *Clavicle fracture*
    D  *Paraspinal cervical tenderness on exam*
    E  *Subgaleal hematoma*

Blunt cerebrovascular injury is rare following blunt trauma. The overall incidence is approximately 1% in centers with aggressive screening protocols. Injuries can occur as a result of severe hyperextension or rotation, direct force to the vessel, or by injury from adjacent fractures (particularly C1–C3). The majority of patients have minimal to no symptoms at presentation. "Symptoms" would include facial hemorrhage, cervical bruit, cervical hematoma, infarct on head CT, or lateralizing neurological deficit. Indications for screening in "asymptomatic" patients are: GCS of 8 or less, presence of diffuse axonal injury, basilar skull fracture, cervical spine fracture, Lefort II or III fractures, direct blow to the neck, and hyperextension injuries (see Table 29.1). An isolated seat belt sign on the neck has not been shown to be an independent risk factor for BCVI following blunt trauma. Similarly, subgaleal hematomas and clavicular fractures have not been found to be risk factors. There is a strong association between cervical and/or skull base fractures and BCVIs (87% in recent studies). Concerning signs would be ecchymosis over the mastoid process (Battle sign), raccoon eyes, and CSF otorrhea. The presence of a skull base fracture in this patient should prompt a CTA of the neck along with other indicated imaging. Conventional angiography may follow.

**Answer: A**

Buch, K., Nguyen, T., Mahoney, E., *et al.* (2016). Association between cervical spine and skull-base fractures and blunt cerebrovascular injury. *European Radiology*, **26** (2), 524–531.

Harrigan, M. R., Hadley, M. N., Dhall, S. S., *et al.* (2013). Management of vertebral artery injuries following non-penetrating cervical trauma. *Neurosurgery*, **72**, 234–243.

7   *Regarding blunt cerebrovascular injuries (BCVI), when would endovascular interventions be considered?*
    A  *Only for Grade 1 and 2 injuries*
    B  *Nonflow limiting dissection with adequate collateral circulation*
    C  *Asymptomatic intra-luminal thrombus*
    D  *Pseudoaneurysm*
    E  *Zone 2 partial transection*

There is very little data regarding the optimal type and duration of treatment for BCVI. Options include anticoagulation, antiplatelet therapy, surgical repair, and endovascular intervention. Grade 1 and 2 injuries can be treated with anticoagulation or antiplatelet therapy alone, as these methods have equivalent efficacy (see Table 29.2). The majority (85%) of low-grade injuries are stable or resolve within 3 months. Repeat imaging is important as a small percentage of Grade 1 (8%) and a larger percentage of Grade 2 lesions (43%) will form a pseudoaneurysm by day 7–10. Grade III injuries (pseudoaneurysms) are less likely to resolve with antithrombotic therapy alone and the risk of thromboembolic complications without treatment can be as high as 43–74%. Complications include distal embolization, obstruction, compression, and bleeding.

**Table 29.2** Injury scale for blunt cerebrovascular injury.

| Grade of injury | Type of injury |
|---|---|
| Grade I | Angiographie appearance of irregularity of vessel wall or dissection with <25% luminal stenosis. |
| Grade II | Injuries in which intraluminal thrombus or raised intimai flap is seen, or dissections or intramural hematomas with luminal narrowing >25%. |
| Grade III | Pseudoaneurysms |
| Grade IV | Vessel occlusion |
| Grade V | Complete vessel transection and free contrast extravasation. |

*Source*: Biffl, W.L., Ray Jr, C.E., Moore, E.E., *et al.* (2002). Treatment-related outcomes from blunt cerebrovascular injuries: importance of routine follow-up arteriography. *Annals of Surgery*, **235** (5), 699–707.

A pseudoaneurysm involving the external carotid artery can cause massive epistaxis. The challenge lies in successfully debulking the aneurysm without occluding the parent artery. Combined coil embolization and stent angioplasty is commonly employed. Stenting mandates the use of dual-platelet therapy for 1 month. Grade IV lesions (occlusions) are unlikely to resolve, however anti-coagulation or antiplatelet therapy should be initiated to prevent propagation of the thrombus. Often there is adequate circulation to maintain cerebral perfusion. Endovascular mechanical thrombolysis is reserved for acutely symptomatic patients. Follow-up imaging is not recommended for Grade IV lesions as they are unlikely to change with time. Grade V lesions (active extravasation) require emergent exploration and surgery.

**Answer: D**

Alderazi, Y.J., Cruz, G.M., Kass-Hout, T., *et al.* (2015). Endovascular therapy for cerebrovascular injuries after head and neck trauma. *Trauma*, **17** (4), 258–269.

Biffl, W.L., Ray Jr, C.E., Moore, E.E., *et al.* (2002). Treatment-related outcomes from blunt cerebrovascular injuries: importance of routine follow-up arteriography. *Annals of Surgery*, **235** (5), 699–707.

Scott, W.W., Sharp, S., Figueroa, S.A., *et al.* (2015). Clinical and radiographic outcomes following traumatic Grade 1 and 2 carotid artery injuries: a 10-year retrospective analysis from a Level I trauma center. The Parkland Carotid and Vertebral Artery Injury Survey. *Journal of Neurosurgery*, **122** (5), 1196–1201.

**8** *What is the most common presenting injury in suicidal hangings?*
  **A** *None*
  **B** *Carotid artery dissection*
  **C** *Laryngotracheal separation*
  **D** *Anoxic brain injury*
  **E** *Fractures of both C2 pedicles*

Hanging is the second most commonly attempted method of suicide in the United States (GSW #1) and carries a 70% mortality rate. The severity of sustained injuries depends on the type and duration of hanging. A judicial or execution-style hanging refers to the body being dropped from a height equal to the height of the person. The fall often causes extreme hyperextension, spinal cord injury, asphyxiation, and death. The unstable C2 pedicle fracture aptly called a Hangman's fracture may not be a pathognomonic as traditionally thought. It is not surprising that there is a different pattern of injuries in suicidal hangings without a fall from height. The soft tissues are compressed causing jugular venous obstruction, hypoxia, and unconsciousness. As the body

relaxes, the weight against the ligature leads to direct tracheal or carotid compression. The overall survival for nonlethal hangings that present to the hospital is favorable at about 90%. There are actually strangulations in the vast majority of cases as they seldom drop the necessary distance to cause an unstable cervical spinal injury with spinal cord injury. Only about one in five patients will have clinical or radiographic evidence of injury other than soft tissue swelling. Anoxic brain injury on CT is seen in 10% of patients. Although not as common, cervical spine injuries are still found in 2–5% of nonjudicial hangings. Laryngeal injuries have been seen in up to 50% of *lethal* hangings (i.e. thyroid cartilage fracture, hyoid bone fracture) but are rarely seen in nonlethal hangings. Although the data is scarce, arterial injury is reportedly found in 0.5–2% of nonlethal hangings. Injuries can range from compressive vasospasm to complete obstruction. In the absence of formal guidelines, most would recommend spinal precautions and immobilization as well as CT of the head and CTA of the neck. Prophylactic intubation is not required however, close monitoring for the progression of airway edema is a consideration. If the patient is unresponsive and airway needs to be obtained, the best method is to perform RSI knowing that unstable cervical fracture is very rare. The next step is CT angiogram and then admission. If the patient is asymptomatic no diagnostic workup is necessary.

**Answer: D**

Chikhani, M. and Winter, R. (2014). Injury after non-judicial hanging. *Trauma*, **16** (3), 164–173.

Gunnell, D., Bennewith, O., Hawton, K., *et al.* (2005). The epidemiology and prevention of suicide by hanging: a systematic review. *International Journal of Epidemiology*, **34** (2), 433–442.

Salim, A., Martin, M., Sangthong, B., *et al.* (2006). Near-hanging injuries: a 10-year experience. *Injury*, **37** (5), 435–439.

**9** *Which of the following is a known complication of complete spinal cord injury?*
  **A** *Infertility in women*
  **B** *Inability to carry a fetus to term*
  **C** *Inability to deliver vaginally*
  **D** *Inability to obtain an erection*
  **E** *Infertility in men*

The reproductive system of both men and women can be affected by spinal cord injury. Women may suffer a temporary interruption of menses, which generally resolves within 6–9 months of injury. However, fertility is preserved and women can carry a fetus to term. Pregnancies of women with SCI can be complicated, most commonly by urinary tract infections, autonomic dysreflexia, and premature labor. Most women can deliver vaginally, although they may require second-stage assistance. In contrast, male fertility is affected at multiple stages. They may suffer from low testosterone, and, while erection is possible, ejaculation is unlikely in the absence of vibrational or electrical stimulation devices. Additionally, spermatogenesis and sperm motility are both decreased after SCI.

**Answer: E**

Cross, L.L., Meythaler, J.M., Tuel, S.M., *et al.* (1991) Pregnancy following spinal cord injury. *The Western Journal of Medicine*, **154** (5), 607–611.

Schopp, L.H., Clark, M., Mazurek, M.O., *et al.* (2006) Testosterone levels among men with spinal cord injury admitted to inpatient rehabilitation. *American Journal of Physical Medicine and Rehabilitation*, **85** (8), 678–684.

Skowronski, E. and Hartman, K. (2008) Obstetric management following traumatic tetraplegia: Case series and literature review. *Australian and New Zealand Journal of Obstetrics and Gynaecology*, **48** (5), 485–491.

**10** *A 29-year-old man is stabbed in the neck; during exploration you note an esophageal as well as a tracheal laceration. Which of the following is the most important principle during repair of these injuries?*

 **A** *Use of nonabsorbable sutures for tracheal repair*
 **B** *Use of two-layered closure of the esophageal repair*
 **C** *Avoidance of drains to prevent erosion into repairs*
 **D** *Interposition of healthy tissue between the esophageal and tracheal repairs*
 **E** *Positive identification of the recurrent laryngeal nerve to rule out injury*

Most tracheal injuries can be closed primarily using an absorbable suture in a single layer. Esophageal injuries should be explored to ensure the entire mucosal defect is addressed. Intraoperative esophagoscopy and insufflation of a nasogastric tube with air or dye can aid in the diagnosis of suspected esophageal injury. Once the injury has been identified it can be repaired in one or two layers with absorbable suture. If there has been significant delay in treatment, or severe tissue destruction, the repair can be protected with a T-tube; esophageal diversion can be performed with a cervical esophagostomy. With these more complex repairs, it is important to place a gastrostomy tube for decompression and a jejunostomy tube for enteral feeds in the postoperative period. All esophageal repairs should be buttressed with healthy tissue; this is of paramount importance if other suture lines are present (i.e. tracheal or vascular repairs). Buttressing can be done with one of the strap muscles or

the sternocleidomastoid (SCM). The SCM has excellent blood supply (thyrocervical trunk, superior thyroid artery, and occipital artery) and can be detached from either end with good results. Wide drainage of all neck explorations is highly recommended. Drains will help prevent hematoma formation, which can lead to acute airway obstruction and can aid in detecting a postoperative leak. Careful posterior approach to the esophagus will help prevent recurrent laryngeal nerve injury, but dissection specifically to identify the nerve is discouraged as it can actually increase the incidence of nerve injury.

**Answer: D**

Biffl, W. L., Moore, E. E., Feliciano, D. V., *et al.* (2015). Western Trauma Association critical decisions in trauma: diagnosis and management of esophageal injuries. *Journal of Trauma and Acute Care Surgery*, **79** (6), 1089–1095.

Britt, L.D. (2007) Penetrating neck trauma, in *Mastery of Surgery*, 5th edn (eds J.E. Fischer and K.I. Bland), Lippincott Williams & Wilkins, Philadelphia PA, pp. 381–386.

**11** *Which of the following statements regarding esophageal injury is the most correct?*

 **A** *Primary repair should be avoided in delayed (>24 hours) injuries*
 **B** *Trauma (penetrating or blunt) is the most common etiology of esophageal injury*
 **C** *Esophagoscopy is highly sensitive and specific for esophageal injury*
 **D** *Cervical injuries have a higher mortality than thoracic or abdominal injuries*
 **E** *Nonoperative management is a reasonable option for the stable patient with a contained perforation*

Despite classical thought, studies have disproven the need to avoid primary repair in injuries presenting more than 24 hours out. The decision to primarily close an injury is determined by the amount of healthy tissue than can be closed without tension. Iatrogenic perforation is by far the most common cause of esophageal injury; trauma accounts for only 5–10% of injuries. Traumatic esophageal perforations are ten times more common in penetrating versus blunt trauma. Esophagoscopy is widely utilized but may have false negative rates up to 25%. If endoscopic results are equivocal, esophagography should follow. Uncontained injuries in the thoracic and abdominal esophagus can freely contaminate the peritoneal, mediastinal, and thoracic cavities leading rapidly to sepsis and death. Mortality is higher in thoracic or abdominal esophageal perforations than cervical injuries. Nonoperative management is an acceptable strategy in select patients. Indications for nonoperative management include hemodynamic stability, contained perforation on imaging studies, absence of distal obstruction, cervical or thoracic location, and minimal systemic signs of infection. Medical management consists of NPO, antibiotics, proton pump inhibitors, and close observation for signs of deterioration. Follow up esophagography is commonly performed in 5–7 days to assess for healing.

**Answer: E**

Biffl, W. L., Moore, E. E., Feliciano, D. V., *et al.* (2015). Western Trauma Association critical decisions in trauma: diagnosis and management of esophageal injuries. *Journal of Trauma and Acute Care Surgery*, **79** (6), 1089–1095.

Wu, J.T., Mattox, K.L., and Wall, M.J. (2007) Esophageal perforations: New perspectives and treatment paradigms. *Journal of Trauma*, **63** (5), 1173–1184.

**12** *A 34-year-old patient with acute quadriplegia following a motor vehicle accident is hypotensive with a heart rate of 55 beats/min. Physical exam is unremarkable, FAST and diagnostic peritoneal lavageare negative. Pelvis and chest x-rays are unremarkable. Two liters of crystalloid are infused with no change in blood pressure. Which of the following is the most likely cause of hypotension?*
 **A** *Spinal shock*
 **B** *Neurogenic shock*
 **C** *Hypovolemic shock*
 **D** *Cardiogenic shock*
 **E** *Obstructive shock*

Hypotension in a trauma patient must be assumed to be hypovolemic shock secondary to blood loss until proven otherwise. In this case, all studies thus far are negative to that effect. Additionally, bradycardia and a negative fluid challenge make hemorrhagic shock less likely. Pneumothorax and tamponade have been ruled out and a massive pulmonary embolus causing obstructive shock is unlikely in this time frame. Cardiogenic shock is a possibility, but significant dysfunction would be unusual in the absence of other signs of thoracic trauma. Spinal shock is a neurologic phenomenon resulting in transient loss of spinal reflexes, and does not cause hypotension. Neurogenic shock occurs in approximately 20% of cervical spinal cord injuries. Loss of sympathetic tone below the level of the injury results in peripheral vasodilation resulting in systemic hypotension. In high cervical spine injuries unopposed vagal tone can also result in bradycardia and decreased cardiac output. Physical exam may reveal warmth and erythema below the level of the injury due to peripheral vasodilation. Patient should be monitored closely in an ICU setting. Treatment should be initiated quickly with fluid resuscitation to maintain mean arterial pressure between 85 and 90 for the first 7 days. Vasopressors and inotropes should be used judiciously to maintain vascular tone and cardiac output. Neurogenic shock generally resolves in 24–72 hours.

**Answer: B**

Guly, H.R., Bouamra, O., and Lecky, F.E. (2008) Trauma audit and research network. The incidence of neurogenic shock in patients with isolated spinal cord injury in the emergency department. *Resuscitation*, **76** (1), 57–62.

Ryken, T.C., Hurlbert, R.J., Hadley, M.N., *et al.* (2013). The acute cardiopulmonary management of patients with cervical spinal cord injuries. *Neurosurgery*, **72**, 84–92.

**13** *A patient requiring intubation for altered mental status has failed several attempts at tracheal intubation via laryngoscopy. What is the next course of action?*
 **A** *Percutaneous tracheostomy*
 **B** *Emergent cricothyrotomy*
 **C** *Supra-glottal airway*
 **D** *Continue attempting tracheal intubation*
 **E** *Percutaneous jet ventilation*

The goal in this situation is not to reach the point of "cannot intubate, cannot oxygenate" (CICO). Hypoxic brain injury occurs between 4 and 6 minutes of apnea and is irreversible after about 6 minutes. The first attempt should be for definitive tracheal access via laryngoscopy. Optimizing the patient's position, preoxygenating with 100% $O_2$ via face-mask, and using the principles of rapid sequence intubation will increase the chances of a successful intubation. Attempts at tracheal intubation should be limited to three or four passes with or without airway adjuncts. Repeated attempts even with experienced personnel are associated with worse outcomes and CICO scenarios. Supra-glottal airway devices (SAD) can buy time to make the next decision: attempt intubation through the device or secure a surgical airway. The laryngeal mask airway (LMA) allows for blind insertion of an endotracheal tube with a success rate of 96%. SADs should not be used in trauma patients with severe facial trauma, suspected airway injury, or external evidence of neck trauma as the point of airway obstruction may be above the glottis, in these cases the next step in management is to proceed immediately with surgical airway. If the patient is still not able to oxygenate, it is necessary to gain surgical access via open or cannula cricothyrotomy. Trans-tracheal jet ventilation (TTJV) is a life-saving maneuver that involves puncturing the cricothyroid membrane and leaving a catheter that can be connecting to high-flow, high concentration oxygen. It is primarily utilized for pediatric patients and is used solely as bridging maneuver to temporarily oxygenate the adult patient.

**Answer: C**

Frerk, C., Mitchell, V.S., McNarry, A.F., *et al.* (2015). Difficult Airway Society 2015 guidelines for management of unanticipated difficult intubation in adults. *British Journal of Anaesthesia*, **115** (6), 827–848.

Boccio, E., Gujral, R., Cassara, M., *et al.* (2015). Combining transtracheal catheter oxygenation and needle-based Seldinger cricothyrotomy into a single, sequential procedure. *American Journal of Emergency Medicine*, **33** (5), 708–712.

14 *A 37-year-old obese male is being evaluated in the Trauma Bay after receiving multiple stab wounds to Zone 2 of the neck. He is hemodynamically stable but complains of pain, dysphagia, and hematemesis. He is taken to the OR for operative exploration however it is difficult to adequately expose and visualize the cervical esophagus. What is the next course of action?*
   A *Adequately drain the area and terminate the operation*
   B *Terminate the operation and obtain a CT head/ neck*
   C *Perform intraoperative esophagoscopy and/or bronchoscopy*
   D *Terminate the operation and observe for worsening of symptoms*
   E *Arrange for endoscopic esophageal stent placement*

The patient has a symptomatic injury to Zone 2 without any hard signs of vascular injury but concerning symptoms for aerodigestive injury. If he was asymptomatic it would be reasonable to admit, observe, and perform serial exams with or without screening CTA. This patient was appropriately explored given his symptoms. Body habitus, radiation, or previous neck surgery may limit intraoperative exposure of the vital structures. Drainage is an important tenant in the repair of esophageal injuries however this patient still requires workup of his suspected injuries. It is reasonable in this situation to procced with on-table esophagoscopy and/or bronchoscopy as clinically indicated. There is increasing evidence that endoscopic stenting is an acceptable option in stable patients with small perforations, however these small case series are limited to iatrogenic or spontaneous (nontraumatic) perforations in the thoracic esophagus, and would not be indicated in this patient where surgical repair could immediately address any injuries identified by esophagoscopy.

**Answer: C**

Biffl, W. L., Moore, E. E., Feliciano, D. V., *et al.* (2015). Western Trauma Association critical decisions in trauma: diagnosis and management of esophageal injuries. *Journal of Trauma and Acute Care Surgery*, **79** (6), 1089–1095.

Sperry, J.L., Moore, E.E., Coimbra, R., *et al.* (2013) Western Trauma Association critical decisions in trauma: penetrating neck trauma. *Journal of Trauma and Acute Care Surgery*, **75** (6), 936–940.

15 *Which of the following maneuvers can decrease the risk of tracheo-innominate fistula?*
   A *Use of stoma sites no lower than the fourth tracheal ring*
   B *Use of open technique*
   C *Use of percutaneous technique*
   D *Use of bronchoscopy*
   E *Use of high pressure, low volume cuff on the tracheostomy tube*

Tracheo-innominate fistula (TIF) is a rare but devastating complication following tracheostomy. It occurs in less than 1% of cases, with a peak incidence in the first 1–2 weeks. The associated mortality rate is as high as 90%. Risk factors include low placement of the stoma, high-riding innominate artery, overinflated cuffs, and older high-pressure, low-volume cuffs. Preventative measures include avoidance of placing the stoma below the fourth tracheal ring, avoidance of neck hyper-extension, maintenance of cuff pressures below 20 mm Hg, and early decannulation. Initial management is to secure an airway, and apply pressure to the bleeding by overinflating the cuff, pulling up on the tracheostomy tube, and direct pressure or packing through the stoma site. Definitive treatment consists of resection of the fistula and ligation or interposition graft of the innominate artery. There is currently no evidence that either open or percutaneous tracheostomy is superior with regard to avoiding TIF. The literature to date on percutaneous tracheostomy reveals few case reports and a single case series consisting of three patients. The single series reported a rate of TIF of 0.3% is comparable to historical rates with open tracheostomy.

**Answer: A**

Grant, C.A., Dempsey, G., Harrison, J., *et al.* (2006) Tracheo-innominate artery fistula after percutaneous tracheostomy: three case reports and a clinical review. *British Journal of Anaesthesia*, **6**, 127–231.

Jamal-Eddine, H., Ayed, A.K., Al-Moosa, A., *et al.* (2008) Graft repair of trachea-innominate artery fistula following percutaneous tracheostomy. *Interactive Cardiovascular and Thoracic Surgery*, 7(4), 654–655.

**16** *A 19-year-old man dives headfirst into a pool, after which he has severe neck pain and presents to the ER. He is neurologically intact. CT scan of his cervical spine is shown in Figure 29.3. What is the most likely diagnosis?*

**A** *Hangman's fracture*
**B** *Jefferson fracture*
**C** *Spinal cord injury without radiologic abnormality (SCIWORA)*
**D** *Atlanto-occipital dissociation (Internal decapitation)*
**E** *Chance fracture*

Spinal cord injury without radiologic abnormality is primarily described in pediatric patients, but has been reported in adults. It is associated with flexion/extension and distraction. CT scans are normal and MRI may find disc herniation or ligamentous injury. Atlanto-occipital dissociation is a rare and frequently fatal injury following violent hyperflexion/hyperextension. It is most common after motor vehicle or auto-pedestrian accidents, and occurs when ligamentous disruption between the skull and spine allows distraction between the skull and C1. The hangman's fracture occurs when violent hyperextension combined with distraction results in fracture of both pedicles of C2. Chance fractures occur when hyperflexion around an axis point anterior to the spine results in compression of the anterior vertebral body with a transverse fracture through the posterior vertebral elements. Jefferson fracture occurs when significant axial load results in compression fracture of the bilateral anterior and posterior arches of C1. The classical pattern has four fractures, however it may also present with two or three fractures. Patients complain of neck pain, but are usually neurologically intact. Treatment is stabilization with HALO, collar, or surgery.

**Answer: B**

Jefferson, G. (1919) Fracture of the atlas vertebra. Report of four cases, and a review of those previously recorded. *British Journal of Surgery*, **7** (27), 407–422.
Yucesoy, K. and Yuksel, K.Z. (2008) SCIWORA in MRI era. *Clinical Neurology and Neurosurgery*, **10**, 429–433.

**17** *A 58-year-old male presented to the trauma center after being struck on his left face with a metal baseball bat. Primary survey is unremarkable. Secondary survey reveals only a swollen left face. CT reveals a right sided C2 pedicle and lamina fracture with transverse foramen involvement (Figure 29.4). Subsequent angiography confirmed a short segment vertebral artery thrombus. What is the most appropriate management of this patient's arterial injury?*

**A** *Arterial angiography and stent placement followed by dual-antiplatelet therapy*
**B** *Antiplatelet therapy, repeat angiography next day*

**Figure 29.3** Axial CT scan of a Jefferson fracture with bilateral anterior and posterior ring disruption.

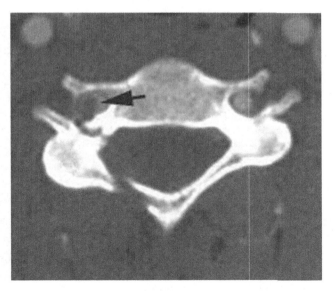

**Figure 29.4** Axial CT scan of C2 vertebrae with right pedicle and lamina fractures (image courtesy of Radiology Key, used by permission).

**C** *Anticoagulation, repeat angiography in 7 days*
**D** *Catheter-directed thrombolysis*
**E** *Thrombectomy with patch angioplasty*

Traumatic injury to the vertebral artery is diagnosed in 0.1% of patients hospitalized for trauma. It is the result of cervical hyperextension, hyperflexion, rotation, or by direct blow. There is a strong association between vertebral artery injuries and C2 fractures (nearly 20%). The Biffl injury scale was proposed in 1999 to organize management-based severity of injury (see question 4). Grade 1 and 2 injuries should be treated with antithrombotic agents if there are no contraindications. Administration of these agents is associated with decreased morbidity and mortality following BCVI. Retrospective studies have failed to show a difference between anticoagulation and antiplatelet therapy. The current evidence recommends heparin (without bolus) and reserves antiplatelet therapy for poor anticoagulation candidates (Level III evidence). The patient should be converted to warfarin for 3 to 6 months with a goal INR between 2 and 3. Followup angiography is recommended after 7 days as management will change in up to 60% of grade 1 and 2 injuries, however injuries are unlikely to be significantly changed within 24 hours. Stent placement is reserved for grade 3 pseudoaneurysm, but has been associated with poor outcomes in previous studies. Surgical approaches to vertebral artery injuries are particularly difficult due to their protected location within the bony vascular canal and as most grade 1 and 2 injuries respond well to antithrombotic treatment complex surgical approaches should be reserved for grade 4 injuries with active hemorrhage.

**Answer: C**

Bromberg, W.J., Collier, B.C., Diebel, L.N., *et al.* (2010). Blunt cerebrovascular injury practice management guidelines: the Eastern Association for the Surgery of Trauma. *Journal of Trauma and Acute Care Surgery*, **68** (2), 471–477.

Ding, T., Maltenfort, M., Yang, H., *et al.* (2010). Correlation of C2 fractures and vertebral artery injury. *Spine*, **35** (12), E520–E524.

**18** *What is true regarding an awake, alert trauma patient without midline cervical tenderness, neurological deficit, or distracting injuries?*
  **A** *Flexion/extension plain films are necessary prior to cervical spine clearance*
  **B** *CT is required in order to clear this patient*
  **C** *CT is not required, but the patient should be evaluated for ligamentous injury by MRI*

**D** *Cervical collar may be safely removed based on the information above*
**E** *Three-view plain film radiographs should be obtained*

Despite the clear transition from plain film radiography to axial CT, controversy still exists regarding the timing of cervical spine clearance. Several clinical studies have shown clear benefits with early cervical collar removal to include less skin breakdown, decreased intracranial pressure after removal, fewer days on mechanical ventilation, and shorter ICU and hospital stays. The recommendation is to remove a cervical collar as soon as clinically feasible, preferably within 24 hours of arrival. The two most commonly used protocols for cervical spine clearance are the NEXUS and Canadian C-spine criteria. NEXUS (National Emergency X-radiography Utilization Study) criteria published in 1992 is a decision-making instrument that requires patients be awake, alert, not intoxicated, have no focal neurological deficit, be free of painful distracting injury, and have no midline cervical spinal tenderness. The validation study boasted a sensitivity of 99%. The Canadian criteria require that patients be greater than 65-years-old, have no numbness or tingling in the extremities, and have a low risk mechanism of injury. They can be cleared if they are pain free and able to rotate their neck 45 degrees left and right. Nonmidline pain, pain that did not limit rotational range of motion, and late-onset pain were not contraindications to clearance. An independent analysis published in the NEJM found the Canadian criteria to be slightly superior in both sensitivity and specificity. With the patient in question, it would be appropriate to clear cervical spine based on clinical exam alone. If there was any suspicion of injury based on the criteria above, the next step would an axial CT with sagittal and coronal reconstructions. In a symptomatic patient with a negative CT scan, it would be reasonable to proceed with MRI to evaluate for ligamentous injury, however MRI is not indicated in the asymptomatic intact patient who meets clinical clearance criteria, or who has had a negative CT scan. Plain film radiography (three view and dynamic flexion/extension) offers no additional information and is inferior to CT and MRI at detecting bony and ligamentous injury. Dynamic flexion/extension imaging also risks patient discomfort as well as additional injury during imaging, and in many centers physician experience with both performing and reading such images is poor.

**Answer: D**

Como, J.J., Diaz, J.J., Dunham, C.M., *et al.* (2009). Practice management guidelines for identification of cervical spine injuries following trauma: update from the Eastern

Association for the Surgery of Trauma Practice Management Guidelines Committee. *Journal of Trauma and Acute Care Surgery*, **67** (3), 651–659.

Stiell, I.G., Clement, C.M., McKnight, R.D., *et al.* (2003). The Canadian C-spine rule versus the NEXUS low-risk criteria in patients with trauma. *New England Journal of Medicine*, **349** (26), 2510–2518.

19 *A patient in a snowmobile accident suffers a "clothesline" injury with a laceration just above the sternal notch, a moderate hematoma, and subcutaneous emphysema. He is unable to lay flat and has a muffled voice. The first priority in management of this patient is:*
   A *Maintenance of cervical spine precautions*
   B *Cricothryoidotomy*
   C *Bronchoscopy*
   D *Intubation*
   E *Operative exploration*

This patient has signs of tracheal injury in a location below the cricoid. Given the respiratory distress, airway management is the first priority. This is best accomplished with orotracheal intubation if possible. Orotracheal intubation will allow bronchoscopic evaluation to localize injury and prevent further trauma to the trachea, which is important if complex reconstruction is required. However, endotracheal intubation is likely to be challenging and should be performed in the operating room so that conversion to open surgical tracheostomy can be performed with sterility and proper equipment and lighting. Cricothyroidotomy is likely to be above the level of the injury in this patient and unlikely to result in a satisfactory airway. It is important to maintain cervical spine precautions until injury can be excluded, but workup should not interfere with diagnosis and treatment of injuries to the airway and vasculature. These patients rarely have an unstable cervical spine injury in the absence of neurologic deficits. While maintaining cervical spine precautions is ideal do not let this hinder in the real priority, which is to obtain an airway. Bronchoscopy is not needed initially and is time consuming on a patient that needs definitive airway soon. Operative exploration is required but needs general anesthesia which means definitive airway management. RSI is the best choice.

**Answer: D**

Gale, S.C. and Mattox, K.L. (2009) Trauma to the head, face, and neck, in *Acute Care Surgery: A Guide for General Surgeons* (eds V.H. Gracias, P.M. Reilly, M.G. McKenney, and G.C. Velmahos), McGraw-Hill, New York, pp. 99–108.

Randall, D.R., Rudmik, L.R., Ball, C.G., and Bosch, JD. (2014) External laryngotracheal trauma: Incidence, airway control, and outcomes in a large Canadian center. *Laryngoscope*, **124** (4), E123–133.

20 *Which one of the following is NOT a preferred emergency airway in a pediatric patient?*
   A *Open cricothyroidotomy*
   B *Needle cricothyroidotomy*
   C *Open tracheostomy*
   D *Supra-glottic airway*
   E *Direct laryngoscopy with endotracheal intubation*

Airway emergencies in pediatric patients are rare but lethal situations. The first attempt to secure the airway should be performed by the most senior operator under optimal conditions and can include advanced airway adjuncts such as bougies, fiberoptic or rigid bronchoscopes, and supra-glottic devices such as laryngeal mask airways (LMAs). The preferred surgical airway is open emergent tracheotomy. Cricothyroidotomy is not recommended for patients under 8 years of age as this is the narrowest portion of the pediatric airway and associated rates of sub-glottic stenosis are high. Instead, a percutaneous catheter or needle cricothyroidotomy and jet insufflation can be used to temporarily oxygenate the patient. Ventilation is necessarily restricted and carbon dioxide levels will predictably rise over time. Conversion to an open tracheostomy or repeated attempt at intubation with advanced airway adjuncts or more experienced personnel should be performed rapidly to prevent accumulation of carbon dioxide.

**Answer: A**

Chatterjee, D., Agarwal, R., Bajaj, L., *et al.* (2016) Airway management in laryngotracheal injuries from blunt neck trauma in children. *Pediatric Anesthesia*, **26** (2), 132–138.

Sabato, S.C. and Long, E. (2016) An institutional approach to the management of the "Can't Intubate, Can't Oxygenate" emergency in children. *Pediatric Anesthesia*, **26** (8), 784–793.

# 30

# Cardiothoracic and Thoracic Vascular Injury

*Leslie Kobayashi, MD and Amelia Simpson, MD*

**1** *Which of the following statements regarding traumatic diaphragmatic hernia (TDH) is true?*
**A** *TDH is more common on the right than the left*
**B** *Left-sided TDHs are associated with a more significant mechanism of injury than the right*
**C** *TDHs due to blunt trauma are smaller than those due to penetrating trauma*
**D** *TDHs are rarely found in association with other injuries*
**E** *TDHs can present in a delayed fashion, months to years after the initial trauma*

A traumatic diaphragmatic hernia occurs as a result of high-energy acceleration–deceleration trauma, or as a direct laceration from a weapon or broken rib. Blunt injuries tend to be large avulsions, while penetrating injuries tend to be smaller lacerations. Injuries can grow over time as viscera migrate into the thoracic cavity due to the normal pressure gradient across the diaphragm. A traumatic diaphragmatic hernia is associated with other injuries in 52–100% of cases. Left-sided injuries are more common accounting for 70% of cases. This is likely due to several factors: the posterolateral aspect of the diaphragm is structurally weak on the left, the right diaphragm is protected by the liver, and it is more difficult to diagnose injuries on the right side. However, right-sided ruptures are associated with more severe injuries and a more severe mechanism. Delay in diagnosis occurs in 30–50% of cases and the delay can range from 7 days to 40 years (average 3–7 years). Mortality ranges from 1–28%, primarily related to associated injuries.

**Answer: E**

Clarke, D.L., Greatorex, G.V., and Muckart, D.J. (2009) The spectrum of diaphragmatic injury in a busy metropolitan surgical service. *Injury*, **40**, 932–937.

Fair, K.A., Gordon, N.T., Barbosa, R.R., *et al.* (2015) Traumatic diaphragmatic injury in the American College of Surgeons National Trauma Data Bank: a new examination of a rare diagnosis. *American Journal of Surgery*, **209**, 864–869.

**2** *In a patient sustaining a stab wound to the left parasternal area, which of the following is the most appropriate way to diagnose cardiac tamponade?*
**A** *Chest x-ray*
**B** *Pulses paradoxus*
**C** *FAST (Focused Assessment with Sonography for Trauma)*
**D** *Friction rub*
**E** *Computed tomography (CT) scan*

The majority of penetrating cardiac injuries are fatal with most, between 60% and 80%, dying at the scene. Overall survival is reported between 19% and 73%. Rapid diagnosis is paramount. Tamponade should be a clinical diagnosis, and a high level of suspicion must be maintained in any penetrating trauma to the parasternal area. The classic (Beck) triad of hypotension, muffled heart sounds, and distended neck veins are often missed in the trauma patient because of the noisy ER setting, and concomitant hypovolemia. Pulsus paradoxus, decreased blood pressure with inspiration, can be difficult to appreciate without the benefit of an arterial tracing, and is present in only 10% of cases. A friction rub is more common with pericarditis than tamponade. A globular heart can be seen on chest x-ray but is neither sensitive nor specific for tamponade. CT scan may reveal pericardial fluid, but should not be performed on patients with suspicion of penetrating cardiac injury. If there is a clinical concern, careful physical exam and FAST should be used to confirm the diagnosis. FAST is rapid, immediately

*Surgical Critical Care and Emergency Surgery: Clinical Questions and Answers*, Second Edition.
Edited by Forrest "Dell" Moore, Peter Rhee, and Gerard J. Fulda.
© 2018 John Wiley & Sons Ltd. Published 2018 by John Wiley & Sons Ltd.
Companion website: www.wiley.com/go/moore/surgical_criticalcare_and_emergency_surgery

available, repeatable, and has a sensitivity nearing 100% in most series.

**Answer: C**

Morse, B.M., Mina, M.J., Carr, J.S., *et al.* (2016) Penetrating cardiac injuries: A 36-year perspective at an urban, Level 1 trauma center. *Journal of Trauma and Acute Care Surgery*, **81** (4), 623–631.

Rozycki, G.S., Feliciano, D.V., Ochsner, M.G., *et al.* (1999) The role of ultrasound in patients with possible penetrating cardiac wounds: a prospective multicenter study. *Journal of Trauma*, **46** (4), 543–552.

3 *In a patient with multiple rib fractures resulting in flail chest which of the following statement is true?*
   A *The majority of patients do not require mechanical ventilation*
   B *Mechanical ventilation is associated with improved mortality*
   C *Age greater than 45 is associated with improved outcome*
   D *PCA is superior to epidural anesthesia*
   E *Mortality is directly related to the flail injury in most patients*

Flail chest occurs when three or more adjacent ribs are fractured in two or more locations, resulting in a segment of chest wall than can move independently. This will result in paradoxical motion of the flail segment with negative pressure respiration. The majority of patients do not require mechanical ventilation. When necessary, mechanical ventilation is associated with worse prognosis and a variety of complications. Pain control and pulmonary toilet are essential in preventing complications associated with flail chest. Several studies have demonstrated the superiority of epidural anesthesia for pain control, prevention of pneumonia, and decreased need for mechanical ventilation. A greater number of rib fractures, development of pneumonia and increasing age are associated with worsened outcomes. Some studies suggesting that ages as low as 45 are associated with increased complications and mortality. When mortality does occur, it is most often due to associated injuries.

**Answer: A**

Battle, C.E., Hutchings, H., and Evans, P.A. (2012) Risk factors that predict mortality in patients with blunt chest wall trauma: A systematic review and meta-analysis. *Injury*, **43** (1), 8–17.

Bulger, E.M., Klotz, P., and Jurkovich, G.J. (2004) Epidural anesthesia improves outcomes after multiple rib fractures. *Surgery*, **136** (2), 426–430.

4 *Hypoxia in flail chest is due to:*
   A *Increased shunt from pulmonary contusion*
   B *Paradoxical chest wall movement*
   C *Change in alveolar diffusion*
   D *Associated hemothorax*
   E *Associated pneumothorax*

Many physiologic changes occur with a flail chest, the paradoxical motion can decrease total lung capacity and functional residual capacity, pain associated with rib fractures can result in splinting and atelectasis, and most importantly the associated lung contusion can lead to ventilation/perfusion mismatch. There is a complex interplay of these pulmonary mechanics that ultimately culminates in increased shunt fraction resulting in hypoxia. Management entails selective mechanical ventilation, multimodal analgesia, and chest physiotherapy. While the mechanical injury to the chest wall undoubtedly contributes to respiratory morbidity, the underlying pulmonary contusion is by far the most important determinant of respiratory status.

**Answer: A**

Athanassiadi, K., Theakos, N., Kalantzi N., *et al.* (2010) Prognostic factors in flail-chest patients. *European Journal of Cardiothoracic Surgery*, **38** (4) 366.

Simon B., Ebert J., Bokhari F., *et al.* (2012) Management of pulmonary contusion and flail chest: An Eastern Association for the Surgery of Trauma practice management guideline. *Journal of Trauma and Acute Care Surgery*, **73** (5), S341–S361.

5 *A chest tube is placed in a 43-year-old woman after a transmediastinal gunshot wound, bloody drainage was minimal, and she is hemodynamically stable. However, you note a continuous air leak. What is the next step in management?*
   A *Place a second chest tube*
   B *Thoracotomy*
   C *Video-assisted thoracoscopic surgery (VATS)*
   D *Bronchoscopy*
   E *Increase the amount of suction on the chest tube*

Air leaks following trauma are common, they may be due to injury of the airways or lung parenchyma, to leaks in the drainage system or from chest wall defects, or as a result of intraparenchymal placement of the chest tube. The presence of a large or continuous air leak immediately after injury may indicate tracheobronchial injury and should be investigated with bronchoscopy. Persistent leaks should also be investigated with bronchoscopy. Proximal tracheobronchial injury should be addressed surgically, and bronchoscopy will aid in diagnosis, as well as localization for preoperative planning. Smaller distal air leaks will generally seal without intervention and rarely require more than tube thoracostomy drainage. If mechanical ventilation is required care should be taken to minimize airway pressures while maintaining oxygenation. Paradoxically, increased suction on the drainage system may keep air leaks open, and as long as the pneumothorax is adequately drained decreasing suction or water sealing the thoracostomy tube may promote sealing.

**Answer: D**

Karmy-Jones, R. and Wood, D.E. (2007) Traumatic injury to the trachea and bronchus. *Thoracic Surgery Clinics*, **17** (1), 35–46.

Livingston, D.H., and Hauser, C.J. (2008) Chest wall and lung, in *Trauma*, 6th edn, (eds, D.V. Feliciano, K.L. Mattox and E.E. Moore), McGraw-Hill, New York, pp. 525–552.

6   With regards to a diaphragmatic injury following penetrating trauma, which of the following exams has the highest sensitivity?
   **A** *CT scan*
   **B** *Magnetic resonance imaging (MRI)*
   **C** *Laparoscopy*
   **D** *Diagnostic peritoneal lavage*
   **E** *Fluoroscopy*

Diaphragmatic injury may complicate as many as 26% of stab and 13% of gunshot wounds. Any patient with penetrating trauma to the area bounded by the nipples superiorly and costal margin inferiorly should be suspected of having a diaphragmatic injury. Injuries are often asymptomatic, and radiographic imaging continues to have poor sensitivity and specificity. A chest x-ray may be normal or nonspecific in up to 50% of cases and sensitivity for CT scan ranges from 14% to 61%. MRI and diagnostic peritoneal lavage have poor sensitivity especially after penetrating trauma. Laparoscopy is the most effective means of both diagnosis and treatment of diaphragmatic injury after penetrating trauma. Sensitivity and negative predictive value are 87.5% and 96.8% respectively.

**Answer: C**

Friese, R.S., Coln, C.E., and Gentilello, L.M. (2005) Laparoscopy is sufficient to exclude occult diaphragm injury after penetrating abdominal trauma. *Journal of Trauma*, **58**, 789–792.

Powell, B.S., Magnotti, L.J., Schroeppel, T.J., *et al.* (2008) Diagnostic laparoscopy for the evaluation of occult diaphragmatic injury following penetrating thoracoabdominal trauma. *Injury*, **39** (5), 530–534.

7   Two days after repair of a stab wound to the heart a patient develops large V waves on the pulmonary artery catheter tracing, which of the following is the most likely explanation?
   **A** *Mitral valve tenea cordae disruption*
   **B** *Post-operative pericarditis*
   **C** *Acute myocardial infarction*
   **D** *Left atrial thrombus*
   **E** *Pulmonary embolus*

Early diastolic pressure waves, or V waves, can be seen with mitral regurgitation and papillary muscle dysfunction. Penetrating cardiac injuries may lacerate or damage both valve leaflets and papillary muscles. Additionally, these internal cardiac injuries may be missed at the time of operation, and are often asymptomatic. In a series of 711 cardiac injuries, valvular injuries were identified in 2.5% of patients. The true incidence is likely higher, but unrecognized because they occur in nonsurvivors and patients without follow-up echocardiography and are not clinically significant. Posttraumatic valvular and papillary muscle injuries generally do not require intervention, but if hemodynamically significant can be repaired electively with valvuloplasty or replacement.

**Answer: A**

Iaizzo, P.A. (2015) *Handbook of Cardiac Anatomy, Physiology, and Devices*, 3rd edn. Springer, New York.

Tang, A., Inaba, K., Branco, B.C., *et al.* (2011) Postdischarge complications after penetrating cardiac injury: a survivable injury with a high postdischarge complication rate. *Journal of the American Medical Association Surgery*, **146** (9), 1061–1066.

8   Which of the following statements regarding subclavian artery injuries is true?
   **A** *Injuries are more common after blunt trauma*
   **B** *Injuries are associated with low overall mortality*
   **C** *There is a concomitant venous injury in approximately 20% of cases*
   **D** *Arterial injury is associated with significantly worse outcome compared to venous injury*
   **E** *Associated neurologic or thoracic injuries are rare affecting <5% of cases*

Subclavian artery injuries are rare and affect less than 3% of all penetrating traumas. Injuries associated with blunt trauma are even more uncommon affecting only 0.4% of patients. These injuries are highly lethal with up to 60% of patients expiring before, or upon presentation to, the hospital. Because of the close association of vital structures in this area, associated injuries are common. Concomitant brachial plexus injuries can affect up to one-third of patients with axillary or subclavian artery injuries, and intrathoracic injuries up to 28%. Concomitant venous injury is seen in 20% of cases, and isolated venous injury is associated with a higher mortality when compared to isolated arterial injury. There may be many reasons for the increased mortality among victims of venous injury including; the inability of the vein to constrict, resulting in increased hemorrhage and air embolus in venous injuries, especially in the hypotensive patient with low intravenous pressure.

**Answer: C**

Sobnach, S., Nicol, A.J., Nathire, H., *et al.* (2010) An analysis of 50 surgically managed penetrating subclavian artery injuries. *European Journal of Vascular and Endovascular Surgery*, **39** (2), 155–159.

Weinberg, J.A., Moore, A.H., Magnotti, L.J., *et al.* (2016) Contemporary management of civilian penetrating cervicothoracic arterial injuries. *Journal of Trauma and Acute Care Surgery*, **81** (2), 303–306.

**9** *Of the following, which is an acceptable management option for a subclavian artery injury?*
   **A** *PTFE or vein interposition graft*
   **B** *Ligation*
   **C** *Placement of a temporary shunt*
   **D** *Angiography and covered stent placement*
   **E** *All of the above*

In repairing subclavian injuries, the operative approach is dictated by the clinical presentation of the patient. Those *in extremis* or in arrest should undergo resuscitative thoracotomy; those who are more stable may undergo median sternotomy with infraclavicular excision for proximal injuries and infraclavicular incision alone for more distal injuries. In unstable patients, ligation can be considered because of the rich collateral blood supply. However, it comes with a significant risk of compartment syndrome and ischemia. The preferred damage-control technique should be temporary arterial shunting. In the stable patient primary repair can be considered in lacerations as a result of stab wounds. However, in most gunshot injuries and in the rare blunt injury tissue loss makes this unfeasible as this vessel has very little mobility and can be very friable. Any existing defect should be bridged with an interposition graft. There is no evidence to suggest the superiority of autologous or artificial graft material and the choice of material should depend on surgeon preference, availability, and condition of the patient. There is growing experience with covered stents for treatment of subclavian artery injuries, primarily pseudoaneurysms, and arteriovenous fistulas. This option should only be used in those patients who present in hemodynamically stable condition with minimal chest tube output.

**Answer: E**

Branco, B.C., Boutrous, M.L., DuBose, J.J., *et al.* (2016) Outcome comparison between open and endovascular management of axillosubclavian arterial injuries. *Journal of Vascular Surgery*, **63** (3), 702–709.

Demetriades, D. and Asensio, J.A. (2001) Subclavian and axillary vascular injuries. *Surgical Clinics of North America*, **81** (6), 1357–1373.

**10** *Which of the following statements regarding the evaluation of a periclavicular gunshot wound is false?*
   **A** *Complete neurologic exam including cranial nerves should be performed in the stable patient*
   **B** *Hemodynamically unstable patients should be explored in the OR immediately*
   **C** *A normal Ankle-Brachial index definitively rules out arterial injury*
   **D** *Traditional angiography can be both diagnostic and therapeutic*
   **E** *CT angiography is an acceptable screening modality in stable patients*

Hemodynamic instability is a hard sign of vascular injury in penetrating trauma and should undergo immediate exploration. Although indications for angiography for both diagnosis and treatment continue to expand hemodynamic instability, critical limb ischemia, and active hemorrhage remain contraindications. In stable patients lacking hard signs of vascular injury physical examination should include a complete neurologic examination of the affected upper extremity as well as cranial nerve examination as there is a high rate of associated injuries to the brachial plexus, sympathetic chain, and cervical nerve roots. Additionally, the Ankle-Brachial Index (ABI) can be performed in stable patients, if the ratio is less than 0.9 further imaging should be performed. Unfortunately, the presence of a normal ABI (>0.9) cannot be relied upon to definitively rule out arterial injury as injuries such as pseudoaneurysm, arterio-venous fistula, and intimal flap may be present with a normal ABI. In all stable patients with suspicion of injury, CT angiography is a viable screening modality. CT angiography has the benefit of speed, ease, and a low rate of complications. It can be performed without an arterial puncture and does not require the presence of an interventional radiology team. It can also be performed with significantly less contrast than traditional angiography and has the benefit of giving additional information on nonvascular structures such as the spine, soft tissues, lungs, and aerodigestive tract.

**Answer: C**

Franz, R.W., Skytta, C.K., Shah, K.J., *et al.* (2012) A five-year review of management of upper-extremity arterial injuries at an urban level 1 trauma center. *Annals of Vascular Surgery*, **26** (5), 655–664.

Seamon, M.J., Smoger, D., Torres, D.M., *et al.* (2009) A prospective validation of a current practice: the detection of extremity vascular injury with CT angiography. *Journal of Trauma*, **67** (2), 238–243.

**11** *Which of the following is an indication for urgent/emergent thoracotomy?*
  **A** *Bloody output from the thoracostomy tube after penetrating trauma*
  **B** *Bloody output from the thoracostomy tube after blunt trauma*
  **C** *Intermittent air leak from the thoracostomy tube*
  **D** *Immediate output of 500 mL of blood from the thoracostomy tube*
  **E** *Immediate output of 2000 mL of blood from the thoracostomy tube*

Indications for thoracotomy following chest trauma, either penetrating or blunt, include thoracic hemorrhage with hypotension, thoracostomy tube output greater than 1500 mL at initial insertion or greater than 250 mL per hour for 3 hours, and unresolved hemothorax with the placement of two intrathoracic chest tubes. Additionally, evidence of major tracheobronchial injuries such as a large continuous air leak or persistent pneumothorax despite adequately placed chest tubes is also an indication for thoracotomy. Immediate thoracotomy, including resuscitative thoracotomy for traumatic arrest, historically was reported to be required in 20–30% of cases. However, most modern trauma series show the need for urgent thoracotomy ranging from 0.5–9%, with a large series including 43,119 patients revealing a 0.5% rate among blunt, and a 2.8% rate among penetrating patients. The need for thoracotomy is higher among penetrating compared to blunt trauma and in military compared to civilian trauma.

**Answer: E**

Loogna, P., Bonanno, F., Bowley, D.M., *et al.* (2007) Emergency thoracic surgery for penetrating, non-mediastinal trauma. *ANZ Journal of Surgery*, **77**, 142–145.

Onat, S., Ulku, R., Avci, A., *et al.* (2011) Urgent thoracotomy for penetrating chest trauma: analysis of 158 patients of a single center. *Injury*, **42** (9), 900–904.

**12** *In penetrating cardiac trauma, injury to which chamber of the heart is associated with the best chance of survival?*
  **A** *Left ventricle*
  **B** *Right ventricle*
  **C** *Left atrium*
  **D** *Right atrium*
  **E** *Intrapericardial aorta*

In penetrating cardiac injuries, there are several favorable prognostic indicators. Stab wounds have a better outcome than gunshot wounds, with mortality ranging from 14–16% compared to 65–81% respectively. Right heart injuries have a better outcome than left-sided injuries presumably due to lower pressures in the right heart, and ventricular injuries have a better prognosis than atrial injuries likely due to the thicker myocardium. The injury with the worst prognosis is the intrapericardial aorta, likely due to the very high pressure and thin wall. The presence of vital signs or cardiac tamponade upon arrival has also been associated with improved survival.

**Answer: B**

Morse, B.M., Mina, M.J., Carr, J.S., *et al.* (2016) Penetrating cardiac injuries: A 36-year perspective at an urban, Level 1 trauma center. *Journal of Trauma and Acute Care Surgery*, **81** (4), 623–631.

Tyburski, J.G., Astra, L., Wilson, R.F., *et al.* (2000) Factors affecting prognosis with penetrating wounds of the heart. *Journal of Trauma*, **48** (4), 587–590.

**13** *Regarding the repair of a cardiac laceration, which of the following is true?*
  **A** *Thoracotomy is preferred over median sternotomy in stable patients*
  **B** *Closure of the pericardium is always recommended*
  **C** *When closing the pericardium, it is important not to leave any defects*
  **D** *Failure to close the pericardium will result in increased postoperative complications*
  **E** *There is generally less postoperative pain and fewer complications after median sternotomy than thoracotomy*

Unstable patients should undergo resuscitative thoracotomy. Patients with suspected cardiac injuries who are stable should be transferred to the operating room immediately. A median sternotomy is the incision of choice because it does not require special positioning, is fast, provides good exposure to the heart, and is associated with less postoperative pain and fewer pulmonary complications than a thoracotomy. Following repair the pericardium is closed, leaving an opening near the base to avoid tamponade in cases of rebleeding. However, acute cardiomegaly may develop due to heart failure or massive fluid resuscitation in many cases, and in these cases, the pericardium should be left open. There does not appear to be any increase in complication rates when the pericardium is left open.

**Answer: E**

Kang, N., Hsee, L., Rizoli, S., *et al.* (2009) Penetrating cardiac injury: Overcoming limits set nature. *Injury,* **40** (9), 919–927.

Morse, B.M., Mina, M.J., Carr, J.S., *et al.* (2016) Penetrating cardiac injuries: A 36-year perspective at an urban, Level 1 trauma center. *Journal of Trauma and Acute Care Surgery,* **81** (4), 623–631.

**14** *Which of the following is an acceptable screening tool for blunt cardiac injury (BCI)?*
   **A** *Trans-esophageal echocardiogram*
   **B** *Trans-thoracic echocardiogram*
   **C** *24-hour Holter monitor*
   **D** *Dobutamine stress test*
   **E** *ECG*

The reported incidence of BCI varies widely from 8–71% due primarily to the wide spectrum of disease, which ranges from mild asymptomatic contusion to free wall rupture. The at-risk population is also broad and includes anyone who has sustained blunt chest trauma. In the hemodynamically stable patient with suspicion of BCI ECG is recommended on admission. If this is normal, there is little risk of BCI. However, sensitivity is not 100%, and, if abnormal, the chance of clinically significant BCI is still quite low. Several studies have demonstrated the utility of troponin-I (Tn-I) as a biomarker of traumatic myocardial injury. However, elevations in Tn-I can occur after both penetrating and blunt trauma in the absence of cardiac injury. To identify patients at highest risk of clinically significant BCI, it is best to combine both ECG and Tn-I. The sensitivity and specificity of Tn-I and ECG, when combined, are 100% and 71% respectively.

**Answer: E**

Clancy, K., Velopulos, C., Bilaniku, J.W., *et al.* (2012) Screening for blunt cardiac injury: an Eastern Association for the Surgery of Trauma practice management guideline. *Journal of Trauma and Acute Care Surgery,* **73** (5 Suppl 4), S301–S306.

Joseph, B., Jokar,T.O., Khalil, M., *et al.* (2016) Identifying the broken heart: predictors of mortality and morbidity in suspected blunt cardiac injury. *American Journal of Surgery,* **211** (6), 982–988.

**15** *Following blunt trauma, the chest x-ray of a patient reveals a wide mediastinum. Which of the following must be excluded?*
   **A** *Thymoma*
   **B** *Thoracic spine fracture*
   **C** *Lymphoma*
   **D** *Teratoma*
   **E** *Mediastinal thyroid gland*

A widened mediastinum can be a result of patient body habitus, positioning, and a variety of pathologies including mediastinal masses. However, in the trauma setting, an acute injury must be first on the differential diagnosis. The three most common traumatic etiologies of widened mediastinum include; sternal fracture, thoracic spine fracture, and aortic disruption. Sternal fracture can be associated with significant blunt cardiac injury, thoracic spine fractures may be unstable, and thoracic aortic injuries are at risk for rupture if not treated. These possible complications mean that diagnosis must be swift and accurate. Errors in technique or positioning or nontraumatic causes of widened mediastinum should be diagnoses of exclusion. The next step in diagnosis should be CT angiography of the chest. This will accurately diagnose aortic injury, associated pulmonary contusion, as well as soft tissue and bony injuries.

**Answer: B**

Bruckner, B.A., DiBardino, D.J., Cumbie, T.C., *et al.* (2006) Critical evaluation of chest computed tomography scans for blunt descending thoracic aortic injury. *Annals of Thoracic Surgery,* **81** (4), 1339–1346.

Gutierrez, A., Inaba, K., Siboni, S., *et al.* (2016) The utility of chest x-ray as a screening tool for blunt thoracic aortic injury. *Injury,* **47** (1), 32–36.

**16** *A resuscitative thoracotomy is indicated in which of the following clinical scenarios?*
   **A** *Absence of vital signs when paramedics arrive*
   **B** *Loss of vitals with cardiopulmonary resuscitation time greater than 15 minutes in penetrating trauma*
   **C** *Loss of vitals with cardiopulmonary resuscitation time greater than 15 minutes in blunt trauma*
   **D** *Loss of vitals with cardiopulmonary resuscitation time greater than 15 minutes in pediatric trauma*
   **E** *Loss of vitals on arrival to the hospital in penetrating trauma*

Resuscitative thoracotomy or emergency department thoracotomy (EDT) is performed to address cardiovascular collapse. It will allow evacuation of hemothorax/pneumothorax, the release of tamponade, repair of cardiac and intrathoracic vessel injuries, evacuation of air embolus, clamping of hilar injuries, cross clamping of the aorta, and performance of open cardiac massage.

Indications for EDT are difficult to clarify and can change from institution to institution. However, in general EDT is indicated for patients with witnessed arrest with cardiopulmonary resuscitation (CPR) less than 15 minutes following penetrating thoracic trauma, witnessed arrest with CPR less than 5 minutes following penetrating nonthoracic trauma, witnessed arrest with CPR less than 5 minutes following blunt trauma, and persistent hypotension due to tamponade or intrathoracic hemorrhage. Outcomes are best with penetrating cardiac injury, followed by penetrating noncardiac thoracic trauma. Outcomes following penetrating abdominal trauma and blunt trauma are poor. Outcomes in children are similar to adults and indications for pediatric EDT are similar to those for adults.

**Answer: E**

Seamon, M.J., Haut, E.R., Van Arendonk, K., *et al.* (2015) An evidence-based approach to patient selection for emergency department thoracotomy: A practice management guideline from the Eastern Association for the Surgery of Trauma. *Journal of Trauma and Acute Care Surgery*, **79** (1), 159–173.

Working Group, Ad Hoc Subcommittee on Outcomes, American College of Surgeons-Committee on Trauma (2001) Practice management guidelines for emergency department thoracotomy. *Journal of the American College of Surgeons*, **193** (3), 303–309.

**17** *Which of the following is not an acceptable treatment for traumatic aortic injury?*
   **A** *Open repair*
   **B** *Endovascular stent graft*
   **C** *Blood pressure control*
   **D** *Temporary intravascular shunt*
   **E** *Video-assisted thoracoscopic surgery (VATS)*

The diagnosis and treatment of traumatic aortic injury has undergone a number of changes in recent years. Two multicenter prospective observational studies revealed almost complete conversion from aortography to CT scan for diagnosis and increasing utilization of stent grafts for treatment. Additionally, when open repair is chosen, bypass is frequently preferred to the clamp-and-sew technique. Open repair is generally performed via posterolateral thoracotomy, although anterolateral thoracotomy may be used for patients who are in extremis, and median sternotomy is used for injuries to the ascending aorta or arch. In addition to open and endovascular repair, nonoperative management with aggressive blood pressure control has become an acceptable treatment option, especially in the elderly patient with multiple comorbidities, or in patients with minor intimal tears.

Shunting is also a viable treatment option in the unstable patient in a damage control situation, although data on patency rates and long-term outcomes are lacking.

**Answer: E**

DuBose, J.J., Leake, S.S., Brenner, M., *et al.* (2015) Contemporary management and outcomes of blunt thoracic aortic injury: a multicenter retrospective study. *Journal of Trauma and Acute Care Surgery*, **78** (2), 360–369.

Inaba, K., Aksoy, H., Seamon, M.J., *et al.* (2015) Multicenter evaluation of temporary intravascular shunt use in vascular trauma. *Journal of Trauma and Acute Care Surgery*, **80** (3), 359–365.

**18** *Which of the following is an acceptable modality for diagnosis of traumatic aortic injury?*
   **A** *CT angiography*
   **B** *Chest x-ray*
   **C** *FAST*
   **D** *Transthoracic echocardiography*
   **E** *PET scan*

Traumatic aortic injury is a rare but potentially lethal complication following thoracic trauma. A chest x-ray has been utilized in the past as a screening exam; however, an x-ray can be normal in up to 33% of patients with traumatic aortic injury, and positive findings are nonspecific. While transesophageal echocardiography has a reported sensitivity of 90–100%, transthoracic echocardiography and FAST have low diagnostic yield and accuracy for aortic injury, especially in the presence of chest-wall injuries. MRI can be used for diagnosis with a sensitivity and specificity of 98%. However, MRI has the drawbacks of poor availability and lengthy exam times outside a monitored critical care setting. The CT scan is increasing in popularity as a screening and diagnostic tool, with sensitivity and specificity ranging from 95–100% in most studies. Additionally, CT scan is widely available in most centers, rapid, easily interpreted, and does not require arterial puncture. Aortography was previously the gold standard; however, it is utilized now primarily for therapy as it is invasive and requires the presence of a specialty angiography team.

**Answer: A**

Bruckner, B.A., DiBardino, D.J., Cumbie, T.C., *et al.* (2006) Critical evaluation of chest computed tomography scans for blunt descending thoracic aortic injury. *Annals of Thoracic Surgery*, **81** (4), 1339–1346.

Khalil, A., Tarik, T., and Porembka, D.T. (2007) Aortic pathology: aortic trauma, debris, dissection, and aneurysm. *Critical Care Medicine*, **35** (8, suppl.), S392–S400.

**19** *A 37-year-old man sustains blunt chest trauma requiring chest tube for drainage of a hemopneumothorax. After placement of the chest tube, there is residual opacification on chest x-ray, subsequent CT scan reveals a retained hemothorax. Which of the following is NOT an acceptable treatment option?*

**A** *VATS drainage/decortication*

**B** *Intrathoracic thrombolysis*

**C** *Thoracotomy with drainage/decortication*

**D** *Increasing suction on the chest tube*

**E** *Placement of a second chest tube with or without image guidance*

Retained hemothorax can complicate the hospital course of 3–8% of patients with traumatic hemothorax. Retained blood may occur as a result of a delay in presentation, delay in diagnosis/treatment, and thoracostomy tube malposition, migration, or occlusion. Retained blood may result in empyema or fibrothorax. The options for treatment include open drainage, video-assisted thoracoscopic drainage, placement of a second drainage tube, and intrapleural thrombolysis. Several studies and a meta-analysis of intrapleural thrombolysis have revealed promising results with complete clinical and radiographic resolution in over 90% of cases in most studies. In contrast, postural drainage, chest physiotherapy, and increased suction on the thoracostomy tube are unlikely to resolve retained hemothoraces.

**Answer: D**

DuBose, J., Inaba, K., Demetriades, D., *et al.* (2012) Management of post-traumatic retained hemothorax: a prospective, observational, multicenter AAST study. *Journal of Trauma*, **72** (1), 11–22.

Stiles, P.J., Drake, R.M., Helmer, S.D., *et al.* (2014) Evaluation of chest tube administration of tissue plasminogen activator to treat retained hemothorax. *American Journal of Surgery*, **207** (6), 960–963.

**20** *For which unstable trauma patient is the use of REBOA contraindicated?*

**A** *30-year-old female with an open book pelvic fracture and SBP of 70 mm Hg after a motorcycle crash*

**B** *55-year-old male with a positive FAST and SBP of 65 mm Hg after a motor vehicle collision*

**C** *25-year-old male with a widened mediastinum on chest x-ray and a SBP of 60 mm Hg after a 30-foot fall.*

**D** *67-year-old female with a positive FAST and lateral compression pelvic fractures and a SBP of 75 mm Hg after a motor vehicle collision*

**E** *There are no absolute contraindications for the use of REBOA in a hemodynamically unstable blunt trauma patient.*

Use of resuscitative endovascular balloon occlusion of the aorta (REBOA) has become an adjunct for temporary hemorrhage control in the hemodynamically unstable trauma patient as a less invasive alternative to a resuscitative thoracotomy with aortic cross-clamping. Some studies have shown efficacy and improved survival for hemorrhage control in patients with truncal hemorrhage in profound shock. Patients with hemorrhage from unstable pelvic fractures and/or intraabdominal etiologies are likely to benefit from placement of REBOA for temporary hemostasis as a bridge to definitive surgical repair. Patients with penetrating chest trauma or possible thoracic aortic injury are considered an absolute contraindication for the use of REBOA.

**Answer: C**

Joseph, B., Ibraheem, K., Haider, A.A., *et al.* (2016) Identifying potential utility of REBOA: An autopsy study. *Journal of Trauma and Acute Care Surgery*, **81** (5), S128–S132.

Moore, L.J., Brenner, M., Kozar, R.A., *et al.* (2015) Implementation of resuscitative endovascular occlusion of the aorta as an alternative to resuscitative thoracotomy for noncompressible truncal hemorrhage. *Journal of Trauma and Acute Care Surgery*, **79** (4), 523–530.

# 31

# Abdominal and Abdominal Vascular Injury

*Leslie Kobayashi, MD and Michelle G. Hamel, MD*

1 *Which of the following is a contraindication to a trial of nonoperative management in liver injury?*
   A *Pediatric patient*
   B *Grade IV injury*
   C *Elderly patient*
   D *Peritonitis*
   E *Penetrating mechanism*

Initially, criteria for nonoperative management (NOM) included Grade I–III injury, intact mental status, age > 65 years, reliable abdominal exam, and transfusion of > 2 units of packed red blood cells. Success rates using these criteria were 80–95%. However, current data indicate that age, grade of injury, mechanism, and even comatose state need not be contraindications for NOM in stable patients. Success rates of up to 40% were reported in stable patients with grade IV and V injuries. Furthermore, no statistically significant differences could be identified among failure rates in patients with a depressed GCS. A study conducted in patients older than 55 revealed a success rate of 97% with NOM. Current contraindications to NOM include hypotension unresponsive to resuscitation, peritonitis, and concomitant injury requiring surgical repair, although controversial patients with liver injury and hypotension who are responders, meaning they respond to fluid resuscitation and/or transfusion with an increase in blood pressure to acceptable levels, may be candidates for angiographic treatment. However, in these patients, there should be a low threshold to convert to laparotomy should they cease responding to resuscitation or have worsening abdominal exam or evidence of ongoing hemorrhage following angiography.

**Answer: D**

Asensio, J.A., Roldán, G., Petrone, P., *et al.* (2003) Operative management and outcomes in 103 AAST-OIS Grades IV and V complex hepatic injuries: trauma surgeons still need to operate, but angioembolization helps. *Journal of Trauma*, **54** (4), 647–654.

Stassen, N.A., Bhullar, I., Cheng, J.D., *et al.* (2012) Nonoperative management of blunt hepatic injury: an Eastern Association for the Surgery of Trauma practice management guideline. *Journal of Trauma and Acute Care Surgery*, **73** (5), S288–S293.

2 *A 34-year-old man is hypotensive after a motorcycle crash. His abdomen is non-tender, his pelvis is unstable, and x-ray demonstrates a severe open book fracture. After receiving 2 L of ringers lactate he is still hypotensive. What is the most immediate next step in management?*
   A *CT scan of the abdomen and pelvis with IV contrast*
   B *Application of a pelvic binder*
   C *Angiography*
   D *Exploratory laparotomy*
   E *Bilateral needle thoracostomy*

If hypotension is present with pelvic fracture, the pelvic ring should be reapproximated as soon as possible. Stabilization devices include pelvic binders, external fixators, and sheets. Binders or sheets are fitted over the anterior superior iliac spines superiorly, and the femoral heads inferiorly. If orthopedic surgeons are available, an external fixation device can be placed to reapproximate the pelvic ring. Stabilization devices close the pelvic ring decreasing pelvic volume to tamponade bleeding. They also stabilize the broken ends of bone preventing further injury to nearby tissues and decrease pain with repositioning and transport. Hemorrhage associated with pelvic fracture can cause significant hypotension and carries a high mortality. The majority of bleeding is from the sacral venous plexus. Occasionally bleeding may be from an arterial source. In stable or semi-stable patients with pelvic hemorrhage, angiography should be considered for diagnostic and therapeutic purposes. If significant

*Surgical Critical Care and Emergency Surgery: Clinical Questions and Answers*, Second Edition.
Edited by Forrest "Dell" Moore, Peter Rhee, and Gerard J. Fulda.
© 2018 John Wiley & Sons Ltd. Published 2018 by John Wiley & Sons Ltd.
Companion website: www.wiley.com/go/moore/surgical_criticalcare_and_emergency_surgery

arterial bleeding is found, selective embolization can be performed. If no arterial bleeding is found, bilateral internal iliac artery embolization can be performed to decrease pelvic inflow. The rich collateral circulation in the pelvis prevents ischemic complications in most patients. Very rarely, complications such as necrosis of pelvic organs or gluteal compartment syndrome can occur. Transfusion of blood products are also a very important aspect of immediate therapy that can be initiated, but stopping bleeding is the highest priority.

**Answer: B**

Cullinane, D.C., Schiller, H.J., Zielinski, M.D., *et al.* (2011) Eastern Association for the Surgery of Trauma practice management guidelines for hemorrhage in pelvic fracture – update and systematic review. *Journal of Trauma*, **71** (6), 1850–1868.

Velmahos, G.C., Chahwan, S., Hanks, S.E., *et al.* (2000) Angiographic embolization of bilateral internal iliac arteries to control life-threatening hemorrhage after blunt trauma to the pelvis. *The American Surgeon*, **66** (9), 858–862.

**3** *A patient sustains a liver injury with a blush noted on CT scan as well as a posterior knee dislocation after a motor vehicle crash. Which of the following is the next best step in management?*
   **A** *Angiography*
   **B** *Operative repair of the dislocated knee*
   **C** *Repeat CT scan of the abdomen*
   **D** *Placement of a traction pin to reduce the knee dislocation*
   **E** *Laparotomy*

Stable patients with any injury grade and evidence of intraparenchymal extravasation of contrast are candidates for angiography and possible embolization. Angioembolization can be used before, after, or instead of, surgery. It is required in 5–6% of patients with liver injury and has a success rate of 80–100%. Complications of embolization are not rare and include hepatic necrosis, abscess, and bile leak. The timing of angiography appears to affect morbidity and mortality, with better outcomes observed in patients undergoing early compared with late angiography. In this patient, there is a second indication for angiography, as it can also be used to diagnose popliteal artery injury, which is associated with knee dislocation.

**Answer: A**

Mohr, A.M., Lavery, R.F., Barone, A., *et al.* (2003) Angiographic embolization for liver injuries: low mortality, high morbidity. *Journal of Trauma*, **55**, 1077–1082.

Wahl, W.L., Ahrns, K.S., Brandt, M.M., *et al.* (2002) The need for early angiographic embolization in blunt liver injuries. *Journal of Trauma*, **52** (6), 1097–1101.

**4** *A patient presents after high-speed motorcycle crash. A pelvis X-ray reveals bilateral pubic rami fractures, and there is blood at the urethral meatus, which of the following should be the next step in management?*
   **A** *Retrograde urethrogram*
   **B** *CT cystogram*
   **C** *Intravenous pyelogram*
   **D** *Diagnostic peritoneal lavage*
   **E** *CT of the bony pelvis*

Urethral injury is rare, occurring in 4–10% of patients with pelvic fractures. Blood at the urethral meatus, perineal hematoma, high riding prostate on rectal exam, and inability to void or gross hematuria are all indicators of urethral injury. When present, suspicion for urethral injury should be high and retrograde urethrogram (RUG) should be performed. This can be done by placing a small foley catheter in the fossa navicularis and partially inflating the balloon or using a non-crushing clamp on the end of the penis to prevent contrast leakage. Approximately 30 mL of full strength contrast is then injected, and ideally, fluoroscopy is used to assess for extravasation, if not available at least two views using plain radiographs should be taken. Ideally, one view will be oblique. While concomitant bladder injury is seen in up to 15% of patients with urethral injury, no attempt should be made to interrogate the bladder or place a foley catheter until a RUG can be performed to rule out urethral injury.

**Answer: A**

Coburn, M (2013) Genitourinary trauma, in *Trauma*, 7th ed. (eds K.L. Mattox and E.E. Moore), McGraw-Hill, New York, pp. 669–708.

**5** *Which of the following is a contraindication to nonoperative management of splenic injury?*
   **A** *Concomitant liver injury*
   **B** *Peritonitis*
   **C** *Hemoperitoneum*
   **D** *Blush on CT scan*
   **E** *Concomitant pelvic fracture*

Rates of success with splenic nonoperative management (NOM) can be as high as 95% for pediatric an 80% for adult populations. There are two strict contraindications for NOM, peritonitis, and hemodynamic instability. Studies have shown acceptable rates of success with NOM in patients with neurologic injury and in patients with concerning CT findings such as high-grade injury, blush, or hemoperitoneum. While these factors increase the risk for failure, they should not be considered strict contraindications to NOM in the stable patient. The addition of angiography with and without embolization has augmented success rates of NOM. Angiography is particularly attractive as an adjunct to NOM in patients with multiple solid organ injuries or concomitant pelvic fracture as it can be diagnostic and therapeutic in these patients with multiple potential sources of hemorrhage.

**Answer: B**

Stassen, N.A., Bhullar, I., Cheng, J.D., *et al.* (2012) Selective nonoperative management of blunt splenic injury: an Eastern Association for the Surgery of Trauma practice management guideline. *Journal of Trauma and Acute Care Surgery*, **73** (5 Suppl. 4), S948–S300.
Wisner, D.H. (2013) Injury to the spleen *Trauma*, 7th ed. (eds K.L. Mattox and E.E. Moore), McGraw-Hill, New York, pp. 561–580.

6   *A patient undergoes laparotomy and hepatorraphy for grade IV liver injury. Postoperatively the patient develops bilious output from his drains. He was made nothing per os (NPO) and started on octreotide he is stable and asymptomatic, but the drainage persists what is the next step in management?*
   **A** *Laparotomy*
   **B** *Endoscopy*
   **C** *Angiography*
   **D** *Endoscopic retrograde cholangiopancreatography (ERCP)*
   **E** *Ultrasound*

Bile leak or biloma formation can complicate the course of 0.5–20% of patients following liver injury. The incidence is slightly higher in operative compared to nonoperative patients and in patients with higher grade injuries. Often these collections are asymptomatic and up to 70% resolve spontaneously. Symptomatic patients with fever, leukocytosis, pain, jaundice, or feeding intolerance, are best treated with image-guided drainage. Percutaneous drainage has a very high success rate. If bilious drainage persists, ERCP with sphincterotomy or stent placement is effective. Surgery can be considered for fluid collections not amenable to percutaneous drainage, or for proximal bile leaks that fail to resolve with ERCP decompression.

**Answer: D**

Kozar, R.A., Moore, F.A., Cothren, C.C., *et al.* (2006) Risk factors for hepatic morbidity following nonoperative management. *Archives of Surgery*, **141**, 451–459.

Kozar, R.A., Moore, J.B., Niles, S.E., *et al.* (2005) Complications of nonoperative management of high-grade blunt hepatic injuries. *Journal of Trauma*, **59** (5), 1066–1071.

7   *Regarding seat belt signs on the abdomen which of the following statements is false?*
   **A** *They are associated with increased mortality*
   **B** *They are associated with lumbar spine fractures*
   **C** *They are associated with pancreatic injury*
   **D** *They are associated with duodenal injuries*
   **E** *They are associated with mesenteric injuries*

The presence of a seat belt sign (SBS) on the abdomen is associated with a significant increase in intra-abdominal injuries. In adult populations, the presence of an SBS increases the risk of intra-abdominal injury twofold to eightfold. An SBS may be even more concerning in pediatric patients where rates of intra-abdominal injury can be increased as much as twelvefold. Hollow viscous, particularly the duodenum, and mesenteric injuries are markedly increased and the threshold to operate on a patient with free fluid and an SBS should be very low. Additionally, pancreatic injury is increased especially in the pediatric population. Lastly, the use of a lap belt without the concomitant use of a shoulder restraint has been associated with chance fracture of the lumbar spine. However, despite increased risk of intra-abdominal injury SBS is not associated with increased mortality. In fact, in a recent study, despite patients with SBS being older, more severely injured and at higher risk of having intra-abdominal injuries, mortality was lower than that of patients without SBS.

**Answer: A**

Bansal, V., Conroy, C., Tominaga, G.T., *et al.* (2009) The utility of seat belt signs to predict intra-abdominal injury following motor vehicle crashes. *Traffic Injury Prevention*, **10**, 567–572.
Sharma, O.P., Oswanski, M.J., Kaminski, B.P., *et al.* (2009) Clinical implications of the seat belt sign in blunt trauma. *American Journal of Surgery*, **75** (9), 822–827.

8   *After falling, a patient is found to have a renal artery injury with thrombosis and ischemia. Which of the following statements regarding renal injury is true?*
   **A** *Hypertension can be an early complication of nonoperative management*
   **B** *Revascularization of the injured kidney generally results in good outcomes*
   **C** *Complications are more common following nephrectomy than nephrorrhaphy*
   **D** *Acute renal failure following nephrectomy is generally permanent*
   **E** *Non-operative management of renal injuries has a high success rate*

Kidney injury occurs in 1–3% of all trauma patients and up to 10% of abdominal traumas. Blunt mechanisms are far more common than penetrating, accounting for approximately 60% of injuries. Blunt trauma to the renal vessels is more likely to result in thrombosis, whereas penetrating trauma more often results in bleeding. Nonoperative management is successful in > 90% of cases. Risk factors for failure include high-grade injuries, large perinephric hematomas, and urinary extravasation. The only absolute contra-indication to nonoperative management is hemodynamic instability. In the cases of renal artery thrombosis, warm ischemia time is the most important determining factor in renal salvage rates. Outcomes are generally disappointing following revascularization and are dismal if revascularization is delayed beyond 6–12 hours. Complications, including recurrence of bleeding, abscess, and urine leak are more common following nephrorrhaphy than nephrectomy. Early complications include re-bleeding, urine leak, and abscess. Late complications include Page kidney, renovascular hypertension, and hydronephrosis. Acute renal dysfunction can occur after traumatic nephrectomy but tends to be transient and self-limited.

**Answer: E**

Coburn, M. (2013) Genitourinary trauma, in *Trauma*, 7th ed. (eds K.L. Mattox and E.E. Moore), McGraw-Hill, New York, pp. 669–708.
van der Wilden, G.M., Velmahos, G.C., Joseph, D.K., *et al.* (2013) Successful nonoperative management of the most severe blunt renal injuries: a multicenter study of the research consortium of New England Centers for Trauma. *Journal of the American Medical Association: Surgery*, **148** (10), 924–931.

9 Which of the following statements regarding blunt pancreatic trauma is true?
   A Pancreatic injury is common following motor vehicle accident
   B Injury is more common in adults than children
   C Associated injuries are uncommon
   D Transection following blunt trauma typically occurs near the mesenteric vessels
   E Duct disruption is common following blunt injury

Pancreatic injury following blunt trauma is uncommon, occurring in less than 2% of abdominal trauma cases. Because they tend to have less intraperitoneal and extra-peritoneal abdominal fat, children tend to be at increased risk of pancreatic injury. The force required to injure this organ is significant, and associated injuries are common, occurring in 70–90% of cases. Anterior-posterior compression of the pancreas against the lumbar spine results

in transection at this location in two-thirds of patients, adjacent and just to the left of the superior mesenteric vessels. While duct integrity is the main determinant of intervention and outcome, major duct injury is rare, occurring in less than 15% of pancreatic injuries, and is much more common following penetrating than blunt trauma. Low-grade injuries require drainage and bowel rest only. If the main duct is injured in the pancreatic tail or body distal to the neck, a distal pancreatectomy is the best treatment. If the duct injury is more proximal options for management include subtotal pancreatectomy, external drainage with postoperative ERCP, and distal drainage with roux-en-Y pancreaticojejunostomy.

**Answer: D**

Biffl, W.L. (2013) Duodenum and pancreas, in *Trauma*, 7th ed. (eds K.L. Mattox and E.E. Moore), McGraw-Hill, New York, pp. 603–619.
Velmahos, G.C., Tabbara, M., Gross, R., *et al.* (2009) Blunt pancreatoduodenal injury: a multicenter study of the Research Consortium of New England Centers for Trauma (ReCONECT). *Archives of Surgery*, **144** (5), 413–419.

10 Regarding iliac vein injuries, which of the following is true?
   A Most blunt injuries can be repaired primarily
   B Mortality is low
   C Mortality and morbidity increase with concomitant arterial injury
   D Compartment syndrome is a common complication following isolated venous injury
   E Post-phlebitic syndrome is an early complication

Iliac vein injury can occur after blunt or penetrating trauma and as a result of iatrogenic injury following pelvic procedures. Mortality can be as high as 70%. Mortality and morbidity are increased with a concomitant arterial injury. Minor lacerations can be repaired primarily, however, more destructive injuries associated with gunshot wounds and blunt trauma most often require ligation. Complications following ligation include extremity edema, compartment syndrome, thromboembolic complications, and outflow ischemia. Leg edema is common after ligation, but compartment syndrome is rare unless there is also an arterial injury or prolonged hypotension. Post-phlebitic syndrome characterized by venous hypertension and incompetence, chronic edema, and ulceration can also occur in the late postoperative period.

**Answer: C**

Oliver, J.C., Bekker, W., Edu, S., *et al.* (2012) A ten-year review of civilian iliac vessel injuries from a single trauma center. *European Journal of Vascular and Endovascular Surgery*, **44** (2), 199–202.

Quan, R.W., Gillespie, D.L., Stuart, R.P., *et al.* (2008) The effect of vein repair on the risk of venous thromboembolic events: a review of more than 100 traumatic military venous injuries. *Journal of Vascular Surgery*, **47**, 571–577.

**11** *Regarding destructive colon injuries, which of the following statements is false?*

  **A** *Blood transfusion >/= 4 units is associated with increased infectious complications*
  **B** *Prophylactic antibiotics should be discontinued after 24 hours*
  **C** *Inappropriate choice of antibiotic is associated with increased infectious complications*
  **D** *Hypotension is associated with increased infectious complications*
  **E** *Primary anastomosis is associated with increased complications compared to colostomy*

Destructive colon injuries have a very high rate of postoperative complications ranging from 20–40%. Complications include ileus, abscess, wound infection, and anastomotic leak. Several factors can significantly increase the rate of complications following surgical repair or resection. A large multicenter prospective observational trial identified severe fecal contamination, transfusion of 4 units of blood or greater, and inappropriate antibiotic prophylaxis as independent predictors of postoperative complications. It also found that the method of repair had no effect on the rate of complications. Several other studies have supported these findings, and additionally identified blood loss greater than 1L, and hypotension as being risk factors for infectious complications. Lastly, several studies have found no additional benefit to continuing antibiotic coverage beyond 24 hours postoperatively regardless of the extent of contamination.

**Answer: E**

Demetriades, D., Murray, J.A., Chan, L., *et al.* (2001) Penetrating colon injuries requiring resection: Diversion or primary anastomosis? An AAST prospective multicenter study. *Journal of Trauma*, **50** (5), 765–775.

Sharpe, J.P., Magnotti, L.J., Weinberg, J.A., *et al.* (2014) Applicability of an established management algorithm for destructive colon injuries after abbreviated laparotomy: a 17-year experience. *Journal of the American College of Surgeons*, **218** (4), 636–641.

**12** *Which of the following retroperitoneal hematomas should be surgically explored?*

  **A** *Zone I hematoma following blunt trauma*
  **B** *Zone II hematoma following blunt trauma*
  **C** *Zone III hematoma following blunt trauma*
  **D** *Retrohepatic hematoma following blunt trauma*
  **E** *Retrohepatic hematoma following penetrating trauma*

Zone I hematomas (Figure 31.1) are centrally located and contain the major abdominal vessels, because of this vascular injury is highly suspected, and Zone I hematomas due to both blunt and penetrating trauma should be explored. Zone II, the lateral upper abdomen, contains the kidneys and renal vessels. Injuries due to blunt trauma in this area are unlikely to require surgical repair and hematomas should be left intact. Zone III is the pelvic retroperitoneum containing the iliac vessels, ureters, rectum and the sacral venous plexus. Following penetrating trauma, major vascular or hollow viscous injuries are common, and all hematomas should be explored. However, this is less likely following blunt trauma, and the risk of releasing venous hemorrhage is high. Most bleeding associated with pelvic fracture following blunt trauma is not amenable to surgical correction and is more likely to respond to interventional techniques or pelvic stabilization. Therefore Zone III blunt hematomas should not be explored. The retrohepatic area contains

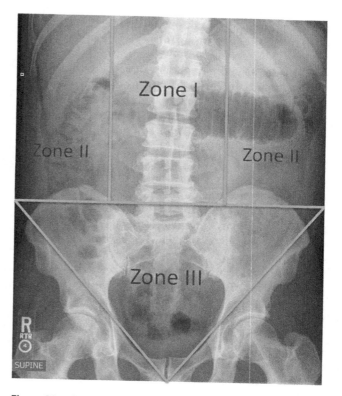

**Figure 31.1** Retroperitoneal zones.

the inferior vena cava (IVC); this area is difficult to access, and injuries to this portion of the IVC are difficult to control. Tamponade is possible even with a major vascular injury in this area, and release of tamponade can result in exsanguinating hemorrhage. Stable hematomas resulting from both penetrating and blunt trauma in this area should not be explored.

**Answer: A**

Buckman, R.F., Pathak, A.S., Badellino, M.M., *et al.* (2001) Injuries of the inferior vena cava. *Surgical Clinics of North America*, **81** (6), 1431–1447.

Dente, C.J. and Feliciano, D.V. (2013) Abdominal vascular injury, in *Trauma*, 7th ed. (eds K.L. Mattox and E.E. Moore), McGraw-Hill, New York, pp. 632–654.

**13** *Of the following, which is/are taken into account when considering damage-control laparotomy and temporary abdominal closure?*
   **A** *Physiologic state*
   **B** *Coagulopathy*
   **C** *Injury burden*
   **D** *Fluid/transfusion requirements*
   **E** *All of the above*

Damage-control surgery (DCS) is a concept originally intended for management of the severely injured exsanguinating trauma patient. It has since been applied to many surgical conditions including nontraumatic abdominal surgery, vascular surgery, and orthopedic surgery. The concept of damage-control laparotomy (DCL) is to stage the treatment of catastrophic injuries or insults into three distinct phases. First, control of acute hemorrhage and contamination, second resuscitation, and third planned re-exploration for definitive treatment of surgical pathology. Indications for DCL include hemodynamic instability, severe medical coagulopathy, acidosis (pH < 7.2), hypothermia (<35 °C), injuries to multiple body cavities, prohibitively long operative time, and massive transfusion requirements. DCL is not without complication, and the decision to convert the goals of laparotomy from definitive care to DCL should not be made based on a single variable but on the global clinical picture. However, the decision to perform DCL should be made early in the procedure, and ideally will precede actual manifestations of the bloody vicious triad (acidosis, coagulopathy, and hypothermia). Severe injury burden, multi-cavitary injury, and poor physiologic reserve should also factor into the decision to pursue DCL. This procedure can be controversial as DCL is associated with complications including ventral hernias and enteric fistulas.

**Answer: E**

Higa, G., Friese, R., O'Keeffe, T., *et al.* (2010) Damage control laparotomy: a vital tool once over utilized. *Journal of Trauma*, **69** (1), 53–59.

Rotondo, M.F., Schwab, W., McGonigal, M.D., *et al.* (1993) Damage control: an approach for improved survival in exsanguinating penetrating abdominal injury. *Journal Trauma*, **35** (3), 375–382.

**14** *Which of the following methods is an option for temporary abdominal closure in primary damage-control surgery?*
   **A** *Whip stitching of the skin*
   **B** *Closure of the skin with towel clips*
   **C** *Vacuum-assisted wound closure*
   **D** *Primary fascial closure*
   **E** *Primary fascial closure with retention sutures*

Any temporary abdominal closure (TAC) must maintain sterility, protect the bowel, prevent evisceration, and prevent adhesions. Additionally, as there may be significant drainage from the abdominal cavity, the closure method must have a means of collecting, removing and quantifying this drainage. Methods that reapproximate fascia or skin may create abdominal compartment syndrome and should be taken into account. There are some surgeons that prefer to approximate the skin over a suction system as it avoids the loss of domain. Fascial closures are usually avoided to preserve it for definitive closure. The two most popular techniques are vacuum-assisted abdominal dressings and the Bogota bag. Vacuum-assisted closure can be performed with commercially available materials or following the Barker method. The Bogota bag uses sterile plastic sutured to the skin to create an abdominal silo. At the time of repeat laparotomy, a number of definitive and TAC methods are available; these include primary closure with or without retention sutures, biologic or artificial graft assisted closure, the previously mentioned TAC methods, as well as devices that attempt to reduce the loss of domain. These devices include the Wittmann Patch, Zipper, and ABRA dynamic fascial closure device. There is also the option of skin closure, or placement of absorbable mesh with a planned ventral hernia. Many physicians also combine methods using a combination of dynamic retention sutures with Barker or another type of vacuum closure system to decrease the loss of abdominal domain.

**Answer: C**

Boele van Hensbroek, P.B., Wind, J., Dijkgraaf, M.G.W., *et al.* (2009) Temporary closure of the open abdomen:

A systematic review on delayed primary fascial closure in patients with an open abdomen. *World Journal of Surgery*, 33 (2), 199–207.

Ribeiro Jnr, M.A., Barros, E.A., de Carvalho, S.M., *et al.* (2016) Open abdomen in gastrointestinal surgery: Which technique is the best for temporary closure during damage control? *World Journal of Gastrointestinal Surgery*, 8 (8), 590–597.

**15** *Following splenectomy for trauma, vaccinations should be sure to include which of the following organisms?*
   **A** Enterobacter aerogenes
   **B** Haemophilus influenzae
   **C** Staphylococcus aureus
   **D** Klebsiella pneumonia
   **E** Pseudomonas aeruginosa

The spleen produces tuftsin and properdin; post-splenectomy patients have diminished immunity and are most at risk of infection from encapsulated organisms. These include *Streptococcus pneumonia, Hemophilus influenzae,* and *Neisseria meningitidis.* Following splenectomy, patients should receive Haemophilus, meningococcal, and pneumococcal vaccinations. Vaccinations are ideally given before surgery. However, this is not possible in trauma patients. There is evidence to suggest vaccinations should be given 14 days following traumatic splenectomy as immunoglobulin titers are highest following vaccination in this period. However, as many patients fail to follow up after trauma, vaccinations should be given at 14 days if possible or before discharge from the hospital.

**Answer: B**

Shatz, D.V., Schinsky, M.F., Pais, L.R., *et al.* (1998) Immune responses of splenectomized trauma patients to the 23-valent pneumococcal polysaccharide vaccine at 1 versus 7 versus 14 days after splenectomy. *Journal of Trauma,* 44 (5), 760–765.

Vercruysse, G.A. and Feliciano, D.V. (2009) The spleen, in *Acute Care Surgery: A Guide for General Surgeons* (eds V.H. Gracias, P.M. Reilly, M.G. McKenney, and G.C. Valmahos), McGraw-Hill, New York, pp. 147–151.

**16** *The second stage of damage-control surgery is aimed at correcting which of the following values?*
   **A** *Acidosis*
   **B** *Alkalosis*
   **C** *Hypercarbia*
   **D** *Hypoxia*
   **E** *Hypernatremia*

Damage-control surgery (DCS) consists of three phases. The first includes operative control of active hemorrhage and gross contamination. The second phase is resuscitation to correct physiologic derangement. The third phase consists of definitive management of injuries and abdominal closure. Patients with severe trauma often present with extreme physiologic derangements including acidosis due to volume losses, hypoperfusion, and anaerobic metabolism; hypothermia; and subsequent coagulopathy. Prolonged surgery with cavitary exposure is likely to exacerbate all of these derangements and contribute to morbidity and mortality. Therefore, the initial surgery should be abbreviated and transfer to the ICU for rewarming, and resuscitation should occur as soon as possible. The goal of resuscitation is to reverse acidosis with the restoration of circulating blood volume using one-to-one plasma-to-red-cell ratios and massive transfusion protocols. Additionally, blankets, forced air warmers, ventilation with warmed humidified air, and warm fluids should be used to correct hypothermia. All of these interventions should help correct hypotension, and reverse coagulopathy. Additionally, evidence of the return of normal physiology such as increased urine output or clearance of elevated lactate levels should occur before starting phase 3 of DCS.

**Answer: A**

Rotondo, M.F., Schwab, W., McGonigal, M.D., *et al.* (1993) Damage control: An approach for improved survival in exsanguinating penetrating abdominal injury. *Journal of Trauma,* 35 (3), 375–382.

Waibel, B.H. and Rotondo, M.F. (2010) Damage control in trauma and abdominal sepsis. *Critical Care Medical,* 38 (9 Suppl), S421–S430.

**17** *Which of the following is currently recommended for the treatment for extra-peritoneal rectal injury?*
   **A** *Prolonged antibiotic course*
   **B** *Pre-sacral drainage*
   **C** *Diverting colostomy*
   **D** *Trans-peritoneal repair*
   **E** *Rectal lavage*

Treatment of extraperitoneal rectal injuries has evolved over the past decades. Traditionally these injuries were treated with the triple approach of diversion, presacral drainage, and rectal lavage. It now appears that this complex and invasive treatment strategy is unnecessary. Comparisons of patients with and without presacral drainage show no benefit in terms of speed of recovery or prevention of abscess or pelvic sepsis. Findings were similar for rectal lavage, with some studies even suggesting worse outcomes with lavage. Similar to other studies of prophylactic antibiotics, prolonged treatment courses do not decrease rates of infectious complications, and most authors only recommend perioperative treatment for 24 hours. While transanal repair may be useful in some patients where injuries are easily accessible, there is no role for trans-peritoneal repair of isolated rectal injuries as this offers no benefit over diversion alone and often results in increased complication rates. Most studies continue to recommend fecal diversion with either open or laparoscopic colostomy.

**Answer: C**

Bosarge, P.L., Como, J.J., Fox, N., *et al.* (2016) Management of penetrating extraperitoneal rectal injuries: an Eastern Association for the Surgery of Trauma Practice Management guideline. *Journal of Trauma and Acute Care Surgery*, **80** (3), 546–551.

Gonzalez, R.P., Phelan, H., Hassan, M., *et al.* (2006) Is fecal diversion necessary for nondestructive penetrating extraperitoneal rectal injuries? *Journal of Trauma*, **61** (4), 815–819.

**18** *A 25-year-old male presents to the trauma bay after high-speed motor vehicle crash. He is hypotensive upon arrival and is intubated for airway protection. His blood pressure initially responds to a fluid bolus. His pelvis is unstable on exam. Chest x-ray demonstrates no hemo- or pneumothorax. FAST exam is negative for any intraabdominal fluid. Pelvic x-ray demonstrates open book pelvic fracture. A pelvic binder is applied, but the patient progressively becomes more hypotensive. His hypotension is unresponsive to blood transfusion. Systolic blood pressure falls to 70, and the patient is tachycardic with a heart rate of 150. The next step in management should be:*

**A** *Proceed with zone I resuscitative endovascular balloon occlusion of the aorta (REBOA)*
**B** *Proceed with zone III REBOA*
**C** *Begin Levophed infusion*
**D** *Immediate transfer to interventional radiology suite for pelvic angiogram and embolization*
**E** *Infuse 1L crystalloid*

For the trauma patient in extremis with noncompressible abdominal or pelvic hemorrhage, REBOA is gaining popularity as an alternative to resuscitative thoracotomy and aortic clamping. Aortic occlusion balloons previously required direct cutdown for femoral artery access, but with the advent of balloons that are compatible with a 7 French sheath, aortic occlusion balloons can now be placed percutaneously with no need to close an arteriotomy. Seldinger technique is utilized to place the

balloon, and confirmation of placement can be done via x-ray. The balloon is inflated in the appropriate zone of the aorta according to injury pattern. Zone I extends from the origin of the left subclavian to the celiac trunk. Inflation of the balloon here is ideal for abdominal hemorrhage. Zone II extends from the celiac to the renal arteries. Inflation of the balloon in zone II should be avoided. Zone III extends from the renal arteries to the bifurcation of the aorta. Inflation in zone III is ideal for hemorrhage from pelvic fractures, or from iliac or femoral arterial hemorrhage. Placement can be confirmed by ultrasound or x-ray. Thoracic hemorrhage is still best treated with thoracotomy. The patient then can be stabilized and transferred to the operating room or interventional radiology for definitive control of hemorrhage.

**Answer: B**

Biffl, W.L., Fox, C.J., Moore, E.E. (2015) The role of REBOA in the control of exsanguinating torso hemorrhage. *The Journal of Trauma and Acute Care Surgery*, **78** (5), 1054–1058.

Martinelli, T., Thony, F., Declety, P., *et al.* (2010) Intra-aortic balloon occlusion to salvage patients with life-threatening hemorrhagic shock from pelvic fractures. *The Journal of Trauma*, **68** (4), 942–948.

**19** *Regarding intra-abdominal hypertension (IAH) and abdominal compartment syndrome (ACS) which of the following statements is true?*

**A** *ACS can affect multiple organ systems including neurologic, cardiac, pulmonary, gastrointestinal, hepatic, and renal*
**B** *Temporary abdominal closure effectively precludes the diagnosis of ACS*
**C** *A bladder pressure of < 20 mm Hg effectively rules out the diagnosis of ACS*
**D** *Physical examination is a reliable method for diagnosing IAH and ACS*
**E** *Non-invasive therapies rarely succeed in treating IAH or ACS*

Abdominal compartment syndrome is defined by the World Society of the Abdominal Compartment Syndrome as sustained IAH >20 mm Hg associated with new organ dysfunction or failure. Intra-abdominal hypertension is defined as a sustained intra-abdominal pressure of 12 mm Hg or greater. Abdominal compartment syndrome can affect many body systems including neurologic, cardiac, pulmonary, gastrointestinal, hepatic, and genitourinary. Risk factors for ACS include severe intra-abdominal trauma, high volume resuscitation, intra-abdominal sepsis, and inflammatory states such as pancreatitis or severe burns. The increasing use of temporary abdominal closure methods may decrease risks of IAH/ACS, however, while ACS is less likely it is not impossible. Patients at high risk for ACS, or those with new onset organ failure should have measurements of their intra-abdominal pressure even if a temporary closure is used. As with other types of compartment syndrome, the absolute value of intra-abdominal pressure is not as important as the perfusion pressure and the clinical picture. A patient may have ACS with organ failure with intra-abdominal pressures below 20 mm Hg, conversely patients with abdominal pressures above 20 mm Hg may not display adverse physiology. The most accurate way to determine intra-abdominal pressure is with intravesicular measurement. Physical examination has a very poor sensitivity even in experienced individuals with sensitivity ranging from 40–60%. Treatment includes adequate sedation, pain control, pharmacologic paralysis, nasogastric decompression, percutaneous catheter decompression, and surgical decompression. Non-invasive methods of treatment especially pharmacologic paralysis and catheter decompression have been shown to be very effective in treating IAH, and even ACS in certain patient populations.

**Answer: A**

Cheatham, M.L., Malbrain, M.L., Kirkpatrick, A., *et al.* (2007) Results from the international conference of experts on intra-abdominal hypertension and abdominal compartment syndrome. II Recommendations. *Intensive Care Medicine*, **33**, 951–962.

Atema, J.J., van Buijtenen, J.M., Lamme, B., and Boermeester, M.A. (2014) Clinical studies on intra-abdominal hypertension and abdominal compartment syndrome. *Journal of Trauma and Acute Care Surgery*, **76** (1), 234–240.

# 32

## Orthopedic and Hand Trauma

*Brett D. Crist, MD and Gregory J. Della Rocca, MD*

**1** *A 45-year-old woman sustains a pelvis fracture (Figure 31.1) and is hypotensive with no other injury. The type of pelvis fracture that application of a pelvic binder or sheet will significantly reduce pelvic volume is:*

**A** *Anterior-posterior compression fracture type 3*
**B** *Lateral compression fracture type 1*
**C** *Vertical shear fracture*
**D** *Lateral compression fracture type 3*
**E** *Anterior-posterior compression fracture type 1*

Commercially available pelvic binders or standard bed sheets have been incorporated into the acute management of pelvic fractures to aid in patient transport and resuscitation. They should be applied at the level of the greater trochanters. The primary function of these devices is to reduce pelvic volume, therefore fractures that do not have increased pelvic volume like lateral compression injuries or vertical shear injuries, pelvic compression devices are unnecessary. APC 1 injuries do not have a significant increase in pelvic volume either. However, APC 3 injuries have a significant increase in pelvic volume and benefit from external compression devices.

Pelvic binders have been shown to generate more compression than sheets and have been thought to more effectively reduce the pelvic volume to an amount similar to the reduction obtained with definitive surgical management. Pelvic binders reduce transfusion requirements, the length of hospital stay and mortality in patients with APC injuries. It is important to remember that sheets can be used instead of commercial binders. Prolonged use of binders or sheets may lead to pressure ulcers and nerve palsies. Regular skin checks should be performed to minimize this risk, particularly in patients that are having large fluid shifts. Furthermore, definitive management of the pelvic ring injury should be performed as early as the patient status allows, to minimize the risk of skin and neurological issues.

**Answer: A**

Langford, J.R., Burgess, A.R., Liporace, F.A., and Haidukewych, G.J. (2013) Pelvic fractures: part 1. Evaluation, classification, and resuscitation. *Journal of the American Academy of Orthopedic Surgeons*, **21** (8), 448–457.
Spanjersberg, W.R., Knops, S.P., Schep, N.W., *et al.* (2009) Effectiveness and complications of pelvic circumferential compression devices in patients with unstable pelvic fractures: a systematic review of literature. *Injury*, **40** (10), 1031–1035.

**2** *An 18-year-old female sustained an Anterior-Posterior Compression type 3 pelvic fracture. She has a pelvic binder in place and remains hemodynamically unstable intraoperatively after splenectomy and 3 units of PRBC and 3 units of FFP. There are no other known sources of uncontrolled bleeding. The next step in resuscitating this patient should include:*

**A** *Transfuse 3 more units PRBC and 3 FFP and reassess*
**B** *Repeat a chest-abdomen-pelvis CT*
**C** *Transfer to angiography for pelvic arterial embolization*
**D** *Perform retroperitoneal packing*
**E** *Repeat head CT*

The most common causes of bleeding associated with pelvic fractures are injuries to the posterior venous plexus and cancellous fracture surfaces (85–90%). Approximately 10–15% of bleeding is associated with injures to branches of the internal iliac system (superior

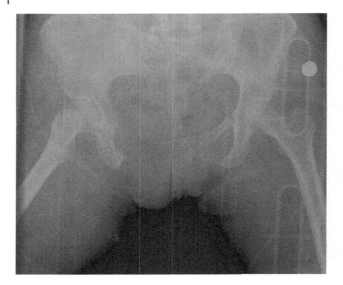

**Figure 32.1**

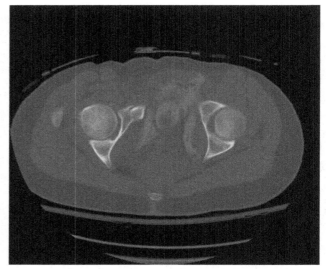

**Figure 32.2**

gluteal or pudendal arteries). Although decreasing the pelvic volume is an important first step, patients that are in the operating room and continue to be hemodynamically unstable after all other known sources of bleeding are addressed should undergo retroperitoneal packing to address the venous and bony bleeding that occurs. Hemodynamically unstable patients should not be transferred to the CT scanner. The patient has already received adequate fluid resuscitation; another source of bleeding must be identified and addressed. Since the patient is already in the operating room and the most likely cause of pelvic bleeding is venous, or fracture surfaces, pre- or retroperitoneal packing should be performed before going to angiography. If continued hypotension occurs after packing and external fixation, then angiography is done to address the probable arterial injury. Following this protocol, only 16.7% of hemodynamically unstable patients required subsequent embolization and there were no mortalities.

**Answer: D**

Langford, J.R., Burgess, A.R., Liporace, F.A., and Haidukewych, G.J. (2013) Pelvic fractures: part 1. Evaluation, classification, and resuscitation. *Journal of the American Academy of Orthopedic Surgeons*, **21** (8), 448–457.

Cothren, C.C., Osborn, P.M., Moore, E.E., et al. (2007) Preperitoneal pelvic packing for hemodynamically unstable pelvic fractures: a paradigm shift. *Jornal of Trauma*, **62** (4), 834–839, 839–842.

**3** *A 25-year-old male sustains a pelvic fracture (Figure 32.2) and has an associated bladder injury. What*

*Young and Burgess fracture type is most commonly associated with a bladder rupture?*
**A** *Vertical shear mechanism*
**B** *Lateral compression mechanism*
**C** *Antero-posterior compression mechanism*
**D** *Combined mechanism*
**E** *Transverse mechanism*

Injuries to the bladder and urethra occur in ~15–20% of patients with pelvic fractures. Bladder injuries are more commonly associated with lateral compression fractures, whereas urethral injuries are more commonly seen in patients with anterior-posterior compression fractures. This pattern makes sense because the fractured rami are forced into the bladder with the lateral compression injuries. Vertical and combined mechanisms are less common causes. A transverse mechanism is not part of the Young and Burgess classification. Mortality may be as high as 34% in patients with bladder ruptures and pelvic fractures. Gross hematuria is the most reliable clinical finding, noted in 95% of pelvic fracture patients with bladder injury, while microscopic hematuria is seen in the remaining 5%.

**Answer: B**

Durkin, A., Sagi, H.C., Durham, R., *et al.* (2006) Contemporary management of pelvic fractures. *American Journal of Surgery*, **192** (2), 211–223.

Fallon, B., Wendt, J.C., and Hawtrey, C.E. (1984) Urological injury and assessment in patients with fractured pelvis. *Journal of Urology*, **131** (4), 712–714.

**4** *A 32-year-old man has an isolated pelvic fracture involving his left hemipelvis and is hemodynamically* *stable. Initial inpatient DVT prophylaxis should consist of:*

**A** *Mechanical prophylaxis and 325 mg aspirin daily*
**B** *Mechanical prophylaxis alone*
**C** *Subcutaneous heparin 5000 units twice daily*
**D** *Low molecular weight heparin within 24 hours*
**E** *Low molecular weight heparin started after 48 hours*

Although it is universal to use DVT prophylaxis in patients with pelvic fractures, the exact protocol used may differ significantly. A systematic review looking at DVT prophylaxis for pelvis and acetabular fractures evaluated 11 studies involving 1760 patients. Due to the limited and poorly controlled data available, no consistent protocol could be recommended except for following published guidelines for the general trauma population. However, low molecular weight heparin started within 24 hours of admission or within 24 hours of hemodynamic stability in patients with pelvic and acetabular fractures had a significantly lower DVT and PE rates when compared to patients started after 24 hours. The 2008 CHEST guidelines do not recommend post-hospital discharge chemoprophylaxis in pelvic fracture patients that can ambulate (although it may be limited), have no other DVT risk factors, and are not undergoing inpatient rehabilitation. This clinical condition was not specifically mentioned in the 2012 CHEST guidelines update.

**Answer: D**

Geerts, W.H., Bergqvist, D., Pineo, G.F., *et al.* (2008) Prevention of venous thromboembolism: American College of Chest Physicians evidence-based clinical practice guidelines (8th edn). *Chest*, **133** (6 Suppl.), 381S–453S.
Slobogean, G.P., Lefaivre, K.A., Nicolaou, S., *et al.* (2009) A systematic review of thromboprophylaxis for pelvic and acetabular fractures. *Journal of Orthopedic Trauma* **23** (5), 379–384.

**5** *Women that sustain pelvic ring injuries are most likely to complain of:*

**A** *Leg length discrepancy*
**B** *Posterior pelvic pain*
**C** *Dyspareunia*
**D** *Genitourinary dysfunction*
**E** *Low back pain*

Although patients that sustain pelvic ring injuries complain of pelvic and low back pain, women have significant risk for pain with sexual intercourse (dyspareunia). Two retrospective reviews show that the incidence of dyspareunia is up to 91% of the time.

Anteroposterior Compression (APC) fractures have the highest incidence – 91%. Women have a high incidence of genitourinary complaints (49%). It is critical to investigate these issues with women that have pelvic ring injuries to address them as able. Of note, women have a more than double rate of having a cesarean section after having a pelvic fracture. The rate of low back pain, posterior pelvic pain, and leg length discrepancy is not different from men.

**Answer: C**

Cannada, L.K. and Barr, J. (2010) Pelvic fractures in women of childbearing age. *Clinical Orthopaedics and Related Research*, **468** (7), 1781–1789.
Vallier, H.A., Cureton, B.A., and Schubeck, D. (2012) Pelvic ring injury is associated with sexual dysfunction in women. *Journal of Orthopedic Trauma*, **26** (5), 308–313.

**6** *A 25-year-old man is struck by a motor vehicle and sustains a Gustilo and Anderson type IIIA open tibia fracture (Figure 32.3). Which of the following will most likely decrease his risk of infection?*

**A** *Operative debridement within 18 hours of injury*
**B** *Operative debridement within 6 hours of injury*
**C** *Antibiotic administration within 24 hours of injury*
**D** *Antibiotic administration within 3 hours of injury*
**E** *Intramedullary nailing of the tibia within 12 hours*

Several factors have been evaluated to look at the risk of infection after open fractures. Of the factors listed, early antibiotic administration is the most appropriate answer. Antibiotic administration within 3 hours of injury significantly reduced the rate of infection in a series of 1104 open fractures compared to patients

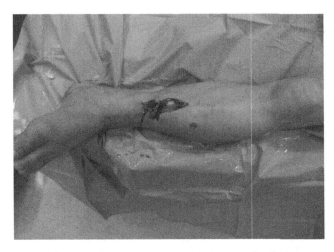

**Figure 32.3** Gustilo and Anderson type IIIA open tibia fracture. A full-color version of this figure appears in the plate section of this book.

receiving antibiotics > 3 hours from injury or no antibiotics at all. The goal should be that the patient receives antibiotics within 3 hours from injury and within 1 hour from admission. The timing of surgical debridement as long as it is within 24 hours has not been shown to reduce infection of open fractures significantly.

**Answer: D**

Pollak, A.N., Jones, A.L., Castillo, R.C., *et al.* (2010) The relationship between time to surgical debridement and incidence of infection after open high-energy lower extremity trauma. *Journal of Bone and Joint Surgery, American Volume*, **92** (1), 7–15.

7 *The same 25-year-old received his antibiotics for his type IIIA open tibia fracture upon arrival to the emergency room. He goes to the operating room within 6 hours for formal debridement and definitive fixation with an intramedullary nail. His traumatic wound is closed primarily. How long should intravenous cefazolin be continued postoperatively?*
   A *24 hours*
   B *48 hours*
   C *72 hours*
   D *12 hours*
   E *6 hours*

The most recent guidelines based on the best available data state that for most open fractures, 24 hours of cefazolin after operative debridement and definitive soft tissue management (closure for this patient) is adequate. Exceptions could be those with significant gross contamination like a type IIIB tibia fracture where 72 hours could be indicated.

**Answer: A**

Halawi, M.J. and Morwood, M.P. (2015) Acute management of open fractures: an evidence-based review. *Orthopedics*, **38** (11), e1025–1033.
Hoff, W.S., Bonadies, J.A., Cachecho, R., and Dorlac, W.C. (2011) East Practice Management Guidelines Work Group: update to practice management guidelines for prophylactic antibiotic use in open fractures. *Journal of Trauma*, **70** (3), 751–754.

8 *A 22-year-old man sustains a Gustilo and Anderson type 2 open tibia and fibula fractures with an 8 cm anteromedial tibial wound without gross contamination and no neurovascular compromise. His GCS score is 7 and is noted to have a left-sided intraparenchymal cerebral hemorrhage. Formal operative irrigation and debridement and stabilization of his open tibia fracture should occur:*

   A *As soon as the OR is ready*
   B *Within 6 hours*
   C *When his head injury allows*
   D *Within 12 hours*
   E *Within 24 hours*

The "6-hour" rule for debridement of open fractures originated from an 1898 presentation by Paul Leopold Frederich where he contaminated guinea pigs with garden mold and stair dust to illustrate the importance of surgical debridement. In this antiquated animal study, debridement of the contaminated wound was less likely to be effective after 6 to 8 hours. Several studies have shown no association between timing of debridement and infection when debridement occurs within 24 hours. Others have shown a difference between debridement within 6 hours and less than 24 hours. However, all of these studies either have flawed study designs or too small a sample size to gain statistical significance. Therefore, emergent debridement is not necessarily supported, but neither is elective debridement. Current practice is based on best evidence and includes debridement of open fractures urgently when the life-threatening emergencies have been addressed, patient's medical condition is stabilized and when the appropriate surgical resources are available.

**Answer: C**

Halawi, M.J. and Morwood, M.P. (2015) Acute management of open fractures: an evidence-based review. *Orthopedics*, **38** (11), e1025–1033.
Werner, C.M., Pierpont, Y., and Pollak, A.N. (2008) The urgency of surgical debridement in the management of open fractures. *Journal of the American Academy of Orthopedic Surgeons*, **16** (7), 369–375.

9 *A 17-year-old boy sustains a distal one-third Gustilo and Anderson type IIIB open tibia fracture with an associated fibula fracture during a motorcycle accident. What finding would push you toward performing a below-knee amputation:*
   A *5 cm of missing tibial bone*
   B *No plantar foot sensation*
   C *Inability to actively dorsiflex the ankle*
   D *No dorsalis pedis pulse*
   E *Transected tibial nerve*

A visibly documented transected tibial nerve is the only answer above that should have a patient consider an amputation. Inability to actively dorsiflex the ankle could be related to the fracture and associated pain. As long as there is an identifiable posterior tibialis pulse, the absence of a dorsalis pedis pulse should not indicate an amputation. Missing 5 cm of tibial bone can be reconstructed with a variety of bone grafting techniques. The lack of plantar foot sensation alone no longer indicates amputation. The Lower Extremity Assessment Project (LEAP) was a multi-center prospective outcome study that involved 601 patients with severe, limb-threatening lower extremity patients that compared limb salvage versus amputation. Of patients in the limb salvage group with a lack of plantar sensation upon admission, 67% had the complete return of plantar sensation within 24 months. There were no significant outcome differences found between the insensate salvage, insensate amputation, and the sensate control groups. The presence or absence of plantar sensation should not be used to direct treatment.

**Answer: E**

Bosse, M.J., McCarthy, M.L., Jones, A.L., *et al.* (2005) The insensate foot following severe lower extremity trauma: an indication for amputation? *Journal of Bone and Joint Surgery, American Volume,* **87,** 2601–2608.

10 *The surgeon taking care of the same 17-year-old with the type 3B open tibia fracture is trying to determine the best antibiotic prophylaxis. He has no medical allergies. The most appropriate antibiotic(s) to start include:*
   A *Vancomycin*
   B *Penicillin*
   C *Gentamicin and Penicillin*
   D *Ancef and Gentamicin*
   E *Vancomycin and Gentamicin*

Antibiotic prophylaxis has been based on the type of open fracture. Type 1, 2 and 3A = 3rd-generation cephalosporin. Type 3B and C = 3rd-generation cephalosporin and aminoglycoside to add gram-negative bacterial coverage. Penicillin is added if there is a concern for anaerobes. Although there are investigations into using 4th-generation cephalosporins only, the current clinical guidelines still follow the classic recommendations.

**Answer: D**

Halawi, M.J. and Morwood, M.P. (2015) Acute management of open fractures: an evidence-based review. *Orthopedics,* **38** (11), e1025–1033.

11 *A 23-year-old man sustains a closed tibial and fibular shaft fracture and is splinted. He has a GCS score of 14 and is complaining of numbness in his leg. He has leg pain that is not improved with IV morphine, loosening of his splint or elevation of his leg; and has increased leg pain with passive flexion and extension*

*of his great toe. His posterior tibialis pulse is 2+/4, and capillary refill is 3 seconds. The next step in this patient's management should include:*
   A *Compartment pressure evaluation*
   B *Perform ankle-brachial indices*
   C *Anesthesia consult for regional nerve block*
   D *Emergent fasciotomies*
   E *IV Toradol and re-examine in 1 hour*

In an awake and alert patient, pain is the earliest and most sensitive clinical sign of compartment syndrome. After the fracture is immobilized in a splint, passive motion of the muscles within the involved compartments (i.e., moving the great toe involves stretching the anterior and deep posterior leg compartments) has been used to correlate with a diagnosis of compartment syndrome. Paresthesia is also an early clinical sign. If these signs develop after splinting, the first step should be loosening any constrictive splint/dressing and elevation of the extremity up to the level of the heart. Elevation above the heart should be avoided to maximize perfusion. Since outcomes associated with compartment syndrome are associated with time to fasciotomy, if clinical signs indicate a high likelihood that the patient has a compartment syndrome, compartment pressure monitoring should be bypassed, and emergent fasciotomies should be performed. Ankle-brachial indices are indicated in knee dislocations and would be too difficult to do in someone with a tibia fracture. Having anesthesia do a regional nerve block would mask an evolving compartment syndrome since pain is the best early indicator. Continued IV pain medication is not indicated if his symptoms and signs are progressing.

**Answer: D**

Frink, M., Hildebrand, F., Krettek, C., *et al.* (2010) Compartment syndrome of the lower leg and foot. *Clinical Orthopaedics and Related Research,* **468** (4), 940–950.
Schmidt, A.H. (2016) Acute compartment syndrome. *Orthopedic Clinics of North America,* **47** (3), 517–525.

12 *If you are sued because a patient has an extremity compartment syndrome, you are most likely to lose if it is associated with a/an:*
   A *Upper extremity injury*
   B *Open fracture*
   C *Eventual amputation*
   D *Delay in fasciotomy*
   E *Associated vascular injury*

Compartment syndrome can have devastating complications that can be avoided with early diagnosis and fasciotomy. Bhattacharyya *et al.* reviewed medical mal-practice claims and identified these risk factors associated with unsuccessful defense and increased liability:

- Physician documentation of abnormal findings on neurological exam but no action was taken
- Poor physician communication
- Increased number of cardinal signs (pain, pallor, pulse-lessness, paralysis, pain with passive stretch)
- Increased time to fasciotomy

**Answer: D**

Bhattacharyya, T. and Vrahas, M.S. (2004) The medical-legal aspects of compartment syndrome. *Journal of Bone and Joint Surgery, American Volume*, **86-A** (4), 864–868.

**13** *A 35-year-old man with a closed right tibia fracture has a GCS score of 8 secondarily to a closed head injury and is intubated. You are concerned about compartment syndrome. His blood pressure is 110/80 mm Hg. His anterior compartment pressure is 55 mm Hg. When undergoing fasciotomies, the fasciotomy incision (Figure 32.4) should be at least how many centimeters (cm) to adequately decompress the involved leg compartment?*
   A *5 cm*
   B *8 cm*
   C *10 cm*
   D *15 cm*
   E *20 cm*

When using dual incision fasciotomies for acute trau-matic leg compartment syndrome, at least 16 cm long was required to decompress the leg compartments. The pressures kept decreasing until the incision reached

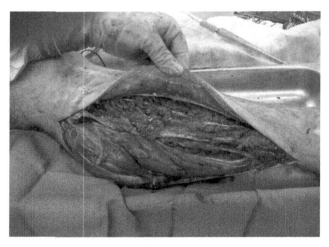

**Figure 32.4** A full-color version of this figure appears in the plate section of this book.

16 cm. Although several different compartment pressure thresholds have been used to determine when fasciotomies should be performed, the current pressure used in tibial fractures is less than a 30 mm Hg difference from the diastolic blood pressure as shown by McQueen *et al.* prospectively. A differential pressure of 30 mm Hg led to no missed cases of acute compartment syndrome and avoided unnecessary fasciotomies. The indication to use invasive compartment pressure monitoring in this patient is the fact that he is obtunded and intubated.

**Answer: E**

Frink, M., Hildebrand, F., Krettek, C., *et al.* (2010) Compartment syndrome of the lower leg and foot. *Clinical Orthopaedics and Related Research*, **468** (4), 940–950.
McQueen, M.M. and Court-Brown, C.M. (1996) Compartment monitoring in tibial fractures. The pressure threshold for decompression. *Journal of Bone and Joint Surgery, British Volume*, **78** (1), 99–104.

**14** *A 20-year-old man was struck by a motor vehicle while walking. He has a large right-knee effusion and has a positive Lachman test (anterior knee laxity at 30° of flexion), posterior drawer test (posterior knee laxity at 90°), and is unstable to varus and valgus stress at 30° of flexion. A lateral knee radiograph shows 7 mm of anterior subluxation of the tibia on the distal femur. His right lower extremity pulse was 1+/4 and is asymmetric. After stabilizing the knee in a long leg splint, his pulse does not change. The next step in management should include:*
   A *Re-evaluation in one hour*
   B *Ankle-brachial index determination*
   C *Duplex ultrasound*
   D *Arteriogram*
   E *Emergent surgery for revascularization of the extremity and external fixation of the knee*

The patient has clinical exam findings of an ACL tear (positive Lachman test), PCL tear (posterior drawer test), and MCL and LCL tears (unstable to varus and valgus stress). Numerous studies have shown that routine angiography after knee dislocation is no longer necessary. Ten studies, including two prospective trials, evaluated 543 patients with knee dislocations and showed that physical exam alone was sufficient to identify clinically significant vascular injuries. Furthermore, many of the vascular injuries associated with knee dislocations are non-flow-limiting arterial intimal tears. Current management of intimal tears in patients with normal vascular examinations includes observation and serial examinations. An arteriogram is indicated in any patient with an abnormal vascular exam. Since this patient had an asymmetric pulse, arteriogram was indicated. The asymmetric pulse also precludes the need for Ankle-Brachial index evaluation. Ultrasound is not indicated in a patient with an acute arterial injury. An arteriogram is indicated before surgery as long as getting the arteriogram does not lead to significant delay. The arteriogram could be done in the operating room before revascularization if resources are available.

**Answer: D**

Levy, B.A., Fanelli, G.C., Whelan, D.B., *et al.* (2009) Controversies in the treatment of knee dislocations and multiligament reconstruction. *Journal of the American Academy of Orthopedic Surgeons,* **17** (4), 197–206.

15 *A 46-year-old morbidly obese (BMI = 50) female sustains a knee dislocation after tripping over her cat. Compared to a 25-year-old male with a BMI of 30 that sustains a knee dislocation after a motor vehicle crash, the morbidly obese patient is less likely to:*
   A *Require an above knee amputation*
   B *Have an associated nerve injury*
   C *Require vascular repair*
   D *Require a formal reduction maneuver*
   E *Have a nerve and vascular injury*

Knee dislocations occur from both high and low energy mechanisms. They are 4 times more likely to occur in males. Around 50% of knee dislocations spontaneously reduce in both patient groups. Patients with a BMI greater than 40 are more likely to sustain a dislocation after activities of daily living. When compared to knee dislocations related to high energy trauma, obese patients with low energy dislocations are more likely to sustain a vascular injury (40%), require a vascular repair (40%) and have both a combined nerve and vascular injury. However, obese patients with low energy dislocations are less likely to require an above knee amputation – 11% vs. ~20%.

**Answer: A**

Azar, F.M., Brandt, J.C., Miller, R.H., 3rd, and Phillips, B.B. (2011) Ultra-low-velocity knee dislocations. *American Journal of Sports Medicine,* **39** (10), 2170–2174.
Boyce, R.H., Singh, K., and Obremskey, W.T. (2015) Acute management of traumatic knee dislocations for the generalist. *Journal of the American Academy of Orthopedic Surgeons,* **23** (12), 761–768.

16 *A 26-year-old male fell 8 feet from a ladder and complains of radial-sided right wrist pain. There's no obvious deformity. He has no other complaints. He did have loss of consciousness with no findings on*

head CT. *Radiographs of the wrist show no obvious fracture. You should treat his wrist pain with:*
   A *CT scan of wrist*
   B *MRI of wrist*
   C *Wrist splint and re-evaluate in 10–14 days*
   D *Orthopedic surgery consult in the ER*
   E *Activities as tolerated*

Wrist pain without acute radiographic findings occur. Radial-sided wrist pain may indicate an occult scaphoid fracture. These can be initially missed up to 60% of the time. If there are no definitive radiographic findings, the best plan is to immobilize the wrist and repeat evaluation – radiographs and clinical exam in approximately 10–14 days. If they still have radial-sided wrist pain, then referral to an orthopedic surgeon is appropriate. Generally, advanced imaging is not indicated acutely in the ER. Activities, as tolerated, may cause displacement of the fracture or poor pain control.

**Answer: C**

Kang, L. (2015) Operative treatment of acute scaphoid fractures. *Hand Surgery,* **20** (2), 210–214.

17 *A 32-year-old right-hand dominant man sustains a table saw injury. He presents with right thumb, index and middle finger amputations through the proximal phalanx. He brought his amputated digits with him. The injury occurred 30 minutes ago. The most appropriate definitive management includes:*
   A *Replantation of all digits*
   B *Replantation of the index finger only and revision amputation of the thumb and middle finger*
   C *Revision amputation of all digits through the metacarpophalangeal joints*
   D *Attempted replantation of the middle finger and revision amputation of the index finger and thumb*
   E *Attempted replantation of the thumb only with revisions amputation of the other digits*

Thumb, multiple digit amputations, and pediatric digit amputations are indications for replantation. Single digit replantation is always indicated for the thumb but is also considered in the other digits if the amputation is distal to the insertion of flexor digitorum superficialis and a sharp mechanism. Amputations secondary to significant crush or avulsion injuries are typically not replantable. Sharp-cut amputations in young and healthy patients are ideal. Maximum ischemia time for digits includes: 12 hours warm and 24 hours cold. However, up to 96 hours, cold ischemia time has been reported for digits.

**Answer: A**

Waikakul, S., Sakkarnkosol, S., Vanadurongwan, V., and Unnanuntana, A. (2000) Results of 1018 digital replantations in 552 patients. *Injury*, **31**(1), 33–40.

Wolfe, V.M. and Wang, A.A. (2015) Replantation of the upper extremity: current concepts. *Journal of the American Academy of Orthopedic Surgeons*, **23** (6), 373–381.

18 *An intoxicated 18-year-old male was thrown from his vehicle in a single vehicle rollover accident. He presents to the trauma bay with a GCS of 14, hemo-dynamically stable and complains of right hip pain. His right leg is flexed, shortened, internally rotated and neurovascularly intact. The most appropriate next step is:*

   A *CT scan of the pelvis*
   B *Attempted closed reduction of his right hip*
   C *AP pelvis radiograph*
   D *Consult Orthopaedic Surgery*
   E *AP right hip radiograph*

The most likely diagnosis is a dislocated right hip. However, closed reduction should not be performed without radiographic evaluation because the acetabulum or femoral head/neck may be fractured as well. Attempted closed reduction before imaging could increase the likelihood of damaging the femoral head or neck. The hip should be reduced as quickly as possible after the AP pelvis radiograph is completed, so going to CT should not be done because the patient is hemodynamically stable and alert. Getting a CT scan would delay diagnosis and reduction. An AP hip radiograph would show the hip dislocation but would not show an associated pelvic or opposite hip injury. Orthopedic surgery should be consulted, but obtaining an AP pelvis radiograph is the first step in making the correct diagnosis.

**Answer: C**

Foulk, D.M. and Mullis, B.H. (2010) Hip dislocation: evaluation and management. *Journal of the American Academy of Orthopedic Surgeons*, **18** (4), 199–209.

19 *A 50-year-old woman fell 5 feet and has a dorsally displaced distal radius fracture with associated volar index and middle finger numbness. The symptoms progress after closed reduction and splinting. The symptoms do not improve with loosening the splint. To minimize the risk of permanent neurological deficits, a carpal tunnel release should be performed:*

   A *Within 24 hours*
   B *Within 48 hours*
   C *Within 2 hours*
   D *Within 12 hours*
   E *Within 6 hours*

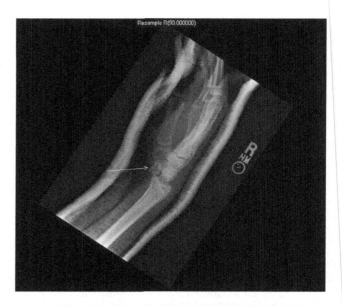

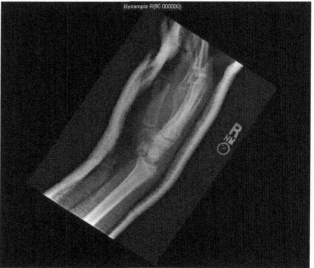

**Figure 32.5** A lateral wrist x-ray with a volarly dislocated lunate (white arrow) indicating a perilunate dislocation.

Nerve injury occurs in ~17% of distal radius fractures with the median nerve most commonly involved. Acute carpal tunnel syndrome occurs most frequently in patients with higher energy and comminuted distal radius fractures. It can also happen in patients that undergo multiple closed reductions. If carpal tunnel symptoms progress after elevation, loosening of the splint and minimizing flexion of the wrist, a carpal tunnel release should be performed *emergently*. Patients undergoing early release have better long-term outcomes than those treated in a delayed manner.

**Answer: C**

Gillig, J.D., White, S.D., and Rachel, J.N. (2016) Acute carpal tunnel syndrome: a review of current literature. *Orthopedics Clinics of North America*, **47** (3), 599–607.

20  *An 18-year-old boy falls 10 feet off of a ladder. He is complaining of right wrist pain. He has significantly limited range of wrist motion and an obvious deformity. Wrist radiographs show no distal radius fracture. The injury that must be ruled out to avoid a poor outcome if diagnosed in a delayed fashion is:*

    **A** *Scapholunate ligament injury*
    **B** *Third metacarpal base fracture*
    **C** *Perilunate dislocation*
    **D** *Scaphoid fracture*
    **E** *Hamate fracture*

Although any of the diagnoses listed above may cause pain and minor deformity in the wrist/carpal area, only a perilunate dislocation (Figure 32.5) will lead to limited wrist range of motion. Up to 25% of perilunate injuries are missed on initial evaluation. A high-quality lateral wrist radiograph is required for diagnosis. To avoid missing these injuries, a normal lateral wrist radiograph will show the lunate and capitate bones located in their fossa. Delay in diagnosis and management leads to poor outcomes and are more likely to require salvage procedures including proximal row carpectomy.

**Answer: C**

Muppavarapu, R.C. and Capo, J.T. (2015) Perilunate dislocations and fracture-dislocations. *Hand Clinic*, **31** (3), 399–408.

# 33

# Peripheral Vascular Trauma
*Amy V. Gore, MD and Adam D. Fox, DO*

**1** *A 19-year-old man arrives by police after sustaining a gunshot wound to the right thigh. He was reportedly hypotensive in the field, however, he is hemodynamically normal on arrival to the trauma bay. Physical examination is notable for a single wound in the medial distal thigh, which is not actively bleeding. Distal pulse evaluation reveals 2+ dorsalis pedis and posterior tibial pulses bilaterally, however, the patient exhibits decreased sensation on the anterior and medial aspect of the thigh. Plain films are significant for a retained foreign body in the lateral aspect of the thigh without evidence of fracture. Which of the following statements is correct?*

**A** *The patient can be safely discharged from the trauma bay without further diagnostic workup as the patient does not have any evidence of vascular "hard signs"*

**B** *Further diagnostic testing for vascular trauma is indicated because the patient has a sensory defect suggestive of femoral nerve injury*

**C** *The patient should be admitted and observed because despite a normal peripheral pulse examination, the patient may have an underlying vascular injury given proximity of his injury to major vessels*

**D** *Further diagnostic testing for vascular trauma is indicated because the patient has a history of hypotension in the field*

**E** *Angiography is indicated because the trajectory of the projectile appears to be in proximity to the major vascular structures in the thigh*

The presence of a vascular "hard sign" (pulsatile bleeding, expanding hematoma, palpable thrill, audible bruit, loss of pulse) is highly specific for major vascular injury and mandates operative exploration, however, absence of hard signs does not reliably exclude injury. In contrast, the "soft signs" of vascular injury (non-expanding hematoma, injury to adjacent nerve, proximity to major blood vessels, unexplained hypotension, or history of prehospital hemorrhage) do not reliably predict major vascular trauma. As delay in operative intervention for a missed injury can potentially be limb-threatening, historically there has been a low threshold for operative exploration when there was any suspicion of vascular injury. High rates of negative exploration lead to liberal use of angiography as an alternative, but this too was associated with a high rate of studies that demonstrated either no injury or injuries that did not require intervention. It is now generally accepted that in the absence of hard signs, patients with a normal peripheral vascular examination do not require further investigation regardless of the presence of soft signs. When angiography is performed under these circumstances, roughly 10% of patients will be found to have an injury, but the natural history of the vast majority of these "minimal vascular injuries" is to resolve without intervention. Physical examination in conjunction with a 24-hour period of observation has been shown to have a false negative rate of less than 1% for major vascular injury, comparable to that of angiography.

**Answer: C**

Ashworth, E.M., Dalsing, M.C., Glover, J.L., and Reilly, M.K. (1988) Lower extremity vascular trauma: a comprehensive, aggressive approach. *Journal of Trauma*, **28** (3), 329–336.

Frykberg, E.R., Crump, J.M., Dennis, J.W., *et al.* (1991) Nonoperative observation of clinically occult arterial injuries: a prospective evaluation. *Surgery*, **109** (1), 85–96.

Frykberg, E.R., Dennis, J.W., Bishop, K., *et al.* (1991) The reliability of physical examination in the evaluation of penetrating extremity trauma for vascular injury: Results at one year. *Journal of Trauma*, **31** (4), 502–11.

*Surgical Critical Care and Emergency Surgery: Clinical Questions and Answers*, Second Edition.
Edited by Forrest "Dell" Moore, Peter Rhee, and Gerard J. Fulda.
© 2018 John Wiley & Sons Ltd. Published 2018 by John Wiley & Sons Ltd.
Companion website: www.wiley.com/go/moore/surgical_criticalcare_and_emergency_surgery

**2** *Regarding the use of diagnostic testing in the evaluation of peripheral vascular trauma, which of the following is correct?*

 A *An arterial pressure index (API) < 0.9 is an indication for operative exploration*

 B *A normal physical examination and an API > 0.9 reliably excludes all vascular injuries*

 C *Compared to CT angiography, conventional angiography is more sensitive and specific*

 D *Compared to CT angiography, conventional angiography is associated with greater costs*

 E *Duplex ultrasound is the single best test for evaluation of peripheral vascular trauma*

The arterial pressure index (API) has gained acceptance in some trauma centers as a useful tool in the evaluation of peripheral vascular trauma. Using Doppler ultrasound, the systolic occlusion pressure is measured in the injured limb and compared to an unaffected limb, usually the contralateral extremity. An API < 0.9 has a 95% specificity and 97% specificity for arterial injury. An abnormal API alone is not an indication for operative exploration, but rather for further diagnostic testing. Having a normal API, however, does not reliably exclude injury; lesions that do not always produce significant interruptions in blood flow, such as intimal flaps and pseudoaneurysms, may not affect the API. These lesions have a < 10% risk of requiring surgical intervention. The API also does not detect venous injury or muscle bleeding, which may contribute to the development of compartment syndrome. When the API is < 0.9, further imaging is warranted. While traditionally, conventional angiography has been used, improvements in computed tomography technology have resulted in CT angiography largely supplanting this technique. Seamon *et al.* and Wallin *et al.* have reported equal sensitivity and specificity of CT angiogram in detecting major vascular injury, but with substantial decreases in time and cost. While duplex ultrasonography is non-invasive, it is less sensitive in the diagnosis of peripheral vascular trauma than angiography and requires the presence of a trained ultrasonographer, which may not be available at all times.

**Answer: D**

Sadjadi, J., Cureton, E.L., Dozier, K.C., *et al.* (2009) Expedited treatment of lower extremity gunshot wounds. *Journal of the American College of Surgeons,* **209** (6), 740–745.

Seamon, M.J., Smoger, D., Torres, D.M., *et al.* (2009) A prospective validation of a current practice: the detection of extremity vascular injury with CT angiography. *Journal of Trauma, Injury, Infection, and Critical Care,* **67** (2), 238–243.

Wallin, D., Yaghoubian, A., Rosing, D., *et al.* (2011) Computed tomographic angiography as the primary diagnostic modality in penetrating vascular injuries: a level I trauma experience. *Annals of Vascular Surgery,* **25** (5), 620–623.

**3** *A 24-year-old man sustained a single stab wound to the right thigh with ensuing pulsatile hemorrhage. A tourniquet was applied to the right lower extremity above the level of the injury by EMS in the field, and he was rapidly transported to the trauma center. Speaking with the patient's family after a successful operative repair, they have concerns about the use of the tourniquet. Which of the following is correct?*

 A *Current advanced trauma life support (ATLS) protocol recommends tourniquet application as the first line of treatment for exsanguinating extremity wounds*

 B *The success rate of hemorrhage control using tourniquets is greater with lower extremity wounds than upper extremity wounds*

 C *Tourniquet application with pressures of 200–250 mm Hg is associated with increased venous bleeding*

 D *Tourniquet application for exsanguinating extremity injury is associated with an amputation rate of nearly 30%*

 E *Neurologic injury is a potential complication of tourniquet application, but is unlikely to occur with tourniquet duration less than 2 hours*

There has been a recent resurgence in interest in the use of tourniquets to control active bleeding from extremity wounds, however, according to current ATLS protocol, direct manual pressure remains the first line of treatment. If a tourniquet is applied, it is important to ensure arterial occlusion, (typically by applying pressures between 200–250 mm Hg) as lower pressures may lead to venous outflow occlusion without arterial inflow occlusion, increasing the amount of venous bleeding. Tourniquets are more successful at controlling hemorrhage from upper extremity wounds than lower extremity wounds (94% versus 71%). The risk of peripheral nerve injury as a result of tourniquet application, while low, appears to be related to the duration of ischemia. In a study of 110 tourniquet applications, Lakstein *et al.* found an overall incidence of peripheral nerve injury of 5.5%, with only one case occurring with a tourniquet time less than two hours. A more recent study by Kragh *et al.* reported a ~ 2% risk of neuropathy in 651 limbs. The amputation rate in this series was ~ 15%.

**Answer: E**

Kragh, J.F., Jr., Littrel M.L., Jones J.A., *et al.* (2011) Battle casualty survival with emergency tourniquet use to stop limb bleeding. *Journal of Emergency Medicine*, **41** (6), 590–597.

Lakstein, D., Blumenfeld, A., Sokolov, T., *et al.* (2003) Tourniquets for hemorrhage control on the battlefield: a 4-year accumulated experience. *The Journal of Trauma*, **54** (5 Suppl.), 221–225.

Passos, E., Dingley, B., Smith, A., *et al.* (2014) Tourniquet use for peripheral vascular injuries in the civilian setting. *Injury*, **45** (3), 573–577.

**4** *You receive notice from pre-hospital providers that a 24-year-old woman with multiple lower extremity stab wounds is en route to your trauma center. She is hypotensive and has pulsatile bleeding from the right groin. Which of the following is not a 'key concept' in her operative management?*

 **A** *Temporary control of bleeding*
 **B** *Extensile exposure*
 **C** *Proximal and distal control of bleeding vessels*
 **D** *Local heparinization*
 **E** *Definitive repair of vascular injury*

Reports of an unstable patient with vascular hard signs and reports of copious blood loss in the pre-hospital setting should prompt providers to secure uncrossmatched blood products and alert the blood bank to the need for activation of a massive transfusion protocol, if one is available. Upon arrival to the trauma bay, assessment should proceed according to guidelines established by ATLS. Temporary control of bleeding refers to arresting hemorrhage prior to operative intervention. While this may be accomplished by direct manual pressure; tourniquets may be useful when direct pressure is not an option secondary to massive tissue destruction. Pulsatile hemorrhage from deep wounds may on occasion be temporized by insertion of a Foley catheter into the tract and inflating the balloon to provide tamponade until the bleeding stops. Ultimately, management of these injuries necessitates operative intervention. Extensile exposure refers to the technique of choosing incisions that can be extended proximally or distally along the course of a vessel, even as this vessel courses through different anatomic regions (e.g., chest to upper extremity). Proximal and distal control of bleeding vessels allows for inspection and repair of the area of injury while hemorrhage is arrested; it is often safest to obtain proximal and distal control outside of the zone of injury using the technique of extensile exposure. While systemic heparinization prior to clamping vessels is ideal, this is often not possible in polytrauma patients who may have other sources of bleeding. Therefore, local heparinization of the extremity prior to distal occlusion must usually suffice.

Whether or not to perform definitive repair at the time of index operation requires consideration of the patient's physiology and concomitant injuries. For patients with competing injury priorities or severely deranged physiology, "damage-control" options must be considered: temporary intraluminal shunting or even arterial ligation ("life over limb") may be the most appropriate option.

**Answer: E**

Feliciano, D.V. (2010) Management of peripheral arterial injury. *Current Opinion in Critical Care*, **16** (6), 602–608.

Hirshberg, A. and Mattlox, K. (2005) *Top Knife*. tfm Publishing Ltd, Shrewsbury, UK.

**5** *While working at an international hospital receiving combat injuries after field hospital stabilization, you receive a 22-year-old soldier who sustained a blast injury to the upper extremity. The trauma surgeon who initially stabilized him discovered a brachial artery injury for which he placed a temporary intravascular shunt. Which of the following statements is correct?*

 **A** *Placement of a temporary intravascular shunt does not require systemic anticoagulation to maintain patency*
 **B** *Temporary intravascular shunting requires the availability of specially manufactured shunting devices*
 **C** *The upper limit of time that a shunt can remain in place is approximately 12 hours*
 **D** *While useful, under conditions of limited resources, temporary intravascular shunts have not been demonstrated to be of value in civilian trauma*
 **E** *While temporary intravascular shunts may be useful as a damage-control technique, up to 25% of shunts will become dislodged with patient transport*

First described for traumatic injury in 1971, temporary intravascular shunt (TIVS) placement has become an invaluable addition to the tool kit of the trauma surgeon. Shunt placement simultaneously arrests hemorrhage and restores distal perfusion, allowing for time to triage other life- and limb-threatening injuries. Because most patients undergoing damage-control techniques such as shunting are not candidates for systemic anticoagulation, heparinization is not generally an option. The use of virtually any available flexible tubing has been described in TIVS placement, from those devices specifically designed for this purpose (such as commercially available Argyle and Javid shunts) to peripheral IV tubing and even nasogastric tubes. There have been case reports describing shunt duration of up to 10 days, however, the absolute upper limit of time a shunt can remain in place is unknown. Beyond the military theatre, temporary intravascular shunts have been employed in civilian trauma. Subramanian *et al.* reported the use of 101 temporary intravascular shunts in 67 patients, with an overall limb salvage rate of 83%. While dislodgement of temporary intravascular shunts is possible this is a rare event, even in combat casualties transported great distances with shunts in place.

**Answer: A**

Dente, C.J., Rasmussen, T.E., Schiller, H.J., *et al.* (2006) The use of temporary vascular shunts as a damage control adjunct in the management of wartime vascular injury. *Journal of Trauma Injury, Infection, and Critical Care,* **61** (1), 12–15.

Granchi, T., Schmittling, Z., Vasquez, Jr. J., *et al.* (2000) Prolonged use of intraluminal arterial shunts without systemic anticoagulation. *American Journal of Surgery,* **180** (6), 493–497.

Inaba, K., Aksoy, H., Seamon, M.J., *et al.* (2016) Multicenter evaluation of temporary intravascular shunt use in vascular trauma. *Journal of Trauma and Acute Care Surgery,* **80** (3), 359–364.

Subramanian, A., Vercruysse, G., Dente, C., *et al.* (2008) A decade's experience with temporary intravascular shunts at a civilian level I trauma center. *Journal of Trauma, Injury, Infection, and Critical Care,* **65** (2), 316–324.

6   *A 17-year-old boy presents at the trauma bay with a slash wound extending from the antecubital fossa proximally onto the forearm. Which of the following statements is not correct?*

   **A** *While vascular hard signs mandate immediate surgical operation, the absence of hard signs does not preclude a major vascular injury*

   **B** *When possible, a thorough neurologic examination of the affected extremity should be performed and documented prior to operation*

   **C** *If, at operation, a brachial artery transection is discovered, synthetic graft is the material of choice for interposition grafting*

   **D** *If, at operation, the ulnar artery is transected, but the radial artery is intact, ligation of the ulnar artery is an acceptable treatment*

   **E** *When a brachial artery injury is associated with a complex orthopedic injury, revascularization prior to orthopedic stabilization is the treatment of choice*

The brachial artery is the most commonly injured artery of the upper extremity, constituting 15–30% of all peripheral arterial artery injuries. While patients with brachial artery injuries typically present with vascular hard signs,

it is possible to have complete transection of the brachial artery while maintaining a radial pulse and perfusion to the hand because of a rich network of collaterals around the elbow. In patients where the diagnosis is uncertain, imaging of the vessel is indicated. Because of the density of nervous structures in the upper extremity and the morbidity associated with loss of function, it is extremely important to perform and document a complete neurologic assessment of the upper extremity prior to operative exploration. This helps assure that neurologic deficits occurring as a result of the extremity injury are not attributed to operative intervention. The most commonly used techniques for upper extremity arterial injuries are primary end-to-end repairs and interposition grafting with saphenous vein graft; size-matched synthetic graft has poor 30-day patency rates. Isolated radial or ulnar artery injuries may be ligated with relative impunity provided that the ipsilateral ulnar or radial vessel is intact and the hand remains well-perfused. Even when repair is undertaken, ultrasound studies demonstrate that only ~50% of repairs remain patent at 30 days. Approximately 50% of patients with injuries to the radial or ulnar artery have postoperative weakness and 12% have postoperative temperature sensitivity, but these morbidity rates appear to be secondary to concomitant nerve injury rather than the treatment approach to arterial injury. Similar to lower extremity vascular injuries associated with complex orthopedic injuries, revascularization of the extremity is the first priority. This may be accomplished with intraluminal shunting as a temporizing measure prior to orthopedic stabilization with definitive vascular repair occurring after orthopedic fixation. Ligation of the brachial artery should not be considered as it is associated with unacceptably high amputation rates.

**Answer: C**

Feliciano, D.V., Mattox, K.L., Graham, J.M., and Bitondo, C.G. (1985) Five-year experience with PTFE grafts in vascular wounds. *Journal of Trauma,* **25** (1), 71–82.

Paryavi, E., Pensy, R.A., Higgins, T.F., *et al.* (2014) Salvage of upper extremities with humeral fracture and associated brachial artery injury. *Injury,* **45** (12), 1870–1875.

Rich, N., Mattox, K., and Hirshberg, A. (2004) *Vascular Trauma,* 2nd edn. Elsevier Saunders, Philadelphia, PA.

7   *In an attempt to stop a crime, a 30-year-old police officer sustains gunshot wounds to the left pelvis and right thigh. On arrival to the trauma bay, he is hypotensive and has pulsatile hemorrhage from the right mid-thigh (Figure 33.1). Which of the following statements is correct?*

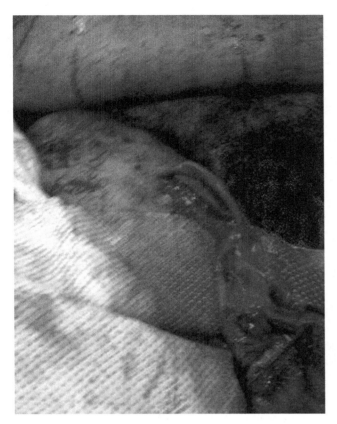

**Figure 33.1** Pulsatile hemorrhage from the right thigh, a vascular "hard sign." A full color version of this figure appears in the plate section of this book.

A *If the patient arrests from this injury in the pre-hospital setting, ED thoracotomy is associated with an approximately 25% chance of survival*

B *Rapid administration of blood and crystalloid prior to operative intervention, with the intent of correcting hypotension prior to operation may be associated with increased survival*

C *Due to concerns for contamination, interposition grafting with synthetic graft material is contraindicated if the trajectory of the bullet may have included the gastrointestinal tract*

D *When compared to open repair, endovascular repair of this injury is associated with decreased morbidity and should be considered the first-line treatment*

E *Completion angiography after repair of vascular injury may reveal technical errors requiring revision in > 10% of cases*

Pre-hospital arrest is a negative prognostic factor for survival in patients undergoing ED thoracotomy, especially with site of injury outside of the thorax. A recent review of 25 years of experience by Rhee *et al.* suggests that survival in the scenario described in answer "A" is

closer to 5%. Administration of fluid and blood products to treat hypotension prior to definitive control of hemorrhage has been shown in at least one randomized controlled trial to be associated with decreased survival; the appropriate treatment of hemorrhagic shock is to stop the bleeding as soon as possible. Interposition grafting using synthetic conduit has been shown to be safe in civilian trauma, even in the presence of a contaminated field. Feliciano *et al.* reported a series of 236 synthetic grafts used to repair traumatic vascular injuries wherein no graft infections were reported in the absence of exposed graft or osteomyelitis. While endovascular repair of penetrating vascular trauma has been reported, it is certainly not the standard of care for patients in hemorrhagic shock and should not be entertained in this situation. Completion angiography reveals technical issues in 10–30% of cases, and in one large series was associated with a decreased rate of amputation.

**Answer: E**

Bickell, W.H., Wall, M.J., Jr, Pepe, P.E., *et al.* (1994) Immediate versus delayed fluid resuscitation for hypotensive patients with penetrating torso injuries. *New England Journal of Medicine*, **331** (17), 1105–1119.

Burlew, C.C., Moore, E.E., Moore, F.A., *et al.* (2012). Western Trauma Association critical decisions in trauma: resuscitative thoracotomy. *Journal of Trauma and Acute Care Surgery*, **73** (6), 1359–1363.

Feliciano, D.V., Mattox, K.L., Graham, J.M., and Bitondo, C.G. (1985) Five-year experience with PTFE grafts in vascular wounds. *Journal of Trauma*, **25** (1), 71–82.

8 *A 25-year-old man with no significant past medial history presents to your trauma center after being involved in a motor vehicle collision in which he was an unrestrained front passenger. He is found to have a posterior dislocation of his right knee with loss of distal pulses.*

*Concerning popliteal artery injuries, which of the following statements is incorrect?*

A *The rate of amputation after popliteal artery injury has declined in both military and civilian series over the past century*

B *Delay in time to revascularization, blunt mechanism of injury, and associated injuries to other body regions are risk factors for amputation in popliteal artery injury*

C *An ABI > 0.9 reliably excludes clinically significant popliteal artery injury after knee dislocation*

D *Due to excellent collateral circulation, popliteal artery injury is associated with a lower rate of amputation when compared to other peripheral arterial injuries*

**E** *In the case of hard signs associated with blunt or complex trauma to the popliteal region, angiography or CT angiography is warranted prior to operative exploration*

Popliteal artery injuries have long been recognized as a condition meriting special consideration because of their unforgiving nature. The rate of limb salvage after these injuries has improved throughout the past century, with amputation rates in recent conflicts reported to be in the range of 12% as compared to approximately 70% during World War I and World War II. In civilian injuries, amputation rates prior to 1980 were reported to be 30%, whereas after 1980 they have been reported to be closer to 15%. Risk factors associated with amputation after popliteal artery injuries include delay to revascularization, blunt mechanism of injury, and concomitant injuries to other body regions. Blunt force injuries to the knee, especially with posterior knee dislocation, are associated with popliteal artery injury. Knee dislocation is associated with a 10–40% incidence of popliteal artery injury, mandating a high index of suspicion. Mills *et al.* reported in a small, prospective study, an API > 0.9 reliably excludes clinically significant popliteal artery injury with a sensitivity of 100%. While an API < 0.9 is an indication for further diagnostic imaging, only 30% of these patients will require operative intervention. Although the popliteal artery is collateralized by the geniculate network around the knee, this is generally not sufficient to maintain perfusion in the absence of popliteal flow; this may in part explain why popliteal artery injuries are associated with higher rates of amputation relative to peripheral vascular injuries at other locations. Although hard signs of vascular injury generally mandate immediate operative intervention, Frykberg advocated imaging of the popliteal artery even in the presence of hard signs associated with blunt or complex trauma, because physical examination may be false positive in up to 87% of these cases.

**Answer: D**

Frykberg, E.R. (2002) Popliteal vascular injuries. *Surgical Clinics of North America*, **82** (1), 67–89.

Keeley, J., Koopman, M., Yan, H., *et al.* (2016). Factors associated with amputation after popliteal vascular injuries. *Annals of Vascular Surgery*, **33**, 83–87.

Levin, P.M., Rich, N.M., and Hutton, J.E. (1971) Collateral circulation in arterial injuries. *American Journal of Surgery*, **102**, 592–599.

Mills, W.J., Barei, D.P., and McNair, P. (2004) The value of the ankle-brachial index for diagnosing arterial injury after knee dislocation: A prospective study. *Journal of Trauma, Injury, Infection, and Critical Care*, **56** (6), 1261–1265.

**9** *A 54-year-old factory worker is hit in the groin by a sharp metal rod, resulting in copious dark red bleeding from the site of injury. At operative exploration, a complete transection of the common femoral vein is discovered. With respect to options for repair for this injury, which of the following statements is correct?*

**A** *Ligation of the femoral vein is associated with a > 25% rate of limb loss*

**B** *When compared to primary repair of this injury, ligation is associated with an equivalent risk of pulmonary thromboembolism*

**C** *Temporary intravascular shunting has no role in the treatment of venous injuries*

**D** *Primary repair of this injury will require systemic anticoagulation to maintain long-term patency*

**E** *Primary repair of this injury is associated with better short-term patency then interposition grafting*

The literature regarding traumatic venous injury is limited to retrospective review and a small number of prospective observational studies, but most experienced surgeons would agree that primary repair should be performed when possible. In unstable patients requiring damage-control surgery, femoral vein ligation is an option for complex venous injuries, and is generally well-tolerated. Approximately 90% of patients will experience lower extremity edema after ligation, but with postoperative use of venous compression stockings, few patients go on to develop severe venous stasis disease. The need for amputation after isolated femoral vein ligation is distinctly uncommon. In the largest series available to date, Quan *et al.* found no difference in pulmonary embolism rates in patients undergoing venous repair versus ligation (3.4% versus 4.2%, p = NS). Temporary intravenous shunting has been employed in both civilian and military settings to allow for life- and limb-saving procedures to occur prior to undertaking complex repair. No strong data exists supporting the use of systemic anticoagulation to promote patency; short-term patency approximates 75% regardless of the type of repair.

**Answer: B**

Kim, J.J., Alipour, H., Yule, A., *et al.* (2016) Outcomes after external iliac and femoral vascular injuries. *Annals of Vascular Surgery*, **33**, 88–93.

Kurtoglu, M., Yanar, H., Taviloglu, K., *et al.* (2007) Serious lower extremity venous injury management with ligation: prospective overview of 63 patients. *American Surgeon*, **73** (10), 1039–1043.

Quan, R.W., Gillespie, D.L., Stuart, R.P., *et al.* (2008) The effect of vein repair on the risk of venous thromboembolic events: a review of more than 100 traumatic military venous injuries. *Journal of Vascular Surgery*, **47** (3), 571–577.

**10** *Regarding fasciotomy for peripheral vascular trauma, which of the following is correct?*

   **A** *Combined arterial and venous injury requires therapeutic fasciotomy*

   **B** *A compartment pressure of > 30 mm Hg is a standard indication for a therapeutic decompressive fasciotomy*

   **C** *Coolness (poikilothermia) of the affected extremity is the most frequently occurring clinical indicator in compartment syndrome*

   **D** *Compartment syndrome can be reliably diagnosed based on physical examination findings*

   **E** *Fasciotomy after peripheral vascular injury is associated with up to a 60% nonclosure rate*

Early diagnosis of compartment syndrome after peripheral vascular injury is of great importance as delays in treatment can lead to increased complications, limb loss, and mortality. While not all patients with peripheral vascular trauma will require fasciotomy, specific clinical scenarios are associated with high rates of developing compartment syndrome and have led some authors to propose guidelines for *prophylactic* fasciotomy. These situations include combined arterial and venous injury, arterial injury in the setting of systemic hypotension, and prolonged (>6 hours) of ischemia time. The diagnosis of compartment syndrome has been made using direct measurement of the compartment pressures. Traditionally, the absolute compartment pressure of > 30 mm Hg has been a trigger for *therapeutic* fasciotomy. More recently, some evidence exists that perfusion may have a role in determining whether a patient will develop a compartment syndrome. To that effect, another approach would be to subtract the intracompartmental pressure (ICP) from diastolic pressure (DBP − ICP). If the value is less than or equal to 30, the patient would require therapeutic fasciotomy. When considering the clinical diagnosis of compartment syndrome, pain has been shown to be the most frequently occurring symptom, but obviously lacks specificity in patients with injured extremities. A high index of suspicion is required for diagnosis, as the sensitivity of clinical indicators alone ranges from 13–19%. Regardless of the indication, it is important to recognize that fasciotomy is not a risk-free procedure; overall, approximately one-third of lower extremity fasciotomies will not be able to be closed by delayed primary intention.

**Answer: B**

Branco, B.C., Inaba, K., Barmparas, G., *et al.* (2011) Incidence and predictors for the need for fasciotomy after extremity trauma: a 10-year review in a mature level I trauma centre. *Injury*, **42** (10), 1157–1163.

Ozkayin, N. and Aktuglu, K. (2005) Absolute compartment pressure versus differential pressure for the diagnosis of compartment syndrome in tibial fractures. *International Orthopedics*, **29**, 396–401.

Velmahos, G.C. and Toutouzas, K.G. (2002) Vascular trauma and compartment syndromes. *Surgical Clinics of North America*, **82** (1), 125–141.

**11** *A 44-year-old man presents to the trauma bay after being run over by a tractor and sustaining a crush injury to his left lower extremity. On physical examination, there is a contaminated open wound on the left thigh with an obvious bony deformity. No pulses are palpable distal to the level of the injury. A plain radiograph reveals a comminuted femur fracture. Regarding the management of this complex injury, which of the following is correct?*

   **A** *The addition of skeletal injury to arterial injury does not confer an increased risk of extremity amputation*

   **B** *Limb salvage rates are equivalent whether revascularization or orthopedic stabilization is performed first*

   **C** *When definitive vascular repair is performed prior to orthopedic stabilization, manipulation of the extremity revision of vascular repair is necessary in the majority of cases*

   **D** *Crush injury, but not severe contamination, is a risk factor for limb loss*

   **E** *In limbs at high risk for amputation, limb salvage and amputation are associated with similar functional outcomes at 2 years*

Patients with combined skeletal and arterial injuries are much more likely to require amputation than patients with either skeletal or arterial injuries alone (15–35% versus 5%, respectively). Recent series suggest that limb salvage rates are highest when revascularization is performed prior to orthopedic stabilization, but definitive vascular repair need not be accomplished at index operation. In the setting of hemodynamic instability, severely unstable or comminuted fractures, or gross contamination, intraluminal shunting should be considered as bridge to definitive vascular repair (Figure 33.2). In the absence of these factors, definitive vascular repair may be undertaken prior to orthopedic stabilization with a less than 7% need for revision after orthopedic fixation. Factors that are associated with limb loss in combination skeletal and arterial injury include extensive soft tissue loss, severe contamination, and associated nerve injury. At 2 years post-injury, patients who underwent limb salvage had similar functional outcomes compared to those who underwent amputation, however, at the cost of higher complication rates and more frequent hospital admissions.

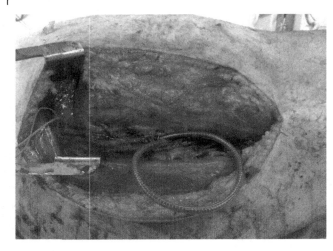

**Figure 33.2** Temporary intravascular shunting of the superficial femoral artery. A full color version of this figure appears in the plate section of this book.

**Answer: E**

Bosse, M.J., MacKenzie, E.J., Kellam, J.F., *et al.* (2002) An analysis of outcomes of reconstruction or amputation of leg-threatening injuries. *New England Journal of Medicine*, **347** (24), 1924–1931.

Cakir, O., Subasi, M., Erdem, K., and Eren, N. (2005) Treatment of vascular injuries associated with limb fractures. *Annals of the Royal College of Surgeons of England*, **87** (5), 348–352.

Liang, N.L., Alarcon, L.H., Jeyabalan, G., *et al.* (2016) Contemporary outcomes of civilian lower extremity arterial trauma. *Journal of vascular Surgery*, **64** (3), 731–736.

Rozycki, G.S., Tremblay, L.N., Feliciano, D.V., and McClelland, W.B. (2003) Blunt vascular trauma in the extremity: diagnosis, management, and outcome. *Journal of Trauma, Injury, Infection, and Critical Care*, **55** (5), 814–824.

**12** *A 22-year-old man presents to the trauma bay with a shotgun wound to the left lower extremity. On physical examination there are multiple punctate wounds from the mid-thigh to the mid-calf. There is no evidence of active bleeding, however, distal pulses in the left foot are absent. Plain films demonstrate innumerable radiopaque foreign bodies consistent with shotgun pellets and no evidence of fracture. Which of the following is not correct?*

**A** *Arterial injuries caused by shotgun wounds are associated with a high rate of concomitant venous injuries*

**B** *Because of the possibility of multi-level injury, angiography should be performed prior to definitive operation*

**C** *This patient is more likely to require multiple operations and have a longer length of stay when compared to patients with handgun wounds*

**D** *Vascular injuries associated with shotgun wounds are associated with a lower rate of amputation than other low-velocity gunshot wounds*

**E** *Pellet embolism via both venous and arterial routes is a known sequelae of vascular injury caused by shotgun wounds*

Shotgun wounds represent a special class of injuries that must be considered separately from other gunshot wounds. Close-range shotgun injuries produce multiple trajectories across the affected body region and are capable of producing massive soft-tissue damage. Combined venous and arterial injures are common following with shotgun injury; a small case series by Bongard *et al.* reported a 100% incidence of venous injuries associated with arterial injuries. A single shotgun blast can create arterial injuries at multiple levels, and delineating the extent of injury before undertaking repair can obviate the need to perform multiple repairs. Despite similar sensitivities in other injury patterns, conventional angiography may be more useful in this situation. CT angiography may be distinctly limited in the evaluation of shotgun wounds due to beam scatter effect from the plethora of retained radiopaque foreign bodies. Patients with shotgun wounds require more operative interventions and have longer lengths of stay compared to those with wounds from other types of guns. The vascular injuries caused by shotgun wounds are associated with a higher rate of amputation than those caused by other low-velocity gunshot wounds (~20% versus 11%). While the overall incidence is unknown, there are dozens of case reports of shotgun pellets embolizing through the venous and arterial circulation with clinical presentation ranging from stroke with hemiparesis to asymptomatic radiographic findings, depending on the ultimate destination of the pellet embolism.

**Answer: D**

Bongard, F.S. and Klein, S.R. (1989) The problem of vascular shotgun injuries: diagnostic and management strategy. *Annals of Vascular Surgery*, **3** (4), 299–303.

Dozier, K.C., Miranda, M.A., Kwan, R.O., *et al.* (2009) Despite the increasing use of non-operative management of firearm trauma, shotgun injuries still require aggressive operative management. *Journal of Surgical Research*, **156** (1), 173–176.

Hafez, H.M., Woolgar, J., and Robbs, J.V. (2001) Lower extremity arterial injury: Results of 550 cases and review of risk factors associated with limb loss. *Journal of Vascular Surgery*, **33** (6), 1212–1219.

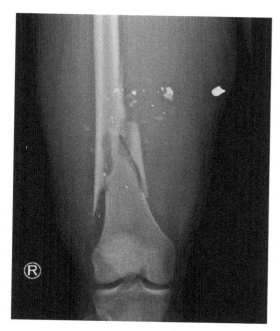

**Figure 33.3**

**13** *A 19-year-old man is brought to the trauma bay via private vehicle with a single gunshot wound to the distal right lateral thigh. DP and PT pulses are palpable on the left, however, only monophasic Doppler signals can be obtained in the right lower extremity. X-ray findings as in Figure 33.3. Which of the following is the most appropriate next step in management?*

**A** *Urgent orthopedic surgery consultation and application of external fixator to re-establish bony alignment*

**B** *CT angiogram to evaluate extent of injury*

**C** *Definitive repair of arterial injury with PTFE graft prior to orthopedic intervention*

**D** *Revascularization with intravascular shunt prior to external fixator application*

**E** *Endovascular repair of the injured artery with covered stent*

The management of concomitant major vascular and musculoskeletal injuries requires coordination between the teams responsible for revascularization and bony fixation. Prompt vascular repair should be undertaken prior to stabilization of orthopedic injuries. Nair *et al.* reported on 117 civilian popliteal artery injuries of which 34 eventually required amputation. Timely resuscitation and revascularization were the only correctable factors associated with improved limb salvage. Depending on the stability of the patient and their other injuries, intravascular shunting may be preferred over definitive repair in the acute setting. Huynh *et al* reported their experience on 57 consecutive lower extremity injuries revascularized with the use of intravascular shunting. 63% of the patients in their series had associated orthopedic injury, two-thirds of which underwent orthopedic fixation after definitive revascularization without complication. Further imaging to determine the extent of injury only delays operative intervention and should not be undertaken. If concern for multiple areas of injury, an on-table angiogram should be performed. While endovascular repair of traumatic peripheral arterial injuries has been reported, it is not standard of care.

**Answer: D**

Huynh, T.T., Pham, M., Griffin, L.W. *et al.* (2006) Management of distal femoral and popliteal arterial injuries: an update. *The American Journal of Surgery*, **192** (6), 773–778.

Nair, R., Abdool-Carrim, A.T.O., and Robbs, J.V. (2000) Gunshot injuries of the popliteal artery. *British Journal of Surgery*, **87** (5), 602–607.

Reuben, B.C., Whitten, M.G., Sarfati, M., *et al.* (2007) Increasing use of endovascular therapy in acute arterial injuries: analysis of the National Trauma Data Bank. *Journal of Vascular Surgery*, **46** (6), 1222–1226.

# 34

# Urologic Trauma and Disorders

*Jeremy Juern, MD and Daniel Roubik, MD*

1 *A 26-year-old man sustains a single through-and-through gunshot wound, with one hole in the right buttock, and the other above the right pubic ramus. There is no blood on digital rectal examination. A CT scan is obtained and shown in Figure 34.1.*

*The patient is taken to the operating room. A Foley catheter is placed and returns bloody urine. Proctoscopy is performed; there is blood in the rectum, and air insufflated via the proctoscope comes out the Foley. Exploratory laparotomy is performed. There is no intra-peritoneal rectal or bladder injury. What is the best next step?*

A *Diverting sigmoid loop colostomy*

B *Bladder exploration*

C *Exploration of retroperitoneal rectum and bladder, closure of adjacent holes, interposition of omentum between the repaired holes, fecal diversion*

D *Nothing further, close the abdomen*

E *End-colostomy*

An isolated retroperitoneal rectal injury is treated with fecal diversion by a colostomy. Penetrating bladder injuries need to be explored with bladder exploration and closure of the holes. When there is a penetrating bladder injury in close proximity to a penetrating rectal injury, the posterior bladder hole and the rectal hole must be closed and healthy tissue such as omentum placed between them. This is true even if the rectal injury is below the peritoneal reflection. Failure to do so has a high rate of colovesical fistula formation. A and E are wrong because the holes in the bladder need to be closed. For an isolated retroperitoneal rectal injury, a diverting loop colostomy would be sufficient. B is wrong because the holes in the rectum must addressed also. D is wrong

because doing nothing will result in drainage of stool and urine into the retroperitoneal space.

**Answer: C**

Crispen, P.L., Kansas, B.T., Pieri, P.G., *et al.* (2007) Immediate postoperative complications of combined penetrating rectal and bladder injuries. *Journal of Trauma*, **62** (2), 325–329.

2 *A 35-year-old man was in a motor vehicle collision. He was found snoring, sprawled out in the front seat. On examination the patient is found to have perineal bruising and blood at the urethral meatus. CT scan of the chest, abdomen, and pelvis finds only a first rib fracture. What is the best next step to workup the urethral finding?*

A *Insert a Foley catheter*

B *Place a condom catheter*

C *Do nothing*

D *Perform a retrograde urethrogram*

E *Cystoscopy in the operating room*

Blood at the urethral meatus is highly suspicious for a urethral injury. A retrograde urethrogram (RUG) should be performed before placing a Foley catheter. A RUG is performed by inserting an 8 Fr Foley catheter into the meatal fossa and inflating the balloon with only 1–2 ml of water. Contrast material is instilled through the catheter, and radiographs or fluoroscopic images are taken. Inserting a Foley catheter (A) is dangerous because it could make the urethral injury worse. At times it may be appropriate for an expert (urologist or experienced trauma surgeon) to attempt one pass, and one pass only,

*Surgical Critical Care and Emergency Surgery: Clinical Questions and Answers*, Second Edition.
Edited by Forrest "Dell" Moore, Peter Rhee, and Gerard J. Fulda.
© 2018 John Wiley & Sons Ltd. Published 2018 by John Wiley & Sons Ltd.
Companion website: www.wiley.com/go/moore/surgical_criticalcare_and_emergency_surgery

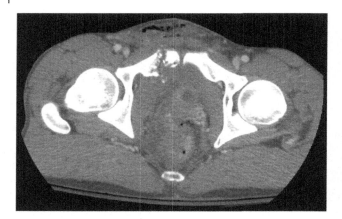

**Figure 34.1**

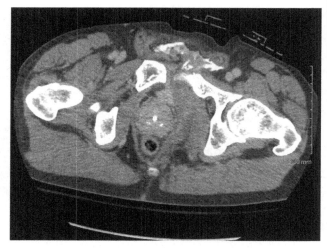

**Figure 34.3**

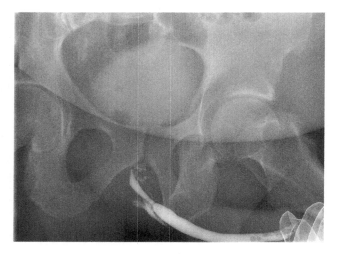

**Figure 34.2**

**3** *57-year-old man is in a motor vehicle collision, and a CT scan is obtained (Figure 34.3). The delayed series shows a pelvic fracture and extra-peritoneal bladder injury. The patient is resuscitated and goes to the operating room two days later for ORIF of the pelvis, including the pubic symphysis. What is the best way of managing his extraperitoneal bladder injury in the operating room?*
    **A** *No bladder repair*
    **B** *Repair of the bladder injury*
    **C** *Foley catheter drainage only*
    **D** *Place percutaneous nephrostomy tubes bilateral*
    **E** *Placement of a suprapubic tube only*

The common consensus is that urinary diversion away from bone hardware is desirable. Therefore, if there is proximity of the fracture site repair to the bladder injury, the bladder injury should be repaired. For that reason, A is wrong. Having only Foley catheter drainage (C) risks urine coming into contact with the hardware. Nephrostomy tubes (D) are unnecessary in this situation. A suprapubic tube (E) might be part of a bladder repair but by itself still risks urine bathing the hardware.

**Answer: B**

Gomez, R.G., Ceballos, L., Coburn, M., *et al.* (2004) Consensus statement on bladder injuries. *BJU International*, **94** (1), 27–32.

of a Foley catheter into the bladder. Placing a condom catheter (B) will not guarantee the flow of urine out of the bladder; it might be blocked by the urethral injury. If nothing is done (C), the patient has a high risk of urinary retention and/or urethral stricture. Cystoscopy (E) may be needed to place a catheter into the bladder, but it is not the best next step.

Figure 34.2 shows a urethral disruption at the junction of the bulbar urethra and the membranous portion of the urethra.

**Answer: D**

American College of Surgeons Committee on Trauma Life Support (2015) *Advanced Trauma Life Support*, 9th edn. Chicago, Elsevier.
Stein, D.M. and Santucci, R.A. (2015) An update on urotrauma. *Current Opinion in Urology*, **25** (4), 323–330.

**4** *A young man sustains a gunshot to the flank. He has a hole in the flank on both the left and the right side of the body. He does not move his lower extremities. There is no missile seen on chest or abdomen x-ray. He is not tender. Foley catheter is placed, and gross hematuria is present. A CT scan is obtained*

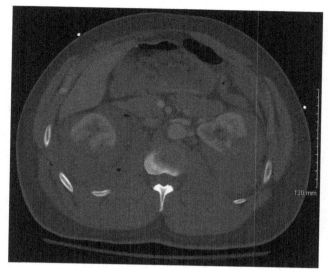

**Figure 34.4**

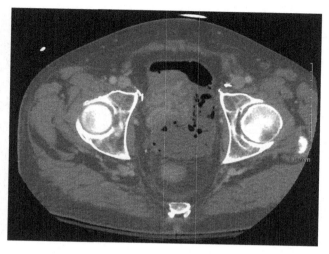

**Figure 34.5**

*(Figure 34.4) with multiple findings, including spleen injury with active extravasation, bilateral kidney injury with active extravasation from the right kidney, and a spinal cord injury. What is the best way to manage this patient?*

**A** *Laparoscopic splenectomy*
**B** *Splenectomy, bilateral nephrectomy*
**C** *Splenectomy, bilateral kidney exploration*
**D** *Splenectomy, no exploration of kidneys unless an obvious expanding hematoma is present.*
**E** *Nonoperative observation*

A penetrating injury to the spleen mandates splenectomy. With any kidney injury, preservation of nephrons is crucial. In this patient with bilateral kidney injuries, it is even more important. On exploration the retroperitoneal hematomas were stable in size and so they were left alone. Follow-up imaging showed minimal urine extravasation that was deemed insignificant by urology. The patient was discharged to spinal cord rehabilitation. A laparoscopic approach (A) would not be appropriate in this penetrating trauma patient. Performing bilateral nephrectomies (B) is too aggressive and would condemn this new paraplegic to potentially lifelong dialysis. Exploring the kidneys (C) is risky because once the hematomas are opened, there is a very high risk of nephrectomy. Nonoperative management (E) of penetrating trauma to the spleen with active extravasation is not appropriate.

**Answer: D**

Shoobridge, J.J., Corcoran, N.M., Martin, K.A., *et al.* (2011) contemporary management of renal trauma. *Reviews in Urology*, **13** (2), 65–72.

Stein, D.M., and Santucci, R.A. (2015) An update on urotrauma. *Current Opinion in Urology*, **25** (4), 323–330.

**5** *A 60-year-old man with bladder cancer undergoes cystoprostatectomy with ileal conduit creation. He recovers and is discharged home. On postoperative day 9 he presents to the ED with severe abdominal pain, elevated WBC, and elevated creatinine. A CT scan was obtained (Figure 34.5). What is the best next step?*

**A** *Loop-o-gram*
**B** *Exploratory laparotomy*
**C** *Digital rectal exam*
**D** *Proctoscopy*
**E** *Admit to floor, start oral antibiotics*

Cystoprostatectomy with ileal conduit creation requires extensive pelvic dissection and a small bowel anastomosis. Either of these locations is at risk for rectal injury or leak. A diverting loop ileostomy may be warranted in the setting of rectal injury. A loop-o-gram (A) is a fluoroscopic study of an ileal conduit and would not be needed. Digital rectal exam (C) would not be contributory. Proctoscopy (D) may aid in diagnosis of a rectal injury, could worsen the injury, and will not provide treatment. This patient has severe sepsis and needs aggressive care, so (E) is wrong.

**Answer: B**

Hemal, A.K., Kolla, S.B., Wadhwa, P., *et al.* (2008) Laparoscopic radical cystectomy and extracorporeal urinary diversion: a single center experience of 48 cases with three years of follow-up. *Urology*, **71** (1), 41–46.

**6** *A 35-year-old man presents to the trauma bay after a motor vehicle collision in which he was ejected from his seat. He was intubated in the trauma bay and ultimately taken to the operating room, where he received 9 L of crystalloid and 6 units of blood. He remained on the ventilator postoperatively. By postoperative day 3, the patient required more aggressive ventilator settings and vasopressor support. He became oliguric with a creatinine of 1.8 mg/dL (baseline 1.0 mg/dL) and developed bilateral pleural effusions. He was also noted to have dependent edema. Other labs in his metabolic panel were within normal limits. How would you best manage his volume status?*

**A** *1 L fluid restriction daily*
**B** *Intermittent hemodialysis*
**C** *Continuous venovenous hemodialysis*
**D** *Continuous venovenous hemofiltration*
**E** *Furosemide*

Continuous renal replacement therapy provides a method of regulating a patient's fluid and electrolyte status in a more physiologic and controlled fashion. This is preferred when a patient is hemodynamically unstable and would likely decompensate from the rapid fluid shifts of intermittent hemodialysis. The main modes of renal replacement therapy are hemodialysis, which focuses on the clearance of solute, and hemofiltration, which focuses on the clearance of solvent or fluid. Combinations and variances of these modes also exist.

The patient above is fluid overloaded, as seen by his worsening pulmonary status, with poor kidney function. Despite his volume status, he still required vasopressor support. Fluid restriction (A) is unlikely to help his volume status, since he has poor urine output. Intermittent hemodialysis (B) would not likely be tolerated in a ventilated patient requiring vasopressors to maintain perfusion. Continuous hemodialysis (C) would not help a patient with otherwise normal electrolytes. Furosemide requires functional kidneys to work so (E) is wrong. This patient requires slow removal of fluid to clear his lungs in the form of continuous hemofiltration

**Answer: D**

Manns, M., Sigler, M.H., and Teehan, B.P. (1998) Continuous renal replacement therapies: an update. *American Journal of Kidney Diseases*, **32**, 185–207.

Mehta, R.L. (2005) Continuous renal replacement therapy in the critically ill patient. *Kidney International*, **67**, 781–795.

Ronco, C., Bellomo, R., and Kellum, J.A. (2002) Continuous renal replacement therapy: opinions and evidence. *Advances in Renal Replacement Therapy*, **9**, 229–244.

**7** *An 18-year-old man is brought to the trauma bay by his friends after he was attempting to slide down a handrail on his skateboard. He had lost his balance, sustained a straddle injury on the rail, and then hit his head on concrete. Friends report loss of consciousness at the scene. Patient has a GCS of 14 due to confusion. He is stable on exam but has blood at the urethral meatus. Retrograde urethrogram demonstrates extravasation. An attempt at gently passing a Foley catheter is unsuccessful. CT scans are performed and shows a small epidural hematoma and a distended urinary bladder in the abdomen. No other injuries are noted. Neurosurgery is consulted. What immediate intervention is recommended for the patient's urethral injury?*

**A** *Urology consult for early urethroplasty*
**B** *Repeat attempt with a Foley catheter and use of traction if successful to approximate the urethral ends*
**C** *Suprapubic catheter*
**D** *Nephrostomy drain placement*
**E** *No intervention required*

Anterior urethral injuries are most common after blunt trauma, such as fall astride injuries or kicks to the perineum, where the bulbar urethra is compressed against the pubic symphysis. Posterior urethral trauma is usually associated with pelvic fractures (72%). Blood at the urethral meatus in noted in 98% of posterior injuries and 75% of anterior urethral injuries. The standard diagnostic modality is retrograde urethrography. Management consists of urinary diversion with either suprapubic catheterization (C) or a trial of early endoscopic realignment (not E). Early urethroplasty (A) is not indicated due to significant spongiosal contusion, which makes debridement difficult. Urinary diversion should be maintained for 2 weeks for partial and 3 weeks for complete ruptures. Another advantage of the suprapubic catheter it to provide an anterograde means of passing a wire for future repair. Nephrostomy drain placement (D) is unnecessary and would not adequately drain the bladder.

**Answer: C**

Brandes, S. (2006) Initial management of anterior and posterior urethral injuries. *Urologic Clinics of North America*, **33** (1), 87–95.

Chapple, C., Barbagli, G., Jordan, G., *et al.* (2004) Consensus statement on urethral trauma. *BJU International*, **93** (9), 1195–1202.

Palminteri, E., Berdondini, E., Verze, P., *et al.* (2013) Contemporary urethral stricture characteristics in the developed world. *Urology*, **81** (1), 191–196.

**8** *31-year-old man presents to the emergency room with complaints of perineal pain and erythema after a perianal abscess was drained recently. He now reports severe pain and erythema extending into his scrotum associated with fever and chills. Physical exam is significant for an erythematous and markedly tender perineum and external genitalia. Patient is also noted to have residual fluctuance near his anus and slight crepitus in the perineum. Labs are significant for WBC of $18 \times 10^9$/L, hemoglobin of 12 g/dL, sodium of 130 mEq/L, creatinine of 1.7 mg/dL, glucose of 200 mmol/L, and a CRP of 220 mg/L. What is the next best step in management?*

**A** *CT scan with IV contrast*
**B** *Admission to the hospital with IV antibiotics alone*
**C** *Incision and drainage of fluctuant area near the rectum with continued trial of PO antibiotics*
**D** *Ultrasound of perineum*
**E** *IV antibiotics with immediate debridement in the OR, with possible orchiectomy*

The above patient has signs and symptoms concerning for a necrotizing soft tissue infection (NSTI) of the perineal region, or Fournier's gangrene. A LRINEC score helps rule out diagnosis of NSTIs when the diagnosis is uncertain. The LRINEC score is calculated using CRP, WBC, hemoglobin, sodium, creatinine, and glucose and has a PPV of only 37.9% and NPV of 92.5%. The above patient has a LRINEC score of 9, which is greater than the threshold of 6 for predicting a NSTI.

This patient requires early and aggressive surgical debridement. When clinical suspicion is high for an NSTI, operative intervention should not be delayed for radiographic imaging (A and D). While radiographic findings may raise concern, surgical exploration is the only way of definitively diagnosing NSTI. Intravenous antibiotics without surgical intervention (B) is associated with a near 100% mortality rate, further emphasizing the importance of aggressive debridement. All affected tissue must be debrided. Incision and drainage is inadequate (C). Patients with Fournier's gangrene may require cystostomy, colostostomy, or orchiectomy depending on the extent of disease. Recommended intravenous antibiotics include: A carbapenem or beta-lactam/beta-lactamase inhibitor PLUS clindamycin (for antitoxin effects) PLUS agent for MRSA (vancomycin, daptomycin, or linezolid)

**Answer: E**

Goldstein, E.J.C., Anaya, D.A. and Dellinger, E.P. (2007) Necrotizing soft-tissue infection: diagnosis and management. *Clinical Infectious Diseases*, **44**, 705–710.
Stevens, D.L., Bryant, A.E., and Hackett, S.P. (1995) Antibiotic effects on bacterial viability, toxin production, and host response. *Clinical Infectious Diseases*, **20** (Suppl 2), S154–S157.
Wong, C.H., Khin, L.W., Heng, K.S., *et al.* (2004) The LRINEC (Laboratory Risk Indicator for Necrotizing Fasciitis) score: a tool for distinguishing necrotizing fasciitis from other soft tissue infections. *Critical Care Medicine*, **32** (7), 1535–1541.

**9** *A 27-year-old man sustained a gunshot wound to the right flank. He is unstable on presentation and is taken to the OR, where a colonic injury was discovered. The patient was left in discontinuity because of hypothermia and acidosis. Negative pressure dressings are applied to the open abdomen, and the patient was taken to the ICU for resuscitation. On postoperative day 2, the patient is hemodynamically stable and is taken to the OR for colon anastomosis. At that time an injury to the lower third of the ureter is noted. What is the next best step in management?*

**A** *Uretero-ureterostomy*
**B** *Ureteral reimplantation with psoas hitch*
**C** *Ureteral reimplantation with Boari flap*
**D** *Proximal ureteral ligation with ureterostomy*
**E** *Autotransplantation*

Ureteral trauma accounts for 1–2.5% of all urinary tract trauma. Gunshot wounds account for 91% of injuries, with stab wounds and blunt trauma accounting for 5% and 4%, respectively. Of all abdominal gunshot wounds, 2–3% have concomitant ureter injury. Hematuria is only seen in 50–75% of patients with ureteral injury. The gold standard is operative exploration and visualization of the ureter. A CT urogram is the preferred diagnostic modality in stable patients.

Intra-operatively, the use of blue intravenous dye, such as indigo carmine or methylene blue, may assist in the detection of ureteral injuries. In a stable patient, definitive repair is preferred if patient condition and expertise allows.

Principles of definitive repair include debridement of necrotic tissue, spatulation of ureteral ends, use of absorbable suture for watertight mucosal approximation, internal stenting, external drainage, and isolation of the injury with peritoneum/omentum. A uretero-ureterostomy (A) is the most common repair, especially in the upper and mid ureters, but should not be performed alone under tension. Transuretero-ureterostomy (anastomosis to contralateral ureter) is also an option in patients with significant injury. Distal ureteral injury often compromises blood supply, making reimplantation into the bladder more favorable. Research does not definitively favor a refluxing (to prevent stenosis) or non-refluxing repair. If there is tension, as in the above scenario, the bladder may be sutured to the ipsilateral psoas tendon to make a psoas hitch (B) to allow for

**Table 34.1** Treatment options, adapted from the European Association of Urology *Guidelines on Urological Trauma*.

| Region of injury | Surgical Repair Options |
| --- | --- |
| Upper ureter | Uretero-ureterostomy |
| | Transuretero-ureterostomy |
| | Uretero-calyxostomy |
| Mid ureter | Uretero-ureterostomy |
| | Transuretero-ureterostomy |
| | Ureteral reimplantation and a Boari flap |
| Lower ureter | Ureteral reimplantation |
| | Ureteral reimplantation with a Psoas hitch |
| Complete | Ileal interposition graft |
| | Autoimplantation |

tension-free anastomosis. A Boari flap (C) is the creation of a tubularized bladder to span long distances. This is more time-consuming and less preferable. When the entire ureter is non-viable, an ileal interposition graft may be used. As a last resort, the kidney may be autotransplanted (E) into the pelvis with anastomosis to the iliac vessels and urinary drainage into the bladder. Table 34.1 shows the treatment options by region of injury.

**Answer:** B

Brandes, S., Coburn, M., Armenakas, N., *et al.* (2004) Diagnosis and management of ureteric injury: an evidence based analysis. *BJU International,* **94** (3), 277–289.

Elliott, S.P. and McAninch, J.W. (2003) Ureteral injuries from external violence: the 25-year experience at San Francisco General Hospital. *Journal of Urology,* **170** (4 Pt 1), 1213–1216.

McGeady, J.B. and Breyer, B.N. (2013) Current epidemiology of genitourinary trauma. *Urologic Clinics of North America,* **40** (3), 323–334.

Patel, V.G. and Walker, M.L. (1997) The role of "one-shot" intravenous pyelogram in evaluation of penetrating abdominal trauma. *The American Surgeon,* **63** (4), 350–353.

Smith, T.G. and Coburn, M. (2013). Damage control maneuvers for urologic trauma. *Urologic Clinics of North America,* **40** (3), 343–350.

Summerton, D.J., Djakovic, N., Kitrey, N.D., *et al.* (2014). *Guidelines on Urological Trauma.* European Association of Urology, Arnhem, The Netherlands.

**10** *34-year-old incarcerated man sustains multiple stab wounds to his left flank after an altercation in prison. In the trauma bay he is hemodynamically stable.*

*CT is consistent with a hilar injury to the spleen, a left renal laceration limited to inferior pole, and an atrophic right kidney. A midline laparotomy is performed for splenectomy, and the retroperitoneum is tense and enlarging. No other intraperitoneal injuries are noted. What is the best approach to the patient's renal injury?*

**A** *No intervention as the retroperitoneum will tamponade any bleeding*

**B** *Abdominal closure with coil embolization of any bleeding vessels with interventional radiology*

**C** *Abdominal closure with repositioning into the right lateral decubitus position for retroperitoneal approach*

**D** *Medialization of the descending colon, exposure of the kidney lateral to medial*

**E** *Midline looping of the renal vessels followed by medialization of the descending colon, exposure of the kidney lateral to medial*

The above patient has abdominal injuries necessitating exploratory laparotomy with retroperitoneal exploration (not A or B). Indications for renal exploration include expanding or pulsatile hematoma, vascular (renal pedicle) injury, and shattered kidney. Relative indications for exploration include devitalized renal segment in the presence of other abdominal injuries. Shariat *et al.* published a nomogram (Figure 34.6) to predict need for exploration in cases of renal trauma using injury grade, trauma type (blunt/stab/gunshot), transfusion need, BUN, and creatinine.

When renal exploration for trauma is indicated, the preferred exposure is through a midline laparotomy for proximal vascular control (not C). Without proximal control, premature decompression of the hematoma may allow for more bleeding (D). To establish proximal control, the transverse colon should be eviscerated superiorly. The small bowel is lifted superiorly and to the right. The aorta is palpated and a vertical incision in the retroperitoneum is made. The dissection is continued to expose the left renal vein running anterior to the aorta (E). The left renal vein is a landmark in locating other renal vessels. Once circumferentially dissected, vessel loops are passed and left loosely in place, using them only when needed for hemostasis. Ideally warm ischemic time will be limited to < 30 minutes. The colon is retracted medially to expose the kidney. Debride all non-viable tissue, as the kidney only requires 1/3 of the parenchyma to sufficiently function. Repair parenchyma and collecting duct lacerations with absorbable suture. Test for leak with methylene blue. The repair should be covered for protection, using Gelfoam or omentum.

**Answer:** E

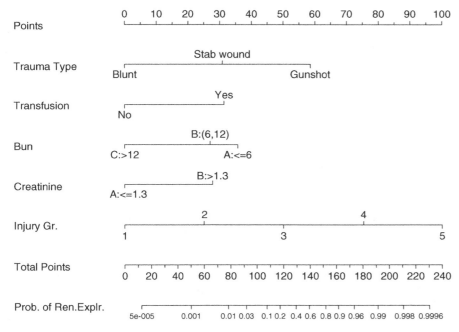

**Figure 34.6** Shariat *et al.* nomogram to predict need for exploration in cases of renal trauma.

Husmann, D.A., Gilling, P.J., Perry, M.O., *et al.* (1993) Major renal lacerations with a devitalized fragment following blunt abdominal trauma: a comparison between nonoperative (expectant) versus surgical management. *Journal of Urology*, **150**, 1774–1777.

Husmann, D.A. and Morris, J.S. (1990) Attempted nonoperative management of blunt renal lacerations extending through the corticomedullary junction: the short-term and long-term sequelae. *Journal of Urology*, **150**, 682–684.

Meng, M.V., Brandes, S.B., and McAninch, J.W. (1999). Renal trauma: indications and techniques for surgical exploration. *World Journal of Urology*, **17** (2), 71–77.

Shariat, S.F., Trinh, Q.D., Morey, A.F., *et al.* (2008) Development of a highly accurate nomogram for prediction of the need for exploration in patients with renal trauma. *Journal of Trauma and Acute Care Surgery*, **64** (6), 1451–1458.

Tillou, A., Romero, J., Asensio, J.A., *et al.* (2001) Renal vascular injuries. *The Surgical Clinics of North America*, **81**(6): 417–430.

## 35

# Care of the Pregnant Trauma Patient
*Ashley McCusker, MD and Terence O'Keeffe, MD*

1 *During the evaluation of pregnant patients who sustain blunt trauma, cardiotocographic monitoring (CTM) for a minimum of 24 hours is recommended for all situations except:*
   A *≥ 3 contractions per hour*
   B *Ejection from the vehicle or motorcycle/pedestrian collisions*
   C *Abdominal or uterine tenderness*
   D *Vaginal bleeding*
   E *Maternal tachycardia*

Cardiotocographic monitoring records both uterine contractions and fetal heart rate, and is one of the mainstays of detecting problems with the fetus or premature labor. A period of monitoring should be considered for every pregnant patient suffering blunt abdominal trauma. Fetal bradycardia or even lack of variability in fetal heart rate indicate distress. If no response to fluid administration, increased maternal oxygen delivery, or maternal repositioning, an emergency delivery should be considered.

Option A represents a fairly low-risk scenario and if all other findings are negative, this patient would not need to be monitored for longer than 4–6 hours. However, if the findings below are present, then this would need to be extended.

Risk factors for fetal loss include: ejection from the vehicle, motorcycle and pedestrian collisions, maternal tachycardia, abnormal fetal heart rate (FHR), lack of restraints, EGA (estimated gestational age) > 35 weeks, ISS > 9, pelvic fractures, need for transfusion, elevated serum lactate on admission, severe traumatic brain injury, and a history of assaults.

Cardiotocographic monitoring for a minimum of 24 hours of CTM is recommended for patients with frequent uterine activity (≥6 contractions per hour), abdominal or uterine tenderness, vaginal bleeding, or hypotension as these are possible signs of placental abruption. Asymptomatic trauma patients should undergo at least 6 hours of CTM prior to considering discharge. These patients should be counseled to observe for decreased fetal movement, vaginal bleeding, abdominal pain, or frequent uterine contractions. Fetal heart tones can be auscultated with a stethoscope beyond 20 weeks EGA and by doppler ultrasound by 12 weeks EGA. Normal fetal heart rate is between 120–160 beats/min. The EGA correlates with fundal height measured from the pubic symphysis, with each centimeter equal to approximately 1 week of gestational age. Twenty weeks of EGA is indicated by a fundal height at the umbilicus. If fundal height and reported EGA do not correlate, this may indicate ruptured uterus or intrauterine hemorrhage.

**Answer: A**

Grabo, D. and Schwab, C.W. (2013) Trauma in pregnant women, in *The Trauma Manual: Trauma and Acute Care Surgery*, 4th edn (eds A.B. Peitzman, M. Rhodes, C.W. Schwab *et al.*), Lippincott Williams and Wilkins, Philadelphia, PA, pp. 228–233.

Knudson, M. and Yeh, D. (2013) Trauma in pregnancy, in *Trauma*, 7th edn (eds K.L. Mattox E.E. Moore and D.V. Feliciano), McGraw-Hill, New York, pp. 709–724.

Lynch, A. (2009) Trauma in pregnancy, in *Trauma Care: Initial Assessment and Treatment in the Emergency Department* (ed. E. Cole), Chichester, Wiley-Blackwell, pp. 231–244.

2 *Premature labor is rare after minor trauma, with an incidence of 1%. Following severe trauma, most patients experience some uterine contractility. In regards to tocolytic medications, which of the following is true?*
   A *Magnesium sulfate can cause hypotension and mental status changes*

*Surgical Critical Care and Emergency Surgery: Clinical Questions and Answers*, Second Edition.
Edited by Forrest "Dell" Moore, Peter Rhee, and Gerard J. Fulda.
© 2018 John Wiley & Sons Ltd. Published 2018 by John Wiley & Sons Ltd.
Companion website: www.wiley.com/go/moore/surgical_criticalcare_and_emergency_surgery

B *Indomethacin may precipitate closing of the fetal PDA, has been associated with oligohydraminos, and may cause bleeding in the trauma patient*
C *Tocolytic medications should not be used in patients with active vaginal bleeding or suspected placental abruption*
D *Calcium channel blockers such as nifedipine may cause hypotension*
E *All of the above*

The most common tocolytic agents used for the treatment of preterm labor are magnesium sulfate, indomethacin, and nifedipine. The tocolytic agents currently used to treat preterm labor appear to be equally efficacious in delaying delivery for at least 48 hours. While magnesium sulfate is associated with maternal toxicity, indomethacin is associated with fetal and neonatal toxicity. For patients in the third trimester who develop contractions or premature labor, betamethasone is administered to accelerate lung maturation in the premature fetus.

While magnesium has remained one of the first line agents for premature labor, it has been associated with both significant hypotension and well as confusion, dizziness, headache, and drowsiness. The patient should be closely monitored while on an infusion of magnesium.

Indomethacin is more commonly used in preterm labor associated with polyhdramnios in early pre-term (<32 weeks) labor. Given the risk of platelet inhibition due to its NSAID effects, it is probably not the first agent in the trauma patient.

Tocolytic medications are utilized in an attempt to delay or prevent actual labor occurring. In patients who have clear indications for surgery or delivery, these drugs should be avoided.

Nifedipine has emerged as an effective and safe alternative tocolytic agent for the management of preterm labor, because of its ability to inhibit contractility in smooth muscle cells by reducing calcium influx into cells. It seems to have a better safety profile on the maternal side than magnesium. However, like all calcium channel blockers, it can cause hypotension and therefore continuous monitoring of the fetal heart rate is recommended as long as the patient has contractions; the patient's pulse and blood pressure should be carefully monitored.

**Answer: E**

Grabo, D. and Schwab, C.W. (2013) Trauma in pregnant women, in *The Trauma Manual: Trauma and Acute Care Surgery*, 4th edn (eds A.B. Peitzman, M. Rhodes, C.W. Schwab, *et al.*), Lippincott Williams and Wilkins, Philadelphia, PA, pp. 228–233.

Knudson, M. and Yeh, D. (2013) Trauma in pregnancy, in *Trauma*, 7th edn (eds K.L. Mattox E.E. Moore, and D.V. Feliciano), McGraw-Hill, New York, pp. 709–724.

Lynch, A. (2009) Trauma in pregnancy, in *Trauma Care: Initial Assessment and Treatment in the Emergency Department* (ed. E. Cole), Wiley-Blackwell, Chichester, UK, pp. 231–244.

3 *Which of the following physiologic changes are associated with pregnancy?*
A *Factors VII, VIII, IX, X, and XII, and fibrinolytic activity are reduced*
B *Auto-regulation of uterine arteries is absent due to their maximal dilation*
C *Uterine blood flow at term is 50 ml/min*
D *Partially compensated respiratory acidosis*
E *Pelvic free fluid during pregnancy is normal; therefore, free fluid on FAST exam is not pathologic*

Pregnancy is normally a hypercoagulable state with physiological changes to prevent hemorrhage during delivery. There is increased production of factors VII, VIII, IX, X, and XII, and fibrinogen, as well as reduced fibrinolytic activity. Due to the enlarged uterus, there is increased pressure on pelvic veins, which may increase the risk of thromboembolic events. As with all trauma patients, the injured pregnant patient has the added thrombotic risk factors of pelvic and lower extremity fractures, immobility, or neurologic injury. Prophylactic doses of enoxaparin, which does not cross the placenta, should be delivered to pregnant trauma patients, as it is more effective and safer than heparin.

After the 12th week of pregnancy, the uterus extends out of the pelvis, rotates slightly to the right, and ascends into the abdominal cavity to displace the intestines laterally and superiorly. Since the viscera are displaced, this can change injury patterns. In the supine position, the uterus compresses the aorta, reducing the pressure in the uterine arteries, which are maximally dilated in pregnancy. Auto-regulation of the arteries is absent; therefore the fetal blood flow is dependent on the maternal MAP and sensitive to maternal hypotension, catecholamines, and vasopressors. The inferior vena cava is also compressed by the uterus when the pregnant patient is in the supine position. This decreases venous return, thereby decreasing cardiac output and causing the blood pressure to decrease. By turning the patient onto her left side with a wedge under the right hip, pressure on aorta and IVC is removed, restoring venous return and increasing cardiac output up to 30%.

At 10 weeks gestation, uterine blood flow is estimated to be about 50 mL/min. With progressive uterine enlargement, uterine blood flow increases dramatically to approximately 500 mL/min at term, constituting up to

17% of the cardiac output. This increases the potential for hemorrhage. Oxytocin 20 U IV is administered for postpartum uterine bleeding.

The chest anatomy changes, largely due to increased levels of progesterone, so as to meet increased oxygen requirements. As the diaphragm is elevated due to the enlarging uterus, the lungs decrease in length and there is an increase in intrathoracic pressure. The rib cage flares out to compensate for the shortening lung length, which needs to be taken into consideration with tube thoracostomy. Functional residual capacity decreases because of a decline in expiratory reserve and residual volumes. Minute ventilation and tidal volume are increased. Respirations may appear deeper and faster, resulting in a reduction in the $PCO_2$ to 30 mm Hg. With an unchanged $PaO_2$ and slight compensatory decrease in plasma bicarbonate levels, the pregnant patient is in a state of compensated respiratory alkalosis. Supplemental oxygen delivery for the mother during resuscitation can dramatically improve the blood oxygen content and reserve for the fetus, due to the difference in fetal hemoglobin-oxygen dissociation curve.

A small amount of pelvic free fluid may be normal during pregnancy. However, this amount is usually between 7–21 mL and is too little to be detected during FAST. FAST is approximately 80% sensitive and 100% specific to detect fluid during pregnancy. Huang *et al.* described a hemoperitoneum scoring system in which fluid in each aspect of the abdominal component of FAST was given one point. If fluid was seen in the pelvis, Morrison's pouch, and left upper quadrant equating 3 points, this was estimated to be over 1 L of intraperitoneal fluid. Therefore, if any fluid is seen on FAST, this should be considered pathologic.

**Answer: B**

Dente, C.J. and Rozycki, G.S. (2013) Surgeon-performed ultrasound in acute care surgery, in *Trauma*, 7th edn (eds K.L. Mattox, E.E. Moore and D.V. Feliciano), McGraw-Hill, New York, pp. 301–321.

Grabo, D. and Schwab, C.W. (2013) Trauma in pregnant women, in *The Trauma Manual: Trauma and Acute Care Surgery*, 4th edn (eds A.B. Peitzman, M. Rhodes, C.W. Schwab, *et al.*), Lippincott Williams and Wilkins, Philadelphia, PA, pp. 228–233.

Huang, M., Liu, M., Wu, J., *et al.* (1994) Ultrasonography for the evaluation of hemoperitoneum during resuscitation: a simple scoring system. *Journal of Trauma*, **36**, 173–177.

Knudson, M. and Yeh, D. (2013) Trauma in pregnancy, in *Trauma*, 7th edn (eds K.L. Mattox, E.E. Moore, and D.V. Feliciano), McGraw-Hill, New York, pp. 709–724.

Lynch, A. (2009) Trauma in pregnancy, in *Trauma Care: Initial Assessment and Treatment in the Emergency Department* (ed. E. Cole), Chichester, Wiley-Blackwell, pp. 231–244.

4 *When the Kleihauer-Betke (KB) test is utilized to detect fetal blood in the maternal circulation, fetal cells are resistant to acid elution of hemoglobin and stain with erythrosine while maternal cells fail to stain. Which of the following is false?*

   **A** *A small amount (1 mL) of Rh-positive fetal blood can sensitize a Rh-negative woman*

   **B** *All Rh-negative pregnant trauma victims should receive 300 mcg of Rh-immune globulin within 72 hours of injury and another 300 mcg for each 30 mL of estimated fetal blood identified in the maternal circulation via the Kleihauer-Betke test*

   **C** *If positive, the KB test should be repeated after 24 hours to identify ongoing fetomaternal hemorrhage*

   **D** *A positive KB test suggests close fetal surveillance*

   **E** *None of the above*

There continues to be a large amount of confusion regarding the use and interpretation of the Kleihauer-Betke (KB) test, particularly in the example of the pregnant trauma patient. This test measures the percent of red cells containing fetal hemoglobin in maternal blood. The KB test should be performed in Rh (D)-negative women who have undergone significant abdominal trauma to determine whether additional doses of anti-D-immune globulin are needed due to a large fetomaternal infusion of blood. If required, all female trauma patients of child-bearing age should receive O negative blood transfusions if needed until cross-matched blood is available. It has been estimated that as little as 0.01 ml of fetal blood can lead to a positive KB test.

Rh-immune globulin dosing will depend on the amount of fetal blood that appears to have entered the circulation, but a single 300 mcg dose is administered to patients who are Rhesus negative and have undergone a significant amount of abdominal trauma

Ongoing evaluation of maternofetal hemorrhage using the KB test can be more sensitive than a single test on admission

A study by Muench *et al.* at the R. Adams Cowley Shock Trauma Center assessed the ability of the KB test to predict uterine contractions and overt preterm labor in the absence of significant maternal or fetal compromise or overt clinical signs. A positive KB test detected all cases of preterm labor. A negative KB test excluded preterm labor. The authors suggested CTM and serial KB testing every 6–12 hours until the KB value decreased, and no need for extended monitoring in patients with a negative KB test.

**Answer: E**

Grabo, D. and Schwab, C.W. (2013) Trauma in pregnant women, in *The Trauma Manual: Trauma and Acute*

348 | Surgical Critical Care and Emergency Surgery


*Care Surgery*, 4th edn (eds A.B. Peitzman, M. Rhodes, C.W. Schwab, *et al.*), Lippincott Williams and Wilkins, Philadelphia, PA, pp. 228–233.

Knudson, M. and Yeh, D. (2013) Trauma in pregnancy, in *Trauma*, 7th edn (eds K.L. Mattox, E.E. Moore and D.V. Feliciano), McGraw-Hill, New York, pp. 709–724.

Lynch, A. (2009) Trauma in pregnancy, in *Trauma Care: Initial Assessment and Treatment in the Emergency Department* (ed. E. Cole), Chichester, Wiley-Blackwell, pp. 231–244.

Muench, M.V., Baschat, A.A., Reddy, U.M., *et al.* (2004) Kleihauer-betke testing is important in all cases of maternal trauma. *Journal of Trauma*, 57 (5), 1094–1098.

5   Neurologic injury in pregnant patients can be challenging. Moderate and severe maternal TBI with GCS < 12 has been shown to adversely affect fetal outcomes. Which of the following is not true regarding management of maternal neurologic injury?

A   Severe hyperventilation can lead to reduced uterine blood flow

B   Hypothermia, mannitol, and hypertonic saline should be avoided in pregnancy

C   Dopamine and dobutamine may not be utilized for blood pressure support

D   Vasopressors compromise placental blood flow due to absent auto-regulation of the uterine arteries

E   Attendant delivery may occur because of unrecognized contractions

The care of the traumatic brain injured pregnant patient should focus on reducing intracranial pressure and replacing maternal hormones depleted due to hypothalamic and pituitary dysfunction. Nutritional support, seizure control, and avoidance of infections and thrombotic complications are required in the care of the pregnant patient with a traumatic brain injury to ensure normal growth and development of the fetus.

Hyperventiliation can result in decreased venous return causing reduced cardiac output.

The care of the traumatic brain injury patient may be focused on reducing intracranial pressure and replacing maternal hormones depleted due to hypothalamic and pituitary dysfunction. and mannitol should be avoided in pregnancy. Hypertonic saline has not been shown to have any adverse fetal affects.

Inotropic agents such as dopamine and dobutamine may be required for blood pressure support in patients in spinal shock. These agents appear to be safe in pregnancy, as they do not reduce uterine perfusion and are not associated with a teratogenic effect on the fetus.

The uterine arteries are maximally dilated in pregnancy. Auto-regulation of the arteries is absent; therefore, the fetal blood flow is dependent on the maternal MAP and sensitive to maternal hypotension, catecholamines, and vasopressors.

Unrecognized contractions in spinal cord injury should be avoided by cardiotocographic monitoring.

**Answer: C**

Grabo, D. and Schwab, C.W. (2013) Trauma in pregnant women, in *The Trauma Manual: Trauma and Acute Care Surgery*, 4th edn (eds A.B. Peitzman, M. Rhodes, C.W. Schwab, *et al.*), Lippincott Williams and Wilkins, Philadelphia, PA, pp. 228–233.

Jain, V., Chari, R., Maslovitz, S., *et al.* (2015) Guidelines for the management of a pregnant trauma patient. *Journal of Obstetrics and Gynaecology*, Canada, 37 (6), 553–571.

Knudson, M. and Yeh, D. (2013) Trauma in pregnancy, in *Trauma*, 7th edn (eds K.L. Mattox, E.E. Moore and D.V. Feliciano), McGraw-Hill, New York, pp. 709–724.

Lynch, A. (2009) Trauma in pregnancy, in *Trauma Care: Initial Assessment and Treatment in the Emergency Department* (ed. E. Cole), Chichester, Wiley-Blackwell, pp. 231–244.

6   Imaging the pregnant trauma patient can lead to concerns. Which statement is true regarding radiation exposure during pregnancy?

A   The maximum permissible radiation dose for fetal exposure is 500 mSv

B   Fetal radiation exposure from a single maternal pelvic CT scan increases the risk of fatal childhood cancer by approximately 2-fold.

C   Exposure during the first eight weeks does not increase the risk of spontaneous abortion, malformations, and mental retardation

D   The radiation risks to the fetus during the first trimester of pregnancy are so high that they outweigh the benefit of timely and accurate diagnosis

E   Three percent of trauma patients who undergoing CT scanning will have an unidentified pregnancy

Ionizing radiation is more harmful to cells that are developing rapidly, such as in a developing fetus, therefore the benefit to imaging any trauma patient should always outweigh the risk of performing the study. In general, routine imaging (other than a FAST ultrasound) is to be avoided in the pregnant trauma patient.

The National Council on Radiation Protection and Measurements has recommended that the maximal permissible radiation dose for fetal exposure during pregnancy is 5 mSv.

The dose exposure from a pelvic CT scan is well within the permissible guidelines, even though it has been estimated to increase the likelihood of fatal childhood cancer by a factor of two.

Early exposure will indeed increase the risk of spontaneous abortion, malformations and mental retardation in the fetus.

Concerns regarding fetal exposure to radiation during investigation for trauma by plain radiography or computed tomographic scanning notwithstanding, it is important to remember that the priority is the mother, and without maternal survival, the fetus will also perish. The benefits of accurate diagnosis always outweigh the fetal risks, in ANY trimester.

It has been estimated that as many as 3% of trauma patients are pregnant, but only approximately 0.3% will be diagnosed during their trauma workup and evaluation.

**Answer: B**

American College of Radiology (2008) ACR practice guideline for imaging pregnant or potentially pregnant adolescents and women with ionizing radiation. *American College of Radiology*, Resolution **26**, 1–15.

Bochicchio, G.V., Napolitano, L.M/, Haan, J., *et al.* (2001) Incidental pregnancy in trauma patients. *Journal of the American College of Surgeons*, **192** (5), 566–569.

Chen, M.M., Coakley, F.V., Kaimal, A., *et al.* (2008) Guidelines for computed tomography and magnetic resonance imaging use during pregnancy and lactation. *Obstetrics and Gynecology*, **112**, 333–340.

Corwin, M.T., Seibert, J.A., Fananapazir, G., *et al.* (2016) JOURNAL CLUB: Quantification of fetal dose reduction if abdominal CT is limited to the top of the iliac crests in pregnant patients with trauma. *American Journal of Roentgenology*, **206** (4), 705–712.

Gilo, N.B., Amini, D., and Landy, H.J. (2009) Appendicitis and cholecystitis in pregnancy. *Clinical Obstetrics and Gynecology*, **52** (4), 586–596.

Raptis, C.A., Mellnick, V.M., Raptis, D.A., *et al.* (2014) Imaging of trauma in the pregnant patient. *Radiographics*, **34** (3), 748–763.

7 *Which of the following is not an indication for emergency Caesarean section in a pregnant trauma patient?*
   A *After 10 minutes of maternal cardiac arrest.*
   B *After 3 minutes of maternal cardiac arrest with ongoing CPR.*
   C *Stable mother with worrisome fetal heart tracing, fetal age 32 weeks.*
   D *Penetrating trauma to the abdomen causing uterine injury in a pregnant patient with a viable, near-term fetus.*
   E *The onset of labor in a pregnant patient with a term (>36 weeks) fetus, in the presence of pelvic fractures related to blunt abdominal trauma.*

An emergency Caesarean section can be accomplished extremely quickly by a skilled operator, and may be used to improve both maternal and fetal mortality and morbidity. Outcomes are optimal in neonates delivered within four minutes after cardiac arrest, as long as delivery can be achieved within one minute for a total time of five minutes following maternal death. Survival is 70% when delivery is achieved in less than five minutes, and survivors are usually neurologically intact, as opposed to 13% survival with 100% neurological morbidity after 5 minutes.

If there has been prolonged CPR, which in the pregnant trauma patient means longer than 5 minutes, the fetal outcomes are uniformly poor, and the procedure is NOT recommended.

Based on the criteria given earlier, the fetus in option B may have a reasonable chance of a good outcome if a C-section can be accomplished rapidly.

A Caesarean section is indicated in a patient with a viable fetus if there is concern for fetal distress, as this will give good outcomes. In the patient in option C, this could be accomplished in a semi-elective fashion, allowing time for any neonatal resuscitation team to be mobilized.

Penetrating trauma to the abdomen in the pregnant female is rare, but can affect up to 8% of all pregnancies. An emergency caesarian section should be performed in the presence of maternal shock, uterine injury, or concern for intra-abdominal injury if the fetus is near term.

Pelvic fractures are not a contra indication for vaginal delivery, according to the American College of Gynecologists, although they acknowledge that a severe, dislocated, or unstable fracture may preclude vaginal delivery.

**Answer: A**

Hill, C.C. and Pickinpaugh, J. (2008) Trauma and surgical emergencies in the obstetric patient. *The Surgical Clinics of North America*, **88** (2), 421–440.

Mirza, F.G., Devine, P.C., and Gaddipati, S. (2010) Trauma in pregnancy: a systematic approach. *American Journal of Perinatology*, **27** (7), 579–586.

Oxford, C.M. and Ludmir, J. (2009) Trauma in pregnancy. *Clinical Obstetrics and Gynecology*, **52** (4), 611–629.

Petrone, P., Talving, P., Browder, T., *et al.* (2011) Abdominal injuries in pregnancy: a 155-month study at two level 1 trauma centers. *Injury*, **42** (1), 47–49.

8 *Which of the following is true regarding the hypercoagulability of pregnancy?*
   A *Pregnancy increases the risk of thrombosis by a factor of ten times*
   B *The risk of arterial thromboembolism is the same as the risk of venous thromboembolism*

C *Normal pregnancy causes an increase in Factors VII, VIII, X, and von Willebrand*

D *Heparin and low-molecular weight heparin can cross the placenta and therefore are not considered safe in pregnancy*

E *Warfarin is transmitted via breast milk and should not be used in a woman developing a peripartum DVT or PE*

The state of pregnancy causes a hypercoagulability which while mostly due to changes in levels of plasma proteins likely also has a mechanical component due to the mechanical obstruction caused by the gravid uterus, as well as increased venous capacitance with decreased venous outflow. Virchow's triad of hypercoagulation, vascular damage, and venous stasis all occur in some fashion or another during pregnancy, which accounts for this increased risk.

Pregnancy increases the risk of thromboembolism by only three to four times, although this is somewhat higher for venous disease at four to five times. The prevalence of VTE in pregnancy is 0.8–2.0 per 1000 pregnancies but it does account for 1.1 deaths per 100 000 pregnancies.

The vast majority of thromboses during pregnancy are venous, with only approximately 20% arising in the arterial system.

It is normal for there to be increases in Factors VII, VIII, X, and von Willebrand factor, and increases in fibrinogen.

Heparin and LMWH do not cross the placenta and are therefore considered the treatment of choice for thromboembolic disease in the pregnant patient, unlike warfarin, which can cross the placenta and is associated with abortion and hemorrhage.

Warfarin is not secreted in the breast milk, however, and can be considered safe in the post-partum period for the treatment of significant VTE.

**Answer: C**

Heit, J.A., Kobbervig, C.E., James A.H., *et al.* (2005) Trends in the incidence of venous thromboembolism during pregnancy or postpartum: a 30-year population-based study. *Annals of Internal Medicine*, **143** (10), 697–706.

James, A.H. (2010) Pregnancy and thrombotic risk. *Critical Care Medicine*, **38** (2 Suppl), S57–63.

9 *Regarding seatbelt use in pregnancy, which of the following statements is correct?*

A *Studies have not demonstrated any significant decline in maternal mortality with the use of seatbelts*

B *Appropriate education has not been demonstrated to improve the use of seatbelts by pregnant woman, as they find the seatbelts too uncomfortable*

C *The correct position for seatbelts in the pregnant woman is under the abdomen, over both anterior superior iliac spines and the pubic symphysis, with the shoulder belt left behind the left shoulder*

D *If a seatbelt is appropriately applied, there is no increased force transmitted to the fetus*

E *Placing the lap belt over the dome of the uterus is associated with uterine and fetal injury*

Pregnant women cite a number of reasons not to use seatbelts in cars, from lack of comfort, fear of injuring the fetus in a crash, to forgetfulness. This increases the risk of noncompliance in the pregnant trauma patient, especially as there is a lot of misinformation that is perpetuated regarding the risk of seatbelts to the uterus in the case of a motor vehicle crash.

The risk of maternal mortality was reduced from 33% to 5% in one early study on seatbelt use in pregnant women, therefore pregnant women should be counseled that seatbelt use is still highly desirable, even if in states where it is not mandatory.

Education has been shown to improve compliance, as it has been shown that only 35–55% of women receive counseling regarding their use during their antenatal visits. A focused prenatal intervention was shown to increase seatbelt use from 70% to 83%.

The correct position for a seatbelt in a pregnant woman is under the abdomen, over both anterior superior iliac spines and the pubic symphysis, with the shoulder belt positioned between the breasts.

Even when the seatbelt is properly applied, there is some suggestion from experimental crash testing that there is increased force transmitted to the fetus. Specifically, the impact of the lap belt on the pelvic bone may lead to fetal head compression and the impact of the backrest in a rear impact collision may result in increased fetal acceleration.

If the lap belt is placed over the dome of the uterus, this is associated with significant morbidity in the event of a crash, and therefore is NOT to be recommended.

**Answer: E**

Crosby, W.M. and Costiloe, J.P. (1971) Safety of lap-belt restraint for pregnant victims of automobile collisions. *New England Journal of Medicine*, **284** (12), 632–636.

Delotte, J., Behr, M., Thollon, L., *et al.* (2008) Pregnant woman and road safety: experimental crash test with post mortem human subject. *Surgical and Radiologic Anatomy*, **30** (3), 185–189.

McGwin, G., Jr, Willey, P., Ware, A., *et al.* (2004) A focused educational intervention can promote the proper application of seat belts during pregnancy. *Journal of Trauma*, **56** (5), 1016–1021.

Vladutiu, C.J. and Weiss, H.B. (2012) Motor vehicle safety during pregnancy. *American Journal of Lifestyle Medicine*, **6** (3), 241–249.

**10** *Intimate partner violence is the most common cause of trauma-related maternal death during pregnancy and is clustered in the third trimester. Which of the following is not a risk factor for pregnancy-related violence?*
   **A** *Low socioeconomic status*
   **B** *Older siblings*
   **C** *Carrying an unwanted/unexpected pregnancy*
   **D** *Low levels of social support*
   **E** *Alcohol or substance abuse*

First-time parenting is a risk factor for pregnancy related violence. Battered pregnant patients have a high rate of fetal loss as well as low fetal birth weight, low maternal weight gain, maternal infections, and anemia. Warning signs while evaluating the pregnant trauma patient include: a history of depression, substance abuse, multiple visits to the ED, delay in seeking medical attention, implausible explanation for injuries, or the presence of an overprotective partner.

Low socioeconomic status unfortunately contributes to poor fetal outcomes on multiple levels, including an increased risk of intimate partner violence.

Having older siblings, while not necessarily protective, is the only one of the factors listed that is *not* associated with an increased risk for pregnant patients to suffer from violence.

Carrying an unplanned/unwanted child can often be a significant source of stress for both the patient and the partner involved, and these tensions can erupt during this period leading to violence, therefore this is a known risk factor.

Low levels of social support, particularly family support, can definitely increase the risk of intimate partner violence, especially if the patient is already in an abused relationship and does not feel that they have options to escape or leave this situation.

Substance abuse, either of drugs or alcohol, while lower than in the general population, unfortunately still occurs in pregnant females, and this risk-taking behavior can often lead to situations putting the person at risk for violence, both from known and unknown individuals.

**Answer: B**

Knudson, M. and Yeh, D. (2013) Trauma in pregnancy, in *Trauma*, 7th edn (eds K.L. Mattox, E.E. Moore, and D.V. Feliciano), McGraw-Hill, New York, pp. 709–724.

**11** *If indicated, how should a perimortem c-section be performed?*

   **A** *Vertical midline abdominal and fascial incision; vertical midline incision of upper uterine segment*
   **B** *Horizontal Pfannenstiel incision 2 cm above the pubic symphysis and transverse fascial incision; horizontal curved incision of lower uterine segment*
   **C** *Horizontal Pfannenstiel incision 2 cm above the pubic symphysis and transverse fascial incision; vertical incision of upper uterine segment*
   **D** *Joel-Cohen incision, a straight lateral incision about two centimeters above the Pfannenstiel location; horizontal curved incision of upper uterine segment*
   **E** *Joel-Cohen incision, a straight lateral incision about two centimeters above the Pfannenstiel location; vertical incision of upper uterine segment*

Although there is still considerable controversy regarding this practice, in a pregnant trauma patient in extremis, with a fetus EGA > 25 weeks and with present fetal heart tones, an emergency C-section should be performed. A concomitant resuscitative thoracotomy may also be considered. The technique for an emergency C-section in the trauma patient varies from the C-section performed on the non-trauma pregnant patient.

Vertical midline abdominal and fascial incisions are made, followed by a vertical midline incision of upper uterine segment. The infant is then removed and suctioned and handed off for further resuscitation. The trauma surgeon then controls bleeding from the placenta, uterus, and other intra-abdominal injuries. While making the vertical uterine incision, care must be taken not to extend it such that the vagina or bladder are injured, which is a reason this vertical incision has fallen out of favor in obstetrics.

The Pfannenstiel incision is more suited to routine obstetrical care, as this does not allow for any operative management of concomitant abdominal injuries, and therefore is not to be recommended in the trauma patient.

Joel-Cohen techniques have been utilized in obstetrics and recently have been compared to the Misgav-Ladach method. The transverse lower uterine incision is more commonly used, as well as extending into a J or T incision to facilitate delivery of a larger infant. Again, this is not to be recommended to the trauma surgeon, particularly those who are not familiar with type of incision and do not practice cesarean sections on a regular basis.

**Answer: A**

Gizzo, S., Andrisani, A., Noventa, M., *et al.* (2015) Caesarean section: could different transverse abdominal incision techniques influence postpartum pain and subsequent quality of life? A systematic review. *PLoS ONE*, **10** (2), e0114190.

Knudson, M. and Yeh, D. (2013) Trauma in pregnancy, in *Trauma*, 7th edn (eds K.L. Mattox, E.E. Moore and D.V. Feliciano), McGraw-Hill, New York, pp. 709–724.

Xavier, P., Ayres-De-Campos, D., Reynolds, A., *et al.* (2005) The modified Misgav-Ladach versus the Pfannenstiel–Kerr technique for cesarean section: a randomized trial. *Acta Obstetricia et Gynecologica Scandinavica*, **84**, 878–882.

**12** *Which of the following is included in the differential diagnosis for altered mental status (AMS) in the pregnant patient?*
   **A** *Acute blood loss*
   **B** *Seizure due to eclampsia*
   **C** *Amniotic fluid embolism*
   **D** *Intracerebral hemorrhage due to HELLP syndrome*
   **E** *All of the above*

Compared to the general trauma patient, the clinician needs to remember not only the usual causes of altered sensorium but in addition, there are specific conditions that are only relevant in the gravid patient. Therefore, all of the answer choices should be considered in the differential diagnosis for AMS in a pregnant patient.

The patient may be suffering from acute blood loss from either an intra-abdominal source or related to either maternofetal hemorrhage or more simply a placental abruption. In its advanced stages, just as in the non-trauma patient, hemorrhagic shock will lead to a dressed mental status.

The precipitating event for the trauma may be a neurologic insult from any disorder on the spectrum of pregnancy induced hypertension. Pre-eclampsia is defined by sustained systolic blood pressure > 160 mm Hg, sustained diastolic blood pressure > 110 mm Hg, proteinuria > 5 g/24 h. Preeclampsia is indicative of decreased placental blood flow and can lead to intrauterine growth retardation. Hypertension should be treated. Magnesium sulfate infusion should be initiated to prevent development of eclampsia, heralded by seizures. The only treatment at that time is delivery of the fetus. Other complications from eclampsia are: intracerebral hemorrhage, acute tubular necrosis, blindness, and disseminated intravascular coagulation.

Amniotic fluid embolism can both lead to hypotension causing decreased cerebral blood flow, resulting in altered mental status. Sudden onset dyspnea, hypoxia, and hypotension may be seen in both pulmonary embolism and amniotic fluid embolism. Of patients with amniotic fluid embolism, 50% will develop DIC.

HELLP syndrome has been known to precipitate intracerebral hemorrhage in rare cases, and although

unlikely should certainly be on the list of differential diagnoses.

**Answer: E**

Knudson, M. and Yeh, D. (2013) Trauma in pregnancy, in *Trauma*, 7th edn (eds K.L. Mattox, E.E. Moore and D.V. Feliciano), McGraw-Hill, New York, pp. 709–724.

Lucia, A. and Dantoni, S.E. (2016) Trauma management of the pregnant patient. *Critical Care Clinics*, **32** (1), 109–117.

**13** *HELLP syndrome can be a life-threatening condition for the mother and fetus. Treatment of HELLP includes:*
   **A** *Delivery if > 34 weeks gestation*
   **B** *Treatment with corticosteroids for improved perinatal outcomes in HELLP with EGA 24–34 weeks*
   **C** *Plasma exchange with FFP if progressive elevation of bilirubin or creatinine > 72 hours after delivery*
   **D** *Platelet transfusion*
   **E** *All of the above*

HELLP syndrome is rare, affecting only 0.6% of pregnant women. Of HELLP cases, 70% occur in the 2nd and 3rd trimesters, while 30% can occur postpartum. Women with postpartum HELLP syndrome have an increased risk of renal failure and pulmonary edema compared to antenatal HELLP development. Criteria for diagnosis include: an elevated LDH > 600 U/L, elevated unconjugated bilirubin > 1.2, elevated transaminases AST > 70 U/L, thrombocytopenia with platelet count < 100, with the presence of schistocytes or burr cells due to microangiopathic hemolytic anemia. Acute fatty liver of pregnancy (AFLP) shares many clinical signs and biochemical changes with HELLP syndrome, but AFLP will also have hypoglycemia and prolonged PTT. Supportive care is achieved with blood pressure control, IV fluids, and transfusion of blood products.

As with severe pre-eclampsia and eclampsia, delivery is indicated for definitive treatment of HELLP syndrome. This should only be done if the condition is severe enough that it is threatening maternal wellbeing, and when the fetus has reached a viable age. Occasionally, a termination may be necessary in order to save the life of the mother.

If the EGA < 34 weeks, betamethasone for fetal lung maturity may be administered and delivery within 48 hours may be performed if there is no maternal or fetal distress. In small retrospective studies, steroids have been shown to have maternal benefits such as quicker recovery of platelet counts, diminished pulmonary edema, inhibited endothelial activation, and reduced endothelial dysfunction, prevention of thrombotic microangiopathic anemia, inhibition of cytokine production. However, in the largest randomized double blinded placebo controlled study of high dose dexamethasone versus placebo, the maternal benefits were not reproduced and the rates of platelets and FFP transfusions were not significantly reduced. Also, long-term maternal and fetal benefits have not been shown. Therefore, high dose dexamethasone is not recommended for maternal treatment of HELLP.

Plasma exchange with FFP should be initiated if progressive elevation of bilirubin or creatinine > 72 hours persists after delivery.

Transfusion of platelets may be required, but thrombocytopenia associated with this condition is usually temporary and self-limited. Platelet counts can decrease even after delivery, but the majority of patients have platelet recovery by the third postpartum day.

**Answer: E**

Haram, K., Svendsen, E., and Abildgaard, U. (2009) The HELLP Syndrome: clinical issues and management. A review. *BMC Pregnancy and Childbirth*, **9**, 8.

Lucia, A. and Dantoni, S.E. (2016) Trauma management of the pregnant patient. *Critical Care Clinics*, **32** (1), 109–117.

Rajasekhar, A., Gernsheimer, T., Stasi, R., *et al.* (2013) *Clinical Practice Guide on Thrombocytopenia in Pregnancy*, American Society of Hematology, Washington, DC.

**14** *Which of the following is false regarding changes in management in the pregnant trauma patient?*

   **A** *Chest tube thoracostomy should be performed 1–2 rib spaces higher than usual*

   **B** *Diagnostic peritoneal lavage should be performed using a SUPRA-umbilical incision*

   **C** *The patient should be tilted to the left after mid-pregnancy to take pressure off the IVC*

   **D** *Every pregnant patient should have a vaginal exam irrespective of the trimester*

   **E** *MRI scans can be used in pregnant patients, even with the addition of Gadolinium contrast*

There are a number of physiologic and anatomical changes that occur in the pregnant female, some of which necessitate changes in management during the initial evaluation and resuscitation. Some are covered in the following sections.

Chest tubes should be placed more superiorly than usual, due to the displacement of the diaphragms in a cephalad direction which increases with the duration of the pregnancy

Should a diagnostic peritoneal aspirate or lavage become necessary, then a supra-umbilical incision should be utilized to avoid damage to the uterus. It also goes without saying that an open approach to this technique should be employed in these circumstances.

As the pregnancy advances, the weight of the gravid uterus can compress the IVC and decrease venous return. The standard practice of extricating all blunt trauma patients onto a long and rigid spine board puts these patients at risk of this complication, especially in the third trimester. In a hypotensive pregnant trauma patient, the first maneuver should be to roll the patient onto their left side, keeping them in spinal alignment if there is continued concern for spinal trauma.

After the fetus weeks is 23 weeks of gestational age, it is important to confirm that placenta previa is NOT present prior to physical examination prompted by bleeding, as this may be a herald bleed that could deteriorate without undue care. A recent or current ultrasound scan should be performed to confirm the absence of this condition prior to either a digital or speculum exam. Urgent obstetrical consultation is highly recommended in these circumstances.

MRI has been shown to be safe and effective in pregnancy, but the length of time taken, lack of ability to provide direct care for the patient during the scan, and the need usually to transport the patient away from the trauma area do not make this modality the imaging type of choice. However, MRI is not currently recommended for pregnant patients in the first trimester due to theoretical concerns regarding fetal development and magnetic fields.

**Answer: D**

Barraco, R.D., Chiu, W.C., Clancy, T.V., *et al.* (2010) Practice management guidelines for the diagnosis and management of injury in the pregnant patient: the EAST Practice Management Guidelines Work Group. *Journal of Trauma*, **69** (1), 211–214.

Jain, V., Chari, R., Maslovitz, S., *et al.* (2015) Guidelines for the management of a pregnant trauma patient. *Journal of Obstetrics and Gynecology Canada*, **37** (6), 553–574.

**15** *One of the most feared complications of trauma in the pregnant patient is placental abruption. Which of the following is true?*

   **A** *The incidence after trauma is comparable to the general pregnant population*

   **B** *Ultrasound findings can be very sensitive in making the diagnosis*

   **C** *Abruption increases the risk of fetal demise by almost nine times*

**D** *A normal platelet count and fibrinogen concentration adequately rules out active abruption*

**E** *Vaginal bleeding is always present in patients presenting with abruption after trauma*

It is thought that the uterus changes its shape slightly when subjected to strong acceleration-deceleration forces, for example, from a motor vehicle crash. As the placenta is not elastic and the amniotic fluid is also not compressible, these acceleration-deceleration forces or direct trauma can cause uterine distortion and result in shear stress at the utero-placental interface. This increases the risk for abruptio placenta, which is one of the most feared complications of pregnancy, as the risk of fetal demise is dramatically increased.

The frequency of abruption is approximately 0.4–1.3% in the general obstetric population, and in all circumstances this is increased following trauma. Depending on the severity of the trauma, and whether the abdomen is involved this may range from 8.5% to as high as over 40%

Unfortunately, ultrasound is helpful only if it does demonstrate a placental abruption, but the sensitivity has been reported to be as low as 40%. If performed, CT and/or MRI scans may be helpful in picking up this condition, but there is no single test that is able to detect this condition with enough accuracy to be relied upon.

The risk to the fetus depends on the degree of placental separation, but in one large study of over 50 000 births, it was estimated that abruption was associated with an 8.9 fold increased risk of stillbirth. This rose to 31.5 if there was a 75% separation between the placenta and the uterus. Given this finding, it is critical to retain a high index of suspicion in these patients for the first 24–48 hours after abdominal trauma

Although disseminated intravascular coagulation is one of the most feared consequences of placenta abruption, it is not common. Normal blood tests do not adequately rule out the diagnosis, and cannot be conclusively relied upon. That being said, serial measurements should form part of the continued monitoring of the patient if the patient is being observed.

Vaginal bleeding can certainly provide further suspicion for abruption, but again may only be about 50% sensitive. Significant abruption can be associated with minimal maternal symptoms, including the absence of vaginal bleeding; therefore, this also cannot be relied upon.

**Answer: C**

Ananth, C.V., Berkowitz, G.S., Savitz, D.A., *et al.* (1999) Placental abruption and adverse perinatal outcomes. *Journal of the American Medical Association*, **282** (17), 1646–1651.

Ananth, C.V. and Kinzler, W.L. (2017) Placental abruption: clinical features and diagnosis, https://www.uptodate.com/contents/placental-abruption-clinical-features-and-diagnosis?source=search_result&search=placental%20abruption%20after%20trauma&selected Title=1~148 (accessed November 11, 2017).

Oyelese, Y. and Ananth, C.V. (2006) Placental abruption. *Obsterics and Gynecology*, **108** (4), 1005–1016.

**16** *All of the following have a role in the routine assessment of fetal well-being except?*
   **A** *Amniocentesis*
   **B** *Admission for observation*
   **C** *FAST exam in the trauma bay*
   **D** *Measurement of the peak systolic velocity of the fetal middle cerebral artery*
   **E** *Fetal heart tracing*

While the focus of care for the pregnant trauma patient should be on ensuring that the mother is stable and uninjured, the next priority will be to assess whether the fetus has suffered any ill effects of the trauma. There are both simple and more complex methods by which this can be achieved, and it is often necessary to obtain an early OB/GYN consultation to help facilitate the necessary investigations and/or monitoring.

While amniocentesis may have a role in the assessment of fetal lung maturity in those patients who start to undergo pre-term labor, it is not performed when the fetus is over 39 weeks as it is unnecessary, and not when the fetus is less than 32 weeks because lung immaturity is highly likely. Given these constraints, and its invasive nature, it is not indicated as part of the routine work-up of a pregnant trauma patient, without signs of premature labor.

Any clinical or laboratory signs of abruption, presence of contractions, and/or other indications of fetal distress (e.g., on fetal heart tracing) should prompt a period of observation for at least 24 hours, which can be extended to 48 hours in patients at high risk for placental abruption.

The FAST exam can detect the presence of blood in the abdominal cavity of the mother, as well as be used to evaluate for the presence of fetal heartbeat and fetal movement. Unfortunately, ultrasound is only about 40% sensitive for the presence of placental abruption in the trauma setting.

In cases of severe fetal anemia following maternal trauma such as placental abruption or severe maternofetal hemorrhage, ultrasound can be used to assess the peak systolic velocity of the middle cerebral artery in the fetus. The ultrasound is looking for a characteristic increase that indicates fetal brain sparing, and can be useful in certain cases where ambiguity exists regarding actual fetal hemorrhage.

The mainstay of fetal assessment is fetal heart tracing, which can be initiated in the trauma bay, and then is often continued in a maternal observation unit or as an inpatient. Close cooperation with the OB/GYN service is essential in patients who have a fetus older than the viability limit, usually considered to be around 23–25 weeks, although the exact age remains controversial.

**Answer: A**

Brown, S. and Mozurkewich, E. (2013) Trauma during pregnancy. *Obstetrics and Gynecology Clinics of North America*, **40** (1), 47–57.

17  Which of the following is false regarding airway management in the pregnant trauma patient?
    A  *Lower doses of succinylcholine are utilized for rapid sequence intubation*
    B  *The tongue is often larger making laryngoscopy more challenging*
    C  *Pre-oxygenation is more important due to the reduced maternal functional residual capacity and increased oxygen demand*
    D  *Awake fiberoptic intubation is the preferred method of intubation in the pregnant patient*
    E  *The oral mucosa and oropharynx are hyperemic and more prone to bleeding with manipulation, making subsequent attempts at intubation harder after an initial failure*

The physiologic and anatomical changes that develop during pregnancy also have an impact on the ease and techniques associated with intubation, so this should be remembered and accounted for. The mother and fetus are more susceptible to hypoxia, and so oxygen should be administered liberally, particularly around the time of intubation.

The placenta also produces pseudocholinesterase, increasing the plasma levels in pregnant patients; therefore the dose of succinylcholine used for intubation should be reduced to achieve the same effect,

The weight gain of pregnancy, contrary to urban myth, is not just on the hips, thighs, and abdomen, but also affects the breasts, the tongue, and causes the oral cavity and oropharynx to have an increased blood supply. This can make direct laryngoscopy significantly more difficult.

Pre-oxygenation prior to intubation of the trauma patient is always important but even more so in this case, where there are two patients, and the tolerance of the fetus for hypoxia is low. In addition, there is decreased functional residual capacity in the mother as well as an increase in oxygen demand. Both of these make oxygen administration even more critical in these patients.

Although awake fiberoptic intubation is certainly an option in the pregnant patient, and should be considered in those cases with a cervical spine fracture, it does not offer significant advantages, and will take significantly longer in addition to requiring specialized equipment.

As stated previously, the weight gain of pregnancy also causes increased blood flow to the mucosa, increasing the changes of bleeding with excessive manipulation. Multiple studies have confirmed that blood in the airway is a risk factor for failure of intubation, therefore gentle manipulation of the oropharynx during each attempt is even more important in this patient population

**Answer: D**

Hill, C.C. and Pickinpaugh, J. (2008) Trauma and surgical emergencies in the obstetric patient. *Surgical Clinics of North* America, **88,** 421–440.
Schneider, R. (2000) Muscle relaxants, in *Emergency Airway Management* (ed. R. Walls), Lippincott Williams & Wilkins, Philadelphia, PA, pp. 121–128.

18  Which of the following laboratories studies would be abnormal in the pregnant trauma patient?
    A  *PCO$_2$ 45 mm Hg*
    B  *Fibrinogen 400 mg/dl*
    C  *Hematocrit 32%*
    D  *WBC 15 000 uL*
    E  *HCO$_3$ 19 mEq/L*

There are multiple changes during the pregnant state, which are designed to help the body cope with the increased metabolic demand, as well as prepare for the blood loss associated with delivery of the fetus. Blood volume increases leading to a relative anemia, both systolic and diastolic blood pressure is lower, there are ECG changes, PaCO$_2$ levels are lower, there may be a leukocytosis, and there is a relative hypercoagulable state. These are all considerations that need to remembered when caring for a pregnant trauma patient.

Progesterone-mediated stimulation of tidal volume results in increased minute ventilation, and a state of mild hypocarbia, with mean PaCO$_2$ of 30 mm Hg, and as low as 25 mm Hg. Because values are lower in pregnancy, a PaCO$_2$ value in the non-pregnant range is concerning.

Most procoagulant factors are increased during pregnancy and may be beneficial for the patient in achieving hemostasis after injury. Fibrinogen may increase as much as 50%, and Low levels of fibrinogen may be consistent with disseminated intravascular coagulopathy (DIC), and suggest placental abruption or other type of hemorrhage.

Due to physiologic anemia of pregnancy hematocrit between 32 and 42 mg/dl is considered normal.

A leukocytosis often exists during pregnancy, and values as high as 25 000/mcL may be normal for a patient while gravid

Lower than normal serum bicarbonate results as compensation for hypocarbia, as there is a compensatory renal excretion of bicarbonate resulting in serum levels of 17 mEq/L to 22 mEq/L, thereby maintaining an arterial pH of 7.40 to 7.45.

**Answer: A**

Brown, S. and Mozurkewich, E. (2013) Trauma during pregnancy. *Obstetrics and Gynecology Clinics of North America*, **40** (1), 47–57.

Yeomans, E.R. and Gilstrap, L.C. (2005) Physiologic changes in pregnancy and their impact on critical care. *Critical Care Medicine*, **33** (10), S256–S.258.

19 *Which of the following statements is true regarding trauma in pregnancy?*
   A *The incidence of trauma during pregnancy is approximately 1–2% of all pregnancies.*
   B *The presence of a pelvic fracture is not an indication per se for Caesarean section at time of delivery*
   C *Assaults are the most common reason for presentation to a trauma center in a pregnant patient*
   D *The leading cause of non-obstetric death during pregnancy is suicide*
   E *Urine toxicology is not indicated during pregnancy due to a very low incidence of drug and alcohol use in these patients.*

Trauma during pregnancy does represent some unique challenges, which is why these patients are regarded as one of the "special" populations within ATLS and therefore it is important to know a little not only about the physiological changes associated with the pregnant state, but also the epidemiology of injuries sustained during this time. Depending on the trauma center, these patients may be encountered on a relatively frequent basis.

Unfortunately the actual incidence of trauma during pregnancy is significantly higher, at approximately 5–7%.

Even in the case of a pregnant patient with a pelvic fracture, up to 80% of patients were able to have a vaginal delivery, so this should not be an absolute indication for a caesarean section in these circumstances.

Motor vehicle collisions account for approximately 55% of all trauma admissions in pregnant women, but assaults follow next, at about 22%, with falls the third most common cause at 21%.

Trauma is unfortunately still the leading cause of non-obstetric death during pregnancy, rather than suicide, which is thankfully fairly rare in this patient population.

Trauma remains the leading cause of death for patients aged between 4–44 irrespective of their pregnant status.

The incidence of drug and alcohol use is in fact lower than in the general population – approximately 5% versus 11.4% for illicit drug use and 9% for alcohol use, but this remains significant enough to be a concern and to be worthy of screening.

**Answer: B**

Brown, S. and Mozurkewich, E. (2013) Trauma during pregnancy. *Obstetrics and Gynecology Clinics of North America*, **40** (1), 47–57.

Connolly, A.M., Katz, V.L., Bash, K.L., *et al.* (1997) Trauma and pregnancy. *American Journal of Perinatology*, **14** (6), 331–336.

Gunter, J. and Pearlman, M. (2001) Emergencies during pregnancy: trauma and nonobstetric surgical conditions, in *Obstetrics and Gynecology: Principles for Practice* (eds F. Ling and P. Duff), McGraw-Hill, New York, p. 253.

Pearlman, M.D., Tintinalli, J.E., and Lorenz, R.P. (1990) Blunt trauma during pregnancy. *New England Journal of Medicine*, **323** (23), 1609–1613.

Substance Abuse and Mental Health Services Administration (2014) Results from the 2013 National Survey on Drug Use and Health: Summary of National Findings and Detailed Tables. At: http://archive.samhsa.gov/data/NSDUH/2013SummNatFindDetTables/Index.aspx (accessed November 11, 2017).

20 *Regarding uterine rupture from trauma, which of the following is false?*
   A *It only occurs after the first trimester, when the uterus has risen out of the pelvis*
   B *Typically involves the uterine fundus*
   C *Clinical presentation varies from uterine tenderness to hypovolemic shock*
   D *Can be diagnosed with ultrasonography*
   E *Most common presentation in laboring patients is an abnormal fetal heart rate pattern*

Uterine rupture is a rare complication of blunt abdominal trauma accounting for approximately 0.6% of all injuries during pregnancy and can result in a maternal mortality rate of up to 10% and nearly universal fetal mortality. It occurs most commonly with rapid deceleration or direct compression injuries and is more frequent in women who have had cesarean deliveries previously.

Traumatic uterine rupture has been reported in all gestational ages, although the risk for uterine rupture tends to increase with advancing gestational age and with increasing severity of direct abdominal trauma.

Approximately three-quarters of cases involve the uterine fundus, but any part of the uterus can be involved, with the extent of injury ranging from serosal hemorrhage to complete disruption of the myometrial wall and extrusion of the fetus.

Presenting signs and symptoms include uterine tenderness, abnormal fetal heart rate patterns, and frank shock. Examination may be remarkable for vaginal bleeding, a rigid abdomen, rebound tenderness, and an asymmetric uterus or fetal parts palpable through the abdomen.

Disruption of the uterus can be diagnosed with ultrasonography, which can detect intraperitoneal hemorrhage, but the accuracy is not high enough for it to be relied upon completely.

The most common sign in an already laboring patient is an abnormal fetal heart rate pattern; therefore cardiotocographic monitoring is vital in patients where there is a high index of suspicion. The actual pattern may be absence of fetal heart rate, decreased fetal heart rate beat-to-beat variability, decelerations, or fetal tachycardia as a result of anemia or hypoxemia.

**Answer: A**

Hill, C.C. and Pickinpaugh, J. (2008) Trauma and surgical emergencies in the obstetric patient. *The Surgical Clinics of North America*, **88** (2), 421–440.

Mirza, F.G., Devine, P.C., and Gaddipati, S. (2010) Trauma in pregnancy: a systematic approach. *American Journal of Perinatology*, **27** (7), 579–586.

Mirza, F.G. and Gaddipati, S. (2009) Obstetric emergencies. *Seminars in Perinatology*, **33** (2), 97–103.

# 36

# Esophagus, Stomach, and Duodenum
*Matthew B. Singer, MD and Andrew Tang, MD*

1 Which statement regarding esophageal anatomy is false?
   A There are three predictable areas of narrowing: the cricopharyngeus muscle, the aortic arch, and the diaphragm
   B The cervical and most distal esophagus lie to the left of midline
   C The left gastric vein provides the principle venous drainage when esophageal varices develop
   D The segmental blood supply to the esophagus arises from the superior thyroid, the intercostals and the left gastric arteries
   E The lower esophageal sphincter is a physiologic rather than an anatomic entity

The esophagus is approximately 25 cm long with inner circular and outer longitudinal muscular layers, and no serosal covering. The upper two-thirds of the esophagus is lined by squamous epithelium, which transitions to columnar epithelium distally. The esophagus is divided into four segments: the pharyngoesophageal segment is between the pharynx and the cervical esophagus. It consists of the superior, middle, and inferior constrictors. The cricopharyngeus muscle is part of the inferior constrictor and serves as the upper esophageal sphincter. The potential space between the inferior constrictor and the cricopharyngeus muscle is the site of Zenker's diverticulum development.

The cervical esophagus is approximately 5 cm long. It begins at the cricopharyngeus muscle and ends at T1. The recurrent laryngeal nerves lie in the grooves between the esophagus and the trachea. The right recurrent laryngeal nerve has a more oblique course and is more prone to anatomic variants. Consequently, surgical access to the cervical esophagus is typically chosen from the left.

The thoracic esophagus begins at T1 and ends at the hiatus. It lies directly posterior to the trachea. Above the level of the tracheal bifurcation, the esophagus courses to the left, behind the bifurcation and the left main-stem bronchus, and descends to the diaphragmatic hiatus left of midline. The left mainstem bronchus and aortic arch create a narrowing of the thoracic esophagus at the level of T4. The bronchoaortic constriction can be visualized during endoscopy as a subtle pulsation along the posterior wall of the esophagus. The lower thoracic esophagus is covered by a flimsy layer of mediastinal pleura to the left, and this location is a common site for Boerhaave's perforation.

The abdominal esophagus begins at the diaphragmatic hiatus, which is the third location of anatomic narrowing. The lower esophageal sphincter is a physiologic entity that does not correspond to any particular anatomic structure. Manometrically, it is detected as a high-pressure zone 3–5 cm long with both intra-abdominal and thoracic components.

Blood supply to the esophagus is segmental. The inferior thyroid artery is the main supply of the cervical esophagus. The proximal thoracic esophagus is largely supplied by the bronchial arteries while branches arising directly from the aorta supply the distal esophagus. The left gastric and inferior phrenic arteries supply the abdominal esophagus.

**Answer: D**

Patti, M.G., Gantert, W., and Way, L.W. (1997) Surgery of the esophagus: anatomy and physiology. *The Surgical Clinics of North America*, 77, 959–970.

2 Which of the following statements regarding Boerhaave's syndrome is false?
   A Endoscopic evaluation of the esophageal tear is an integral part of diagnosis
   B The full-thickness esophageal tear is typically located in the left posterolateral aspect of the lower

*Surgical Critical Care and Emergency Surgery: Clinical Questions and Answers*, Second Edition.
Edited by Forrest "Dell" Moore, Peter Rhee, and Gerard J. Fulda.
© 2018 John Wiley & Sons Ltd. Published 2018 by John Wiley & Sons Ltd.
Companion website: www.wiley.com/go/moore/surgical_criticalcare_and_emergency_surgery

esophagus approximately 2–3 cm above the gastroesophageal junction

C Mackler's triad of vomiting, lower chest pain, and subcutaneous emphysema is seen in up to two-thirds of patients with Boerhaave's syndrome

D The underlying pathophysiology involves uncoordinated esophageal contraction against a closed pylorus distally and cricopharyngeus muscle proximally

E Upper GI bleeding frequently accompanies Boerhaave's syndrome

Boerhaave's syndrome is postulated to result from forceful esophageal contractions against a closed cricopharyngeus muscle and pylorus. The resultant sudden increase in intraluminal pressure creates a transmural esophageal tear, typically located in the left posterolateral aspect of the distal esophagus, 2–3 cm above the gastroesophageal junction. Meckler's triad of vomiting, lower chest pain, and subcutaneous emphysema is only present in up to two-thirds of patients, and therefore cannot be heavily relied on for diagnosis. The diagnostic test of choice is an esophagram.

When a perforation is suspected, water-soluble contrast is the initial agent used. It has a sensitivity of 80% in detecting intrathoracic esophageal perforations. If a perforation is not identified by gastrografin, the study should be repeated with thin barium, which has a sensitivity of 90% for intrathoracic perforations. Endoscopic evaluation of the esophageal tear adds little additional diagnostic value, and air insufflation can potentially enlarge the injury and further spread bacterial contamination.

The treatment of choice in Boerhaave's syndrome identified within 24 hours in a stable patient is primary repair in two layers with tissue buttressing through a laparotomy or left thoracotomy. Boerhaave's syndrome, in contrast to a Mallory-Weiss tear, is not typically associated with significant upper gastrointestinal bleeding.

**Answer: A**

Brinster, C.J., Singhal, S., Lee, L., *et al.* (2004) Evolving options in the management of esophageal perforation. *Annals of Thoracic Surgery*, **77** (4), 1475–1483.

Vial, C.M. and Whyte, R.I. (2005) Boerhaave's syndrome: diagnosis and treatment. *The Surgical Clinics of North America*, **85** (3), 515–524.

3 Which statement regarding esophageal perforation is most accurate?

A In spite of recent advances in the diagnosis and treatment of esophageal perforation, recent series demonstrate mortality as high as 80%

B Iatrogenic injury accounts for the majority of esophageal perforations

C High mortality rates seen in patients with penetrating esophageal injuries are directly related to severe mediastinitis

D In hemodynamically normal patients, free perforations of the thoracic esophagus can be successfully managed with chest drainage and antibiotics alone

E Esophageal perforation from food bolus impedance is frequently associated with untreated achalasia

While esophageal perforation has historically been associated with a mortality as high as 80%, recent improvements in imaging technology and critical care have contributed to improvements in morbidity and survival. The majority of esophageal perforations (approximately 60% in most series) are iatrogenic in nature, most commonly resulting from endoscopic therapy for strictures or achalasia. The exact mortality attributable to esophageal perforation in the setting of blunt or penetrating trauma is unknown due to its rarity as well as the impact of associated mediastinal and thoracic injuries on outcome.

Free esophageal perforation is a contraindication to conservative management since it represents an uncontrolled source of sepsis. However, small contained perforations with little or no mediastinal contamination may be amenable to non-operative management including endoscopic therapy or endoluminal stenting.

Achalasia is an esophageal motility disorder characterized by a failure of normal relaxation of the lower esophageal sphincter in response to bolus transport. Pneumatic dilatation for achalasia carries a perforation risk of 4–6%. Achalasia alone is not associated with spontaneous esophageal perforation.

**Answer: B**

Carrott, P.W. and Low, D.E. (2011) Advances in the management of esophageal perforation. *Thoracic Surgical Clinics*, **21** (4), 541–555.

4 What is the antibiotic regimen of choice for a patient on long-standing proton pump inhibitor therapy with suspected esophageal perforation from balloon dilation of a benign esophageal stricture?

A Cefazolin, piperacillin/tazobactam

B Cefazolin, fluconazole

C Vancomycin, piperacillin/tazobactam

D Piperacillin/tazobactam, fluconazole

E Vancomycin, piperacillin/tazobactam, fluconazole

Esophageal perforation can lead to overwhelming mediastinal sepsis and multisystem organ failure. Appropriate antibiotic administration is of paramount importance in addition to prompt therapeutic intervention. The proximal and mid esophagus are thought to harbor mostly transient bacteria and yeasts. By contrast, the distal esophagus contains a moderately diverse microbiome dominated by *Streptococcus*. Broad spectrum intravenous antibiotics that provide coverage for aerobes and anaerobes should be administered intravenously. Choices include ampicillin/sulbactam, piperacillin/tazobactam, or a carbapenem.

Antifungal coverage (e.g., fluconazole) is warranted in select cases. These include patients who have received broad-spectrum antimicrobial agents prior to perforation, patients on long-term antacid therapy, patients with human immunodeficiency virus infection, patients who have received steroids or other immunosuppressive therapy prior to perforation, and/or patients who fail to improve after several days of appropriate antibacterial therapy.

**Answer: D**

Bennett, J.E., Dolin, R., and Blaser, M.J. (2014) *Principles and Practice of Infectious Diseases*, Elsevier Health Sciences, Chicago.

Sepesi, B., Raymond, D.P., and Peters, J.H. (2010) Esophageal perforation: surgical, endoscopic and medical management strategies. *Current Opinion in Gastroenterology*, **26** (4), 379–383.

5 *Which of the following statements most accurately describes the management of a Mallory-Weiss tear?*
   A *The primary treatment modality is arteriography with trans-catheter embolization*
   B *Most Mallory-Weiss tears will stop bleeding with resuscitation and observation alone*
   C *Endoscopic epinephrine injection is less effective than hemoclip placement in controlling hemorrhage from a Mallory-Weiss tear*
   D *Rebleeding has been reported in up to 50% of patients after successful initial endoscopic therapy*
   E *Surgical intervention for a Mallory-Weiss tear is necessary in approximately 20% of cases*

Mallory-Weiss tear is a common cause of upper gastrointestinal bleeding and typically presents as hematemesis after an initial episode of vomiting without blood. It is defined as a mucosal laceration at the gastroesophageal junction or gastric cardia, usually caused by retching or forceful vomiting. Many factors have been associated with the development of Mallory-Weiss tears, including alcohol use, use of aspirin and warfarin, paroxysms of coughing, pregnancy, heavy lifting, straining, seizures, blunt abdominal trauma, colonic lavage, and cardiopulmonary resuscitation. Most Mallory-Weiss tears stop bleeding spontaneously. A minority of cases require endoscopic treatment.

Definitive diagnosis is confirmed by flexible upper endoscopy, which reveals a single mucosal tear in most cases. Endoscopic therapies that employ epinephrine injection, hemoclip placement, and band ligation have all been used with equal success to achieve primary hemostasis. Rebleeding is observed in up to 6% of patients after initial endoscopic therapy. Angiography with selective transcatheter embolization is another effective treatment option. However, it is not the first-line therapy due to the increased cost and higher local (hematoma, bleeding, arteriovenous fistulas) and systemic (acute kidney injury, ischemia) complications.

Surgery for hemorrhage refractory to endoscopic and angiographic therapies accounts for less than 3% of cases. It is performed through a longitudinal proximal anterior gastrotomy with oversewing the tear with absorbable sutures. Ligation of the descending branch of the left gastric artery should be considered.

**Answer: B**

Loffroy, R., Rao, P., Ota, S., *et al.* (2010) Embolization of acute nonvariceal upper gastrointestinal hemorrhage resistant to endoscopic treatment: results and predictors of recurrent bleeding. *Cardiovascular and Interventional Radiology*, **33** (6), 1088–1100.

Tjwa, E.T.T.L., Holster, I.L., and Kuipers, E.J. (2014) Endoscopic management of nonvariceal, nonulcer upper gastrointestinal bleeding. *Gastroenterology Clinics of North America*, **43** (4), 707–719.

6 *For a patient with a penetrating zone II neck wound with suspected cervical esophageal injury, which of the following statements is false:*
   A *Clinical findings of esophageal injury are unreliable*
   B *Upper endoscopy is an accurate method of diagnosis*
   C *Negative fluoroscopic esophagography with water soluble contrast should be followed by a confirmatory study using thin barium*
   D *CT esophagography is an acceptable method of evaluating a patient with altered mental status*
   E *Immediate operative cervical exploration is contraindicated in the absence of confirmatory diagnostic testing*

Clinical findings of esophageal injury are unreliable, identifying just 80% of injuries in the cervical esophagus. Evaluation for esophageal injuries involves esophagoscopy and esophagography. Contemporary literature demonstrates that flexible videoendoscopy is very accurate in experienced hands. If endoscopic findings are equivocal, esophagography should follow. The standard technique for contrast esophagography is to first administer water-soluble contrast. It is absorbed rapidly from the mediastinum and thus will not cause mediastinal fibrosis. Because this property also compromises the study's sensitivity, a "negative" water-soluble contrast study result should be followed by a confirmatory study using thin barium.

As an alternative to fluoroscopic esophagography, helical CT esophagography has been proposed and seems to be very accurate, with the advantages of avoiding the need for additional transportation to the fluoroscopy suite and the active participation of a radiologist as well as the potential for misinterpretation of the live images. Furthermore, it allows a contrast study in patients who are unable to actively participate (e.g. those who are intubated or mentally altered), as the contrast may be administered via a tube.

Given the difficulty in imaging the upper cervical esophagus and the potential for pulmonary edema if contrast is aspirated, the clinician must weigh the risks versus the benefits of immediate operative cervical exploration. The operative morbidity of cervical exploration is low enough that it is difficult to justify any complications related to nonoperative management.

**Answer: E**

Biffl, W.L., Moore, E.E., Feliciano, D.V., *et al.* (2015) Western Trauma Association critical decisions in trauma: diagnosis and management of esophageal injuries. *Journal of Trauma and Acute Care Surgery,* **79** (6), 1089–1095.

7  *Which of the following statements regarding operative repair of a cervical esophageal injury is most accurate?*
   A *Buttressing a primary repair with vascularized tissue is recommended, especially in the setting of concomitant tracheal injury*
   B *The cervical esophagus is best approached via an incision along the medial border of the right sternocleidomastoid muscle.*
   C *There is no role for intraoperative endoscopy during cervical esophageal repair*
   D *Primary repair is contraindicated in patients whose injury occurred more than 24 hours prior to presentation*
   E *The use of methylene blue in the identification of small esophageal perforations has fallen out of favor*

The cervical esophagus is approached via an incision along the medial border of the left sternocleidomastoid muscle; a cervical collar incision can be used if bilateral cervical exploration is planned. The esophagus should be exposed and circumferentially examined to identify all

injuries. Endoscopy is recommended intraoperatively to aid in identifying a perforation that might be obscured by hematoma; to evaluate the opposite side to help identify a through-and-through injury; and to insufflate air following repair to assess for a leak. In addition, endoscopy can identify esophageal pathology that may have contributed to perforation or may be associated with a postoperative leak (e.g., malignancy or stricture). Methylene blue administration can also help identify multiple or small perforations such as in the setting of shotgun wounds.

The principles of esophageal repair include debridement of contaminated and necrotic material, closure of the defect, and control of esophageal drainage. The classical tenet of performing primary repair when less than 24 hours from perforation and avoiding primary repair when more than 24 hours has been disproven in clinical studies. Primary repair of cervical esophageal injuries can be performed when there is an ability to get a closure of healthy tissue without tension.

The esophagus should be debrided to healthy tissue and repaired with a single- or double-layer closure using absorbable or non-absorbable suture (there are no studies comparing the techniques). Some recommend non-absorbable suture with knots on the outside to avoid granuloma formation, but this has not been subjected to rigorous evaluation.

One element that is widely recommended is to buttress the repair with vascularized tissue. In the neck, it is simplest to buttress with sternocleidomastoid or strap muscle. This is particularly important when there is concomitant tracheal or carotid artery injury.

**Answer: A**

Biffl, W.L., Moore, E.E., Feliciano, D.V., *et al.* (2015) Western Trauma Association critical decisions in trauma: diagnosis and management of esophageal injuries. *Journal of Trauma and Acute Care Surgery,* **79** (6), 1089–1095.

8  *Which of the following statements about peptic ulcer disease is true?*
   A *The pathophysiology of duodenal ulcer formation is related to acid hyper-secretion rather than* Helicobacter pylori *infection*
   B *Use of non-steroidal anti-inflammatory drugs has a more pronounced effect on ulcer formation in the stomach compared to the duodenum*
   C *Peptic ulcer disease is the second most common cause of upper gastrointestinal bleeding behind stress gastritis*
   D *Angiography has no defined role in the treatment of bleeding peptic ulcers*

**E** *Three-point ligation of the right gastric artery is a proven method of controlling bleeding from a posterior wall duodenal ulcer*

Gastric and duodenal ulcers are the most common cause of upper gastrointestinal bleeding. Ninety percent of duodenal ulcers and 70% of gastric ulcers are associated with *Helicobacter pylori*. Identified in 1982, this gram-negative bacterium disrupts the mucosal barrier and causes inflammation of the mucosa of the stomach and duodenum.

Another common cause of peptic ulcer disease is consumption of non-steroidal anti-inflammatory drugs (NSAIDs), which inhibit cyclooxygenase, leading to impaired mucosal defenses via decreased mucosal prostaglandin synthesis. Use of NSAIDs has a more pronounced effect on the stomach than on the duodenum, with a fortyfold increase in gastric ulcers and an eightfold increase in duodenal ulcers.

In the setting of bleeding from a peptic ulcer, upper endoscopy represents first line therapy. Angiography is now considered second-line treatment (before surgery) in the 5–10% of patients who are unresponsive to medical and endoscopic treatment. Bleeding should be localized by selective catheterization of the most likely artery involved. Factors predicting the need for operative intervention include failure of endoscopy or angiography and ongoing hemodynamic instability.

Surgical options include oversewing of the ulcer, three-point ligation of the gastroduodenal artery in the case of posterior wall duodenal ulcers, vagotomy and pyloroplastly, vagotomy and antrectomy, and highly selective vagotomy.

**Answer: B**

Feinman, M. and Haut, E.R. (2014) Upper gastrointestinal bleeding. *The Surgical Clinics of North America*, **94** (1), 43–53.

Rotondano, G. (2014) Epidemiology and diagnosis of acute nonvariceal upper gastrointestinal bleeding. *Gastroenterology Clinics of North America*, **43** (4), 643–663.

**9** *A 35-year-old man presents with 12 hours of severe epigastric pain that has progressed to diffuse abdominal tenderness. His vital signs include: temperature 101.7 °F, hear rate of 115 beats/min, blood pressure of 110/65 mm Hg. A CT scan demonstrates periduodenal inflammation with free air and free fluid. Which statement about his treatment is false?*

**A** *Surgical options include patch closure and postoperative* H. pylori *eradication*

**B** *Surgical options include patch closure and highly selective vagotomy*

**C** *Patch closure without an acid reduction procedure is sufficient for patients whose duodenal perforation is clearly associated with NSAID use*

**D** *Large diameter perforation is a common cause of conversion from laparoscopic to open repair*

**E** *Non-operative management consisting of nil per os, nasogastric decompression and broad spectrum antibiotics is the safest option in patients with hemodynamic instability from sepsis*

Perforation is the second most common complication of duodenal ulcer after bleeding. Pneumoperitoneum is demonstrated in 80% of upright chest X-rays, and therefore its absence should not exclude this diagnosis. Surgical options for duodenal perforation include simple patch closure alone if the underlying pathophysiology does not involve *H. pylori* or acid hypersecretion, as in the case of NSAID use. If *H. pylori* or acid hypersecretion is suspected, an acid reduction procedure is not always necessary, particularly in patients who have not been placed on *H. pylori* or acid reduction therapies.

In the current era, proton pump inhibitors and $H_2$-blockers have been shown to achieve over 90% symptom resolution. *H. pylori* treatment is an imperative component of therapy. It expedites ulcer healing and reduces the likelihood of ulcer recurrence. An acid reduction procedure is appropriate in stable patients who are medically noncompliant or refractory to medical therapy.

Nonresective procedures such as highly selective vagotomy or truncal vagotomy and pyloroplasty have higher recurrence rates when compared to resective procedures, however they are also associated with lower morbidity and mortality rates. In the setting of duodenal perforations, resective procedures including antrectomy are discouraged due to the duodenal inflammation and the resultant increased risk of duodenal stump leak in the case of Billroth II or anastomotic leak in the case of Billroth I.

Recent reports indicate that in the era of effective acid suppression and *H. pylori* treatment, definitive ulcer surgery in the emergent setting may not be necessary. In recent years, minimally invasive techniques for the management of duodenal ulcer disease and its complications have been shown to be safe and technically feasible. Several studies have demonstrated decreased postoperative analgesia requirements, decreased incidence of wound infection, shorter hospital stays, and earlier return to work. In a recent review of 56 papers, laparoscopy was associated with a 12.4% conversion rate, mainly due to the diameter of the perforation.

Hemodynamic instability in the setting of perforated viscus is an indication for urgent resuscitation and surgical septic source control, not nonoperative management.

**Answer: E**

Bertleff, M.J.O.E. and Lange, J.F. (2010) Laparoscopic correction of perforated peptic ulcer: first choice? A review of literature. *Surgical Endoscopy*, 24 (6), 1231–1239.

Sarosi, G.A., Jr, Jaiswal, K.R., Nwariaku, F.E., *et al.* (2005) Surgical therapy of peptic ulcers in the 21st century: more common than you think. *American Journal of Surgery*, **190** (5), 775–779.

**10** *A 50-year old cachectic Korean woman with known stage 4 gastric cancer presents with progressive oral intolerance and weight loss. An upper gastrointestinal series demonstrates high-grade gastric outlet obstruction. Which of the following statements about management of malignant gastric outlet obstruction is true?*

   **A** *Gastrojejunostomy is the current standard of care for patients with malignant gastric outlet obstruction*

   **B** *Endoscopic stenting is contraindicated in malignant gastric outlet obstruction due to the risk of biliary sepsis from ampullary obstruction*

   **C** *Compared to endoscopic stenting, gastrojejunostomy is associated with a higher proportion of late complications including recurrent obstruction and cholangitis*

   **D** *Compared to gastrojejunostomy, endoscopic stenting is associated with better short-term outcomes as well as shorter hospital length of stay*

   **E** *Nasogastric decompression and nil per os will resolve malignant gastric outlet obstruction in 60% of patients*

Gastric outlet obstruction is a well-recognized complication of upper gastrointestinal tract malignancies. It is most commonly associated with gastric and pancreatic cancers, although it is also seen with lymphomas, ampullary and biliary cancers. The mean survival in this group of patients is 3–4 months. The ideal palliative procedure should quickly establish oral tolerance, have few complications, short hospital stays, and does not adversely impact survival.

Traditionally the open gastrojejunostomy has been the standard of care. However, it is associated with complication rates in the range of 20–50%, most commonly related to postoperative hemorrhage. Endoscopically placed, self-expanding stents have been used to restore gastrointestinal continuity in esophageal, duodenal and colonic malignancies. The available data comparing endoscopic stents to gastrojejunostomy does not favor one method over the other, and the choice of procedure is patient dependent.

The patients with endoscopic stents have shorter hospital stays, faster relief of obstructive symptoms, and fewer early complications. However, patients with gastrojejunostomies have fewer recurrences of obstructive symptoms. Laparoscopic gastrojejunostomy is gaining popularity for its equivalence in achieving symptom relief compared to open gastrojejunostomies, in addition to shorter hospital stays and possibly earlier initiation of oral tolerance.

**Answer: D**

Ly, J., O'Grady, G., Mittal, A., *et al.* (2010) A systematic review of methods to palliate malignant gastric outlet obstruction. *Surgical Endoscopy*, **24** (2), 290–297.

Miyazaki, Y., Takiguchi, S., Takahashi, T., *et al.* (2016) Treatment of gastric outlet obstruction that results from unresectable gastric cancer: Current evidence. *World Journal of Gastrointestinal Endoscopy*, **8** (3), 165–172.

**11** *After repair of several small bowel enterotomies in a 35-year-old victim of multiple gunshot wounds, you are left with a 60% disruption of the gastroesophageal junction. The patient remains hemodynamically normal throughout the operation requiring 2 units of packed red blood cell transfusions. What is the optimal management of this injury?*

   **A** *Left anterolateral thoracotomy, resection of the gastroesophageal segment, intrathoracic esophagogastric anastomosis*

   **B** *Debridement of injury with primary closure*

   **C** *Segmental resection with intraabdominal anastomosis*

   **D** *Segmental resection, intra-abdominal anastomosis and Nissen fundoplication*

   **E** *Staple off the distal esophagus, gastrostomy and jejunostomy*

Esophageal injuries account for less than 1% of patients admitted following trauma. The majority of traumatic perforations require operative management with the intention of primary repair. However, in the presence of hemodynamic instability or delayed diagnosis where intense inflammation precludes safe primary anastomosis, simple drainage with or without stapling above and below the esophageal injury is most prudent.

Primary repair of a destructive injury involving more than 50% of luminal circumference will result in stricture. In such cases segmental resection with tissue buttressing provides the most leak-proof anastomosis. The cervical esophagus can be buttressed with the sternocleidomastoid or other strap muscles. Pleura, intercostal muscles or the pericardium can buttress the thoracic esophagus. Of note, it is not advisable to buttress the esophagus circumferentially as the scar tissue formation will lead to an unyielding extrinsic stricture.

In the abdomen, the omentum or various forms of fundoplications are options. In this case of a destructive gastroesophageal junction disruption, the injury can be relatively easily accessed from the abdomen, through the hiatus. Further mobilization can be achieved through blunt transhiatal dissection in order to gain adequate length for a tension free anastomosis.

**Answer: D**

Bufkin, B.L., Miller, J.I., and Mansour, K.A. (1996) Esophageal perforation: emphasis on management. *Annals of Thoracic Surgery*, **61** (5), 1447–1452.

Richardson, J.D. (2005) Management of esophageal perforations: the value of aggressive surgical treatment. *American Journal of Surgery*, **190** (2), 161–165.

**12** *With regard to corrosive substance ingestion, which of the following statements are true?*

   **A** *After caustic ingestion, the esophagus is at the highest risk for perforation within the first 24 hours*

   **B** *Blind passage of nasogastric tube with gastric lavage should be immediately performed in order to reduce gastric exposure to the caustic substance*

   **C** *Milk or activated charcoal should be used to neutralize corrosive substances in the stomach*

   **D** *Steroids have been shown to decrease the rate of esophageal stricture formation*

   **E** *Early endoscopy is the gold standard in evaluating esophageal caustic injuries and should be performed with 12–48 hours*

Caustic ingestion is the leading toxic exposure in children and the second most common in adults after analgesic ingestion. The extent of tissue damage depends on the type, quantity, and concentration of ingested substance, and the duration of exposure. Acids cause coagulation necrosis, with eschar formation that may limit substance penetration and injury depth. Conversely, alkalis combine with tissue proteins and cause liquefactive necrosis and saponification, and penetrate deeper into tissues, helped by a higher viscosity and a longer contact time through the esophagus. Additionally, alkali absorption leads to thrombosis in blood vessels, impeding blood flow to already damaged tissue.

Esophagogastroduodenoscopy is considered crucial and usually recommended in the first 12–48 hours after caustic ingestion, though it is safe and reliable up to 96 hours after the injury; gentle insufflation and great caution are mandatory during the procedure. Contraindications to endoscopy are a radiologic suspicion of perforation or supraglottic or epiglottic burns with edema, which may be a harbinger of airway obstruction and an indication for endotracheal intubation or tracheostomy.

Gastric lavage and induced emesis are contraindicated because of the risk of re-exposure to the corrosive agent and additional injury to the esophagus. The effectiveness of milk and water either as antidotes or to dilute the corrosive agents has never been proven. pH neutralization, with either a weak acid or base, is not recommended for fear of an exothermic reaction, which may increase the damage. Milk and activated charcoal are contraindicated as they may obscure subsequent endoscopy.

A nasogastric tube may be placed to prevent vomiting and as stent in severe circumferential burns, but it should not be placed blindly because of the risk of esophageal perforation.

The utility of corticosteroid is controversial. A meta-analysis of studies between 1991 and 2004, and an additional analysis of the literature over a longer period from 1956 to 2006 did not find any benefit of steroid administration in terms of stricture prevention.

**Answer: E**

Contini, S. and Scarpignato, C. (2013) Caustic injury of the upper gastrointestinal tract: a comprehensive review. *World Journal of Gastroenterology*, **19** (25), 3918–3930.

**13** *Which of the following statements correctly describes the treatment of a hemodynamically normal, asymptomatic 5-year-old child who presents one hour after accidental ingestion of a liquid cleaning substance?*

   **A** *Upper endoscopy should be performed within 24 hours to evaluate the extent of injury*

   **B** *Administration of ipecac is contraindicated*

   **C** *In lieu of upper endoscopy, this patient can undergo contrast radiography performed with water-soluble contrast followed by thin barium to evaluate for esophageal injury*

   **D** *The patient should be placed on a proton pump inhibitor infusion for 3 days*

   **E** *Due to the high risk of stricture formation, a gastrostomy should be performed for enteral nutrition and retrograde dilations*

As a general rule, caustic ingestions are accidental in children and suicidal attempts in adults. Initial assessment should begin with a determination of airway patency. The administration of ipecac is contraindicated following a caustic ingestion because of potential re-exposure of the esophageal mucosa to the caustic agent.

Indications for endoscopy include any patient with stridor, all intended suicidal ingestions, any symptomatic patient, and those with oropharyngeal burns. Endoscopy is not necessary in asymptomatic children who have ingested only small amounts of caustic material.

The classification of caustic injury is based on endoscopic findings. First-degree injury is limited to the mucosa and are associated with very low immediate and long-term complication rates. Second-degree injury is transmucosal and further subclassified into IIA and IIB based on patchy ulcerations versus circumferential injury. As in first-degree injury, grade IIA is not associated with stricture formation. However, grade IIB will have invariable rates of progression to strictures. Third-degree injury is managed with a low threshold for aggressive operative intervention as the transmural injury may result in mediastinitis or peritonitis.

The management algorithm for grade IIB and III injuries consist of *nil per os*, antibiotics to reduce oropharyngeal flora, gastric acid suppression and either intravenous or enteral nutrition. In addition, gastrostomies should be considered as a conduit for enteral feeding and future retrograde dilations.

**Answer: B**

Kay, M. and Wyllie, R. (2009) Caustic ingestions in children. *Current Opinion in Pediatrics*, **21** (5), 651–654.

14 *A 50-year-old man presents to the emergency department with severe epigastric pain and nausea with an inability to vomit. Attempts at passing a nasogastric tube fail due to resistance at 20 cm from the incisors. Which statement regarding the patient's condition is true?*
   A *Endoscopic detorsion of the incarcerated paraesophageal hernia should be attempted*
   B *Acute strangulation is seen in approximately 30% of patients with paraesophageal hernias*
   C *Mesh closure of the hiatal repair have been associated with erosion and fibrotic strictures*
   D *Repair of a strangulated paraesophageal hernia through a left thoracotomy yields superior results compared to the transabdominal approach*
   E *The addition of an antireflux procedure to paraesophageal hernia repair is associated with high rates of dysphagia*

Paraesophageal hernias develop due to attenuation of the phrenoesophageal ligament thus allowing for the intrathoracic migration of abdominal contents. The location of the gastroesophageal junction serves as the reference point for determining the four types of hiatal hernias. Type I is the most common and involves herniation of the gastroesophageal junction into the mediastinum. Most patients are asymptomatic, however, surgical repair should be offered to symptomatic patients. Type II is a true paraesophageal hernia in which the gastroesophageal junction is in its anatomical subdiaphragmatic

location, however, the gastric fundus herniates through the patulous hiatus alongside the esophagus. Type III is a combination of Types I and II with herniation of the gastroesophageal junction and stomach into the chest. Type IV hernia is a complex entity where the herniation includes the stomach as well as other abdominal organs.

In contrast to the previous belief that all paraesophageal hernias should undergo elective repair regardless of symptoms, new studies suggest that the risk of strangulation is around 1% per year. Currently, it is acceptable to offer surgical correction on the basis of significant symptoms and perhaps younger age (< 60 years of age). Epigastric pain, the inability to vomit and failure to pass a nasogastric tube are together known as Borchardt's triad and suggest an incarcerated intrathoracic stomach. In this surgical emergency, endoscopy has no diagnostic or therapeutic role.

Transthoracic, transabdominal, or laparoscopic approaches have all been described with similar long-term results in the elective setting although thoracotomy is associated with higher postoperative morbidity. In the setting of strangulated paraesophageal hernias, the transabdominal approach is most prudent given the shorter operative time and possible need for subtotal gastrectomy. The patulous esophageal hiatus should be closed with non-absorbable sutures and a fundoplication should be created.

The reinforcement of prosthetic mesh is gaining popularity as some studies have shown the practice to reduces the incidence of recurrence. However, it is associated with complications including erosions, fibrotic strictures and dysphagia. These risks are theoretically reduced by the usage of bioprosthetic mesh although the long-term data are lacking.

**Answer: C**

Oleynikov, D. and Jolley, J.M. (2015) Paraesophageal hernia. *The Surgical Clinics of North America*, **95** (3), 555–565.

15 *A hemodynamically normal 16-year-old boy is found to have an obstructive duodenal hematoma on CT performed for blunt assault. He remains nil per os and continues to have bilious nasogastric tube output of 2.5 L per day, four days after admission. What is the most accepted management of his duodenal obstruction?*
   A *Nil per os, nasogastric decompression and total parenteral nutrition until resolution of the duodenal obstruction*
   B *Operative drainage of the duodenal hematoma*
   C *CT-guided percutaneous aspiration of the duodenal hematoma*

**D** *Gastrostomy tube placement with expectant management of the duodenal hematoma*
**E** *Endoscopic duodenal stent placement*

Although the incidence of duodenal hematoma is unclear, it is recognized as a rare complication particularly following blunt trauma, endoscopic biopsies or peptic ulcer disease. Much of the data regarding this subject are limited to small case series in the pediatric population, however, extrapolations are made for the treatment of adults.

It is believed that the rich blood supply of the duodenum accelerates hematoma resorption and protects against the late development of fibrosis and stenosis. Available data suggest that most of the symptomatic duodenal hematomas resolve in 7–10 days. Therefore, expectant management is advocated for up to two weeks after which operative hematoma evacuation is considered.

More recently, case reports of ultrasound or CT-guided percutaneous drainage have shown that these techniques can be safe and effective alternatives to operative evacuation.

**Answer: A**

Clendenon, J.N., Meyers, R.L., Nance, M.L., *et al.* (2004) Management of duodenal injuries in children. *Journal of Pediatric Surgery*, **39**, 964–968.

Peterson, M.L., Abbas, P.I., Fallon, S.C., *et al.* (2015) Management of traumatic duodenal hematomas in children. *Journal of Surgical Research*, **199** (1), 126–129.

**16** *A 26-year-old man presents to the emergency department after sustaining a stab wound to the right upper quadrant with omental evisceration. At laparotomy, he is found to have an injury at D2 measuring less than 50% of the duodenal circumference. A tension-free transverse repair is not possible. In the setting of hemodynamic stability, what is the best option for management of this patient?*
   **A** *Close the injury in a longitudinal orientation*
   **B** *Debride back to healthy tissue and create a Roux-en-Y duodenojejunostomy*
   **C** *Divide and mobilize the duodenum to create a duodenoduodenostomy*
   **D** *Perform pancreaticoduodenectomy*
   **E** *Staple off the duodenum proximal to the injury and perform temporary abdominal closure*

The duodenum is primarily a retroperitoneal structure and is relatively well protected; consequently, injuries to the duodenum are uncommon, representing less than 2% of all abdominal injuries. Although uncommon, the consequences of duodenal injury can be devastating.

Unstable patients with suspected intra-abdominal injuries should undergo emergent laparotomy, while hemodynamically normal patients with significant blunt trauma generally undergo CT scan. If the initial CT scan shows periduodenal air in addition to fluid or stranding, the safest (most conservative) approach is immediate laparotomy.

If the patient is demonstrating evidence of severe physiologic compromise in the form of acidosis, coagulopathy, and hypothermia, the decision to proceed with damage control should be made early. In these scenarios, hemorrhage should be controlled, and simple closure of the duodenum should be performed. The bile duct may be ligated or, if possible, cannulated and externally drained.

If the patient remains stable in the operating room, duodenal repair may be undertaken. Transverse repair is preferred to avoid luminal narrowing. For more extensive lacerations, duodenal mobilization with duodenoduodenostomy may be necessary. If tension-free repair is not possible and the defect is less than 50% of the duodenal circumference, the edges of the duodenal injury should be debrided back to healthy bleeding tissue, and a limb of jejunum brought up to the defect to create a Roux-en-Y duodenojejunostomy. This is a fairly robust repair and can tolerate moderate contamination in the field.

**Answer: B**

Malhotra, A., Biffl, W.L., Moore, E.E., *et al.* (2015) Western Trauma Association critical decisions in trauma: diagnosis and management of duodenal injuries. *Journal of Trauma and Acute Care Surgery*, **79** (6), 1096–1101.

**17** *Which statement about* Helicobacter pylori *testing is true?*
   **A** *Serologic testing is the most expensive of the non-endoscopic tests*
   **B** *The use of proton pump inhibitors does not reduce the sensitivity of the urease breath test*
   **C** *The monoclonal antibody test detects serum* H. pylori *antigens*
   **D** *Urea breath test can be used to confirm* H. pylori *eradication*
   **E** *Random biopsies are taken from the stomach for culture and histologic assessment*

Testing for *H. pylori* falls into of two categories: endoscopic or non-endoscopic. Among the three non-endoscopic methods, serologic testing which examines for serum IgG antibody to *H. pylori* is the most widely available and least expensive. However, the overall sensitivity and specificity of the several commercially available quantitative assays is 85% and 70% respectively.

In addition, the presence of IgG antibody for months after *H. pylori* eradication makes this test suboptimal for assessing treatment response. The urea breath test utilizes *H. pylori's* intrinsic urease activity in converting orally administered $^{13}$C-labeled or $^{14}$C-labeled urea into measurable radiolabeled carbon dioxide. The test is 95% sensitive and specific. The fecal antigen test detects *H. pylori*-specific antigen in the stool with the use of either monoclonal or polyclonal antibodies.

For both the urea breath test and the fecal stool antigen test, the patient should be off proton pump inhibitors for 2 weeks, $H_2$-blockers for 24 hours, and avoid antimicrobials for four weeks before testing since these medications may suppress the infection and reduce the test sensitivity.

All endoscopic methods begin with biopsy of the gastric antrum. The tissue can then be processed for histologic evaluation for the presence of *H. pylori* and associated gastritis. *H. pylori* can also be cultured from the antral tissue, although facilities with such capabilities are not widely available. The urease based method entails placing the biopsy specimen in a solution of urea and pH-sensitive dye. In the presence of active infection, the urease converts urea into ammonium, which alkalinizes the solution and changes its color. The test is 95% sensitive and 90% specific, but the aforementioned medications should be avoided.

In the United States, the recommended treatment of *H. pylori* infection consists of a 10–14-day course of two antibiotics plus a proton-pump inhibitor or a bismuth preparation.

**Answer: D**

Patel, K.A. and Howden, C.W. (2015) Update on the diagnosis and management of *Helicobacter pylori* infection in adults. *Journal of Clinical Gastroenterology*, **49** (6), 461–467.

**18** Which statement regarding gastric Dieulafoy's lesion is true?
   A Dieulafoy's lesions are associated with up to 20% of non-variceal upper gastrointestinal hemorrhages
   B It is caused by erosion of a submucosal arterio-venous malformation
   C Epigastric pain is a common finding among patients with bleeding gastric Dieulafoy's lesions
   D Sucralfate has been shown to decrease the incidence of hemorrhage from Dieulafoy's lesion
   E The gastric erosions associated with Dieulafoy's lesions are usually less than 5 mm

Dieulafoy's lesion is an abnormally large, tortuous, submucosal artery (1–3 mm) that erodes through the gastric mucosa. They are thought to account for 0.3–7% of non-variceal upper gastrointestinal hemorrhages but may be under recognized. Patients typically present with painless and massive, but intermittent hematemesis. The diagnosis of Dieulafoy's lesion can be difficult due to the relatively small size of the mucosal erosion (2–5 mm) that is surrounded by normal appearing gastric mucosa. Esophagogastroduodenoscopy is the diagnostic and treatment modality of choice, and can identify up to 80% of lesions. The various modalities used to treat variceal bleeding can be used for Dieulafoy's lesions, including multipolar electrocoagulation, injection sclerotherapy, band ligation and endoscopic clipping. In cases refractory to endoscopic therapy, angioembolization is second line therapy. One of the greatest challenges in the surgical management of Dieulafoy's lesion is identification of this intraluminal lesion. However, endoscopic tattooing and intraoperative endoscopic transillumination of the lesions can facilitate both open and laparoscopic gastric wedge resection.

**Answer: E**

Baxter, M. and Aly, E. (2010) Dieulafoy's lesion: current trends in diagnosis and management. *Annals of the Royal College of Surgeons England*, **92** (7), 548–554.

**19** A 34-year-old woman who is one-day status post laparoscopic Roux-en-Y gastric bypass is persistently tachycardic at 130 beats/min. Her blood pressure is 115/70 mm Hg, and her respiratory rate is 25 breaths/min. Her abdomen is mildly tender. An arterial blood gas obtained on room air is pH 7.32/pCO2 32/pO2 98/HCO3 25/BE-0.5. Upper gastrointestinal series with gastrografin and thin barium does not demonstrate a leak. What is the next step in management?
   A Continue observation for another 24 hours
   B Discharge the patient with follow up in two weeks
   C Repeat upper gastrointestinal series with full strength barium
   D Operative exploration to rule out a leak
   E CTPA to rule out pulmonary embolism

Despite the apparent decreased incidence over time, anastomotic leak remains an important cause of overall morbidity and mortality after primary stapled bariatric procedures. Identified risk factors include male gender, increased weight, multiple comorbidities and revision surgery. The clinical presentation of anastomotic leak may be subtle or delayed in obese patients, making the diagnosis challenging in many patients.

Once signs and symptoms develop, prompt diagnosis and treatment of a leak may minimize the inflammatory and septic sequelae.

Routine postoperative upper gastrointestinal series with gastrografin is associated with a sensitivity of 22% for detecting a leak, and the sensitivity of CT scans is around 40%. Laparoscopic or open re-exploration is an appropriate diagnostic option, regardless of the feasibility of obtaining a postoperative imaging test, when an anastomotic leak is suspected. Re-exploration is characterized by a higher sensitivity, specificity, and accuracy than any other postoperative test to assess for leak and should be considered the definitive assessment for the possibility of a leak. Although invasive and not without potential difficulty or morbidity, several studies have reported that re-exploration is a well-tolerated intervention compared with the consequences of peritonitis, excessive inflammatory response, sepsis, organ failure, and mortality, which may develop when diagnosis and treatment of a leak are delayed.

**Answer: D**

Kim, J., Azagury, D., Eisenberg, D., *et al.* (2015) ASMBS position statement on prevention, detection, and treatment of gastrointestinal leak after gastric bypass and sleeve gastrectomy, including the roles of imaging, surgical exploration, and nonoperative management. *Surgery for Obesity and Related Disorders*, **11** (4), 739–748.

# 37

## Small Intestine, Appendix, and Colorectal
*Vishal Bansal, MD and Jay J. Doucet, MD*

**1** *A 72-year-old woman presents to the ED with acute left lower quadrant abdominal pain. Her past medical history is significant only for mild hypertension. On exam, she is febrile to 38.2°C with focal rebound tenderness in her left lower quadrant. She has a WBC of 12 000 /mm³. Abdominal CT imaging reveals a thickened sigmoid with a 3.0 cm × 3.0 cm peri-sigmoid colon abscess with a very small pocket of extra-luminal air in the pelvis. The next step in management should be:*

**A** *Exploration, sigmoidectomy with descending end-colostomy (Hartmann's procedure)*

**B** *Exploration with sigmoidectomy, primary colorectal anastomosis*

**C** *Exploration with sigmoidectomy, primary colorectal anastomosis, and loop ileostomy*

**D** *Resuscitation, broad spectrum IV antibiotics and percutaneous drainage of the abscess*

**E** *Resuscitation, broad spectrum IV antibiotics, colonoscopy for likely colon carcinoma on this admission*

Complicated diverticulitis will often require operative intervention and depending on the Hinchey staging system, a morbid two-stage procedure may be avoided. Hinchey I is defined as colonic inflammation with associated pericolic abscess; stage II includes inflammation with pelvic abscess; stage III is purulent peritonitis, and stage IV is fecal peritonitis. This patient has Hinchey I diverticulitis, where IV antibiotics with percutaneous abscess drainage offers a chance for a future colonoscopy to rule out malignancy (four to six weeks later) and a planned one-stage sigmoidectomy with primary anastomosis. For patients with persistent, unresolving symptoms, pelvic sepsis or patients who are immunocompromised, sigmoidectomy and diversion should be considered, although a single-stage operation with intraoperative colonic lavage and primary anastomosis has been reported in these patients.

**Answer: D**

Aydin, H.N., Tekkis, P.P., Remzi, F.H., *et al.* (2006) Evaluation of the risk of a nonrestorative resection for the treatment of diverticular disease: the Cleveland Clinic diverticular disease propensity score. *Diseases of the Colon and Rectum*, **49** (5), 629–639.

Schilling, M.K., Maurer, C.A., Kollmar, O., and Büchler, M.W. (2001) Primary vs. secondary anastomosis after sigmoid resection for perforated diverticulitis (Hinchey Stage II and IV): A prospective outcome and cost analysis. *Diseases of the Colon and Rectum*, **44** (5), 699–703.

**2** *An 86-year-old male nursing home resident with severe dementia presents to the ER with a four-day history of constipation and a distended abdomen. His vital signs and laboratory studies are unremarkable. His abdominal x-ray reveals a "coffee-bean" sign of his sigmoid colon with dilated transverse and descending colon. The patient underwent successful endoscopic decompression of his sigmoid volvulus and was observed in the hospital. On the second hospital day the patient had a return of abdominal distention with evidence of a recurrent sigmoid volvulus. The patient should undergo:*

**A** *Exploration, sigmoidectomy with descending end-colostomy (Hartmann's procedure)*

**B** *Exploration with detorsion of the sigmoid and sigmoidopexy*

**C** *Repeat endoscopic decompression through rigid proctoscopy*

**D** *Exploration with sigmoidectomy and primary colorectal anastomosis*

**E** *Laparoscopic detorsion of the sigmoid with sigmoidopexy*

*Surgical Critical Care and Emergency Surgery: Clinical Questions and Answers*, Second Edition.
Edited by Forrest "Dell" Moore, Peter Rhee, and Gerard J. Fulda.
© 2018 John Wiley & Sons Ltd. Published 2018 by John Wiley & Sons Ltd.
Companion website: www.wiley.com/go/moore/surgical_criticalcare_and_emergency_surgery

In a stable patient without evidence of bowel ischemia, endoscopic decompression is the first-line therapy for a sigmoid volvulus. However, a 40–50% recurrence rate is expected and the timing can vary from immediate to a recurrence several years following the initial volvulus. In the face of a recurrent sigmoid volvulus, operative intervention is the treatment of choice. Even though there are several reports in the literature documenting the possibility of sigmoidectomy with primary anastomosis, in this institutionalized patient with evidence of a dilated descending colon without the ability for preoperative colonic cleansing, a Hartmann's procedure with end-colostomy is the best therapeutic option offering the quickest chance of recovery and minimal complications.

**Answer: A**

Grossmann, E.M., Longo, W.E., Stratton, M.D., *et al.* (2000) Sigmoid volvulus in Department of Veterans Affairs medical centers. *Diseases of the Colon and Rectum,* **43** (3), 414–418.

Oren, D., Atamanalp, S.S., Aydinli, B., *et al.* (2007) An algorithm for the management of sigmoid colon volvulus and the safety of primary resection: Experience with 827 cases. *Diseases of the Colon and Rectum,* **50**, 489–497.

**3** *A 48-year-old man undergoes successful renal transplantation for end-stage renal disease. He is maintained on prednisone and tacrolimus for immunosuppression. Four weeks post-transplant he developed diarrhea, increasing pain, and abdominal distention and presents to the ED. He denied any history of nausea or vomiting, but continues to have diarrhea. He has a temperature of 38.0°C, a pulse of 96 beats/min and blood pressure of 129/64 mm Hg. His abdomen was markedly distended and minimally tender to palpation with a white cell count of 21 000 /mm³. A CT of the abdomen and pelvis reveals dilated large bowel from cecum to splenic flexure, with a cecal diameter of 9 cm and pneumatosis within the cecal wall. The next best step in management is:*

A *Admit, resuscitate, empiric IV metronidazole, and send stool for* C. difficile *toxin*

B *Exploratory laparotomy and right hemicolectomy and primary anastomosis*

C *Exploratory laparotomy and subtotal colectomy with end-ileostomy*

D *Exploratory laparoscopy*

E *Admit, resuscitate, NPO, send stool for* C. difficile *toxin and begin metronidazole pending results*

*Clostridium difficile* (*C diff*) colitis has increased in incidence and severity since the early 2000s. The emergence of hypervirulent *C diff* strains, which can cause death within 48 hours of onset of symptoms, has required more urgent surgical consultation and decision making. Severe *C diff* colitis is defined as (WBC > 15 000 cells/microL, albumin < 3 g/dL, and/or a creatinine level ≥ 1.5 times the premorbid level). Initial therapy is usually with oral vancomycin, but in patients with ileus, intravenous metronidazole can be added. Vancomycin enemas can be added in patients not responding to standard therapies, but there is a risk of colon perforation. Fidaxomicin and fecal transplants have been used in patients with recurrent *C diff*, but their use in severe *C diff* colitis is not defined.

Retrospective review of severe cases due to the hypervirulent strain showed colectomy was most beneficial for immunocompetent patients aged ≥ 65 years with a white blood cell count ≥ 20 000 cells/microL and/or a plasma lactate between 2.2 and 4.9 mEq/L. Surgery is also advisable with peritoneal signs, severe ileus, or toxic megacolon.

The recommended procedure for *C diff* colitis is subtotal colectomy (removal of the entire colon with ileostomy, without removal of the rectum). Four series describe the use of various colectomies for *C diff* colitis. One series of 14 patients undergoing surgery for severe *C diff* colitis, nine patients survived, of whom eight had subtotal colectomy and one had a right hemicolectomy. Four of the five patients who died had undergone left hemicolectomy; death presumably due to residual disease as the ongoing source of sepsis. Primary anastomosis is avoided until the acute inflammation has resolved.

A recently described procedure is diverting loop ileostomy and colonic lavage as alternative procedure to colectomy in the treatment of severe, complicated *C diff* colitis. In 42 patients, reduced mortality was observed among patients who underwent loop ileostomy and colonic lavage, compared with the historical controls who underwent colectomy (19 versus 50%; odds ratio 0.24; p = 0.006). Intraoperative colonic lavage with warmed polyethylene glycol solution via loop ileostomy is performed followed by postoperative antegrade instillation of vancomycin flushes via the ileostomy. Preservation of the colon was achieved in 93% of patients. However, there has been no randomized, controlled study to validate this approach.

This patient has severe *C diff* colitis plus radiologic evidence of toxic megacolon and moreover, is highly immune suppressed, which may blunt peritoneal signs and abdominal tenderness. Sub-total colectomy is indicated. Laparoscopic exploration is not an effective option since the external appearance of the colon may seem normal.

**Answer: C**

Berman, L., Carling, T., Fitzgerald, T.N., *et al.* (2008) Defining surgical therapy for pseudomembranous colitis with toxic megacolon. *Journal of Clinical Gastroenterology*, **42** (5), 476–480.

Koss, K., Clark, M.A., Sanders, D.S., *et al.* (2006) The outcome of surgery in fulminant Clostridium difficile colitis. *Colorectal Disease*, **8** (2), 149–154.

Neal, M.D., Alverdy, J.C., Hall, D.E., *et al.* (2011) Diverting loop ileostomy and colonic lavage: an alternative to total abdominal colectomy for the treatment of severe, complicated Clostridium difficile associated disease. *Annals of Surgery*, **254** (3), 423–429.

**4** *A 42-year-old woman presents to the ED with right lower quadrant pain. She is afebrile with pain to palpation to her right lower quadrant. Her abdominal CT imaging reveals a thickened appendix with pelvic fluid. A diagnosis of acute appendicitis was made. During laparoscopy thick omental and peritoneal mucinous caking was noted throughout the abdomen, with significant pelvic ascites. The next step in management should be:*

**A** *Conversion to an open appendectomy through a McBurney incision*

**B** *Midline laparotomy, appendectomy, omentectomy, and peritoneal tumor debulking*

**C** *Proceed with laparoscopic appendectomy*

**D** *Abort procedure and consult hospice services*

**E** *Laparoscopic peritoneal biopsy and aspiration of ascites*

This patient likely has pseudomyxoma peritonei, a rare and controversial disease which likely arises from either the appendix or the ovary. Depending on the nature of the disease and the patient's overall health, surgical debulking is the treatment of choice with possible hyperthermic intra-operative peritoneal chemotherapy. These techniques have been shown to effect survival to nearly 40% in 5 years. In this clinical scenario, where laparoscopy has already commenced, peritoneal tissue and a peritoneal aspirate may help in grading. Given the extensive nature and relative high morbidity of these operations, it would not be advisable to perform any further operation until a detailed discussion is held with the patient and their family.

**Answer: E**

Sugarbaker, P.H., Alderman, R., Edwards, G., *et al.* (2006) Prospective morbidity and mortality assessment of cytoreductive surgery plus perioperative intraperitoneal chemotherapy to treat peritoneal dissemination of appendiceal mucinous malignancy. *Annals of Surgical Oncology*, **13** (5), 635–644.

Sugarbaker, P.H. and Chang, D. (1999) Results of treatment of 385 patients with peritoneal surface spread of appendiceal malignancy. *Annals of Surgical Oncology*, **6** (8), 727–731.

**5** *A 28-year-old man undergoes a laparoscopic appendectomy secondary to suspected appendicitis. The patient is discharged home on postoperative day one without complication. Final pathology of the appendix reveals an 0.8 cm carcinoid tumor at the tip of the appendix. The next step in management is:*

**A** *Exploratory laparotomy, omentectomy, right hemicolectomy, intraoperative hyperthermic chemotherapy*

**B** *Completion right hemicolectomy*

**C** *Observation, no additional operation is required*

**D** *Six-month imatinib (Gleevec) adjuvant therapy followed by completion right hemicolectomy*

**E** *Six-month adjuvant therapy with imatinib only*

Carcinoid tumors are rare gastrointestinal tumors, the majority of which are found on the appendix. These tumors may appear as a dense mass on CT imaging, resembling a fecolith, and thus are often found incidentally on pathology when the suspected diagnosis is appendicitis. Malignant potential as well as risk of metastasis is directly related to size. Carcinoid tumors of the appendix < 1 cm are treated by simple appendectomy. Tumors > 1 cm should also undergo an extended-right hemicolectomy. In this patient, with an 0.8 cm carcinoid of the appendix, no additional operation besides an appendectomy is needed, since there is a low probability of recurrence in this lower stage. Imatinib therapy may be effective in gastrointestinal stromal tumors but does not have a role in treating carcinoid tumors.

**Answer: C**

Landry, C.S., Woodall, C., Scoggins, C.R., *et al.* (2008) Analysis of 900 appendiceal carcinoid tumors for a proposed predictive staging system. *Archives of Surgery*, **143** (7), 664–670.

Roggo, A., Wood, W.C., and Ottinger, L.W. (1993) Carcinoid tumors of the appendix. *Annals of Surgery*, **217** (4), 476–480.

**6** *An 18-year-old man arrives at the trauma bay via EMS after sustaining a single stab wound to the epigastrium. The patient is awake and orientated and complains of abdominal pain. Breath sounds and chest X-ray are normal. Blood pressure is 100/60 mm Hg and heart rate 126 beats/min with respirations 26 breaths/min. He has a tender abdomen. FAST ultrasound exam shows fluid in Morrison's pouch. The patient is taken quickly for exploratory laparotomy. On opening his abdomen, about 500 mLs of blood is noted in the abdomen. A through-and-through penetrating injury of the mid-transverse colon is noted. An expanding hematoma is noted at the base of the transverse mesocolon and the inferior margin of* *the pancreas. You suspect a superior mesenteric artery (SMA) injury, obtain proximal control of the aorta at the hiatus by clamping or REBOA, and perform a Mattox maneuver to expose the SMA. You find an injury of the SMA just proximal to the middle colic artery. Regarding this SMA injury:*

A *This is a zone 1 SMA injury and the SMA can be ligated without risk of ischemia*

B *Most SMA injuries are sharp partial-transections and can be repaired by lateral arteriorrhaphy*

C *This is a zone 4 SMA injury and ligation of this SMA injury will likely result in only localized ischemia of the intestine*

D *Most deaths after laparotomy for SMA injury are due to short-gut syndrome*

E *This is a zone 2 injury and has an overall mortality of 43%*

Injuries to the SMA are highly lethal; the typical reported survival rate of patients with isolated superior mesenteric vein injuries is 48–52%. Most laparotomy deaths for SMA injuries are due to exsanguination. Patients typically have multiple associated injuries. Patients undergoing primary repair have higher survival rates (63%) and lesser numbers of associated vascular and nonvascular injuries; whereas those undergoing ligation have a smaller survival rate (40%) and higher number of associated vascular and nonvascular injuries. Only about 40% of injuries can be repaired by lateral arteriorrhaphy. The zones of the SMA are as follows:

Zone 1: Aorta to inferior pancreatico-duodenal artery, mortality about 100%.
Zone 2: Inferior pancreatico-duodenal artery to middle colic artery, mortality about 43%
Zone 3: Distal to mid-colic artery, about 25% mortality.
Zone 4: Segmental branches, about 25% mortality.

Ligation should be considered in unstable patients with existing bowel ischemia. Ligation in zone 1 and 2 is likely to result in extensive bowel ischemia with a risk of death or short-gut syndrome. Ligation in zone 3 and 4 is associated with a moderate risk of gut ischemia. Damage-control may be obtained in patients with hypothermia, coagulopathy or acidosis by temporary stenting with an intraluminal vascular shunt. Reconstruction can then be accomplished at a later laparotomy with a saphenous vein or PTFE interposition graft. A second-look laparotomy at 24 hours to asses for bowel ischemia is mandated by most authors.

**Answer: E**

Asensio, J.A., Britt, L.D., Borzotta, A., *et al.* (2001) Multiinstitutional experience with the management of superior mesenteric artery injuries. *Journal of the American College of Surgeons*, **193** (4), 354–366. Erratum in *Journal of the American College of Surgeons*, **193** (6), 718.

Asensio, J.A., Petrone, P., Garcia-Nuñez, L., *et al.* (2007) Superior mesenteric venous injuries: to ligate or to repair remains the question. *Journal of Trauma*, **62** (3), 668–675.

7 *A 91-year-old man with severe dementia presents to the ED from his nursing home with constipation and abdominal distention for the last eight days. The patient's past medical history is remarkable for hypertension and dementia. His abdomen is distended but non-tender. His laboratory studies are unremarkable. Abdominal x-ray reveals a markedly distended ascending, transverse and descending colon with no visible air in the sigmoid or rectum. The next step in management is:*

A *Urgent exploratory laparotomy for toxic megacolon*

B *Loop sigmoid ostomy for managing chronic pseudo-obstruction*

C *Decompressive rectal tube*

D *IV neostigmine for colonic pseudo-obstruction*

E *Gastrografin enema*

Colonic pseudo-obstruction (Ogilvie's syndrome) commonly occurs in hospitalized or immobilized patients. Narcotic use, prolonged bed rest, electrolyte abnormalities and other medications can contribute to developing this adynamic condition. These patients rarely require operative intervention. A rectal tube usually does not help with decompression since the adynamic colon is usually proximal. Endoscopic colonoscopy may be helpful to decompress the dilation. Neostigmine has been shown to induce colonic motility and relieve the pseudo-obstruction. However, because of significant bradycardia and transient asystole, neostigmine should not be used in patients with known heart block or significant cardiovascular disease. All medical and endoscopic treatment should only be utilized when a mechanical obstruction, such as tumor, can be ruled out. Of the choices above, this is best accomplished by gastrografin enema.

**Answer: E**

Ponec, R.J., Saunders, M.D., and Kimmey, M.B. (1999) Neostigmine for the treatment of acute colonic pseudo-obstruction. *New England Journal of Medicine*, **341** (3), 137–141.
Strodel, W.E. and Brothers, T. (1989) Colonoscopic decompression of pseudo-obstruction and volvulus. *Surgical Clinics of North America*, **69** (6), 1327–1335.

8 *A 63-year-old woman is undergoing chemotherapy for lymphoma. She presents to the emergency department with severe right sided abdominal pain. She has no previous surgical history. On exam she is tender on the right side of her abdomen with mild guarding. She is febrile to 38.2°C and her white count is 0.9 /mm³*

with 30% neutrophils. All other laboratory values are unremarkable. A CT scan reveals a moderately dilated and thickened ileum, right and transverse colon. What is the most appropriate management?

A  Urgent exploratory laparotomy for toxic megacolon

B  Colonoscopy to rule out colonic ischemia

C  Ileo-cecectomy with ileostomy and mucus fistula

D  IV fluid resuscitation, NPO, and IV gram-negative, gram-positive and anaerobic antibiotic coverage

E  Outpatient management with oral broad-spectrum antibiotics

Neutropenic enterocolitis, or typhlitis, is a rare yet well-described complication of chemotherapy causing transmural bowel wall inflammation of the ileum, and most commonly involves the right colon. The exact pathophysiology of this condition is not completely known. Typical presentation is right-sided abdominal pain with peritoneal signs, fever, and neutropenia. Diagnosis is made clinically and should be confirmed using abdominal CT, which usually shows bowel wall edema and thickening of the terminal ileum and ascending colon. Treatment should entail cessation of chemotherapy, aggressive fluid resuscitation, bowel rest, and broad-spectrum antibiotics targeting colonic flora. Granulocyte-colony stimulating factor may play a role to improve the neutropenia. Surgical exploration in these cases is usually not indicated unless the patient has evidence of colonic perforation or sepsis.

**Answer: D**

Kirkpatrick, I.D. and Greenberg, H.M. (2003) Gastrointestinal complications in the neutropenic patient: characterization and differentiation with abdominal CT. *Radiology*, **226** (3), 668–674.

Kunkel, J.M. and Rosenthal, D. (1986) Management of the ileocecal syndrome. Neutropenic enterocolitis. *Diseases of the Colon and Rectum*, **29** (3), 196–199.

**9**  A 39-year-old man is brought to the emergency department after a pistol gunshot wound to the right flank. On examination by the trauma team he is awake and alert with good air entry and a normal chest x-ray. His blood pressure is 130/80 mm Hg with a respiratory rate of 26 breaths/min and heart rate of 110 beats/min. There is a single gunshot wound located in the right anterior axillary line at the level of the umbilicus. He has no comorbidities. His abdomen is very tender. He is brought to the operating room for exploratory laparotomy. You find a right zone II retroperitoneal hematoma that when opened by mobilizing the right colon medially reveals a grade I injury of the right kidney as well as a through-and-through destructive right colon injury. The patient has no other injuries. His blood loss is about 500 mLs. He is hemodynamically normal with a temperature of 36 °C. You perform repair of the kidney with a pledgeted-suture. What is the appropriate management of the colon injury?

A  Primary resection only

B  Primary resection with diverting loop ileostomy

C  Right colostomy

D  Primary resection and exteriorization with "drop-back" in 5–7 days

E  Right ileocolectomy and ileocolic anastomosis.

EAST trauma guidelines suggest that patients with low-energy penetrating intraperitoneal colon wounds that are destructive (involvement of > 50% of the bowel wall or devascularization of a bowel segment) can undergo resection and primary anastomosis if they are:

- Hemodynamically normal without evidence of shock (sustained pre- or intraoperative hypotension as defined by SBP < 90 mm Hg)
- Have no significant underlying disease
- Have minimal associated injuries (PATI < 5, ISS < 25, Flint grade < 11)
- Have no peritonitis

Patients with shock, underlying disease, significant associated injuries, or peritonitis should have destructive colon wounds managed by resection and colostomy. This patient has a kidney injury which might raise concern for an intra-abdominal urine leak which might cause the anastomosis to fail, however a grade I kidney injury should be reparable without significant leak. Colostomy is unnecessary. Exteriorization was popular in the 1960s and 1970s but has been abandoned. There is no need to resect more colon (i.e., right ileocolectomy) than that actually visibly injured if a safe, tension-free anastomosis can be obtained.

**Answer: A.**

EAST (1998) EASTPractice Parameter Workgroup for Penetrating Colon Injury Management; Penetrating Colon Injuries, Management of – Practice Management Guideline East.org. At: http://www.east.org/education/practice-management-guidelines/penetrating-colon-injuries-management-of- (accessed November 11, 2017).

Sharpe, J.P., Magnotti, L.J., Weinberg, J.A., et al. (2012). Adherence to a simplified management algorithm reduces morbidity and mortality after penetrating colon injuries: a 15-year experience. *Journal of the American College of Surgeons*, **214** (4), 591–598.

**10**  A 64-year-old otherwise healthy woman presents with significant lower GI bleeding for the last 12 hours. Her systolic blood pressure is 80 mm Hg, pulse of

*100 beats/min, and her physical exam is unremarkable except for gross blood-per-rectum. Her current hematocrit is 28%. What is the next step in management?*

A *Urgent exploration, subtotal colectomy and ileostomy*

B *Urgent exploration, procto-colectomy and ileostomy*

C *Resuscitation with IV fluid, blood and nasogastric lavage*

D *Urgent colonoscopy*

E *Resuscitation with IV fluid, blood and abdominal CT scan*

Severe lower GI bleeding can lead to profound shock and circulatory collapse. First-line therapy is aggressive resuscitation and appropriate transfusion with correction of coagulopathy as needed. Nearly 15% of lower GI bleeding is caused by upper GI sources, therefore expeditious gastric lavage is important. More than 70% of lower GI bleeding ceases spontaneously, therefore urgent laparotomy without localization of the source of hemorrhage should only be undertaken when the patient is in extremis. In hemodynamically normal patients, colonoscopy is the procedure of choice following resuscitation. If the source of bleeding cannot be localized, nuclear RBC scanning or angiography may be useful followed possibly by capsule endoscopy.

**Answer: C**

Elta, G.H. (2001) Urgent colonoscopy for acute lower-GI bleeding. *Gastrointestinal Endoscopy*, **29**, 227–234.

Laine, L. and Shah, A. (2010) Randomized trial of urgent vs. elective colonoscopy in patients hospitalized with lower GI bleeding. *American Journal of Gastroenterology*, **105** (12), 2636–2641.

11 *A 73-year-old man is admitted to the hospital with a history of bright red blood-per-rectum for the last 4 days. The patients past medical history is significant for diabetes and a myocardial infarction 1 year ago which resulted in coronary bypass grafting. He is taking metformin, atenolol, and a baby aspirin. His heart rate is 92 beats/min with a blood pressure of 105/73 mm Hg. His physical exam is unremarkable except for gross blood on rectal examination. His laboratory findings reveal a hematocrit of 24%. Colonoscopy reveals a large, bleeding, fungating tumor in the descending colon. Abdominal CT imaging reveals two 2 cm lesions in the right lobe of the liver suspicious for metastasis. Which is the next best step in management?*

A *Left colectomy with right liver lobectomy*

B *Left colectomy with primary colonic anastomosis*

C *Transfusion to correct anemia followed by neoadjuvant chemo-radiation therapy*

D *Endoscopic fulguration of bleeding tumor followed by neoadjuvant chemotherapy*

E *Left colectomy and end-colostomy*

Hemorrhage from colon cancers are commonly encountered. As with any hemorrhage, resuscitation and stabilization is paramount. In this specific patient, only surgical resection will offer definitive control of ongoing hemorrhage irrespective of distant metastasis. Resection of the tumor with a left hemicolectomy and primary anastomosis is the procedure of choice. Given the relatively small size of the liver metastasis, this patient would benefit from neoadjuvant chemotherapy (FOLFOX combination of: 5-fluorouracil/folinic acid, leucovorin, and oxaliplatin) before surgical resection. It is possible that FOLFOX therapy alone may offer the best treatment for the liver.

**Answer: B**

Hebbar, M., Pruvot, F.R., Romano, O., *et al.* (2009) Integration of neoadjuvant and adjuvant chemotherapy in patients with resectable liver metastases from colorectal cancer. *Cancer Treatment Review*, **35** (8), 668–675.

12 *A 45-year-old male Jehovah's Witness with diabetes presents to the ED with right lower quadrant pain for three days and tenderness to abdominal palpation, fever to 38.2°C and a WBC of 12 000 /mm³. An abdominal CT scan shows a thickened appendix, appendiceal fecolith, and small amount of pelvic fluid. A diagnosis of appendicitis is made. What is the next step in management?*

A *Broad spectrum IV antibiotics, non-operative observation, interval appendectomy in 6 weeks*

B *Broad spectrum IV antibiotics, with percutaneous drainage of pelvic fluid, interval appendectomy in 6 weeks*

C *Appendectomy*

D *Oral ciprofloxacin and metronidazole, inpatient observation*

E *Outpatient therapy with oral ciprofloxacin and metronidazole*

With the emergence of percutaneous drainage techniques and data suggesting that antibiotic therapy is as efficacious as operative management for appendicitis, one may be confused with these various management strategies. Data supporting antibiotic treatment for appendicitis must be taken with caution, since these reports exclude septic patients and patients with known early perforation. There is also a 15% reported failure rate of nonoperative management, ultimately requiring appendectomy. Given the free pelvic fluid in this patient's CT scan, a partial perforation of the appendix is likely. In this case, operative appendectomy is the treatment of choice. Percutaneous drainage should be reserved for perforation without a visible appendix and adequate fluid or abscess for drainage. The operative approach is either laparoscopic or an open approach with mostly equivalent outcomes.

**Answer: C**

Styrud, J., Eriksson, S., Nilsson, I., *et al.* (2006) Appendectomy versus antibiotic treatment in acute appendicitis. a prospective multicenter randomized controlled trial. *World Journal of Surgery*, **30** (6), 1033–1037.

Varadhan, K.K., Humes, D.J., Neal, K.R., and Lobo, D.N. (2010) Antibiotic therapy versus appendectomy for acute appendicitis: a meta-analysis. *World Journal of Surgery*, **34** (2), 199–209.

**13** *A 23-year-old man presents with a 24-hour history of increasing crampy abdominal pain, nausea, vomiting, and a CT scan showing dilated small bowel with a transition point in the terminal ileum. Past medical history is unremarkable; he has had no previous surgery. On examination, he has mild abdominal distension, no peritoneal signs and frequent bowel sounds. He has a while blood cell count (WBC) of 12 300 /mm³. After explanation of likely diagnoses and informed consent, he is taken to the operating room for laparotomy. The operative findings are shown in Figure 37.1, with food impacted in the large diverticulum. This congenital condition is associated with what other mechanical cause of bowel obstruction?*

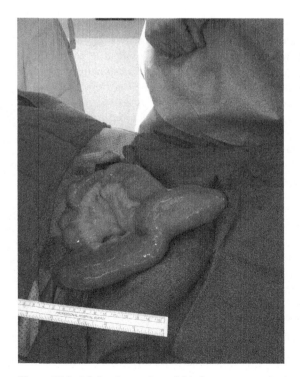

**Figure 37.1** A full color version of this figure appears in the plate section of this book.

A *Mesodiverticular band*
B *Ileocecal intussusception*
C *Terminal ileitis*
D *Hirschsprung's disease*
E *Cecal volvulus*

The operative photograph shows a large Meckel's diverticulum with obstruction due to impaction with food. Meckel's diverticulum can also present with bowel obstruction due to internal hernia caused by interposition of a small bowel loop between the diverticulum and a persistent mesodiverticular band. Meckel's diverticulum is an embryologic remnant of the omphalovitelline duct and its features can be recalled by the "rule of 2s": present in 2% of the population, usually about 2 feet (60 cm) proximal to the ileocecal valve and malignancy is present in 2% of specimens. Meckel's diverticulum can also present with other symptoms, most notably upper gastrointestinal bleeding caused by the presence of ectopic gastric, pancreatic, or other mucosa with leads to ulceration and bleeding. This diagnosis should be entertained in patients with an obscure source of gastrointestinal bleeding. Management is by resection of the diverticulum and adjacent intestinal segment. Meckel's diverticulum does not increase the risk of ileocecal intussusception. Terminal ileitis may cause obstructive symptoms but is readily identified by contrast CT scanning. Hirschsprung's disease can cause colonic obstruction due to a distal colonic aperistaltic segment with aganglionosis; this is not associated with Meckel's diverticulum. There is no association between Meckel's diverticulum and cecal volvulus.

**Answer: A**

Sagar, J., Kumar, V., and Shah, D.K. (2006) Meckel's diverticulum: a systematic review. *Journal of the Royal Society Medicine*, **99** (10), 501–505.

Tavakkolizadeh, A., Whang, E., Ashley, S.W., *et al.* (eds) (2009) *Schwartz's Principles of Surgery*, 9th edn, McGraw-Hill, New York.

**14** *A 52-year-old man with a history of hepatocellular carcinoma presents with a three-day history of nausea, vomiting, and crampy abdominal pain. He has had no bowel movements since the onset of symptoms. On examination he has diffuse, mild abdominal tenderness, no peritoneal signs, and obvious abdominal distension. Bowel sounds are infrequent. His past medical history is remarkable only for a liver resection two years ago and a course of trans-arterial chemoembolization (TACE) of a recurrent liver tumor four weeks ago. Lab work shows a white blood cell (WBC) count of 9200 /mm³, ALT*

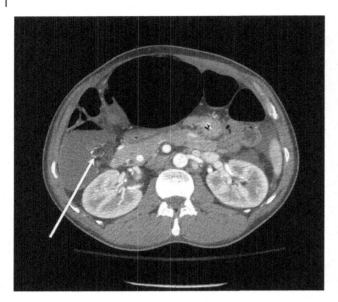

**Figure 37.2**

of 192 units/L, AST of 178 units/L and is otherwise unremarkable. Representative abdominal imaging studies are shown in Figure 37.2. What is the best initial management of this patient?
A Placement of a nasogastric tube, NPO status and observation with serial abdominal examinations
B Colonoscopy
C Laparoscopic cecopexy
D Laparotomy and cecostomy
E Laparotomy and ileocecal resection

The imaging shows a cecal volvulus. Cecal volvulus occurs in younger patients who are less-debilitated than those presenting with sigmoid volvulus. The acute presentation is best treated by resection of the redundant segment of colon in those patients that can tolerate the procedure and may be required if ischemic intestine is discovered. Flexible sigmoidoscopy is successful in over 50% of cases of sigmoid volvulus, but decompressive colonoscopy is almost never successful in cecal volvulus. Cecopexy would appear to have less risk as no colonic resection or anastomosis would be required, however the recurrence rate is high and would place the patient at risk of recurrent volvulus with risk of perforation or reoperation. Cecostomy has been performed as a percutaneous, laparoscopic, endoscopic or open procedure. It is associated with a high rate of serious complications such as leak, perforation or missed intestinal ischemia and has no advantage over colostomy or ileostomy at laparotomy.

**Answer: E**

Bullard, D.K.M. and Rothenberger, D.A. (2010) Colon, rectum, and anus, in *Schwartz's Principles of Surgery*, 9th edn, (eds. F.C. Brunicardi, D.K. Andersen, T.R. Billiar, *et al.*), McGraw-Hill, New York, pp. 219–314.
Madiba, T.E. and Thomson, S.R. (2002) The management of cecal volvulus. *Diseases of the Colon and Rectum*, **45** (2), 264–267.

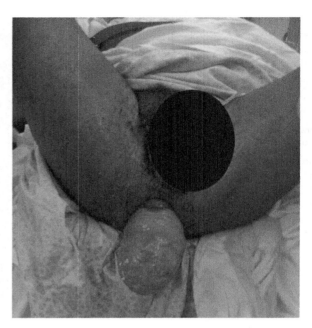

**Figure 37.3** A full color version of this figure appears in the plate section of this book.

15 A 62-year-old man presents to the emergency department with the condition shown in Figure 37.3. He is a resident of a nursing home due to cognitive defects after a disabling traumatic brain injury that occurred six years previously. Other medical history reveals type II diabetes managed with oral antihyperglycemic agents. According to his attendants, this condition also occurred about six weeks ago. The nursing home physician was able to reduce the mass into the rectum after pouring sugar on it. This therapy was repeated with this episode and was unsuccessful. The mass is dusky in color and has an area of ulceration. It has apparently been present for more than 18 hours on this occasion. The patient has normal vital signs and appears to be in moderate distress with perineal pain. Laboratory results are unremarkable. What is the next best step in management of this condition, if attempted reduction in the emergency department is unsuccessful?
A Operating room reduction under general anesthesia
B Altemeier procedure
C Laparotomy and sigmoidopexy (Ripstein procedure)
D Laparoscopic sigmoid resection
E Sigmoid colostomy

This patient has a large rectal prolapse. Reduction of the prolapse can allow conversion of a surgical emergency into a delayed procedure. Prolonged prolapse and dependency of the prolapsed segment can lead to congestion of the exposed rectum, which can make reduction impossible. Gentle circumferential pressure usually allows reduction, however use of topically osmotically active agents such as powdered sugar may allow a previously irreducible prolapse to be reduced. If monitored sedation does not allow reduction, then general anesthesia may allow reduction. Irreducible rectal prolapse is uncommon and leads to a decision for an emergent perineal versus abdominal procedure. The Altemeier procedure is a perineal procto-colectomy, which avoids a laparotomy but has a higher recurrence rate than abdominal procedures. The perineal incision of the Altemeier can also cause complications such as bleeding, infection, and dehiscence. If the patient can tolerate a laparotomy, abdominal procedures have the lowest rates of recurrence when the excess colon is resected rather than simply anchoring with sacral sutures or a mesh sling (Ripstein procedure). Colostomy is reserved for complications such as bowel necrosis, perforation, or failure of prior procedures. It is important to recognize that this condition is associated with pelvic floor dysfunction, and the associated incontinence is not managed by resection of bowel alone.

**Answer: A**

Bullard, D.K.M. and Rothenberger, D.A. (2010) Colon, rectum, and anus, in *Schwartz's Principles of Surgery*, 9th edn, (eds. F.C. Brunicardi, D.K. Andersen, T.R. Billiar, *et al.*), McGraw-Hill, New York, pp. 219–314.

Jones, O.M., Cunningham, C., and Lindsey, I. (2011) The assessment and management of rectal prolapse, rectal intussusception, rectocoele, and enterocoele in adults. *British Medical Journal*, **342**, c7099.

16 *A 54-year-old female nurse practitioner presents with crampy abdominal pain of 60 hours duration, associated with nausea and vomiting. Her last bowel movement was 24 hours ago. She has a past history of being admitted 22 days ago after a freeway motor vehicle collision. She recalls that she had a seat-belt mark across her mid-abdomen and significant abdominal pain. A CT scan of the abdomen was done during that admission and she was told she had "minor internal bleeding." Her abdominal pain gradually improved and she was discharged five days later. She undergoes laparotomy and the intraoperative findings are seen in Figure 37.4. What is the diagnosis?*

A *A "bucket-handle" tear of the small bowel mesentery which has led to a segment of ischemic ileum and internal small bowel hernia*

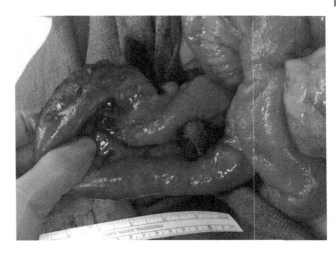

**Figure 37.4** A full color version of this figure appears in the plate section of this book.

B *Mesenteric ischemia caused by arterial embolism from an aortic injury*

C *Antibiotic-associated enteritis caused by recent administration of broad-spectrum antibiotics*

D *Small bowel perforation caused by compression of a closed-loop of small bowel by the seat belt*

E *Regional enteritis, consistent with Crohn's disease in the terminal ileum*

After blunt abdominal trauma, a CT scan revealing intraperitoneal fluid without an attributable solid organ source should be considered evidence of a mesenteric injury. When blunt trauma is associated with an abdominal seat belt mark, the diagnosis should also be considered. Multi-detector CT scan with IV contrast may show the mesenteric injuries and small bowel ischemia and/or edema, but is reader-dependent. Early exploration is the optimal management. Seat belts, while reducing traffic accident fatalities and serious injuries, can cause mesenteric injuries by shearing forces that may tear the small bowel from its supporting mesentery. The small bowel may then become ischemic, which may lead to perforation or stricture, which may present in a delayed fashion. The mesenteric defect is a possible source for an internal hernia as small bowel may become trapped or twisted within the fenestration. Figure 37.4 shows a strictured segment of ischemic ileum with an accompanying mesenteric defect that caused bowel obstruction due to internal hernia. Perforation from seat belt injury can also occur, but would be associated with peritonitis, abdominal sepsis, or abscess. Early prediction of bowel injury via the Bowel Injury Prediction Score (BIPS) was achieved in a retrospective series of patients with CT diagnosis of mesenteric injury after blunt abdominal trauma. Three predictors (admission CT scan grade of mesenteric injury, white blood cell count, and abdominal tenderness) were used to create a new bowel injury score, with a score of 2 or greater being strongly associated with bowel injury. Antibiotic-associated enteritis is typically a colitis; the small bowel is usually not inflamed although it may become edematous with severe pancolitis. Aortic injuries from trauma are most commonly associated with delayed aortic rupture, not embolism.

**Answer: A**

McNutt, M.K., Chinapuvvula, N.R.., Beckmann, N.M., *et al.* (2015) Early surgical intervention for blunt bowel injury: the Bowel Injury Prediction Score (BIPS). *Journal of Trauma and Acute Care Surgery*, **78** (1), 105–111.

Ng, A.K., Simons, R.K., Torreggiani, W.C., *et al.* (2002) Intra-abdominal free fluid without solid organ injury in blunt abdominal trauma: an indication for laparotomy. *Journal of Trauma*, **52** (6), 1134–1140.

**17** *A 54-year-old man presents with a history of one week of increasing abdominal pain, which is made worse with meals. He notes some abdominal bloating and his bowel movements have been normal. On examination he has mild diffuse abdominal tenderness without peritoneal signs. He relates no prior abdominal surgery, and he has a past history of non-traumatic deep venous thrombosis of his left leg 3 years ago for which he took coumadin for six months. A CT scan was obtained and is shown in Figure 37.5. What is the appropriate initial therapy for this condition?*

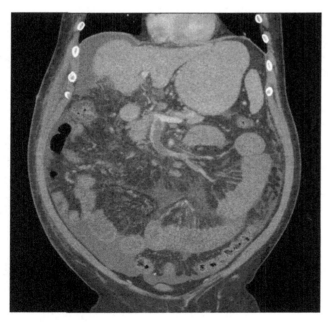

**Figure 37.5**

**A** *Intravenous heparin, followed by coumadin*
**B** *Mesenteric angiography*
**C** *Exploratory laparotomy*
**D** *Low-molecular-weight heparin*
**E** *Trans-jugular intrahepatic portal-caval shunt (TIPS)*

This patient has mesenteric venous ischemia, associated with portal vein and superior mesenteric vein thrombosis. While this condition has a slower progression than mesenteric arterial ischemia, the diagnosis is typically delayed, and may lead to extensive intestinal infarction, short-gut syndrome, or death. The condition is usually associated with portal or mesenteric vein thrombosis. Patients may have cirrhosis or a thrombotic disorder such as protein C or S deficiency, factor V Leiden or antithrombin III deficiency. Hematologic workup for a prothrombotic condition is indicated. Management in cases when bowel infarction is not suspected is by anticoagulation, intravenous heparin being the first choice in case of non-response and subsequent need for an urgent procedure. Angiography will not show the mesenteric venous anatomy significantly better than CT scanning with intravenous contrast. Laparotomy is performed when peritonitis and bowel infarction are suspected. TIPS is used to reduce risk of variceal bleeding from portal hypertension, but its use in mesenteric venous ischemia is not defined.

**Answer: A**

Harnik, I.G. and Brandt, L.J. (2010) Mesenteric venous thrombosis. *Vascular Medicine*, **15** (5), 407–418.

Tavakkolizadeh, A., Whang, E.E., Ashley, S., *et al.* (2010) Small intestine, in *Schwartz's Principles of Surgery*, 9th edn, (eds. F.C. Brunicardi, D.K. Andersen, T.R. Billiar, *et al.*), McGraw-Hill, New York, pp.279–298.

**18** *You are consulted regarding a 78-year-old woman who presented with left lower quadrant pain and a single episode of dark red blood-per-rectum 4 hours ago. She is afebrile and is hemodynamically normal and in normal sinus rhythm. Lab work reveals a WBC count of 13 000 /mm³ with 80% segmented neutrophils and a hemoglobin of 11 g/dL. Her past medical history reveals a remote cholecystectomy, type II diabetes, and she takes clopidogrel for a suspected transient ischemic attack three years ago. Abdominal examination reveals tenderness in the left lower quadrant without peritoneal signs. On rectal examination, dark red blood is seen on a gloved finger. Pulses are palpable in all extremities. A CT scan with intravenous contrast was obtained, which reveals a 4 cm infrarenal aortic aneurysm, and some* *bowel wall thickening in the sigmoid colon. The inferior mesenteric artery is not visualized. What is the appropriate initial management?*

**A** *Intravenous antibiotics, observation*

**B** *Colonoscopy*

**C** *Mesenteric angiogram*

**D** *Vascular surgery consult for endovascular stenting*

**E** *Laparotomy and sigmoid resection*

This patient has a presentation typical of ischemic colitis, which is typified by abdominal pain accompanied by lower gastrointestinal bleeding. Most mild-to-moderate cases will resolve under observation as the affected sigmoid colon develops collateral circulation. Severe cases resemble small bowel mesenteric ischemia with abdominal pain out-of-proportion to findings on examination. Some patients may develop frank necrosis of the colon and therefore close follow-up examinations are required. Antibiotics reduce pain and fever symptoms caused by poor gut wall integrity. CT scans with intravenous contrast will reveal mucosal edema, and "thumb-printing" of the affected colon. Colonoscopy will confirm the diagnosis, but is unnecessary in this case. Mesenteric angiography will not add significantly to the CT findings. A late complication is ischemic stricture (10–15%), which can be confirmed by a contrast study or colonoscopy, and may require sigmoid resection.

**Answer: A**

Bullard, D.K.M. and Rothenberger, D.A. (2010) Colon, rectum, and anus, in *Schwartz's Principles of Surgery*, 9th edn, (eds. F.C. Brunicardi, D.K. Andersen, T.R. Billiar, *et al.*), McGraw-Hill, New York, pp. 219–314.

Feuerstadt, P. and Brandt, L.J. (2010) Colon ischemia: recent insights and advances. *Current Gastroenterology Reports*, **12** (5), 383–390.

**19** *A 61-year-old man presents to the ED with pain at the umbilicus for one day, nausea, and he has vomited twice today. He is known to be cirrhotic with a history of hepatitis C and alcoholism, and he has ascites for which he takes spironolactone. He has had two prior trans-jugular intrahepatic portocaval shunt (TIPS) procedures. On examination, he has a protuberant umbilicus and some erythema around the umbilicus. The ED resident states she attempted to reduce the mass but was unsuccessful. The patient has a white blood cell count of 14 000 /mm³, hemoglobin of 11 g/dL, platelets of 72 000 /mm³, AST and ALT are within normal limits, INR of 1.6, total bilirubin of 1.9 mg/dL, and albumin of 2.9 g/dL. A CT scan shows a proximal bowel obstruction with a transition point at the umbilicus, and there appears*

*to be bowel within the umbilicus. Moderate ascites is also noted. Reduction of the umbilical mass with moderate pressure fails. What is the optimal management of this patient provided no bowel resection is required?*

**A** *Laparoscopy, reduction of hernia, intraperitoneal composite mesh umbilical repair*

**B** *Open umbilical hernia repair with polypropylene mesh*

**C** *Open umbilical hernia with biologic mesh*

**D** *Open umbilical hernia repair without mesh*

**E** *Open umbilical hernia repair, without mesh, and placement of paracentesis catheter*

This is a patient with advanced cirrhosis and ascites. These patients typically have umbilical hernias and little omentum, which is a setup for incarcerated or strangulated umbilical hernias with trapped bowel. Laparotomy in such patients is associated with significant mortality. Umbilical hernia repair in these patients has a high failure rate, and indeed the objective is often to reduce subsequent complications rather than obtain definitive hernia repair. Breakdown of the umbilical repair and uncontrolled ascites leakage from the wound is a morbid complication. Mesh repair has not shown to lessen hernia recurrence rates in such patients, and may risk mesh-related complications such as mesh infection and bowel perforation. Placement of a paracentesis catheter or drain in the peritoneal space may prevent the postoperative reaccumulation of tense ascites, allowing the umbilical wound an opportunity to heal without tension. Refractory cases may need a functioning TIPS prior to attempted repair.

**Answer: E**

Deveney, K.E. (2009) Hernias and other lesions of the abdominal wall, in *Current Diagnosis and Treatment: Surgery*, 13th edn (ed. G.M. Doherty), McGraw-Hill, New York, pp. 724–736

Telem, D.A., Schiano, T., and Divino, C.M. (2010) Complicated hernia presentation in patients with advanced cirrhosis and refractory ascites: management and outcome. *Surgery*, **148** (3), 538–543.

**20** *A 28-year-old man presents to the emergency department with a complaint of severe anal pain of 2 days duration. Surgery is consulted with a referring diagnosis of "hemorrhoids." The patient is very uncomfortable and cannot sit. He relates no prior episodes or prior history of anorectal problems. His past medical history reveals a childhood appendectomy and a history of asthma that is infrequent. On examination there is a small round bluish mass, about 8 mm* in diameter in a left-lateral position at the anal verge. This is very tender on palpation. The remainder of the examination is unremarkable. What is the best management of this condition?

**A** Excision under local anesthesia
**B** Observation, Sitz baths, oral analgesics
**C** Hemorrhoid banding
**D** Examination under general anesthesia, formal high ligation and hemorrhoid excision.
**E** Incision and expression of hematoma.

A wide variety of anorectal conditions are referred to surgeons as "hemorrhoids," however severe pain is not a common feature of hemorrhoids. Severe pain occurs when patients have thrombosis of prolapsed internal hemorrhoids or a thrombosed external pile. This patient has a thrombosed external pile, also known as a perianal hematoma. It is believed to be caused by rupture of a blood vessel in the sensitive perianal skin, possibly due to straining, and is not associated with prolapsing hemorrhoidal tissue. American Board of Surgery procedure log data indicates most graduating surgical residents have never treated this condition, despite its frequency. It is best managed by excision under local anesthesia, which relieves the painful stretching of the skin by the hematoma, and does not leave remnant skin tags as when incision and expression are performed. The hematoma within the pile will become organized and adherent to the skin within 72 hours of onset of symptoms. After 48–72 hours of onset of symptoms, incision of the hematoma and expression of the clot becomes difficult, making excision the preferred management. The other options listed are for treatment of internal hemorrhoids.

**Answer: A.**

Bullard, D.K.M. and Rothenberger, D.A. (2010) Colon, rectum, and anus, in *Schwartz's Principles of Surgery*, 9th edn, (eds. F.C. Brunicardi, D.K. Andersen, T.R. Billiar, *et al.*), McGraw-Hill, New York, pp. 219–314.
Sneider, E.B. and Maykel, J.A. (2010) Diagnosis and management of symptomatic hemorrhoids. *The Surgical Clinics of North America*, **90** (1), 17–32.

**21** A 42-year-old man trips at a construction site, falling onto a steel rebar rod which penetrates the perineum, 2 cm lateral the right of the anus. In the trauma bay the patient is hemodynamically normal. Chest x-ray, pelvis x-ray and FAST exam are negative. He has blood on digital rectal exam. He has no other injuries or comorbidities. The wound in the perineum is packed with saline-soaked gauze and the patient is brought to the CT scanner. CT scan demonstrates that the wound track traverses the rectum from

right-to-left below the levator muscles. There does not appear to be any intraperitoneal fluid. The patient is brought to the operating room and under general anesthesia, examination of the perineum and rectum and rigid sigmoidoscopy is performed. There appear to be two lacerations on the right and left side of the rectum 10–12 cm above the anal verge. What is the appropriate management of this injury?

**A** Trans-anal primary repair of the injuries alone
**B** Diverting sigmoid loop colostomy
**C** Diverting sigmoid loop colostomy with distal limb washout
**D** Diverting sigmoid loop colostomy with presacral drain placement
**E** Endoscopic placement of trans-anal vacuum-assisted closure sponge devices (Endosponge®)

The management of extraperitoneal rectal injury has evolved slowly over the past 40 years. The concern for these injuries is the development of pelvic sepsis which can lead to significant morbidity and mortality. The traditional triple-contrast CT scan can be replaced by CT tractography. Workup of these injuries includes anosigmoidoscopy and examination under anesthesia. During the Vietnam era, extraperitoneal penetrating trauma was commonly managed with diversion accompanied by pre-sacral drain placement and distal limb washout. However, the literature and current guidelines do not support the routine use of presacral drains or distal limb washout. The incidence of pelvic sepsis in modern series is quite low regardless of approach. Routine diversion of extraperitoneal rectal injury such as with a loop colostomy is recommended in an attempt to avoid pelvic sepsis. Trans-anal repair of injuries alone has not been described in any significant series. New techniques for using trans-anal endoscopic placement of vacuum assisted closure sponge devices have been described for management of prolonged colorectal anastomotic leaks, but not for acute rectal trauma.

**Answer: B**

Bansal, V., Reid, C.M., Fortlage, D., *et al.* (2014) Determining injuries from posterior and flank stab wounds using computed tomography tractography. *American Surgeon*, **80** (4), 403–407.
Bosarge, P.L., Como, J.J., Fox, N., *et al.* (2016) Management of penetrating extraperitoneal rectal injuries: An Eastern Association for the Surgery of Trauma practice management guideline. *Journal of Trauma and Acute Care Surgery*, **80** (3), 546–551.

**22** You are consulted by the ED for a 29-year-old man who has a rectal foreign body. On plain imaging, the *object appears to be a glass jar. The ED physician has attempted removal after administering morphine and was unsuccessful. The patient relates no prior surgery and is otherwise healthy. Vital signs are normal and the patient is afebrile. On examination, the patient is obese, and the metal lid of the jar is palpable high in the rectum on rectal examination. There is no free air on plain X-rays. Your next step should be:*

**A** *Reattempt extraction under deep sedation and perianal local anesthesia with a second operator*

**B** *Attempt removal under general anesthesia in the operating room*

**C** *Laparotomy with patient in stirrups; operator pulling from below as second operator pushes from above*

**D** *Flexible colonoscopy*

**E** *Rigid sigmoidoscopy*

Rectal foreign bodies are a common presenting complaint in the emergency department, and most of these can be removed without undue difficulty, especially if appropriate sedation is accompanied by local anesthesia.

A second operator gently pushing on the object if it is palpable in the abdomen, above the pelvic brim, may be helpful. Objects that cannot be removed in this manner may be impacted high in the rectum and cannot be easily turned to follow the sacral curve. Laparotomy may be required in such cases, although it may not be necessary to open the colon if the object can be manipulated through the sacral curve from above. Flexible colonoscopy or rigid sigmoidoscopy are performed after removal of the object to look for evidence of bowel injury, along with careful review of imaging for free air. Discovery of a transmural injury into the extraperitoneal rectal space requires diversion of the fecal stream, in the same manner that penetrating extraperitoneal injury such as after gunshot injury is managed.

**Answer: A**

Bullard, D.K.M. and Rothenberger, D.A. (2010) Colon, rectum, and anus, in *Schwartz's Principles of Surgery*, 9th edn, (eds. F.C. Brunicardi, D.K. Andersen, T.R. Billiar, *et al.*), McGraw-Hill, New York, pp. 219–314.

Goldberg, J.E. and Steele, S.R. (2010) Rectal foreign bodies. *The Surgical Clinics of North America*, **90** (1), 173–184.

# 38

## Gallbladder and Pancreas
*Matthew B. Singer, MD and Andrew Tang, MD*

**1** *A hepaticojejunostomy is performed immediately after intraoperative identification of a transected common bile duct during laparoscopic cholecystectomy (Strasberg E1). Which of the following statement is most accurate?*
   **A** *In experienced hands, the anastomosis has a 90% long-term patency rate*
   **B** *The patient will likely require anastomotic revision within 3 years due to stricture*
   **C** *Approximately 75% of bile duct injuries are recognized intraoperatively*
   **D** *An end-to-end anastomosis has a lower stricture rate than a hepaticojejunostomy*
   **E** *Immediate bile duct reconstruction should be delayed for 72 hours to allow for proximal bile duct dilation*

More than 750 000 laparoscopic cholecystectomies are performed annually in the United States. Laparoscopic cholecystectomy offers several advantages over open cholecystectomy, including less pain, fewer wound infections, improved cosmesis, decreased activation of inflammatory mediators, and an earlier return to normal activities. The only potential disadvantage to laparoscopic cholecystectomy is a higher incidence of major bile duct injury. Several large population-based studies indicate that the incidence of major bile duct injury is 0.3–0.5%, which is higher than the 0.1–0.2% incidence reported with open cholecystectomy.

A minority of bile duct injuries are recognized during the index cholecystectomy, only about 25% in most series. There are several factors that facilitate recognition of intraoperative injury, but the most important is a change in the surgeon's awareness to suspect and/or evaluate for a bile duct injury. Immediate cholangiography is imperative to clarify the anatomy should a ductal injury be suspected.

In general, debridement and primary anastomosis are not recommended. The undiseased common bile duct is narrow which makes the anastomosis challenging and prone to a higher stricture rate. The tenets of a successful biliary surgical repair include: anastomoses to healthy bile duct tissue, single-layer anastomoses using fine monofilament absorbable suture, tension-free anastomoses, Roux-en-Y hepaticojejunostomy with a 40–60 cm retrocolic Roux limb and an experienced biliary surgeon. Several studies have shown that bile duct reconstruction performed by experienced hepatobiliary surgeons have up to a 90% long-term patency rate.

**Answer: A**

Stewart, L. (2014) Iatrogenic biliary injuries. *Surgical Clinics of North America*, **94** (2), 297–310.

**2** *Which of these patients should undergo prophylactic cholecystectomy for asymptomatic gallstones?*
   **A** *55-year-old man with end-stage renal disease on the kidney transplant waiting list*
   **B** *25-year-old African American man with sickle cell anemia*
   **C** *35-year-old woman with a complete cervical spinal cord injury*
   **D** *50-year-old man with short bowel syndrome who is dependent on total parenteral nutrition*
   **E** *85-year-old woman with moderately well-controlled diabetes*

Management of asymptomatic gallstones in solid organ transplant patients has been controversial. Convincing data exist to support the decision for expectant management of asymptomatic cholelithiasis in kidney and pancreas transplant patients. Risks and disease progression among patients with heart and lung transplants, however,

*Surgical Critical Care and Emergency Surgery: Clinical Questions and Answers*, Second Edition.
Edited by Forrest "Dell" Moore, Peter Rhee, and Gerard J. Fulda.
© 2018 John Wiley & Sons Ltd. Published 2018 by John Wiley & Sons Ltd.
Companion website: www.wiley.com/go/moore/surgical_criticalcare_and_emergency_surgery

appear different. These patients are recommended to undergo prophylactic cholecystectomy.

Hemoglobinopathies including sickle cell disease cause hemolysis and formation of pigment stones. More than 55% of patients with sickle cell disease have gallstones by the age of 22 years and up to 75% of these patients develop symptoms. Symptom differentiation between biliary colic, cholecystitis, and sickle cell crisis can be difficult. As such, prophylactic cholecystectomy is frequently recommended in this population.

Risk of spinal cord injury is approximately two to three times greater among patients with spinal cord injury compared to the general population. In spite of this, the risk of symptomatic progression is the same as the general population. Thus, expectant management should be advocated in this population.

Reports from the early era of parenteral nutrition among chronically ill patients, almost half of whom required emergency open cholecystectomy, suggested routine ultrasound surveillance and consideration for early prophylactic cholecystectomy. In retrospect, the high rate of morbidity in that population was likely the result of a delay in diagnosis for a relatively new pathophysiologic diagnosis. Modern understanding of hepatobiliary complications from parenteral nutrition precludes cholecystectomy in the asymptomatic patient.

A historic report described increasing rates of severe cholecystitis among patients with diabetes presenting with cholecystitis. Subsequent studies failed to identify diabetes as an independent risk factor for adverse outcomes. Thus, prophylactic cholecystectomy for asymptomatic cholelithiasis in patients with diabetes is not recommended.

**Answer: B**

Cameron, J.L. and Cameron, A.M. (2013) *Current Surgical Therapy*, Elsevier Health Sciences, Philadelphia, PA.

3   Which statement is most accurate regarding early (<7 days) versus delayed laparoscopic cholecystectomy for acute cholecystitis?
   A Delayed laparoscopic cholecystectomy has a higher rate of conversion to open cholecystectomy
   B Early laparoscopic cholecystectomy has a higher incidence of bile duct injuries
   C Patients who undergo early laparoscopic cholecystectomy have a shorter length of hospital stay compared to the delayed group
   D Delayed laparoscopic cholecystectomy is associated with longer operating time
   E A higher incidence of wound infection is associated with delayed laparoscopic cholecystectomy

Controversy exists between the timing of cholecystectomy for acute cholecystitis. Some surgeons advocate "cooling down" patients with acute cholecystitis who present beyond seven days with antibiotics, fluid maintenance, and *nil per os*. They cite the theoretical increased risk of inflammation-induced obliteration of anatomy which increases the likelihood of bile duct injury, operative blood loss, and potentially associated with a higher conversion rate. However, such concerns are unsubstantiated in several randomized clinical trials comparing the outcomes between the two approaches. A Cochrane review that examined seven studies of high methodological quality found no difference in conversion rate or bile duct injury rate between cholecystectomies performed within or beyond seven days. The authors then conducted a meta-analysis using six of the seven randomized clinical trials, which in addition to the same findings as the Cochrane review, also found the total hospital stay to be shorter by four days for the early cholecystectomy group.

**Answer: C**

Gurusamy, K.S., Davidson, C., Gluud, C., and Davidson, B.R. (2013) Early versus delayed laparoscopic cholecystectomy for people with acute cholecystitis. *Cochrane Database of Systematic Reviews*, **30**(6).

4   A 45-year-old man with alcohol-induced pancreatitis has been intubated in the intensive care unit for three days. His current vital signs include: temperature 100.3°F, heart rate 110 beats/min, blood pressure 140/70 mm Hg. His abdominal exam reveals mild epigastric tenderness. His white blood cell count is 14 000 and his amylase is 527. What is the optimal plan for nutritional support?
   A Initiate total parenteral nutrition (TPN) and convert to enteral nutrition only after his abdomen is non-tender
   B Initiate TPN and convert to enteral nutrition only after his amylase and lipase have normalized
   C Begin nasoenteric feeding
   D Continue nil per os for seven days and initiate nasoenteric feeding if the patient remains intubated
   E Continue nil per os for seven days and initiate TPN if the patient still has abdominal pain

In patients with severe acute pancreatitis, it is recommended to initiate enteral nutrition via a nasoenteric tube within the first 72 hours of hospitalization. A 2012 meta-analysis of 381 patients with severe acute pancreatitis confirms the benefit of enteral versus parenteral feeding. With two groups randomly assigned to receive each variation of nutrition, those with enteral feeding bene-fitted in mortality, infection, organ failure, and had a lower surgical rate. Nasojejunal feeding has long been preferred, although there is evidence that nasogastric feeding has similar clinical efficacy. Although evidence shows a preference toward enteral feeding, if the patient is unable to tolerate it or not meet nutritional goals, parenteral nutrition should be initiated while maintaining a slow rate of enteral feeding.

**Answer: C**

Janisch, N.H. and Gardner, T.B. (2016) Advances in management of acute pancreatitis. *Gastroenterology Clinics of North America*, **45** (1), 1–8.

Yi, F., Ge, L., Zhao, J., *et al.* (2012) Meta-analysis: total parenteral nutrition versus total enteral nutrition in predicted severe acute pancreatitis. *Internal Medicine*, **51** (6), 523–530.

**5** *A 67-year-old woman who has been hospitalized for seven days undergoes endoscopic retrograde cholangiopancreatography and biliary stent placement for a benign biliary stricture. On postprocedure day three she develops fevers, right upper quadrant pain, and jaundice. Which of the following is an appropriate empiric antibiotic regimen?*
 **A** *Cefuroxime*
 **B** *Cefepime*
 **C** *Meropenem and metronidazole*
 **D** *Piperacillin/tazobactam and metronidazole*
 **E** *Piperacillin/tazobactam, metronidazole, and vancomycin*

The Infectious Disease Society of America identifies four distinct patient populations with biliary infection and recommends the following recommend initial empiric treatment regimens:

1) Community-acquired acute cholecystitis – mild to moderate: cefazolin, cefuroxime, or ceftriaxone
2) Community-acquired acute cholecystitis – severe, or in patients with advanced age, or in immunocompromised patients: imipenem-cilastatin, meropenem, doripenem, piperacillin-tazobactam, ciprofloxacin, levofloxacin, or cefepime, each in combination with metronidazole
3) Acute cholangitis following bilio-enteric anastamosis of any severity: imipenem-cilastatin, meropenem, doripenem, piperacillin-tazobactam, ciprofloxacin, levofloxacin, or cefepime, each in combination with metronidazole
4) Health care-associated biliary infection of any severity: imipenem-cilastatin, meropenem, doripenem, piperacillin-tazobactam, ciprofloxacin, levofloxacin, or cefepime, each in combination with metronidazole, vancomycin added to each regimen

**Answer: E**

Solomkin, J.S., Mazuski, J.E., Bradley, J.S., *et al.* (2010) Diagnosis and management of complicated intra-abdominal infection in adults and children: guidelines by the Surgical Infection Society and the Infectious Diseases Society of America. *Clinical Infectious Diseases*, **50** (2), 133–164.

**6** *Which of the following is not a risk factor for cholesterol stone formation?*
 **A** *Female sex*
 **B** *Advancing age*
 **C** *Sickle cell disease*
 **D** *Rapid weight loss*
 **E** *Obesity*

Women are twice as likely as men to form gallstones, a process related to female sex hormones, birth control medications, parity, and hormone replacement therapies. The increased levels of estrogen and progesterone lead to cholesterol hypersecretion and gallbladder stasis.

The risk of developing gallstones increases markedly with advancing age. After 40 years of age, the incidence of gallstones increases by 1–3% per year. With increasing age, hepatic cholesterol secretion is increased, cholesterol saturation increases, and bile acid synthesis is decreased.

Sickle cell disease is a strong risk factor for the formation of pigment stones, not cholesterol stones.

Obesity is an epidemic in developed nations and is a strong risk factor for gallstone disease. This factor may be, in part, caused by the increased activity of 3-hydroxy-3-methylglutaryl–coenzyme A reductase, the rate-limiting enzyme in cholesterol synthesis, leading to increased cholesterol synthesis in the liver and secretion into the bile.

Bariatric surgery patients with rapid postoperative weight loss develop gallstones in 30–71% of cases. The incidence of gallstones is highest within the first two years after surgery. Most of these stones are asymptomatic. The mechanism for increased lithogenesis in bariatric patients is unclear.

**Answer: C**

O'Connell, K. and Brasel, K. (2014) Bile metabolism and lithogenesis. *Surgical Clinics of North America*, **94** (2), 361–375.

**7** Which statement regarding biliary anatomy is false?

    **A** The most common hepatic arterial variant is a replaced right hepatic artery

    **B** The right hepatic artery arises from the superior mesenteric artery in 20% of patients

    **C** The common bile duct and the pancreatic duct form a common channel in 70% of patients

    **D** The 3 and 9 o'clock arteries that supply the common bile duct are branches of the proper hepatic artery

    **E** The right anterior sectoral duct drains Couinaud's segments 5 and 8

The right and left lobes of the liver are defined by Cantlie's line, which corresponds to an imaginary line between the gallbladder fossa and the inferior vena cava. The left lobe is then divided into a medial (segment 4) and lateral sections (segments 2 and 3), separated by the umbilical fissure that is in continuity with the falciform ligament. The right lobe is divided into the anterior (segment 5 and 8) and the posterior sections (6 and 7). Each section is subdivided into the inferior (segments 5 and 6) and superior (7 and 8) segments.

Normally, the cystic artery branches from the right hepatic artery. Its location is fairly constant within Calot's triangle, which is bordered medially by the common hepatic duct, the cystic duct inferiorly and the inferior edge of the right lobe superiorly. The 3 and 9 o'clock arteries are major axial vessels that run along the medial and lateral borders of the supraduodenal common bile duct in locations implied by their names. They arise inferiorly from the anterior and posterior superior pancreaticoduodenal, gastroduodenal, and retroportal arteries, and above from the right and left hepatic and cystic arteries. Given the locations of the 3 and 9 o'clock arteries, choledochotomies should be created longitudinally through an area devoid of vessels, leaving the fascial envelope intact.

The CBD invariably lies to the right of the proper hepatic artery, and both structures lie anterior to the portal vein. In most cases, the right hepatic artery then courses posterior to the common hepatic duct as it ascends to supply Couinaud's segments 5-8.

The most common hepatic vascular variant occurring in 20% of patients is a replaced or accessory right hepatic artery arising from the superior mesenteric artery. The variant right hepatic artery can be palpated in the hepatoduodenal ligament posterior to the CBD and portal vein. In 15% of patients, a replaced or accessory left hepatic artery courses through the gastrohepatic ligament as it branches from the left gastric artery.

**Answer: D**

Keplinger, K.M. and Bloomston, M. (2014) Anatomy and embryology of the biliary tract. *Surgical Clinics of North America*, **94** (2), 203–217.

**8** A 75-year-old nursing home resident presents with two days of nausea, vomiting, and abdominal pain. His vital signs include: temperature of 100.2°F, heart rate 110 beats/min, blood pressure 159/90 mm Hg. An abdominal series reveals pneumobilia, small bowel air fluid levels and a 5 cm opacification in the right lower quadrant. Which statement regarding his treatment is true?

    **A** Gallstone ileus recurs in 30% of patients who undergo enterolithotomy alone

    **B** The cholecystoenteric fistula must be repaired either at the time of the enterolithotomy or as a second stage operation due to the low likelihood of spontaneous closure

    **C** The patient should be managed conservatively given the likelihood of spontaneous stone passage

    **D** Resection of the obstructed small bowel segment and enterolithotomy have similar complication rates

    **E** The one-stage procedure is associated with a higher mortality than enterolithotomy alone

Gallstone ileus accounts for 1-4% of mechanical small bowel obstructions and up to 25% of bowel obstructions in patients over 65 years. The process starts with gallstone impaction which leads to ischemia and pressure necrosis at the interface between the gallbladder and adjacent viscera. The duodenum is the site of cholecystoenteric fistula formation in over 80% of cases. Stone passage is dependent on the size of the stone and the intestinal luminal diameter. It is generally believed that stones less than 2 cm will pass spontaneously. Those greater than 5 cm are likely to be impacted, typically in the terminal ileum in cases of small bowel fistulas, or the sigmoid colon in cases of colonic fistulas.

The clinical presentation is characteristic of bowel obstruction. Most gallstones are not radiopaque enough to be easily detected on plain abdominal radiographs. Rigler's triad of abdominal radiograph findings (pneumobilia, small bowel air fluid levels and an ectopic gallstone) is only present in 50% of patients. The sensitivity and specificity of CT scan for the detection of gallstone ileus is 93% and 100% respectively.

Controversy exists regarding the optimal management of gallstone ileus. Three options exist: enterolithotomy alone, a one-stage procedure consisting of enterolithotomy with cholecystectomy and fistula repair, or a two-stage procedure including enterolithotomy followed in 4–6 weeks by cholecystoenteric fistula takedown. Enterolithotomy alone is the most commonly performed procedure.

Gallstone ileus is thought to recur in only 5% of patients and cholecystoenteric fistulas are though to close spontaneously in 50% of cases. In the largest review to date, Reisner and Cohen found a mortality rate of 17% for the one-stage procedure compared to 12% for enterolithotomy alone. Enterolithotomy is performed by milking the obstructing stone proximally to unaffected bowel where the longitudinal enterotomy and stone extraction take place. The enterotomy is then closed transversely to avoid luminal narrowing. Small bowel resection and anastomosis is another option when the impacted stone has created irreversible damage to the bowel wall. However, this approach is associated with particularly high anastomotic leak rates.

**Answer: E**

Nuño-Guzmán, C.M., Marín-Contreras, M.E., Figueroa-Sánchez, M., and Corona, J.L. (2016) Gallstone ileus: clinical presentation, diagnostic and treatment approach. *World Journal of Gastrointestinal Surgery*, **8** (1), 65–76.

**9**  *Which statement regarding the treatment of gall-stone-related disease during pregnancy is true?*
   **A** *Symptomatic cholelithiasis should be managed non-operatively during pregnancy*
   **B** *Cholecystitis during the first trimester should be "cooled off" with antibiotics, followed by cholecystectomy in the second trimester*
   **C** *Due to the low risk of recurrent symptoms, no intervention should be undertaken for choledocholithiasis during pregnancy*
   **D** *Common bile duct exploration is preferred over endoscopic retrograde cholangiopancreatography in the management of choledocholithiasis during pregnancy due to the risk of radiation exposure*
   **E** *Laparoscopic cholecystectomy is associated with decreased risk of spontaneous abortion and preterm labor when compared to open cholecystectomy*

Complications from gallstone disease represent the second most common nonobstetric condition requiring operative management during pregnancy after appendicitis. It has been reported that approximately 40% of patients presenting with symptomatic cholelithiasis intrapartum require cholecystectomy during that pregnancy. When a decision for operative management is made, the options include either a laparoscopic or an open approach. The benefits of a laparoscopic approach in pregnant patients are similar to nonpregnant patients and include: reduced morbidity, reduced postoperative narcotic requirements, shorter hospital stay and earlier mobilization. A 2016 meta-analysis of 11 studies with over 10 000 patients found that laparoscopic cholecystectomy is associated with fewer maternal and fetal complications compared to open cholecystectomy. Additionally, it was found that laparoscopic cholecystectomy can be safely performed in all trimesters of pregnancy.

Choledocholithiasis represents another complication of gallstone disease that may arise during pregnancy. While maternal and fetal death as a consequence of complications of choledocholithiasis is uncommon, relapse of symptoms is common and is found to occur in 58–72% of cases, usually associated with repeated hospitalizations. It is, therefore, recommended that endoscopic retrograde cholangiopancreatography (ERCP) be performed when choledocholithiasis arises to minimize risk of relapse. ERCP has been performed during pregnancy for over two decades and, when performed appropriately, appears to be safe, with maternal outcomes similar to those in a nonpregnant cohort and with no significant fetal adverse outcomes.

**Answer: E**

Chan, C.H.Y. and Enns, R.A. (2012) ERCP in the management of choledocholithiasis in pregnancy. *Current Gastroenterology Reports*, **14** (6), 504–510.
Sedaghat, N., Cao, A.M., Eslick, G.D., and Cox, M.R. (2016) Laparoscopic versus open cholecystectomy in pregnancy: a systematic review and meta-analysis. *Surgical Endoscopy*, **31** (2), 673–679.

**10**  *An abdominal ultrasound incidentally identifies a 0.8 cm polypoid gallbladder lesion in a 45-year-old man. What is the next step in management?*
   **A** *Laparoscopic cholecystectomy*
   **B** *Open cholecystectomy with intraoperative frozen section*
   **C** *Extended cholecystectomy with hepatic segment IVB and V resection and portal lymphadenectomy*
   **D** *CT scan with IV contrast*
   **E** *Observation with repeat ultrasound in 6 months*

The estimated prevalence of gallbladder polyps varies by the demographics of the studied population, but it is generally considered to be around 5%. The current accepted classification divides these polyps into neoplastic (adenomas, carcinoma in situ) and non-neoplastic, with the non-neoplastic polyps accounting for about 95% of these lesions. Any gallbladder polyp that is felt to be symptomatic should be removed from a patient otherwise fit for surgery. In asymptomatic patients, solitary sessile polyps greater than 10 mm in patients over age 50 should be considered for cholecystectomy, particularly in patients with cholelithiasis and primary sclerosing cholangitis, as these characteristics represent risk factors for malignancy. Gallbladder polyps that are not resected should be followed with serial ultrasound examinations. Clear guidelines on a screening interval are not available, and individual patient characteristics need to be considered. However, recent studies support a screening interval of every 6–12 months, to be continued for as long as 10 years.

**Answer: E**

Gallahan, W.C. and Conway, J.D. (2010) Diagnosis and management of gallbladder polyps. *Gastroenterology Clinics of North America*, **39** (2), 359–367.

**11** *A 45-year old immigrant from Southeast Asia presents with cholangitis and jaundice. Ultrasound reveals multiple intrahepatic stones. Which of the following is not an advisable treatment option?*
   **A** *Hepaticocutaneous jejunostomy (Hudson Loop)*
   **B** *Roux-en-Y hepaticojejunostomy*
   **C** *Percutaneous transhepatic cholangiocatheterization with biliary drainage and choledoscopic stone removal*
   **D** *Hepatic resection if stones are confined to one anatomical region*
   **E** *Endoscopic retrograde cholangiopancreatography*

Hepatolithiasis is characterized by the presence of stones within the intrahepatic bile ducts proximal to the right and left hepatic ducts. This condition is rare in Western countries but has an incidence of 2–25% in China, Taiwan, Korea, and Japan. Hepatolithiasis is benign in nature, but the prognosis is poor due to an association with recurrent cholangitis, biliary strictures, liver abscesses, and liver atrophy or cirrhosis. The hepatoliths are typically brown pigment stones formed in association with states of prolonged partial biliary tract obstruction such as primary sclerosing cholangitis, biliary strictures and biliary parasites.

Endoscopic retrograde cholangiopancreatography is associated with a high failure rate due to biliary stricture imposed access difficulty and the extensive nature of stone formation. Percutaneous transhepatic cholangiography allows for repeated fluoroscopically guided stone extraction with steerable stone baskets, or with percutaneous choledochoscopy. Surgical options include Roux-en-Y hepaticojejunostomy after intraoperative choledochoscopic guided stone clearance. A hepaticocutaneous jejunostomy, otherwise known as a Hudson Loop, involves a long Roux limb that extends from the hepaticojejunostomy to the anterior abdominal wall. This construct allows for future endoscopic access to the biliary tree should stone disease recur or for treatment of biliary strictures. If the hepatolithiasis is limited to a single lobe or segment of the liver, and associated with significant biliary stricture or atrophy, then hepatic resection may be indicated.

**Answer: E**

Kim, H.J., Kim, J.S., Joo, M.K., *et al.* (2015) Hepatolithiasis and intrahepatic cholangiocarcinoma: a review. *World Journal of Gastroenterology*, **21** (48), 13418–13431.
Pitt, H.A., Venbrux, A.C., Coleman, J., *et al.* (1994) Intrahepatic stones: the transhepatic team approach. *Annals of Surgery*, **219** (5), 527–537.

**12** *Gallbladder cancer limited to the lamina propria (stage T1a) was found in the cholecystectomy specimen. What is the next step?*
   **A** *Referral to radiation and medical oncology*
   **B** *Re-operation for radical cholecystectomy*
   **C** *CT of the abdomen and pelvis for cancer staging*
   **D** *Endoscopic retrograde cholangiopancreatography and endoscopic ultrasound*
   **E** *Observation*

Gallbladder cancer remains a relatively rare malignancy with a highly variable presentation. Gallbladder cancer is the most common biliary tract malignancy with the worst overall prognosis. From a surgical perspective, gallbladder cancer can be suspected preoperatively, identified intraoperatively, or discovered incidentally on final surgical pathology. Up to half of all gallbladder cancers are diagnosed pathologically after cholecystectomy for presumed benign disease.

It is well recognized that T1a tumors require no further management beyond simple cholecystectomy, assuming negative resection margins. The prognosis for Tis and T1a tumors is good, with 85–100% cured after simple cholecystectomy. However, if preoperative suspicion for cancer exists such as in the case of large polyps, then open cholecystectomy is recommended in order to minimize the risk of gallbladder perforation with tumor spillage and port site metastasis.

**Answer: E**

Wernberg, J.A. and Lucarelli, D.D. (2014) Gallbladder cancer. *Surgical Clinics of North America*, **94** (2), 343–360.

**13** *A 45-year-old woman is recovering from a three-week intensive care unit course complicated by acute respiratory distress syndrome and acute renal failure secondary to necrotizing pancreatitis. Over the past 48 hours, she has been spiking fevers to 102°F and now has a white blood cell count of 14 000. A CT of the abdomen demonstrates an 8 cm rim-enhancing fluid collection with an air-fluid level near the pancreatic tail. Which is the most appropriate next step in management?*
   **A** *Observation with repeat CT scan in 2 weeks*
   **B** *Antimicrobial administration with aerobic, anaerobic, and fungal coverage*

C *Percutaneous aspiration of the fluid collection*
D *Percutaneous retroperitoneal drain placement*
E *Open necrosectomy*

The traditional approach to the treatment of necrotizing pancreatitis with secondary infection of necrotic tissue is open necrosectomy to completely remove the infected necrotic tissue. This invasive approach is associated with high rates of complications (34–95%) and death (11–39%) and with a risk of long-term pancreatic insufficiency. As an alternative to open necrosectomy, less invasive techniques, including percutaneous drainage, endoscopic (transgastric) drainage, and minimally invasive retroperitoneal necrosectomy, are increasingly being used. These techniques can be performed in a so-called "step-up" approach.

A landmark 2010 study by the Dutch Pancreatitis Study Group showed that the minimally invasive step-up approach, as compared with primary open necrosectomy, reduced the rate of the composite end point of major complications or death, as well as long-term complications, health-care resource utilization, and total costs, among patients who had necrotizing pancreatitis and confirmed or suspected secondary infection. With the step-up approach, more than one third of patients were successfully treated with percutaneous drainage and did not require major abdominal surgery.

**Answer: D**

da Costa, D.W., Boerma, D., van Santvoort, H.C., *et al.* (2014) Staged multidisciplinary step-up management for necrotizing pancreatitis. *British Journal of Surgery*, **101** (1), e65–79.
van Santvoort, H.C., Besselink, M.G., Bakker, O.J., *et al.* (2010) A step-up approach or open necrosectomy for necrotizing pancreatitis. *New England Journal of Medicine*, **362** (16), 1491–1502.

**14** *A 38-year-old woman passenger involved in a motor vehicle collision undergoes laparotomy for a small bowel mesenteric injury with active contrast extravasation seen on CT scan. After the bleeding is controlled, inspection of the lesser sac reveals a major contusion with hematoma formation at the head of the pancreas. What is the next best step in the management of this injury?*
A *Closure of the abdomen*
B *Closure of the abdomen after placement of a closed suction drain adjacent to the head of the pancreas*
C *Closure of the abdomen followed by endoscopic retrograde cholangiopancreatography*

D *Exploration of the hematoma to assess for pancreatic duct injury*
E *Pancreaticoduodenectomy*

The AAST classifies pancreatic injuries on a grading scale of I–V. The injury described above corresponds to Grade I. When Grade I and II injuries are discovered intraoperatively, the vast majority can be treated with surgical hemostasis and drainage. Even capsular tears that are not bleeding are not repaired and may be simply drained with closed suction drainage. Drainage is used liberally because many minor appearing injuries will drain for several days. Unnecessary attempts at repair of lacerations without evidence of ductal disruption can result in late pseudocyst formation, whereas the vast majority of controlled, minor pancreatic fistulae are self-limited and easily managed with soft closed suction drains. The drains are usually removed within a few days, as long as the amylase concentration in the drain is less than that of serum. If amylase levels are elevated, drainage is continued until there is no further evidence of pancreatic leak.

**Answer: B**

Biffl, W.L., Moore, E.E., Croce, M., *et al.* (2013) Western Trauma Association critical decisions in trauma: management of pancreatic injuries. *Journal of Trauma and Acute Care Surgery*, **75** (6), 941–946.

**15** *A 24-year-old restrained driver presents to the emergency department after losing control of his vehicle and driving into a concrete wall. CT scan of his abdomen reveals a large peripancreatic fluid collection. He is taken to the operating room for exploratory laparotomy which reveals a disruption of the pancreatic duct at the neck of the pancreas. Definitive treatment of this injury includes which of the following?*
A *Placement of two closed suction drains*
B *Temporary abdominal closure followed by postoperative endoscopic retrograde cholangiopancreatography*
C *Distal pancreatectomy*
D *Central segmental pancreatectomy with distal pancreaticojejunostomy*
E *Pancreaticoduodenectomy*

Injuries to the pancreas present a significant challenge, for a number of reasons. First, while the deep, central position of the pancreas affords the organ some degree of protection, its retroperitoneal location confounds the clinical detection of injury. Second, physiologic functions contribute to a disturbingly high incidence of complications following injury, and morbidity is exacerbated by delays in diagnosis and treatment. Third, the infrequency of these injuries has resulted in a lack of significant management experience among practicing trauma surgeons.

The primary non-operative diagnostic modality for pancreatic injury is CT scanning. Findings may be subtle, particularly when the imaging is performed within 12 hours of injury. CT scan evidence of pancreatic transection or extensive peri-pancreatic fluid warrants laparotomy. These findings are associated with a higher risk of pancreatic ductal disruption, which is the major determinant of prognosis.

The anatomic division between the head and body of the pancreas is the neck, where the superior mesenteric artery (SMA) and superior mesenteric vein (SMV) pass behind the pancreas. This anatomic division will provide an estimated 50% of pancreatic tissue. Ductal injuries at or distal to the neck are treated definitively with distal pancreatectomy.

**Answer: C**

Biffl, W.L., Moore, E.E., Croce, M., *et al.* (2013) Western Trauma Association critical decisions in trauma: management of pancreatic injuries. *Journal of Trauma and Acute Care Surgery*, **75** (6), 941–946.

16  *A 45-year-old man is admitted for severe alcohol-induced pancreatitis. A CT scan demonstrates non-enhancement in 45% of the pancreatic body and tail. Which statement regarding antibiotic prophylaxis in necrotizing pancreatitis is most accurate?*

　　**A** *Antibiotic prophylaxis used in conjunction with an antifungal agent is associated with the least infectious complications*

　　**B** *Prophylactic antibiotics should be started on all patients with pancreatic necrosis*

　　**C** *Prophylactic antibiotics should be started within 24 hours of admission*

　　**D** *Antibiotic prophylaxis should be started in patients who demonstrate progression to pancreatic necrosis on serial contrast enhanced CTs*

　　**E** *Antibiotic prophylaxis does not reduce mortality or protect against infected necrosis*

Necrotizing pancreatitis develops in about 15% of patients with pancreatitis and accounts for mortality ranging from 12 to 35%. The associated mortality has a bimodal distribution with multisystem organ failure implicated in the early phase while pancreatic or peri-pancreatic infections account for much of the late deaths. The prevalent practice of antibiotic prophylaxis directed against common causative enteric organisms such as *E. coli*, Klebsiella, Enterobacter and Bacteroides does not appear to reduce the incidence of late infectious complications. Rather, several recent studies have documented an increase in gram-positive and Candida isolates from infected pancreatic aspirates, possibly due to the prevalent use of prophylactic antibiotics.

A multicenter prospective randomized, double blinded, placebo-controlled trial with 100 participants with greater than 30% pancreatic necrosis showed no difference in the incidence of pancreatic and peri-pancreatic infections, the number of surgical interventions, or mortality between those who received meropenem and placebo. A Cochrane review of 7 studies involving 404 patients randomly assigned to receive prophylactic antibiotics or placebo likewise concluded that there is no difference in the rate of infectious complications. The preponderance of available evidence does not support antibiotic prophylaxis for pancreatic necrosis.

**Answer: E**

Jafri, N.S., Mahid, S.S., Idstein, S.R., *et al.* (2009) Antibiotic prophylaxis is not protective in severe acute pancreatitis: a systematic review and meta-analysis. *The American Journal of Surgery*, **197** (6), 806–813.

Villatoro, E., Mulla, M., and Larvin, M. (2010) Antibiotic therapy for prophylaxis against infection of pancreatic necrosis in acute pancreatitis. *Cochrane Database Systemic Reviews*, **12** (5).

# 39

## Liver and Spleen

*Cathy Ho, MD and Narong Kulvatunyou, MD*

1 *Which of the following statements about the current management of blunt liver trauma is not true?*
   A *Nonoperative management is often appropriate*
   B *Operative management is indicated for hemodynamic instability and associated organ injury*
   C *A patient with a grade V injury always requires operative intervention*
   D *Angiographic embolization can be useful adjunct in both operative and nonoperative management*
   E *An anatomic lobar resection is not required for most injuries*

Nonoperative management of hepatic trauma is often appropriate. It can be performed with a 77–100% success rate, as long as the patient remains hemodynamically within a normal range and does not have any other associated intra-abdominal injuries. Although the failure rate is increased with higher grade injuries, most grade IV, and V injuries may still be successfully managed nonoperatively. In a nonoperative patient, angiographic embolization (AE) can be an adjunct in liver injuries that contains an arterio-venous fistula or have ongoing bleeding. AE can also be of assistance in operative cases where bleeding may be difficult to access and control. An anatomic lobar resection is rarely required for blunt hepatic trauma.

**Answer: C**

Asensio, J.A., Demetriades, D., Chahwan, S., *et al.* (2000) Approach to the management of complex hepatic injuries. *Journal of Trauma*, **48** (1), 66–69.
Green, C.S., Bulger, E.M., and Kwan, S.W. (2015) Outcomes and complications of angioembolization for hepatic trauma: a systematic review of the literature. *Journal of Trauma and Acute Care Surgery*, **80** (3), 529–537.
Malhotra, A.K., Fabian, T.C., Croce, M.A., *et al.* (2000) Blunt hepatic injury: a paradigm shift from operative to

non-operative management in the 1990s. *Annals of Surgery*, **231** (6), 804–813.

2 *Which of the following is incorrect regarding liver abscess?*
   A *Both pyogenic and amebic abscess have similar clinical presentation*
   B *Both pyogenic and amebic abscess require drainage*
   C *Amoebic abscesses are caused by* Entamoeba histolytica
   D *The most common source of a pyogenic liver abscess is a biliary source*
   E *Antibiotic of choice for amoebic abscess is metronidazole*

In the United States, pyogenic liver abscesses are much more common than amoebic abscesses; however, the clinical presentation for both is similar. Amoebic abscesses are caused by *Entamoeba histolytica*. One must obtain a thorough history of traveling to the endemic areas – Central America, Southeast Asia, and so on – and diagnosis is confirmed by a serologic test. Amebic abscesses do not require drainage because they respond effectively to metronidazole. Pyogenic abscess treatment requires antibiotic administration, source control, and likely drainage. Ascending suppurative cholangitis is the most common identifiable cause of pyogenic abscess.

**Answer: B**

Cameron, J.L. (2008) *Current Surgical Therapy*, 9th edn, Mosby, Philadelphia, PA.

3 *An 8-year-old girl is taken to the emergency department after being struck by a car. She landed on her right side. On arrival, she is alert with a systolic blood pressure of 110 mm Hg after 500 mL of crystalloids.*

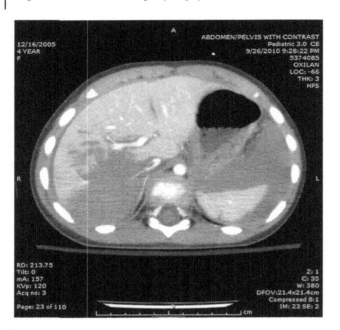

**Figure 39.1**

*She has bilateral breath sounds. Her vital signs have remained normal. The computed tomography (CT) scan in Figure 39.1 is obtained. The most appropriate next step would be:*

A *Laparotomy*

B *Diagnostic peritoneal lavage (DPL)*

C *Angiography*

D *Admission for observation*

E *Laparoscopy*

The image is an abdominal computed tomography (CT) that shows a grade IV liver injury without contrast extravasation. Nonoperative management of blunt liver injuries in patients with normal hemodynamics is recommended with greater than 90% success. Diagnostic peritoneal lavage will confirm the presence of blood but will not add any information helpful in the management of this patient. Laparoscopy may benefit this patient later in her course if she develops significant hemoperitoneum or biliary ascites but has no role in initial management once the diagnosis has been made. While some authors recommend angiography in all high-grade liver injury, it is not an absolute indication especially when the CT does not show any evidence of active bleeding (a "blush") or arterio-venous fistula. While the CT looks as if the liver injury is severe and there is a lot of blood in the abdomen, in hemodynamically normal patients, observation is the first course of action, the CT should make one cautious and careful monitoring and follow-up is required.

**Answer: D**

Duane, T.M., Como, J.J., Bochicchio, G.V., *et al.* (2004) Reevaluating the management and outcomes of severe blunt liver injury. *Journal of Trauma*, **57**, 494–500.

Kozar, R.A., Moore, J.B., Niles, S.E., *et al.* (2005) Complications of non-operative management of high-grade blunt hepatic injuries. *Journal of Trauma*, **59**, 1066–1071.

4 *Which of the following is incorrect regarding hydatid disease of the liver?*

A *It is caused by parasitic* Echinococcus *whose definitive host is a cat*

B *A unique ultrasound or computed tomography characteristic is a calcified cyst wall, but diagnosis can be confirmed by serology*

C *Chemotherapeutic benzimidazole compound derivatives should be given 1–4 days preoperatively before and continued post-procedurally*

D *Percutaneous aspiration, injection, and re-aspiration (PAIR) is a possible treatment option*

E *Before surgically entering the cyst, the operative field should be protected with scolicidal agent-soaked gauzes to prevent contamination*

Hydatid disease of the liver is uncommon. It is caused by parasitic *Echinococcus*, which has dogs as its definitive hosts. Humans come in contact by ingesting contaminated food infested with parasites. Signs and symptoms are vague, but ultrasound, and computed tomography have the unique characteristic of a cyst with a calcified wall. Medical therapy alone with benzimidazole agent results in incomplete resolution as 70% will have a recurrence. Treatment must be combined with PAIR (percutaneous aspiration, injection, and re-aspiration) or surgical cystectomy. It is important that operative field be protected with scolicidal agent-soaked gauzes, usually 20% normal saline, to prevent spillage and contamination.

**Answer: A**

Alonso, C.O., Moreno, G.E., Loinaz, S.C., *et al.* (2001) Results of 22 years of experience in radical surgical treatment of hepatic hydatid cyst. *Hepatogastroenterology*, **48**, 235–239.

Gavara, C.G., Lopez-Andujar, R., Ibanez, T.B., *et al.* (2015) Review of the treatment of liver hydatid cysts. *World Journal of Gastroenterology*, **21** (1), 124–131.

Gil-Grande, L.A., Rodriguez-Caabeiro, F., Prieto, J.G., *et al.* (1993) Randomized controlled trial of efficacy of albendazole in intra-abdominal hydatid disease. *Lancet*, **342**, 1269–1275.

5 *A 24-year-old woman continues to have persistent abdominal pain one month after her motor vehicle collision in which she suffered a liver injury. The computed*

*tomography (CT) shows a biloma. Attempted CT-guided drainage was unsuccessful. What would be the next step of management?*

A *Exploratory laparotomy and hepatectomy*

B *Exploratory laparotomy and debridement of necrotic parenchyma*

C *Laparoscopy with drainage*

D *Drainage and endoscopic retrograde cholangiopan-creatography (ERCP) with sphincterotomy*

E *Somatostatin and observe*

Patients with high-grade liver injuries have an increased risk of developing post-injury biloma as a complication. In general, CT-guided drainage is the initial treatment of choice for a patient who is asymptomatic, and it is usually successful. However, if unsuccessful, endoscopic retrograde cholangiopancreatography (ERCP) with sphincterotomy and stent insertion reduces the biliary ductal pressure, and shortens the time to resolution of the biloma. Laparoscopic insertion of a drain has been described for early management of grade III and IV liver injury, but not for the management of biloma. Hepatectomy and debridement are not indicated for this patient and is probably too radical an option at this time. Somatostatin use for this indication has not been shown to be effective.

**Answer: D**

Duane, T.M., Como, J.J., Bochicchio, G.V., *et al.* (2004) Reevaluating the management and outcomes of severe blunt liver injury. *Journal of Trauma*, **57**, 494–500.

Green, C.S., Bulger, E.M., and Kwan, S.W. (2015) Outcomes and complications of angioembolization for hepatic trauma: a systematic review of the literature. *Journal of Trauma and Acute Care Surgery*, **80** (3), 529–537.

Kozar, R.A., Moore, J.B., Niles, S.E., *et al.* (2005) Complications of non-operative management of high-grade blunt hepatic injuries. *Journal of Trauma*, **59**, 1066–1071.

6 *A 13-year-old girl suffered a grade V liver injury from a motor vehicle collision. Three weeks later she presents to the emergency department complaining of abdominal pain and hematemesis. Her vital signs are stable, and her abdominal exam is unremarkable. Upper endoscopy showed no obvious bleeding source. What would be the most appropriate next step in the management of this patient?*

A *Assure the mother of the patient that her symptoms will pass*

B *Prescribe H₂-blocker and ask her to see her primary physician the following day*

C *Obtain serial ultrasound examinations*

D *Laparotomy*

E *Angiography*

Fifty percent of high-grade (IV–V) blunt liver injuries may develop delayed complications such as those seen in this patient. This patient developed hemobilia: bleeding into the biliary tree from a hepatic pseudoaneurysm resulting in gastrointestinal bleeding. The clinical triad for hemobilia is jaundice, abdominal pain, and gastrointestinal bleeding. However, this triad is only seen 20% of the time. The patient's clinical history of hepatic injury and presentation of GI bleeding is enough to suspect hemobilia. The diagnosis and treatment option of choice is angiography and embolization. Prescribing of H₂ blockers will not treat the pseudoaneurysm that is causing the hemobilia. Ultrasound will not definitively diagnose the problem, and while it is not invasive, it will not treat the underlying problem. Because angiography can be curative and is relatively less invasive than surgery, the first approach should be angiography.

**Answer: E**

Carrillo, E.H., Spain, D.A., and Wohltmann, C.D. (1999) Interventional techniques are useful adjuncts in non-operative management of hepatic injuries. *Journal of Trauma*, **46**, 619–622.

Carrillo, E.H., Wohltmann, C., and Richardson, J.D. (2001) Evolution in the treatment of complex blunt liver injuries. *Current Problems in Surgery*, **38**, 1–60.

Schouten van der Velden, A.P., de Ruijter, W.M., Janssen, C.M., *et al.* (2010) Hemobilia as a late complication after blunt abdominal trauma: a case report and review of the literature. *Journal of Emergency Medicine*, **39** (5) 592–595.

7 *A 47-year-old patient was involved in a motorcycle collision. On arrival to the trauma bay, he was hypotensive with a positive FAST (focused assessment by sonography for trauma). He was emergently taken to the operating room for laparotomy. Intra-operatively he was found to have liver cirrhosis. Which of the following statements is not true concerning trauma patients with cirrhosis in comparison to those without cirrhosis?*

A *They have double the complication rate in comparison to noncirrhotic patients*

B *They have prolonged intensive care unit and hospital stay*

C *Their mortality is not affected by the presence of cirrhosis*

D *The mortality is higher in subset of cirrhotic patients who undergo abdominal surgery*

**E** *The presence of cirrhosis is a criterion for a trauma team activation*

Cirrhosis probably represents 1% of all trauma admission annually. The literature on cirrhosis and trauma is, however, limited. A study by Georgiou *et al.*, which represents the largest series, demonstrates mortality and morbidity rates are significantly increased (12% versus 6%, 10% versus 4%), respectively. Surviving cirrhotic patients have an increased intensive care unit and overall hospital length of stay when compared to noncirrhotic patients. A subset of patients who underwent abdominal surgery in this series has a 40% mortality rate, in comparison to 15% for noncirrhotic patients. The wide-ranging systemic abnormalities in physiology mean that a minor trauma can be significant; hence, a trauma patient who has a known history of cirrhosis is a criterion for a transfer to the trauma center with trauma team activation.

**Answer: C**

Georgiou, C., Inaba, K., Teixeira, P.G., *et al.* (2009) Cirrhosis and trauma are a lethal combination. *World Journal of Surgery*, **33** (5), 1087–1092.

Talving, P., Lustenberger, T., Okoye, O.T., *et al.* (2013) The impact of liver cirrhosis on outcomes in trauma patients: a prospective study. *Journal of Trauma and Acute Care Surgery*, **75** (4), 699–703.

Wahlstrom, K., Ney, A.L., Jacobson, S., *et al.* (2000) Trauma in cirrhotics: survival and hospital sequelae in patients requiring abdominal exploration. *American Surgery*, **66**, 1071–1076.

**8** *Concerning liver anatomy, which of the following statement is not true?*
  **A** *Morphologic anatomy: The liver is divided into two lobes divided by the falciform ligament*
  **B** *Functional anatomy: The liver is divided into segments based on the distribution of portal pedicles and hepatic veins*
  **C** *Right liver is divided anteromedially and posterolaterally by the plane drawn by the right hepatic vein*
  **D** *Left liver is divided into anterior and posterior by the plane drawn by the left hepatic vein*
  **E** *Quadrate lobe (segment IV) is a part of the left lobe*

To deal successfully with liver surgery, one must understand liver anatomy. Liver anatomy can be described by morphologic and functional anatomy. Morphologically, the liver is divided by a line drawn between the gallbladder and the inferior vena cava, giving rise to the anatomical right and left lobes. Functionally, the liver is divided based on hepatic veins and portal pedicles distribution, giving rise to the Couinaud's eight segments (Figure 39.2).

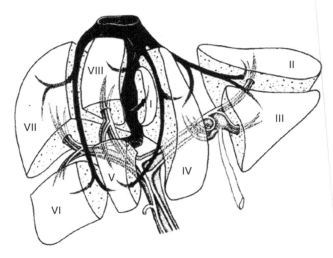

**Figure 39.2** Couinaud's eight segments of the liver. *Source:* Reproduced from Tsugawa, K., Koyanagi, N., Hashizume, M., *et al.* (2002) Anatomical resection for severe blunt liver trauma in 100 patients: significant differences between young and elderly. *World Journal of Surgery*, **26**, 544–549 with the kind permission of Spring Science and Business Media.

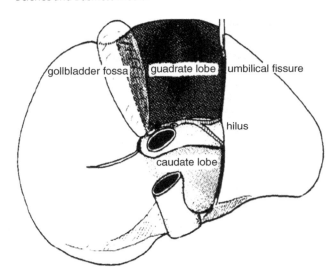

**Figure 39.3** *Source:* Reproduced from Bismuth, H. (1982) Surgical anatomy and anatomical surgery of the liver. *World Journal of Surgery*, **6**, 3–9 with the kind permission of Spring Science and Business Media.

The middle hepatic vein runs along the main fissure, which divides the liver into the right and left (not lobe, to prevent confusion with anatomical lobe). The right hepatic vein runs and divides the right liver into the anteromedial (segment V, VIII) and the posterolateral (segment VI, VII) segments. Similarly, the left hepatic vein runs and divides the left liver into anterior (segment IV, III) and posterior (II) segments. Quadrate lobe (segment IV) (Figure 39.3) is a part of the left lobe and lies to the right of the falciform ligament.

**Answer: A**

**Table 39.1** Classification of hepatic tumors.

| Benign | Malignant |
|---|---|
| Hepatic adenoma | Hepatocellular carcinoma |
| Focal nodular hyperplasia | Hepatic angiosarcoma |
| Hemangioma | Hepatic metastasis |
| | Hepatic cholangiocarcinoma |

**9** *Which of the following statement is not true regarding liver tumor?*

**A** *Hepatic adenoma is a benign tumor and often associated with women of child-bearing age who are taking oral contraceptives*

**B** *Focal nodular hyperplasia (FNH) is a malignant tumor that is characterized by central scarring*

**C** *Hepatic hemangioma is the most common hepatic benign tumor and characterized by early enhancement of the periphery*

**D** *Hepatic angiosarcoma is a rare malignant tumor seen in children*

**E** *Hepatocellular carcinoma is associated with history of viral or alcohol hepatitis, and elevated alpha-fetoprotein is diagnostic*

Distinguishing hepatic tumors as benign or malignant is important in liver management (see Table 39.1). History and radiographic findings will help guide the diagnosis and management. Hepatic adenoma is a benign tumor that is seen in women of childbearing age and who are taking oral contraceptives. They often present with abdominal pain because of their size. They require resection because of symptomatic pain, and they can degenerate into hepatocellular carcinoma. Focal nodular hyperplasia (FNH) is a benign tumor that is sometimes difficult to distinguish from hepatic adenoma, except for the radiographic characteristic of central scarring. They do not require resection. Hepatic hemangioma is the most common benign hepatic lesion. It has a CT scan characteristic of early enhancement of periphery. It may require resection when it is associated with large size and abdominal pain. Hepatic angiosarcoma is a rare malignant tumor seen primarily in children. It is highly vascular on CT scan and treatment is resection. Finally, hepatocellular carcinoma is a malignant tumor that is frequently seen in patient with hepatitis. It requires surgical resection, and an elevated alpha-fetoprotein is diagnostic.

**Answer: B**

Cameron, J.L. (2008) *Current Surgical Therapy*, 9th edn, Mosby, Philadelphia, PA.

Yun, E.J., Choi, B.I., Han, J.K., *et al.* (1999) Hepatic hemangioma: contrast-enhancement pattern during arterial and portal venous phases of spiral CT. *Abdominal Imaging*, **24**, 262–266.

**10** *Which of the following has not been shown to be a reliable criterion predicting increased mortality for a non-transplant surgery in a patient with cirrhosis?*

**A** *Age*

**B** *American Society of Anesthesiologists (ASA) physician status*

**C** *Emergency operation*

**D** *Model end-stage liver disease (MELD) score*

**E** *APACHE II score*

Cirrhosis of the liver is associated with increased morbidity and mortality when the patient must undergo an operation. Appreciating the risk factor may help clinicians make better decisions if the risk outweighs the benefit. Several studies have shown that increasing age, ASA class IV and V, emergency operation, and MELD score are reliable risk factors predicting peri-operative morbidity and mortality (Table 39.2). APACHE II score, although used for predicting prognosis of a broad range of critically ill patients, has not performed well in cirrhotic patients because of the lack the liver function components (bilirubin, albumin). The MELD score, calculated from serum creatinine, total serum bilirubin, and international normalized ratio (INR) for prothrombin time, dialysis requirement, and serum sodium has been found to be reliable not only just in the allocation of livers for transplantation, but also for risk assessment of non-transplant elective and emergency operation as well.

**Answer: E**

Kamath, P.S. and Kim, W.R. (2007) Advanced Liver Disease Study Group. The model for end-stage liver disease (MELD). *Hepatology*, **45**, 797–805.

Teh, S.H., Nagorney, D.M., Stevens, S.R., *et al.* (2007) Risk factors for mortality after surgery in patients with cirrhosis. *Gastroenterology*, **132**, 1261–1269.

**Table 39.2** MELD estimated three-month mortality.

| Age | Estimated three-month mortality (%) |
|---|---|
| 40 | 71.3 |
| 30–39 | 52.6 |
| 20–29 | 19.6 |
| 10–19 | 6.0 |
| 9 or less | 1.9 |

Ziser, A., Plevak, D.J., and Wiesner, R.H. (1999) Morbidity and mortality in cirrhotic patients undergoing anesthesia and surgery. *Anesthesiology*, **90**, 42–53.

**11** Which of the following statement is incorrect regarding splenic anatomy?

A It has three constant ligament attachments including splenogastric, splenorenal, and splenocolic ligament

B Splenorenal ligament contains the short gastric vessels that need to be ligated when performing the splenectomy

C When mobilizing colon splenic flexure, splenocolic ligament is responsible for the tear of splenic capsule

D The main blood supply derives from the splenic artery which is derived from the celiac artery

E The venous drainage is through the splenic vein which joins the superior mesenteric vein to become a portal vein

The spleen has three constant ligament attachments (splenogastric, splenorenal, and splenocolic) that must be divided when performing a splenectomy. There may often be additional ligament attachments including splenophrenic and splenoomental. Most ligament attachments are avascularized except the splenogastric, which contains the short gastric vessels. Splenocolic can sometimes be vascularized. The spleen derives dual blood supplies from the main splenic artery and the short gastric. The venous drainage follows the same arterial path.

**Answer: B**

Fraker, D.L. (2006) Splenic disorders, in *Greenfield's Surgery: Scientific Principles and Practice* (eds M.W. Mulholland, K.D. Lillemore, G.M. Doherty, *et al.*), Philadelphia, PA, Lippincott Williams & Wilkins, pp. 1220–1250.

**12** A 26-year-old man with autoimmune hemolytic anemia has failed medical therapy and requires a splenectomy. The most likely location for an accessory spleen would be the

A Greater omentum

B Splenic hilum

C Small bowel mesentery

D Tail of the pancreas

E Splenocolic ligament

The accessory spleen is a common anomaly, occurring in up to 20% of the population. However, it can occur in up to 30% of patients with a hematologic disorder. If splenectomy is indicated as a treatment for hemolytic anemia, then a thorough search for accessory spleens must be accomplished; otherwise, it can lead to a relapse. Approximately 80% of accessory spleens are located within the splenic hilum or its vascular pedicle. Other areas include the greater omentum, tail of the pancreas, splenocolic ligament, small bowel mesentery, and ovary.

**Answer: B**

Fraker, D.L. (2006) Splenic disorders, in *Greenfield's Surgery: Scientific Principles and Practice* (eds M.W. Mulholland, K.D. Lillemore, G.M. Doherty, *et al.*), Philadelphia, PA, Lippincott Williams & Wilkins, pp 1220–1250.

**13** A 23-year-old man diagnosed with idiopathic thrombocytopenic purpura (ITP) failed medical therapy and has a platelet count of 20 000/$mm^3$. He now requires a splenectomy. Which of the following best predicts that he will have a favorable response to a splenectomy?

A Time since diagnosis

B Response to glucocorticoids

C HIV status

D Age

E Preoperative platelet count

Idiopathic thrombocytopenic purpura (ITP) is an autoimmune disorder resulting in low platelets counts secondary to the development of IgG antiplatelets antibodies. In adults, it tends to affect more women than men. It is usually a diagnosis of exclusion after other causes have been ruled out. It can be associated with other chronic immune conditions such as HIV infection. Initial therapy consists of oral glucocorticoids. Intravenous immunoglobulin is usually reserved for refractory cases associated with bleeding. Splenectomy is indicated for the failure of medical management. Several preoperative indicators have been suggested for predicting a positive response to splenectomy, including short interval between diagnosis and operation, the initial response to glucocorticoid therapy, positive HIV status, high preoperative platelet count, and young age. Young age was the strongest predictor of a positive response.

**Answer: D**

Duperier, T., Brody, F., Feisher, J., *et al.* (2004) Predictive factors for successful laparoscopic splenectomy in patients with immune thrombocytopenic purpura. *Archives of Surgery*, **139**, 61–66.

Kojouri, K., Vesely, S.K., Terrell, D.R., *et al.* (2004) Splenectomy for adults patients with idiopathic thrombocytopenic purpura: a systemic review to assess long-term platelet count responses, prediction of response, and surgical complication. *Blood*, **104**, 2623–2634.

Patel, N.Y., Chilsen, A.M., Mathiason, M.A., *et al.* (2012) Outcomes and complications after splenectomy for hematologic disorders. *American Journal of Surgery*, **204**, 1014–1020.

**14** *A 17-year-old boy presents with several months of increasing left upper quadrant discomfort. Computed tomography (CT) demonstrates a large 7 cm splenic cyst. The single best treatment would be:*
A *Non-steroidal anti-inflammatory agents*
B *Percutaneous aspiration*
C *Angiographic embolization*
D *Partial splenectomy*
E *Total splenectomy*

Splenic cysts overall are uncommon. Approximately 75% of all splenic cysts are post-traumatic in nature and are truly pseudocysts. Primary cysts are generally classified as parasitic, congenital, and neoplastic, and the treatment is based on the type. Parasitic cysts (*Echinococcus*) are treated medically, followed by resection. Neoplastic cysts require splenectomy. Congenital or post-traumatic cysts can be observed if they are asymptomatic, however, if symptomatic, they should be treated with partial splenectomy. A partial splenectomy resulting in greater than 25% residual spleen is immunologically protective to the patient. Asymptomatic cysts over 5 cm in diameter should also be treated with partial splenectomy, primarily to rule out a neoplasm. The patient in this question is symptomatic and has a cyst greater than 5 cm.

**Answer: D**

Hansen, M.B. and Moller, A.C. (2004) Splenic cysts. *Surgical Laparoscopy Endoscopy & Percutaneous Techniques*, **14**, 316–322.

Ingle, S.B., Hinge, C.R., and Patrike, S. (2014) Epithelial cysts of the spleen: a mini review. *World Journal of Gastroenterology*, **20** (38) 13899–13903.

Morgenstern, L. (2002) Nonparasitic splenic cysts: pathogenesis, classification, and treatment. *Journal of the American College of Surgeons*, **194** (3), 306–314.

**15** *A 26-year-old woman presents with two weeks of increasing vague left upper quadrant abdominal pain. A computed tomography (CT) shows a 2.5 cm splenic aneurysm. Which of the following is true about this medical condition?*
A *This condition is best observed in this patient*
B *Artery embolization offers the most definitive treatment*

C *Surgical splenectomy should be considered in this patient as there is increasing risk of rupture*
D *This condition is more common in men than women*
E *The treatment is the same for a 45-year-old who lacks any symptoms*

Splenic artery aneurysm is very uncommon, but it is the third most frequent abdominal artery to undergo aneurismal changes (most common abdominal aneurysms: aortic and iliac). Women are 4:1 more likely to have splenic artery aneurysms. There is an increasing risk of rupture for this patient at this young childbearing age and surgical intervention is recommended. An aneurysm can be addressed by ligation, excision, or revascularization, and these options can be performed with or without splenectomy. The recommendation is not true in an elderly patient whose pathophysiology is related to atherosclerotic changes and, if the patient is asymptomatic, no surgical intervention is required. Endovascular intervention such as embolization or covered stent placement has been described but is not well proven and is generally reserved for patients unfit for surgical intervention.

**Answer: C**

Abdulrahman, A., Shabkah, A., Hassanain, M., and Aljiffry, M. (2014) Ruptured spontaneous artery aneurysm: a case report and review of the literature. *International Journal of Surgery Case Reports*, **5**, 754–757.

Lambert, C.J. and Williamson, J.W. (1990) Splenic artery aneurysm: a rare cause of upper gastrointestinal bleeding. *American Journal of Surgery*, **56**, 543–545.

**16** *A 34-year-old man was involved in a motorcycle accident. On arrival, his initial systolic blood pressure (SBP) was 80/50 mm Hg but subsequently improved to 120/65 mm Hg after 2 L of normal saline bolus. His Glasgow coma scale (GCS) was 13. He was taken to the computerized scan (CT). His head CT showed depressed skull fracture with a subdural hematoma. While being transported back to the trauma bay, he again became hypotensive with SBP 85/50 mm Hg. His abdominal CT scan is shown in Figure 39.4. What would be the most appropriate treatment for this patient?*
A *Administer 2 L of normal saline and continue to observe*
B *Administer 2 units of O- and continue to observe*
C *Arterial embolization by interventional radiologist*
D *Administer 2 units of O- and take the patient directly to surgery*
E *Type and cross and wait for radiologist report*

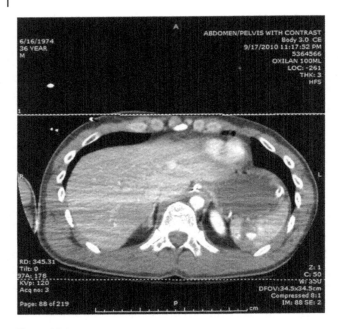

**Figure 39.4**

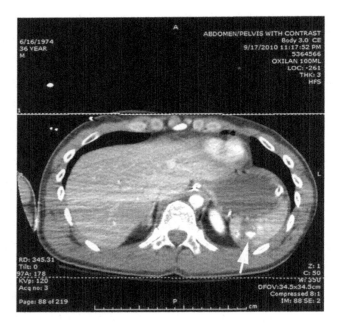

**Figure 39.5**

This patient has a blush (arrow) on the CT scan (Figure 39.5), which indicates active contrast extravasation. Although he has a transient response to fluid resuscitation, he should be taken emergently to surgery and two units of O– should be transfused. Any further delay may further compromise his traumatic brain injury. Contacting and mobilizing an interventional radiology team would take time and is usually not as expedient as the surgical approach. Although the patient's blood

pressure normalized, to prevent secondary traumatic brain injury from any future episodes of hypotension, rapid definitive treatment is wise. It does not put the patient at risk of hypotension and bleeding due to the splenic injury. If the patient did not have a concomitant head injury and the patient's blood pressure was hemodynamically normal, and the institution has rapid access to interventional radiology, then embolization may have been an alternative.

**Answer: D**

Haan, J.M., Bochicchio, G.V., Kramer, N., and Scalea, T.M. (2005) Nonoperative management of blunt splenic injury: a 5-year experience. *Journal of Trauma*, **58** (3), 492–498.

Thompson, B.E., Munera, F., Cohn, S.M., *et al.* (2006) Novel computed tomography scan scoring system predicts the need for intervention after splenic injury. *Journal of Trauma*, **60** (5), 1083–1086.

17 *Which of the following is true regarding angioembolization and splenic injury?*
   A *AAST splenic injury grading system has a high correlation with the success and failure of nonoperative management*
   B *Angioembolization does not alter the success rate of nonoperative management*
   C *Superselective distal embolization is associated with less splenic infarct, as compared to the proximal embolization*
   D *The presence of contrast extravasation followed by the absence of a blush on a delay or "washout" phase of the CT scan is indicative of pseudoaneurysm*
   E *Angioembolization has a success rate of 60%*

For blunt splenic injury, nonoperative management has a success rate of approximately 90% in the modern series. However, the AAST splenic injury grading system does not take into account the presence of splenic vascular injury, which manifests itself as a blush on a modern CT scan. As a result, there is a poor correlation between the grading system. The presence of a "blush" implies active extravasation or a post-traumatic pseudoaneurysm or arterio-venous malformation. However, unlike active hemorrhage, pseudoaneurysms or arteriovenous fistulas have a "wash-out" from the parenchyma and becomes isodense relative to normal parenchyma during the delay or "washout" phase. The addition of angioembolization in the management of blunt splenic injury has improved the success rate of non-operative management, especially in the group who are hemodynamically stable. Proximal embolization is associated with lower incidence of splenic infarct because of collateralization for the short gastric, and overall the success rate of angioembolization has improved to 73–100% in the most current series.

**Answer: D**

Gavant, M.L., Schurr, M., and Flick, P.A. (1997) Predicting clinical outcome of non-surgical management of blunt splenic injury: using CT to reveal abnormalities of splenic vasculature. *American Journal of Roentgenology*, **168**, 207–212.

Raikhlin, A., Baerlocher, M.O., Asch, M.R., and Myers, A. (2008) Imaging and transcatheter arterial embolization for traumatic splenic injuries: review of the literature. *Canadian Journal of Surgery*, **51** (6), 464–472.

18  *Which of the following is a contraindication to non-operative management of splenic trauma?*
   A  *Contrast extravasation*
   B  *Associated intra-abdominal injuries*
   C  *Abnormal hemodynamic status*
   D  *Patient is a Jehovah's Witness*
   E  *Subcapsular splenic hematoma*

An abnormal hemodynamic status that is unresponsive to resuscitation is an indication that this patient must go to the operating room. On the other hand, the presence of contrast extravasation may be amendable to angiographic embolization so as long as the patient remains hemodynamically within the normal range and there is ample time to mobilize an endovascular team. The presence of other associated intra-abdominal injuries is not contraindicated for a nonoperative management, but serial abdominal exam must be performed to exclude blunt hollow viscus injury. A Jehovah's Witness with splenic injury is not treated differently from other patients aside from transfusion of blood products.

**Answer: C**

Peitzman, A.B., Harbrecht, B.G., Rivera, L., *et al.* (2005) Failure of observation of blunt splenic injury in adults: variability in practice and adverse consequences. *Journal of the American College of Surgeons*, **201**, 179–187.

Peitzman, A.B., Heil, B., Rivera, L., *et al.* (2000) Blunt splenic injury in adults: multi-institutional study of the Eastern Association for the Surgery of Trauma. *Journal of Trauma*, **49**, 177–187.

19  *Splenectomy is not the recommended treatment option in which of the following diseases?*
   A  *Immune (idiopathic) thrombocytopenic purpura (ITP)*
   B  *Thrombotic thrombocytopenic purpura (TTP)*
   C  *Felty's syndrome*
   D  *B-Thalassemia*
   E  *Spherocytosis*

Immune (idiopathic) thrombocytopenic purpura (ITP) is a diagnosis of exclusion. HIV, pregnancy, drugs, and systemic lupus erythematosus can produce similar syndromes. Platelets are normally produced. Primary treatment is glucocorticoid or gamma globulin. However, if medical therapy fails, splenectomy is performed.

Thrombotic thrombocytopenic purpura (TTP) classically presents with thrombocytopenia, fever, hemolytic anemia, renal disease, and central nervous system dysfunction, and is quite similar to hemolytic uremic syndrome. Plasmapheresis is the treatment of choice.

Felty's syndrome is the clinical triad of thrombocytopenia, cutaneous leg ulcers, and rheumatoid arthritis. The syndrome is not well understood, but sometimes patients will benefit from splenectomy if medical therapy fails.

Both B-thalassemia and spherocytosis are genetic disorders that result in abnormal red blood cells. Splenectomy can provide the treatment of choice if medical therapy fails.

**Answer: B**

Swain, J.M. and Schlinkert, R.T. (2004) Thrombocytopenia and other hematologic disorders, in *Mayo Clinic Gastrointestinal Surgery* (eds K.A. Kelly, M.G. Sarr, and R.A. Hinder), W.B. Saunders, Philadelphia, PA, pp. 365–374.

20  *Which of the following statement is not true about overwhelming postsplenectomy infection (OPSI)?*
   A  *The risk occurs within the first two to three years after the splenectomy*
   B  *Pneumococcal infection is the most common cause of OPSI*
   C  *It is more common after splenectomy for the underlying hematological diseases*
   D  *The vaccination is targeted against encapsulated organisms such as pneumococcus, H. Influenza, and N. meningococcus*
   E  *Hyposplenic diseases like sickle cell disease, celiac disease, and dermatitis herpetiformis can result in impaired immunity just like post-splenectomy*

In the early 1950s, it was noticed that neonates with hematological disease who required splenectomy had a very high subsequent risk of serious infection. However, the actual incidence is not known. Initially it was believed that it only occurred within the first two to three years but, as shown in a study by Waghorn and Mayon-White, it could occur from as early as 24 days to as late as 59 years after splenectomy, and it can affect patients of any age, from 18 months old to 85 years old. It is more common in hematological patients, probably because of their underlying suppressed immunity. Currently, vaccination against encapsulated bacteria *Pneumococcus, H. influenzae, N. meningococcus*, as well as viral influenza, is given, usually before the patient is being discharged from the hospital. The most common cause of OPSI is pneumococcal infection. Several medical conditions including sickle disease, celiac disease, and dermatitis herpetiformis behave like an asplenic condition; hence, the clinician must beware of the same risk.

**Answer: A**

Theilacker, C., Ludewig, K., Serr, A., *et al.* (2016) Overwhelming post-splenectomy infection: a prospective multicenter cohort study. *Clinical Infectious Diseases*, **62** (7), 871–878.

Waghorn, D.J. and Mayon-White, R.T. (1997) A study of 42 episodes of overwhelming post-splenectomy infection: is current guidance for asplenic individuals being followed? *Journal of Infection*, **35**, 289–294.

Wisner, D.H. (2004) Injury to the spleen, in *Trauma*, 5th edn (eds E.E. Moore, D.V. Feliciano, and K.L. Mattox), McGraw-Hill, New York, p. 681.

# 40

## Incarcerated Hernias

*Cathy Ho, MD and Narong Kulvatunyou, MD*

**1** *A 34-year-old man presents to the emergency department with acute onset of right groin pain, nausea, and vomiting. The symptoms occurred after he tried to lift a heavy box. Physical examination shows abdominal distension and a right groin mass that is tender to palpation. What is the most appropriate management for this patient?*
A *Prescribe ibuprofen for pain and ask him to see his primary physician the following day*
B *Attempt to reduce the hernia and then discharge home*
C *Premedicate the patient, attempt to reduce the hernia, and then instruct him to never lift heavy boxes*
D *Premedicate the patient, attempt to reduce the hernia and then scheduled for an elective hernia repair*
E *Surgical evaluation for an emergency repair*

There is no consensus whether one should ever attempt to reduce a hernia. However, if there are signs and symptoms suggesting intestinal obstruction, it would be unsafe to discharge the patient. A hernia can be repaired in many different ways as well as at different times, but the main focus should be possible incarceration and bowel obstruction. He has an increased risk of recurrence with possible strangulation and its associated morbidity.

**Answer: E**

Akinci, M., Ergul, Z., Kulah, B., *et al.* (2010) Risk factors related with unfavorable outcomes in groin repairs. *Hernia*, **14**, 489–493.

Harissis, H.V., Douitsis, E., and Fatouros, M. (2009) Incarcerated hernia: to reduce or not to reduce. *Hernia*, **13**, 263–266.

Kulah, B., Kulacoglu, I.H., Oruc, M.T., *et al.* (2001) Presentation and outcome of incarcerated external hernias in adults. *American Journal of Surgery*, **181** (2), 101–104.

**2** *A 62-year-old woman presents to the emergency department with acute onset of umbilical pain. She has nausea but no vomiting. Examination of the umbilicus shows the overlying skin to have reddish discoloration, and it is associated with tenderness to palpation. The most appropriate management is:*
A *Prescribe pain medication and then discharge*
B *Prescribe antibiotic and then discharge*
C *Obtain ultrasound to rule out urachal cyst*
D *Obtain CT-guided biopsy since this is probably a Sister Mary Joseph node*
E *Surgical repair*

Because of the sudden onset of periumbilical pain in association with discoloration of skin and tenderness, the differential diagnosis of skin cellulitis, infected urachal cyst, or other benign conditions are unlikely. Reduction of incarceration and repair of the umbilical hernia should be considered immediately.

**Answer: E**

Kulah, B., Kulacoglu, I.H., Oruc, M.T., *et al.* (2001) Presentation and outcome of incarcerated external hernias in adults. *American Journal of Surgery*, **181** (2), 101–104.

Tufaro, A.P. and Campbell, A.K. (2008) Incisional, epigastric, and umbilical hernias, in *Current Surgical Therapy*, 9th edn (ed. J.L. Cameron), Mosby, Philadelphia, PA, pp. 573–576.

*Surgical Critical Care and Emergency Surgery: Clinical Questions and Answers*, Second Edition.
Edited by Forrest "Dell" Moore, Peter Rhee, and Gerard J. Fulda.
© 2018 John Wiley & Sons Ltd. Published 2018 by John Wiley & Sons Ltd.
Companion website: www.wiley.com/go/moore/surgical_criticalcare_and_emergency_surgery

**3** *Three borders that define the femoral ring (hernia) are:*
  **A** *Inferior epigastric vessels, inguinal ligament, conjoined tendon*
  **B** *Inferior epigastric vessels, inguinal ligament, spermatic cord*
  **C** *Inferior epigastric vessels, inguinal ligament, femoral vessels*
  **D** *Lacunar ligament, inguinal ligament, femoral vessels*
  **E** *Conjoined tendon, inguinal ligament, femoral vessels*

A femoral hernia is bordered superiorly by the inguinal ligament, laterally by a femoral vein, and medially by the lacunar ligament. The lacunar ligament is a crescent ligament made of a reflection of the external oblique aponeurosis that connects the inguinal (Poupart's) ligament to the pectineal (Cooper's) ligament. Understanding this anatomy is important for the repair and to prevent recurrence. The repair may be performed by suturing the conjoined tendon to the Cooper ligament (McVay repair), by using the mesh plug technique, or by open versus laparoscopic pre-peritoneal repair technique.

The inferior epigastric vessel, conjoined tendon, and inguinal ligament define the border that represents a direct hernia.

**Answer: D**

Alimoglu, O., Okan, K.I., Dasiran, F., *et al.* (2006) Femoral hernia: a review of 83 cases. *Hernia*, **10**, 70–73.
Sandblom, G., Haapaniemi, S., and Nilsson, E. (1999) Femoral hernias: a register analysis of 588 repairs. *Hernia*, **3**, 131–134.

**4** *In contrast to an inguinal hernia, a femoral hernia:*
  **A** *Is often associated with an elective operation*
  **B** *Is more common in men*
  **C** *Is often associated with intestinal resection*
  **D** *Age is not the risk factor associated with increased morbidity*
  **E** *Clinical presentation is always obvious*

Dahlstand *et al.* studied 3980 femoral hernias from the national Swedish Hernia Registry and found that femoral hernias, in comparison to inguinal hernias, are more commonly associated with an emergency operation (36% versus 5%), and a bowel resection (23% versus 5%). In both the Dahlstand *et al.* and Alimoglu *et al.* series, femoral hernias are more common in women (60–70%). Femoral hernias often present as a mass below the inguinal ligament, which can be confused with a lymph node, lipoma, and so on. Increasing age is a risk factor for perioperative morbidity and mortality for both femoral and inguinal hernias, particularly under an emergency operation.

**Answer: C**

Alimoglu, O., Okan, K.I., Dasiran, F., *et al.* (2006) Femoral hernia: a review of 83 cases. *Hernia*, **10**, 70–73.
Dahlstand, U., Wollert, S., Nordin, P., *et al.* (2009) Emergency femoral hernia repair: a study based on a national register. *Annals of Surgery*, **249**, 672–676.

**5** *A 50-year-old man with advanced hepatitis C cirrhosis with Child–Turcotte–Pugh class C and a model of end-stage liver disease (MELD) score of 15 presents to the emergency department complaining of fluid leaking from his umbilicus. Examination shows an umbilical hernia with skin excoriation and fluid leakage but no evidence of infection. His abdominal exam is benign. Which is incorrect regarding the management of this patient?*
  **A** *He should not undergo operative repair due to his high perioperative risk*
  **B** *He should undergo operative repair with a preoperative transjugular intrahepatic portosystemic shunt (TIPS) placement*
  **C** *Intraoperative drain does not prevent wound complication*
  **D** *He should be evaluated for a possible liver transplant*
  **E** *His postoperative complication includes worsening encephalopathy*

Operative repair should be considered; however, the definitive guideline for the management of this condition is lacking. Regardless, it has an associated high short-term and long-term mortality. Several experts suggest a preoperative TIPS to help control the ascites and minimize the wound complication. However, there is a lack of level-1 evidence. Several authors also recommend leaving a drain, but then again there is no level-1 evidence to support or reject this approach. Worsening encephalopathy, wound complications, and liver decompensation are among the usual postoperative complications. As a result, this patient should be considered for a possible liver transplant.

**Answer: A**

Belghiti, J. and Durand, F. (1997) Abdominal wall hernia in the setting of cirrhosis. *Seminars in Liver Disease*, **17**, 219–226.
Coelho, J.C., Claus, C.M., Campos, A.C., *et al.* (2016) Umbilical hernia in patients with liver cirrhosis: a

surgical challenge. *World Journal of Gastrointestinal Surgery*, **8** (7), 476–482.

Telem, D.A., Schiano, T., and Divino, C.M. (2010) Complicated hernia presentation in patients with advanced cirrhosis and refractory ascites: management and outcome. *Surgery*, **148** (3), 538–543.

**6** *Which of the following is not considered a principle for the repair of an incisional hernia?*
   **A** *Patient optimization by improving nutrition and ceasing smoking*
   **B** *Wound preparation by reducing the wound bioburden*
   **C** *Midline wound reapproximation if possible using a component separation*
   **D** *Immediate reconstruction should always be considered*
   **E** *Use of appropriate reinforcement material in a patient at increased risk of recurrence*

The Ventral Hernia Working Group (VHWG) convened in September 2008 to develop principles and guidelines for the management of ventral hernias, using an evidence-based approach. These guidelines include: optimizing the patient's condition by improving nutrition and smoking cessation, wound preparation by reduction of wound bioburden, fascial midline reapproximation with or without component separation, and usage of appropriate reinforcement material in high-risk ventral hernia repair. Reduction of bioburden means excision of all devitalized or infected tissue. If it cannot be done in one stage, immediate reconstruction should be delayed.

**Answer: D**

Breuing, K., Butler, C.E., Ferzoco, S., *et al.* (2010) Incisional ventral hernias: review of the literature and recommendations regarding the grading and technique of repair. *Surgery*, **148**, 544–558.

**7** *Which of the following regarding component separation is not true?*
   **A** *Requires incision and release of the posterior rectus sheath as well as the lateral external oblique release*
   **B** *Lateral skin and subcutaneous tissue mobilization is always required*
   **C** *Achieving midline approximation is the goal*
   **D** *It is often associated with an increased incidence of skin and fat necrosis*
   **E** *To minimize hernia recurrence at the epigastrium, the rectus muscle should be mobilized above the costal margin*

Ramirez *et al.* first described the component separation in 1990 and it consisted of the posterior rectal sheath

release and the lateral external oblique release. To perform the external oblique release, one often has to mobilize the skin and subcutaneous tissue laterally. This maneuver often leads to a disruption of the blood supply to skin and fat, which results in an increased postoperative wound complication.

Several modifications to preserve the "peri-umbilical perforators" includes a bilateral inguinal approach with subfascial dissection. This maneuver allows the avoidance of excessive lateral mobilization of the skin and subcutaneous tissue and hence minimizes the disruption of the blood supply and postoperative wound complications

**Answer: B**

Clarke, J.M. (2010) Incisional hernia repair by fascial component separation: results in 128 cases and evolution of technique. *American Journal of Surgery*, **200**, 2–8.

Ramirez, O.M., Ruas, E., and Dellon, A.L. (1990) Component separation method for closure of abdominal wall defects: an anatomic and clinical study. *Plastic and Reconstructive Surgery*, **86**, 519–526.

**8** *Which of the following is not true regarding a parastomal hernia?*
   **A** *A higher incidence is associated with loop colostomy compared to end-colostomy*
   **B** *Repair includes relocation, aponeurotic repair, or repair with prosthetic mesh*
   **C** *Incidence may be as high as 50%*
   **D** *A new large pore light weight mesh with decreasing polypropylene content has shown promise in decreasing the incidence of a para-colostomy hernia in a recent randomized trial*
   **E** *A "sublay" or retro-muscular technique has been proposed to decrease the incidence of intestinal obstruction*

A para-colostomy hernia is a complicated issue with which an acute care surgeon may have to deal. The incidence can be as high as 50% and is higher with an end-colostomy. Just as with the risk of development of an incisional hernia, the incidence of developing a parastomal hernia is associated with obesity, smoking, and diabetes. Several recent randomized studies have suggested utilization of a new lightweight large pore with decrease polypropylene content prosthetic mesh in a "sublay" position (between the peritoneum and posterior fascia) may help decrease the incidence of a para-colostomy hernia.

**Answer: A**

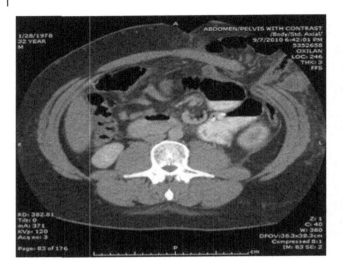

**Figure 40.1**

Glascow, S.C. (2016) Parastomal hernia: avoidance and treatment in the 21st century. *Clinics in Colon and Rectal Surgery*, **29**, 277–284

Reinhard, K., Klinge, U., and Schumpelick, V. (2000) The repair of large parastomal hernias using a midline approach and a prosthetic mesh in the sublay position. *American Journal of Surgery*, **179**, 186–188.

Serra-Aracil, X., Moreno-Matias, J., Darnell, A., *et al.* (2009) Randomized, controlled, prospective trial of the use of a mesh to prevent parastomal hernia. *Annals of Surgery*, **249**, 583–587.

**9** *A 32-year-old man underwent multiple small bowel resections with primary anastomoses and a left colectomy with an end-colostomy after a gunshot wound to the abdomen. He had been doing relatively well until postoperative day 17 when he develops abdominal pain, nausea, and vomiting. His colostomy is not producing stool. He is afebrile, and his abdominal exam shows distension and fullness around the colostomy. Computed tomography (CT) scan of the abdomen is obtained and is shown In Figure 40.1. What is the diagnosis?*

**A** *Intra-abdominal abscess*

**B** *Small bowel obstruction secondary to adhesion*

**C** *Small bowel obstruction secondary to a para-colostomy hernia*

**D** *Large bowel obstruction secondary to a mal functioning colostomy*

**E** *CT scan showed no abnormality*

This patient developed clinical signs and symptoms of a postoperative small-bowel obstruction. The CT showed distended small-bowel loops (Figure 40.2, arrow) and an incarcerated para-colostomy hernia (arrow head).

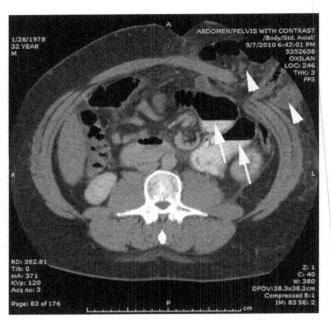

**Figure 40.2**

Clinical exam of fullness around the colostomy and this CT finding should prompt reexploration and repair of a para-colostomy hernia. Intraoperative findings showed 20 cm of incarcerated para-colostomy hernia with a proximal small-bowel obstruction. An early parastomal hernia, especially with incarceration, as in this case, is quite unusual. A technical error from the initial operation resulted in an excessively large stoma that allowed the small bowel to herniate through. A large-bowel obstruction is unlikely as the CT showed a normal colon. Small-bowel obstruction secondary to adhesion is also unlikely considering that patient has been doing relatively well and acutely developed a small bowel obstruction picture. The CT scan did not show an obvious fluid collection, so intra-abdominal abscess is also unlikely.

**Answer: C**

Serra-Aracil, X., Moreno-Matias, J., Darnell, A., *et al.* (2009) Randomized, controlled, prospective trial of the use of a mesh to prevent parastomal hernia. *Annals of Surgery*, **249**, 583–587.

Tam, K.W., Wei, P.L., Kuo, L.J., and Wu, C.H. (2010) Systemic review of the use of a mesh to prevent parastomal hernia. *World Journal of Surgery*, **34**, 2723–2729.

**10** *A 69-year-old man with a history of COPD presents with a 24-hour history of abdominal distension and emesis. Physical examination reveals abdominal distension with hypoactive bowel sounds and a* *tender mass in the left groin below the inguinal ligament. During groin exploration, an incarcerated femoral hernia is found. The bowel is not viable and required resection. The preferred repair of the hernia would be*

**A** *Bassini repair*

**B** *Lichenstein repair*

**C** *Shouldice repair*

**D** *Cooper's ligament repair*

**E** *Mesh plug in femoral canal*

A Bassini repair involves reconstruction of the floor by suturing the transversalis fascia, the transverses abdominis, and the internal oblique muscle to the inguinal ligament. The Shouldice, which used to be the standard repair, is similar but is done in multiple layers. Both are tension repairs. The Lichenstein repair uses mesh and is considered a tension-free repair, which is viewed as a gold standard. These repairs, however, do not address the femoral canal defect.

The mesh-plug technique was developed by Gilbert and then modified by Rutkow and Robbins, Milikan, and others. The technique involves placing a piece of mesh into the defect of the internal ring for an indirect hernia, the neck of the defect for a direct hernia, or into the femoral canal in a femoral hernia and secured in place with stitches. However, it is not recommended in this case because of the contamination and a possible mesh infection.

A Cooper's ligament repair (McVay repair) addresses the femoral canal defect by suturing Cooper's ligament to the conjoined tendon.

**Answer: D**

Deveney, K.E. (2006) Hernias and other lesions of abdominal wall, in *Current Surgical Diagnosis and Treatment*, 12th edn (ed. G.M. Doherty), New York, McGraw-Hill, pp. 765–778.

# 41

# Necrotizing Soft Tissue Infections and Other Soft Tissue Infections

*Jacob Swann, MD and LTC Joseph J. DuBose, MD*

1 *Which of the following signs or symptoms of necrotizing soft tissue infection (NSTI) are present in the vast majority of patients?*
   A *Bullae*
   B *Crepitus*
   C *Gas on radiograph*
   D *Skin necrosis*
   E *None of the above*

Proposed "hard signs" of necrotizing soft tissue infection include bullae, crepitus, gas in the tissues on radiographic imaging, hypotension with systolic blood pressure less than 90 mm Hg, or skin necrosis (Figure 41.1). The presence of these signs or symptoms certainly aids a rapid diagnosis of this infectious process. However, hard signs of NSTI are often absent on presentation with studies documenting that less than 50% of patients who have had definitive diagnosis of NSTI established actually presented with hard signs of these infections.

**Answer: E**

Hussein, Q.A. and Anaya, D.A. (2013) Necrotizing soft-tissue infections. *Critical Care Clinics*, **29**, 795–806.

2 *Which statement is most true of complicated skin and soft tissue infections (cSSTIs):*
   A *They are associated with very low risk for life- or limb-threatening infection*
   B *They can best be treated by surgical incision alone*
   C *They can be treated on an outpatient basis with careful follow-up*
   D *They require initial empiric antimicrobial therapy with coverage for MRSA*
   E *They are rarely associated with comorbid conditions*

As opposed to uncomplicated SSTIs—such as simple abscesses, cellulitis, or furuncles—which are associated with low risk for life- or limb-threatening infection, complicated SSTIs include infections of the deep soft tissue requiring significant surgical intervention, infected ulcers, infected burns, and major abscesses. Patients with complicated SSTIs require hospitalization for treatment and commonly have significant underlying disease conditions that complicate response to treatment. Early initial empiric antibiotic coverage for these patients should include coverage for MRSA.

**Answer: D**

Lipsky, B.J., Moran, G.J., Napolitano, L.M., *et al.* (2012) A prospective, multicenter, observational study of complicated skin and soft tissue infections in hospitalized patients: clinical characteristics, medical treatment, and outcomes. *BioMed Central Infectious Diseases*, **12** (227), 1–11.

3 *The most definitive method available to accurately diagnose the presence of necrotizing soft-tissue infection (NSTI) is:*
   A *Erythema and pain*
   B *Magnetic resonance imaging*
   C *The presence of an elevated white blood cell count and hyponatremia*
   D *Surgical exploration*
   E *Hyponatremia in the setting of fever and an elevated white blood cell count*

Erythema and pain may be present but are not specific to necrotizing infections. MRI may demonstrate soft-tissue edema or fluid, but these findings do not prove the presence of NSTI and may also occur in any condition causing edema. The presence of an elevated WBC and hyponatremia, even in the setting of fever, are not specific to NSTI. The definitive diagnosis requires surgical incision carried down to the fascia and muscle (Figure 41.2).

**Answer: D**

*Surgical Critical Care and Emergency Surgery: Clinical Questions and Answers*, Second Edition.
Edited by Forrest "Dell" Moore, Peter Rhee, and Gerard J. Fulda.
© 2018 John Wiley & Sons Ltd. Published 2018 by John Wiley & Sons Ltd.
Companion website: www.wiley.com/go/moore/surgical_criticalcare_and_emergency_surgery

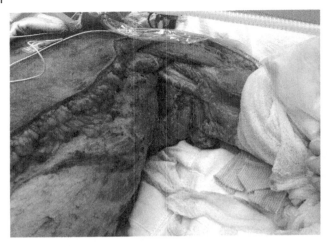

**Figure 41.1** Trunk and extremity necrotizing soft-tissue infection. Head at top of photo, left arm to right of photo.

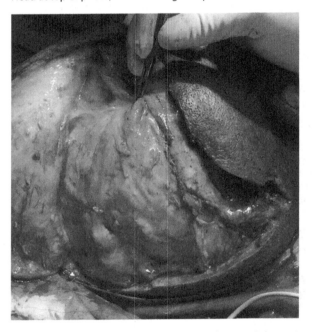

**Figure 41.2** Scalp necrotizing soft-tissue infection; right ear is to the right, face anteriorly.

Hakkarainen, T.W., Kopari, N.M., Pham, T.N., *et al.* (2014) Necrotizing soft tissue infections: review and current concepts in treatment, systems of care, and outcomes. **51** (8), 344–362.

4   *What factor has been identified as an independent predictor of both treatment failure and hospital mortality among MRSA soft-tissue infections?*
   A *Type I diabetes mellitus*
   B *Failure to initiate early and appropriate antibiotics*
   C *Delay of initial surgical intervention*
   D *Patient age*
   E *None of the above*

Appropriate and timely antibiotic therapy improves treatment outcomes for SSTIs caused by MRSA. Studies have demonstrated that initiation of therapy within 48 hours improves treatment outcomes and failure to initiate antimicrobial therapy within 48 hours of presentation is an independent predictor of treatment failure. Additionally, among patients admitted to the hospital for MRSA sterile-site infections, it has been shown that inappropriate antibiotics are an independent risk factor for hospital mortality.

All of the other factors—diabetes, delay in surgical intervention, and patient age—are likely to be contributory, but these have not been identified as independent predictors of treatment failure and hospital mortality.

**Answer: B**

Ostermann, H., Blasi, F., Medina, J., *et al.* (2014) Resource use in patients hospitalized with complicated skin and soft tissue infection in Europe and analysis of vulnerable groups: the REACH study. *Journal of Medical Economics*, **17** (10), 719–729.

5   *Which antibiotic choice is least appropriate for patients with complicated severe skin and soft-tissue infections (cSSTIs) and evidence of toxic shock syndrome?*
   A *Vancomycin*
   B *Linezolid*
   C *Clindamycin*
   D *Amoxicillin*
   E *Daptomycin*

The selection of antimicrobials to treat cSSTIs should include those that inhibit toxin production, particularly among patients with evidence of toxic shock syndrome. Toxic shock syndrome is commonly present in patients with streptococcal and staphylococcal infections. Beta-lactams, such as amoxicillin, may actually enhance the toxin production of some classes of secreted staphylococcal peptides and should be avoided. In contrast, clindamycin and linozelid have the ability to inhibit toxin production by suppressing translation of toxin genes for *S. aureus* and by directly inhibiting synthesis of group A streptococcal toxins. Vancomycin and daptomycin are other appropriate choices for utilization, but they do not have the same demonstrated ability to inhibit toxin production.

**Answer: D**

Ramakrishnan, K., Salinas, R.C., Agudelo Higuita, N.I. (2015) Skin and soft tissue infections. *American Family Physician*, **92** (6), 474–483.

Stevens, D.L., May, Y., Salmi, D.B., *et al.* (2007) Impact of antibiotics on expression of virulence-associated exotoxin genes in methicillin-sensitive and methicillin-resistant Staphylococcus aureus. *Journal of Infectious Diseases*, **195**, 202–211.

**6**  *What laboratory values have been identified as risk indicators for necrotizing fascitis?*
  **A**  *Total white blood cell count*
  **B**  *Hemoglobin*
  **C**  *Glucose*
  **D**  *Sodium*
  **E**  *All of the above*

The laboratory risk indicator for necrotizing fasciitis (LRINEC) score was initially developed in a retrospective observational study of 145 patients with necrotizing fasciitis and 309 patients with cellulitis (see Table 41.1). This score uses C-reactive protein, total white blood cell count, hemoglobin, sodium, creatinine, and glucose levels. In the initial study, a score of ≥6 had a positive predictive value of 92% for the detection of necrotizing

**Table 41.1** The Laboratory Risk Indicator for Necrotizing Fascitis (LRINEC) score.

| Variable, Units | Score |
| --- | --- |
| **C-reactive protein, mg/L** | |
| <150 | 0 |
| ≥150 | 4 |
| **Total white cell count, cells per mm$^3$** | |
| <15 | 0 |
| 15–25 | 1 |
| >25 | 2 |
| **Hemoglobin, g/dL** | |
| >13.5 | 0 |
| 11–13.5 | 1 |
| <11 | 2 |
| **Sodium, mmol/L** | |
| ≥135 | 0 |
| <135 | 2 |
| **Creatinine mg/dL** | |
| ≤1.6 | 0 |
| >1.6 | 2 |
| **Glucose, mg/dL** | |
| ≤180 | 0 |
| >180 | 1 |

The maximum score is 13; a score of ≥6 should raise suspicion of necrotizing fascitis, and a score of ≥8 is strongly predictive of this disease.

fascitis. Several subsequent cohort studies have validated the utility of the LRINEC in diagnosing necrotizing soft-tissue infections.

**Answer: E**

Borschitz, T., Schlicht, S., Siegel, E., *et al.* (2015) Improvement of a clinical score for necrotizing fasciitis: "pain out of proportion" and high CRP levels aid the diagnosis. *PLoS One*, **10** (7), e0132775.
Wong, C.H., Khin, L.W., Heng, K.S., *et al.* (2004) The LRINEC (Laboratory Risk Indicator for Necrotizing Fasciitis) score: A tool for distinguishing necrotizing fasciitis from other soft tissue infections. *Critical Care Medicine*, **32** (7), 1535–1541.

**7**  *The most common identifiable cause of severe soft-tissue infections is:*
  **A**  *Clostridial infections*
  **B**  *Methicillin-resistant Staphylococcus aureus infections*
  **C**  *Methicillin-sensitive Staphylococcus aureus infections*
  **D**  *Acinetobacter infections*
  **E**  *Streptococcal infections*

In a recent prospective multicenter US study, MRSA was the most common identifiable cause of SSTI. *S. aureus* was isolated from 76% of patients who had SSTIs. The prevalence of MRSA was 59% overall and ranged from 15% to 74% by ED. The spectrum of skin infections caused by community acquired MRSA is wide and can range from simple cutaneous abscesses to large abscesses and more severe forms of soft-tissue infections.

**Answer: B**

Espositi, S., Noviello, and S., Leone, S. (2016) Epidemiology and microbiology of skin and soft tissue infections. *Current Opinion in Infectious Diseases*, **29** (2), 109–115.

**8**  *The most common cause of necrotizing fascitis and myonecrosis is:*
  **A**  *Group A Streptococcus*
  **B**  *Clostridium perfringens*
  **C**  *Polymicrobial infection*
  **D**  *Methicillin sensitive Staphylococcus aureus*
  **E**  *Fungal infections*

Necrotizing fasciitis and myonecrosis are *most* commonly caused by aerobic and anaerobic organisms as part of a polymicrobial infection that may include *Staphylococcus aureus*. Other common causes include group A Streptococcus and *Clostridium perfringens*. The most predominant organisms isolated in case series have been community-acquired MRSA, accounting for one-third of isolates from a recent retrospective review.

Necrotizing STIs are commonly categorized into three specific types based upon the microbiologic etiology of the infection: Type 1, or polymicrobial; Type 2, or group A streptoccal; and Type 3, gas gangrene, or clostridial myonecrosis.

**Answer: C**

Endorf, W.F., Cancio, L.C., and Klein, M.B. (2009) Necrotizing soft-tissue infections: clinical guidelines. *Journal of Burn Care and Research*, **30** (5), 769–775.

**9** *Vibrio infections are uncommon but potentially serious causes of necrotizing soft-tissue infections that should be particularly suspected among patients with:*
   **A** *History of simple soft tissue community acquired MRSA infections*
   **B** *History of exposure to sea water or shellfish*
   **C** *History of dog bite*
   **D** *History of a recent wooden splinter*
   **E** *None of the above*

Vibrio and Aeromonas species are uncommon causes of NSTIs. Vibrio species thrive in aquatic environments, particularly sea water and in shellfish. Aeromonas species are also rare causes of NSTIs that are associated with contact with fresh or brackish water, soil, or wood. The contact history and rapid onset of SSTIs can alert providers to infections from these organisms. At least 64 different species of bacteria can be present in dog saliva; thus, infections from canine bites are most likely polymicrobial. Infections associated with splinters are, likewise, most commonly polymicrobial.

**Answer: B**

Horseman, M.A. and Surani, S. (2011) A comprehensive review of *Vibrio vulnificus*: an important cause of severe sepsis and skin and soft-tissue infection. *International Journal of Infectious Diseases*, **15** (3), e157–e166.

**10** *Which of the following is true about the use of negative-pressure wound therapy (NPWT) devices in the setting of necrotizing soft tissue infections?*
   **A** *NPWT use negates the need for adequate debridement of dead tissues*
   **B** *NPWT use has been validated by prospective randomized trials*
   **C** *NPWT use decreases mobility post-operatively*
   **D** *NPWT use has been associated with decreased time to wound closure*
   **E** *NPWT therapy is associated with increased patient discomfort*

Several reports have documented the utility of NPWT for managing patients who have acute NSTIs. NPWT has been associated with reduced time for wound care, improved patient comfort, greater mobility, reduced drainage, and decreased time to wound closure compared to traditional wet-to-dry dressings. Although no prospective randomized trials have yet been conducted to compare NPWT to traditional techniques, it can be considered, particularly for larger wounds and those patients requiring liberal use of conscious sedation and general anesthesia for wound care. The use of VAC has not been validated in prospective randomized trials to date.

**Answer: D**

Chennamsetty, A., Khourdaji, I., Burks, F., *et al.* (2015) Contemporary diagnosis and management of Fournier's gangrene. *Therapeautic Advances in Urology*, **7** (4), 203–215.

**11** *The potential benefit of intravenous immunoglobulin (IVIG) therapy for treating NSTIs is related to*
   **A** *Improve glucose control in acute illness*
   **B** *Bacterocidal activity*
   **C** *Increased IL-1 production*
   **D** *Improved tolerance of sepsis-related hypotension*
   **E** *Binding of Gram-positive organism exotoxins*

While the use of IVIG for treatment of NSTIs remains controversial, the potential benefit of this intervention is related to the binding of Gram-positive organism exotoxins. The clinical studies that have been completed are not randomized, blinded trials; however, some show evidence of improved outcomes with IVIG treatment. The treatment should be restricted, however, to critically ill patients who have either staphylococcal or streptococcal NSTIs.

**Answer: E**

Alejandria, M.M., Lansang, M.A., Dans, L.F., *et al.* (2002) Intravenous immunoglobulin for treating sepsis and septic shock. *Cochrane Database Systematic Reviews*, **1**.
Darabi, K., Abdel-Wahab, O., and Dzik, W.H. (2006) Current usage of intravenous immunoglobulin and the rationale behind it: The Massachusetts General Hospital data and review of the literature. *Transfusion*, **46**, 741–753.
Norrby-Teglund, A., Muller, M.P., Mcgeer, A., *et al.* (2005) Successful management of severe group A streptococcal soft tissue infections using an aggressive medical regimen including intravenous polyspecific immunoglobulin together with a conservative surgical approach. *Scandinavian Journal of Infectious Diseases*, **37** (3), 166–172.

**12** *Which of the following is TRUE regarding hyperbaric oxygen (HBO) therapy for necrotizing soft tissue infections (NSTIs)?*

**A** *The use of HBO has been validated by large prospective randomized control trials*

**B** *HBO use has been shown to significantly decrease mortality after NSTIs*

**C** *HBO use decreases the number of debridements required for treatment of NSTIs*

**D** *HBO use decreases hospital length of stay after NSTIs*

**E** *HBO use does not decrease the duration of antibiotic use after for NSTIs*

The benefit of HBO as an adjunctive treatment for NSTIs remains controversial with no prospective randomized clinical trials having been performed to date. Retrospective reviews have failed to demonstrate a significant decrease in mortality, number of debridements required, length of hospital stay, or duration of antibiotic use following HBO use.

**Answer: E**

Levett, D., Bennett, M.H., and Millar, I. (2015) Adjunctive hyperbaric oxygen for necrotizing fasciits." *The Cochrane Database of Systemic Reviews*, **15**, 1.

**13** *Diabetic foot infections (DFIs) can be a cause of severe SSTIs. These patients:*

**A** *Never present with severe sepsis or septic shock*

**B** *Rarely require surgical abscess drainage or debridement*

**C** *Rarely require vascular examination for improved arterial flow*

**D** *May sometimes require amputation for source control of infection*

**E** *A and C*

Diabetic foot infections can, and do, cause severe SSTIs. These patients can present with severe sepsis and septic shock, frequently require surgical abscess drainage and debridement, often require vascular evaluation for improved arterial flow, and can require amputation for source control.

**Answer: D**

Lipsky, B.A., Berendt, A.R., Cornia, P.B., *et al.* (2012) 2012 Infectious Disease Society of America clinical practice guideline for the diagnosis and treatment of diabetic foot infections. *Clinical Infectious Diseases*, **54** (12), e132–e173.

**14** *The predominant pathogens identified among diabetic foot infections are:*

**A** *Aerobic Gram-positive cocci*

**B** *Gram-negative rods*

**C** *Fungal pathogens*

**D** *Obligate anerobic pathogens*

**E** *Gram-positive rods*

Aerobic Gram-positive cocci (especially *S. aureus*) are the predominant pathogens in diabetic foot infections. Patients with chronic wounds or who recently have received antimicrobial therapy may also be infected with Gram-negative rods, and those with foot ischemia or gangrene may have obligate anaerobic pathogens. Special attention to the potential of concurrent osteomyelitis and the need for potential vascular reconstruction for ischemic arterial disease must be paid in this population.

**Answer: A**

Anakwenze, O.A., Milby, A.H., Gans, I., *et al.* (2012) Foot and ankle infections: diagnosis and management. *Journal of the American Academy of Orthopaedic Surgeons*, **20** (11), 684–693.

**15** *An 18-year-old girl presents to the ED with a five-day history of a painful tooth and fevers, followed by 12 hours of progressive neck swelling and mental status changes. WBC is 19,000/mm. CT demonstrates evidence of deep cervical infection with evidence of necrotic changes in the cervical musculature and significant edema. Which of the following is false regarding this process?*

**A** *This represents a type I NSTI*

**B** *Airway obstruction is rarely a concern in these patients*

**C** *Surgical drainage is a pillar of therapy for this patient*

**D** *Common causative organisms include Fusibacterium*

**E** *Odontogenic infections are the most common cause of these infections*

Cervical necrotizing fasciitis is a type 1 NSTI that is caused by bacterial penetration into the fascial compartments of the head and neck, resulting in a rapidly progressive infection with life-threatening airway obstruction. It is most often associated with odontogenic infection and is likely to require antibiotics and surgical intervention. Airway obstruction is common; early intubation and airway protection should always be considered. Both Ludwig's angina (submandibular space infection) and cervical necrotizing fasciitis are usually caused by mouth anaerobes—such as *Fusobacterium* species—anaerobic Streptococcus, Peptostreptococcus, Bacteroides, and spirochetes, which are usually susceptible to penicillin and clinidamycin.

**Answer: B**

Derber, C.J. and Troy, S.B. (2012) Head and neck emergencies: bacterial meningitis, encephalitis, brain abscess, upper airway obstruction, and jugular septic thrombophlebitis. *Medical Clinics of North America*, **96** (6), 1107–1126.

16  *Invasive zygomycosis has been demonstrated in an ICU patient with onset of profound sepsis and necrotizing soft tissue infection. Initial treatment should include all of the following except:*
A  *Surgical debridement*
B  *Pressor support and resuscitation per the Surviving Sepsis guidelines*
C  *Amphotericin B or equivalent liposomal formulation*
D  *An Echinocandin class of anti-fungal medications*
E  *Broad-spectrum antibiotics*

When invasive zygomycosis has been demonstrated, amphotericin B or equivalent liposomal formulation should be initiated, along with surgical debridement and appropriate supportive care per the Surviving Sepsis guidelines. The liposomal fomulation allows higher dosing with less nephrotoxicity. Echonocandins have no *in vitro* activity against zygomycetes and should be avoided. Posaconazole, which has broad spectrum activity against zygomycetes may be considered for combination therapy or as a step-down therapy for patients who have responded to amphotericin B. Broad-spectrum antibiotics are started empirically and then tapered (or stopped in this instance) once the causative organism(s) is identified.

**Answer: D**

Austin, C.L., Finley, P.J., Mikkelson, D.R., *et al.* (2014) Mucormycosis: a rare fungal infection in tornado victims. *Journal of Burn Care and Research*, **35** (3), e164–e171.

Prasanna Kumar, S., Ravikumar, A., and Somu, L. (2014) Fungal necrotizing fasciitis of the head and neck in 3 patients with uncontrolled diabetes. *Ear, Nose, and Throat Journal*, **93** (3), E18–E21.

Sun, Q.N., Fothergill, A.W., McCarthy, D.I., *et al.* (2002) In vitro activities of posaconazole, itraconazole, voriconazole, amphtericin B, and fluconazole against 37 clinical isolates of zygomycetes. *Antimicrobial Agents and Chemotherapy*, **46**, 1581–1582.

17  *A 54-year-old diabetic man, who has an anaphylactic allergy to penicillin, presents to the ED with bullae along the right lower extremity, hypotension, and mental status changes. WBC is 24,000/mm$^3$ and the patient has a temperature of 103.0°F. The decision is made to proceed to the operating room for surgical exploration and potential debridement. What initial antibiotic choices are not appropriate for this penicillin-allergic patient?*
A  *Ampicillin*
B  *Clindamycin*
C  *Aminoglycoside with appropriate renal dosing*
D  *Metronidazole*
E  *Ciprofloxacin*

The initial antibiotic therapy should be broad enough to cover diverse and various causative agents. High-dose penicillin G or ampicillin should be used to cover for potential Clostridium, Streptococcus, and Peptostreptoccos infections. Anaerobes such as Bacteroides, Fusobacterium and Peptostreptococcus should also be covered with clindamycin or metronidazole. Clindamycin is also effective in treating group A beta-hemolytic Streptococcus by suppressing exotoxins. Clindamycin is the drug of choice for patients with allergies to penicillin. Gram-negative coverage can be achieved by adding an aminoglycoside, a third- or fourth-generation cephalosporin, a floroquinolone, or a carbapenem. Alternatively, penicillin or ampicillin can be replaced by piperacillin-tazobactam or ticaricillin-clavulanate to include Gram-negative coverage. Given this patient's history of anaphylactic response to penicillin, ampicillin is not a viable option in this scenario.

**Answer: A**

Burnham, J.P., Kirby, J.P., and Kollef, M.H. (2016) Diagnosis and management of skin and soft tissue infections in the intensive care unit: a review. *Intensive Care Medicine*, **42** (12), 1899–1911.

## 42

# Obesity and Bariatric Surgery
*Gregory Peirce, MD and LTC Eric Ahnfeldt, DO*

**1** *Which of the following statements is true regarding the classification of body mass index in kg/m² (BMI)?*

**A** *A BMI of 20 is considered underweight*
**B** *A BMI of 28 is considered normal weight*
**C** *A BMI of 32 is considered Class I obesity*
**D** *A BMI between 40 and 50 is considered super obese*
**E** *A BMI of > 50 is considered Class II obesity*

BMI is defined as weight in kilograms divided by height in meters squared. An individual will fall into one of the classifications below according to BMI. Obesity is defined as having a BMI > 30 (Table 42.1). Complications associated with obesity often begin at a BMI of 30. Patients with Class 1 obesity have been shown to live shorter and have a decreased quality of life. In fact, the American Society for Metabolic and Bariatric Surgery has recommended bariatric surgery as an option for Class I obesity. The prevalence of obesity continues to increase in the United States, with a faster growth seen in the higher obesity classes. From 2000 to 2005, the prevalence of Class I, II, III and IV obesity grew 24%, 39%, 52%, and 75% respectively.

**Answer: C**

ASMBS Clinical Issues Committee (2013) Bariatric surgery in class I obesity. *Surgery for Obesity and Related Diseases*, **9**, e1–e10.

Sturm, R. (2007) Increases in morbid obesity in the USA: 2000–2005. *Public Health*, **121** (7): 492–496.

World Health Organization (2000) *Obesity: preventing and managing the global epidemic.* Report of a WHO Consultation. WHO Technical Report Series 894. World Health Organization, Geneva.

**2** *Which of the following is true concerning obesity and pulmonary physiology when compared to non-obese individuals?*

**A** *Obese individuals have increased chest wall compliance*
**B** *Obese individuals have no change in lung volumes*
**C** *Obese individuals have lower rates of oxygen consumption*
**D** *Obese individuals have a higher respiratory rate*
**E** *Obese individuals have a decreased work of breathing*

Obese individuals have a decreased chest wall compliance due to accumulation of adipose tissue in the abdomen, on the chest wall, and between the ribs. They have reduced lung volumes – specifically a decrease in expiratory reserve volume and functional residual capacity. Due to the increased work to breath and move, obese individuals have increased metabolic demands, and as such have a higher rate of oxygen consumption and carbon dioxide production. To meet these demands, obese individuals have a higher respiratory rate and minute ventilation.

**Answer: D**

Jubber, A.S. (2004) Respiratory complications of obesity. *International Journal of Clinical Practice*, **58**, 573–580.

Kuchta, K.F. (2005) Pathophysiologic changes of obesity. *Anesthesiology Clinics of North America*, **23**, 421–429.

Levi, D., Goodman, E.R., Patel, M., and Savransky, Y. (2003) Critical care of the obese and bariatric surgical patient. *Critical Care Clinics*, **19**, 11–32.

*Surgical Critical Care and Emergency Surgery: Clinical Questions and Answers*, Second Edition.
Edited by Forrest "Dell" Moore, Peter Rhee, and Gerard J. Fulda.
© 2018 John Wiley & Sons Ltd. Published 2018 by John Wiley & Sons Ltd.
Companion website: www.wiley.com/go/moore/surgical_criticalcare_and_emergency_surgery

**Table 42.1** BMI classification.

| Classification | BMI (kg/m$^2$) |
| --- | --- |
| Underweight | <18.5 |
| Normal | 18.5–24.9 |
| Overweight | 25–29.9 |
| Obese | ≥30 |
|   Class I | 30–34.9 |
|   Class II (moderately obese) | 35–39.9 |
|   Class III (severely obese) | 40–49.9 |
|   Class IV (super obese) | ≥50 |

3  *You are caring for a patient who was involved in a motor vehicle collision. She has bilateral femur fractures, bilateral humerus fractures, and no other injuries. She remains intubated after an orthopedic surgery. Her height is 5 feet and 0 inches (152 cm), and her weight is 220 lbs (100 kg). Her BMI is 43 kg/m$^2$. Which of the following is the most appropriate initial tidal volume setting?*

A  *250 mL/breath*
B  *350 mL/breath*
C  *450 mL/breath*
D  *550 mL/breath*
E  *650 mL/breath*

Ventilator tidal volumes are based on ideal body weight (IBW). Even though this patient is physically obese and large, she has a relatively small thoracic cavity being 5 feet tall. There are several methods of calculating IBW. The method of Devine is a simple and easy method to remember, and is shown below. This patient's IBW is 100 lbs (45.5 kg). Using lung protective ventilation (6–8 mL/kg), her tidal volume would be between 273 mL and 364 mL.

**Answer: B**

Devine, B.J. (1974) Gentamicin therapy. *Drug Intelligence and Clinical Pharmacy*, **8**, 650–655. Levi, D., Goodman, E.R., Patel, M., and Savransky, Y. (2003) Critical care of the obese and bariatric surgical patient. *Critical Care Clinics*, **19**, 11–32.

4  *You are caring for a patient who was involved in a motor vehicle collision. She has bilateral femur fractures, bilateral humerus fractures, and no other injuries. She remains intubated after an orthopedic surgery. Her height is 5 feet and 0 inches (152 cm), and her weight is 220 lbs (100 kg). Her BMI is 43 kg/m$^2$. Her postoperative course is complicated by ARDS and pneumonia and is unable to extubate during the first week following surgery. You decide she would benefit from a tracheostomy. Which of the following is true?*

A  *Complication rates of percutaneous verses open tracheostomy in the obese population are similar*
B  *Morbid obesity is an absolute contra-indication to percutaneous tracheostomy*
C  *Complication rates of percutaneous tracheostomy are clearly higher for obese patients compared with lean individuals*
D  *There is little benefit to doing a percutaneous tracheostomy in the operating room for morbidly obese patient as opposed to doing it in the intensive care unit*
E  *The cervical spine must be cleared prior to attempting a percutaneous tracheostomy in obese individuals*

Morbid obesity was considered a relative contraindication to performing a percutaneous tracheostomy. However, recent evidence shows no difference in complication rate in the open compared with the percutaneous population. In fact, there is conflicting data in the literature with regard to whether obese patients have a higher complication rate when compared to lean individuals. If one is concerned that a percutaneous tracheostomy may be difficult due to body habitus, difficult airway, and a large amount of pretracheal tissue, it is prudent to perform the percutaneous tracheostomy in the operating room. Doing so in that environment will ensure that an anesthesia provider is present if an airway is lost, and that a difficult percutaneous tracheostomy can be converted to an open tracheostomy if necessary. Cervical spine clearance, while desirable, is not absolutely necessary prior to percutaneous tracheostomy as long as appropriate spinal precautions are taken.

**Answer: A**

Heyrosa, M.G. (2006) Percutaneous tracheostomy: A safe procedure in the morbidly obese. *Journal of the American College of Surgeons*, **202**, 618–622.

5  *You are the on-call provider for the surgical intensive care unit. A bariatric surgeon just finished with a Roux-en-Y gastric bypass on a 55-year-old female with a history of obstructive sleep apnea (OSA) and you are to assume ICU care. Which of the follow is true regarding OSA in the obese population?*

A  *OSA is over diagnosed in the obese population*
B  *Less than 50% of the obese population have OSA*
C  *All bariatric patients with OSA should be admitted to the ICU for observation postoperatively*
D  *Bariatric patients with OSA using CPAP at home do not need to use CPAP in the hospital postoperatively*
E  *All bariatric patients should initially be monitored with continuous pulse oximetry*

OSA is present in at least 50% of the obese population and is under diagnosed. Bariatric patients are at increased risk of apnea and death from OSA in the immediate postoperative period due to the anesthesia and narcotics. The American Society of Metabolic and Bariatric Surgery (ASMBS) recommends that patients who use CPAP at home, also be placed on CPAP in the immediate postoperative period. The ASMBS also recommends the use of pulse oximetry monitoring and states that the majority of these patients do not require an ICU setting.

**Answer: E**

ASMBS guideline. (2012) Peri-operative management of obstructive sleep apnea. *Surgery for Obesity and Related Diseases*, **8**, e27–e32.

Gross, J.B. (2006) Practice guidelines for the perioperative management of patients with obstructive sleep apnea: a report by the American Society of Anesthesiologists Task Force on Perioperative Management of patients with obstructive sleep apnea. *Anesthesiology*, **104** (5), 1081–1093.

6   *You are consulted by the emergency room to see a 40-year-old woman with peritonitis. She had a Roux-en-Y gastric bypass 6 months ago. Her preoperative BMI was 45 (kg/m²), and her current BMI is 39. She has been taking multivitamins, metformin, and takes ibuprofen regularly for joint pain. She has stopped drinking alcohol, but continues to smoke. What is the most likely cause of her abdominal pain?*

   A  *Internal hernia*
   B  *Perforated ulcer*
   C  *Perforation of a gastro-gastric fistula*
   D  *Obstruction of her jejuno-jejunal anastomosis resulting in proximal perforation*
   E  *Acute cholecystitis*

A marginal ulcer at the jejunal border of the gastrojejunal anastomosis is a known complication after Roux-en-Y gastric bypass. These occur as a result of acidic gastric secretions injuring the jejunum. Risk factors for development of a marginal ulcer include ulcerogenic medications (such as NSAIDS), smoking, tissue ischemia, tension on the gastrojejunal anastomosis, and *Helicobacter pylori* infection. This patient likely has a marginal ulcer as she continues to smoke and is taking ibuprofen. While she could have an internal hernia with bowel ischemia, this is less likely as an internal hernia more often occurs in those with a more significant weight loss.

**Answer: B**

Patel, R.A., Brolin, R. E., and Gandhi, A. (2009) Revisional operations for marginal ulcer and Roux-en-Y gastric bypass, *Surgery for Obesity and Related Diseases*, **5**, 317–322

7   *The above patient has free air on abdominal plain films. Which of the following is not an appropriate treatment plan?*

   A  *Repair of defect with an omental or jejunal patch*
   B  *Primary closure with absorbable suture*
   C  *Gastric pouch and gastro-jejunal anastomosis resection with esophago-jejunostomy*
   D  *Wide drainage of the anastomotic area if unable to re-approximate or patch*
   E  *Resection and revision of the gastro-jejunal anastomosis*

A perforated marginal ulcer can be treated with a laparoscopic or open approach. If amenable to primary closure, this can be done with absorbable suture. If not amenable to closure, options include patching with an omental or jejunal patch, or widely draining the area. If the ulcer is thought to be caused by ischemia, resection and revision of the anastomosis is appropriate. Resection of the gastric pouch and gastro-jejunal anastomosis followed by creation of an esophago-jejunostomy would only be done if there was not enough gastric pouch remaining – as this is a more challenging anastomosis to create.

**Answer: C**

Racu, C. and Mehran, A. (2010) Marginal ulcers after roux-en-y gastric bypass: pain for the patient … pain for the surgeon. *Bariatric Times*, **7**, 23–25.

8   *A 35-year-old woman status post Roux-en-Y gastric bypass 8 months ago presents with epigastric pain, cholelithiasis, a common bile duct of 0.5 cm diameter, and pericholecystic fluid. Which of the following should be performed during the surgery?*

   A  *Run the bowel from terminal ileum to the jejuno-jejunal anastomosis*
   B  *Inspect gastric pouch and remnant to assess for a gastro-gastric fistula*
   C  *Perform an intraoperative cholangiogram*
   D  *Perform an upper endoscopy assessing for a marginal ulcer*
   E  *Perform a leak test on the gastro-jejunal anastomosis*

Gallstones tend to form with rapid weight loss. Therefore, cholelithiasis is common in the bariatric population. The common bile duct should be cleared when performing a cholecystectomy in a Roux-en-Y gastric bypass patient who has evidence of choledocholithiasis. Clearing the common bile duct of stones trans-orally with an endoscope is difficult with the anatomic configuration of a bypass surgery. Therefore, the best opportunity is at the initial operation. Often a cholecystectomy will be done at the initial bariatric surgery if the patient has gallstones – whether symptomatic or not.

**Answer: C**

Lombard, M., Green, J., Beckingham, I., *et al.* (2008) Guidelines on the management of common bile duct stones (CBDS). *Gut: Journal of the British Society of Gastroenterology,* **57** (7) 1004–1021.

9 *You perform a laparoscopic intraoperative cholangiogram in the above patient and find three large gallstones in the common bile duct. Which of the following is the least appropriate management option?*

 A *A laparoscopic trans-cystic common bile duct exploration*
 B *Close and follow the patient clinically for signs of biliary obstruction*
 C *An open common bile duct exploration*
 D *A trans-gastric ERCP*
 E *Ask a college for assistance or advice on how to remove the gallstones*

Choledocholithiasis should be cleared intraoperatively if found in a Roux-en-Y gastric bypass patient. Treatment options include performing a laparoscopic transcystic common bile duct exploration, an open common bile duct exploration, or an ERCP performed through the gastric remnant. The transgastric ERCP involves creation of an anterior gastrotomy in the remnant stomach to allow passage of the side-viewing endoscope into the duodenum. This can be performed during laparoscopic or open surgery.

**Answer: B**

Snauwaert, C., Laukens, P., Dillemans, B., *et al.* (2015) Laparoscopy-assisted transgastric endoscopic retrograde cholangiopancreatography in bariatric Roux-en-Y gastric bypass patients. *Endoscopy International Open,* **3** (5), E458–E463.

10 *A 43-year-old woman presents to the emergency room with a 4-day history of erythema and tenderness over her gastric band port site. She is 8 years post gastric*

*band placement and recently had it filled with 2 mL. What is the most likely cause of her symptoms?*

 A *Infection of the subcutaneous port from recent access*
 B *Cellulitis*
 C *Irritation from loss of subcutaneous adipose tissue and the proximity of the port to the skin*
 D *Band erosion*
 E *Breakdown of the band catheter and leakage of fluid into the subcutaneous tissue*

Evidence of an infection at the gastric band port site is a band erosion until proven otherwise. After a band erodes through the stomach, the first sign can often be an infection at the port site. This is due to luminal gastric secretions and bacteria tracking along the band catheter from the stomach to the port.

**Answer: D**

Angrisani, L., Furbetta, F., Doldi, S.B., *et al.* (2003) Lap band adjustable gastric banding system: the Italian experience with 1863 patients operated on 6 years. *Surgical Endoscopy,* **17** (3), 409–412.
Fielding, G.A., Rhodes, M., and Nathanson, L.K. (1999) Laparoscopic gastric banding for morbid obesity. Surgical outcome in 335 cases. *Surgical Endoscopy,* **13** (6), 550–554.
Rubenstein, R.B. (2002) Laparoscopic adjustable gastric banding at a U.S. center with up to 3-year follow-up. *Obesity Surgery,* **12** (3), 380–384.
Weiner, R., Blanco-Engert, R., Weiner, S., *et al.* (2003) Outcome after laparoscopic adjustable gastric banding – 8 years' experience. *Obesity Surgery,* **13** (3), 427–434.

11 *For the above patient, which of the following is the best treatment option?*

 A *Total gastrectomy with esophago-jejunal anastomosis*
 B *Antibiotics and removal of the access port and placement of a new one at separate location on the abdomen*
 C *Port removal, catheter removal, band removal, abdominal washout, and coverage of the band tract with omentum, and wide drainage*
 D *Removal of the band and conversion to a Roux-en-Y gastric bypass*
 E *Admission with for IV antibiotics and serial abdominal examinations*

This patient has a band erosion demonstrating itself as infection of the subcutaneous port. This can be confirmed endoscopically. She needs removal of the whole device. Of the options given, the safest treatment would be to remove the device (port, catheter and band) and cover any visible defect with omentum. In 4 to 6 months, the patient will likely be able to undergo another bariatric surgery if desired. An additional surgical option would be to make a distal gastrotomy and remove the band through the lumen of the stomach, washout and drainage.

**Answer: C**

Angrisani, L., Furbetta, F., Doldi, S.B., *et al.* (2003) Lap Band adjustable gastric banding system: the Italian experience with 1863 patients operated on 6 years. *Surgical Endoscopy*, **17** (3), 409–412.

Fielding, G.A., Rhodes, M., and Nathanson, L.K. (1999) Laparoscopic gastric banding for morbid obesity. Surgical outcome in 335 cases. *Surgical Endoscopy*, **13** (6), 550–554.

Rubenstein, R.B. (2002) Laparoscopic adjustable gastric banding at a U.S. center with up to 3-year follow-up. *Obesity Surgery*, **12** (3), 380–384.

Weiner, R., Blanco-Engert, R., Weiner, S., *et al.* (2003) Outcome after laparoscopic adjustable gastric banding – 8 years' experience. *Obesity Surgery*, **13** (3), 427–434.

**12** *The emergency room calls you about a 47-year-old man who had a gastric band placed 5 years ago. For dinner, he was unable to swallow food or even keep liquids down. He has not had his band volume adjusted for several years. His physical exam and labs are normal. A chest X-ray centered at the diaphragm shows the band to be in proper position. What is the next best course of action?*

**A** *Laparoscopic band removal*
**B** *Removal of all the band fluid by accessing the port*
**C** *Upper gastro-intestinal swallow study*
**D** *Admission, IV fluid, NPO and NG tube drainage of the esophagus*
**E** *Endoscopic dilation of the stricture*

This patient is having poor PO tolerance due to stricture at the band. This can usually be relieved by removal of band fluid. This is done at bedside by accessing the port using a Huber needle. Once the fluid is removed, a bedside swallow can be performed and if tolerated the patient can be discharged.

**Answer: B**

Weiner, R., Blanco-Engert, R., Weiner, S., *et al.* (2003) Outcome after laparoscopic adjustable gastric banding – 8 years' experience. *Obesity Surgery*, **13** (3), 427–434.

**13** *A 50-year-old woman was admitted to your service with acute cholecystitis which you successfully treated surgically. She had a Roux-en-Y gastric bypass 8 years ago. Preoperatively, she was noted to have a hemoglobin of 8. She has not been seeing any physician and is not taking any medications or supplements. Concerning her workup and treatment for anemia, which of the following is true?*

**A** *An EGD and colonoscopy are not necessary*
**B** *Iron supplementation will assist if her mean corpuscular volume (MCV) is 110*
**C** *Cobalamin (Vitamin B12) supplementation should be started for microcytic anemia*
**D** *Folate (Vitamin B9) deficiency may result in macrocytic anemia and neurologic symptoms*
**E** *She may need a referral to hematology for treatment of refractory anemia*

Postoperative anemia is a common complication after a Roux-en-Y gastric bypass. This is most commonly due to malabsorption of needed nutrients. However, in this patient an EGD should be performed to rule out a marginal ulcer and a colonoscopy performed to rule out colon cancer. Iron deficiency anemia results in a microcytic anemia with an MCV of less than 80. Both cobalamin (Vitamin B12) and folate deficiencies result in a macrocytic anemia (MCV > 100)—however, only Vitamin B12 deficiency will result in neurologic symptoms. A referral to hematology for intravenous iron supplementation is often needed if the patient remains anemic after appropriate supplementation.

**Answer: E**

Davies, D.J., Baxter, J.M., and Baxter, J.N. (2007) Nutritional deficiencies after bariatric surgery. *Obesity Surgery*, **17**, 1150–1158.

Schweitzer, D.H. and Posthuma, E.F. (2008) Prevention of vitamin and mineral deficiencies after bariatric surgery: evidence and algorithms. *Obesity Surgery* **18**, 1485–1488.

**14** *Concerning nutrients and the location of absorption within the gastro-intestinal tract, which of the following is true?*

**A** *Iron is mostly absorbed in the duodenum*
**B** *Calcium is mostly absorbed in the jejunum and ileum*
**C** *Folate is mostly absorbed in the jejunum*
**D** *Vitamin B12 is mostly absorbed in the duodenum*
**E** *Bile salts are mostly absorbed in the jejunum*

Lack of essential nutrients is common after bariatric surgery. Iron is mostly absorbed in the duodenum. Poor iron absorption is due both to ingested food bypassing the duodenum and decreased gastric acid secretions. The acid secretion reduces iron from $Fe^{3+}$ to the more absorbable $Fe^{2+}$. Most calcium is absorbed in the duodenum and proximal jejunum. Hypocalcemia can be due to bypass of the duodenum and decreased Vitamin D. Folate and Vitamin B12 are absorbed in the terminal ileum. Vitamin B12 deficiency can occur secondary to decreased intrinsic factor secretion. Bile salts and fat-soluble vitamins are absorbed in the terminal ileum. All patients after bariatric surgery should take a daily multivitamin and should be followed with frequent laboratory assessment of important nutrients.

**Answer: A**

Davies, D.J., Baxter, J.M., and Baxter, J.N. (2007) Nutritional deficiencies after bariatric surgery. *Obesity Surgery*, **17**, 1150–1158.
Schweitzer, D.H. and Posthuma, E.F. (2008) Prevention of vitamin and mineral deficiencies after bariatric surgery: evidence and algorithms. *Obesity Surgery* **18**, 1485–1488.

**15** *A 55-year-old man was discharged from the hospital on postoperative day 2 after a Roux-en-Y gastric bypass. He returns to the emergency room with chest pain and difficulties breathing. His oxygen saturations are stable after being placed on 6 L/min of oxygen. Of the following, what is the most appropriate next step in management?*

**A** *Intravenous antibiotics*
**B** *Cardiac catheterization*
**C** *CTA scan of the chest*
**D** *Upper gastro-intestinal swallow study*
**E** *Chest x-ray*

Pulmonary embolus is the most common cause of mortality in the acute setting following a bariatric surgery. This is best diagnosed with a CTA of the chest. A chest x-ray is not sensitive when evaluating for a pulmonary embolus. Treatment with antibiotics would only be appropriate if he present with signs of sepsis or anastomotic leak. A myocardial infarction is certainly possible, and this would best be diagnosed first with an EKG and cardiac enzymes. However, an MI would be less likely than a PE at this time. A prompt CTA should be performed followed by heparin if positive. If the patient were unstable with difficulties oxygenating, heparin should be started empirically.

**Answer: C**

Gagner, M., Milone, L., Young, E., and Broseus, A. (2008) Causes of early mortality after laparoscopic adjustable gastric banding. *Journal of the American College of Surgeons*, **206**, 664–649.
Mason, E.E., Renquist, K.E., Huang, Y.H., *et al.* (2007) Causes of 30-day bariatric surgery mortality: with emphasis on bypass obstruction. *Obesity Surgery*, **17**, 9–14.

**16** *A 40-year-old man is 5 years post laparoscopic retrocolic Roux-en-Y gastric bypass. He has lost 120 pounds. He presented to the emergency room complaining of epigastric pain. The emergency room performed a CT scan which shows moderately dilated small bowel. The mesenteric vessels also appear to rotate in a circular fashion in the axial plane. What is the most likely cause of his symptoms?*

**A** *Small bowel herniation between the Roux limb and the mesocolon*
**B** *Small bowel herniation through the small bowel mesenteric defect*
**C** *Intussusception of the small bowel at the jejuno-jejunal anastomosis*
**D** *Small bowel herniation through the mesocolic defect*
**E** *Obstruction from adhesive disease*

Internal hernias are a common complication after Roux-en-Y gastric bypass surgery. Usually these occur after a significant amount of weight loss as the mesenteric fat thins and the potential space for a hernia develops. Internal hernias often present with epigastric pain, small bowel dilation and CT imaging showing a "swirl sign" of the mesenteric vessels and small bowel in the upper quadrants. With a retrocolic bypass, 3 potential spaces are created. Small bowel can hernia through the mesocolic defect, between the Roux limb mesentery and the biliopancreatic limb mesentery, or between the Roux limb and the mesocolon (Petersen's defect). The rates of these hernias are reported at 67%, 21%, and 7.5% respectively. Use of an antecolic Roux limb eliminates the potential for herniation through the mesocolic defect.

**Answer: D**

Jeansonne, L.O., Morgenthal, C.B., White, B.C., and Lin, E. (2007) Internal hernia after laparoscopic gastric bypass: a review of the literature. *Bariatric Times*. April 26.

**17**  *For the above patient, what is the best technical approach to reduce an internal hernia?*

   **A**  *Run the bowel from the terminal ileum to the jejuno-jejunostomy*
   **B**  *Find the jejuno-jejunal anastomosis and from there assess the potential spaces for a hernia*
   **C**  *Run the bowel from the gastro-jejunostomy to the jejuno-jejunostomy*
   **D**  *Run the bowel from the ligament of Treitz to the jejuno-jejunostomy*
   **E**  *Begin with a laparotomy on all patients, as exposure is inadequate during laparoscopy*

The herniated small bowel is likely distal to the jejuno-jejunostomy (the alimentary limb). This is often reduced simply by running the bowel proximally from the terminal ileum. After reduction of the small bowel and running the alimentary limb to the jejuno-jejunostomy, the Roux limb and biliopancreatic limb should also be inspected for viability. Afterwards, the hernia defect should be closed. Running the bowel from the gastro-jejunostomy will likely not reduce the hernia as this segment of bowel is usually not involved. Finding the ligament of Treitz initially will be very difficult as there will likely be herniated and dilated bowel in this area. Initially finding the jejuno-jenunal anastomosis is of little help because proper identification of each segment is not possible without completely running the bowel. The anatomy can often be identified laparoscopically, follow by successful reduction of the hernia and repair of the defect. Conversely, conversion to a laparotomy may be necessary if one is unable to identify the proper anatomy or reduce and repair the hernia.

**Answer: A**

Jeansonne, L.O., Morgenthal, C.B., White, B.C., and Lin, E. (2007) Internal hernia after laparoscopic gastric bypass: a review of the literature. *Bariatric Times*. April 26.

**18**  *A 25-year-old woman is one week post Roux-en-Y gastric bypass. She has had worsening abdominal pain for which she came into the emergency room. Laboratory values obtained by the emergency room show an elevated lipase. An acute abdominal series shows dilated small bowel. What is the most likely cause of her symptoms?*

   **A**  *Internal hernia*
   **B**  *Obstruction at the jejuno-jenunostomy*
   **C**  *Gastro-jejunostomy stricture*
   **D**  *Obstruction from adhesions*
   **E**  *Pancreatitis*

Acute postoperative obstruction after a Roux-en-Y gastric bypass is most likely due to obstruction at the jejuno-jejunal anastomosis from a technical error. This is best diagnosed with a CT scan that may demonstrate dilation of the Roux limb, the biliopancreatic limb, or both. Obstruction of the biliopancreatic limb may result in pancreatitis. Obstruction from an internal hernia or from adhesions is less likely to occur in the acute setting. A gastro-jejunal stricture would not result in dilated small bowel distally.

**Answer: B**

Capella, R.F., Iannace, V.A., and Capella, J.F. (2006) Bowel obstruction after open and laparoscopic gastric bypass surgery for morbid obesity. *Journal of the American College of Surgeons*, **203**, 328–335.

Koppman, J.S., Li, C., and Gandsas, A. (2008) Small bowel obstruction after laparoscopic Roux-en-Y gastric bypass: a review of 9527 patients. *Journal of the American College of Surgeons*, **206**, 571–584.

**19**  *Which of the following is true regarding postoperative enteric leaks after a Roux-en-Y gastric bypass?*

   **A**  *Leaks from the jejuno-jejunostomy are usually diagnosed earlier than those from the gastro-jejunostomy*
   **B**  *A late sign of a leak is often persistent tachycardia above 120 beats/minute*
   **C**  *Failure to promptly return to the operating room is the most common cause of preventable morbidity or mortality after bariatric surgery*
   **D**  *Two thirds of those found to have a leak will have a normal UGI and CT scan*
   **E**  *Drain amylase levels do not assist with diagnosis of a leak*

Diagnosing a postoperative leak in the bariatric population can be very difficult. This is in part due to an unreliable abdominal exam due to body habitus and the poor sensitivity in imaging studies. One third of those with leaks will have a normal UGI and CT scan. Tachycardia is common in those with an enteric leak – however, it is not specific to a leak. Other causes of tachycardia include pain, dehydration, bleeding, myocardial infarction, and pulmonary embolus. If a drain is left, elevated drain amylase levels can be an early indicator of a leak. A high index of suspicion is needed to diagnose an enteric leak and if suspected the safest course of action is to return to the operating room. Failure to promptly return to the operating room in the setting of an enteric leak is the number one cause of preventable major long-term morbidity and death after bariatric surgery.

**Answer: C**

Capella, R.F., Iannace, V.A., and Capella, J.F. (2006) Bowel obstruction after open and laparoscopic gastric bypass surgery for morbid obesity. *Journal of the American College of Surgeons*, **203**, 328–335.

Koppman, J.S., Li, C., and Gandsas, A. (2008) Small bowel obstruction after laparoscopic Roux-en-Y gastric bypass: a review of 9527 patients. *Journal of the American College of Surgeons*, **206**, 571–584.

# 43

## Thermal Burns, Electrical Burns, Chemical Burns, Inhalational Injury, and Lightning Injuries

*Joseph J. DuBose, MD and Jacob Swann, MD*

1  *Which of the following is false regarding the initial resuscitation of burn victims?*
   A *Ineffective resuscitation will result in shock among patients with >20% total body surface area burn involvement*
   B *Delays in resuscitation beyond 2 hours have not been associated with increased mortality*
   C *Consequences of over-resuscitation include the need for fasciotomy*
   D *Overresuscitation may be associated with conversion of superficial into deep burns*
   E *Abdominal compartment syndrome may result from over-resuscitation*

Without effective and rapid initiation of resuscitation, hypovolemia and shock will develop in patients with burns >15-20% total body surface area (TBSA) burns. Delay in fluid resuscitation beyond 2 hours of burn injury increases mortality and morbidity after these injuries. Consequences of overresuscitation following burns include pulmonary edema, conversion of superficial into deep burns, the need for fasciotomy (including unburned limbs), and abdominal compartment syndrome.

**Answer: B**

Cancio, L. (2014) Initial assessment and fluid resuscitation of burn patients. *Surgical Clinics of North America*, **94**, 741–754.

2  *Burn shock pathophysiology is marked by:*
   A *Neurogenic shock*
   B *High pulmonary artery occlusion pressure*
   C *Decreased cardiac output*
   D *Decreased systemic vascular resistance*
   E *Increased intravascular volume*

Burn shock is the result of distributive and hypovolemic shock, manifested by intravascular volume depletion, low pulmonary artery occlusion pressure, elevated systemic vascular resistance, and depressed cardiac output. Reduced cardiac output is a combined result of decreased plasma volume, increased afterload, and decreased contractility. Impaired cardiac contractility is likely caused by circulating mediators such as tumor necrosis factor and impaired cellular calcium levels.

**Answer: C**

Rae, L., Fidler, P., and Gibran, N. (2016) The physiologic basis of burn shock and the need for aggressive fluid resuscitation. *Critical Care Clinics of North America*, **32**, 491–505.

3  *All of the following are sequelae of initial burn injury except:*
   A *Loss of vessel wall integrity with leakage into the interstitium*
   B *Increased intravascular colloid osmotic pressure*
   C *Decreased circulating plasma volume*
   D *Depressed cardiovascular function*
   E *Massive edema formation*

Following burn injury, capillary leak promotes protein and osmotic loss into the interstitial space. This—in turn—decreases intravascular colloid osmotic pressure. The outcome of the dramatic pouring of fluids, electrolytes, and proteins into the interstitium is reflected in the loss of circulating plasma volume, hemoconcentration, massive edema formation, decreased urine output, and depressed cardiovascular function.

**Answer: B**

Rae, L., Fidler, P., and Gibran, N. (2016) The physiologic basis of burn shock and the need for aggressive fluid resuscitation. *Critical Care Clinics of North America*, **32**, 491–505.

Swanson, J., Otto, A., and Gibran, N. (2013) Trajectories to death in patients with burn injury. *Journal of Trauma and Acute Care Surgery*, **74** (1), 282–288.

4  *How much fluid should routinely be given to the acutely burned patient?*
   **A**  *2 liters of crystalloid over one hour for every patient*
   **B**  *1 mL/kg of lactated Ringer's for 24 hours*
   **C**  *2 mL/kg per percentage body surface area burned of albumin for the first 24 hours*
   **D**  *2 to 4 mL/kg per percentage body surface area burned of 7.5% hypertonic saline for the first 24 hours*
   **E**  *2 to 4 mL/kg per percentage body surface area burned of lactated Ringer's for the first 24 hours, half of which is given in the first 8 hours*

Although several resuscitation formulas exist, the Parkland formula is the Consensus formula used by the American Burn Association in the Advanced Burn Life Support Curriculum. This formula calls for 4 mL/kg per percentage TBSA, describing the amount of lactated Ringer's solution required in the first 24 hours after burn injury, where "kg" represents the patient's weight, and percentage TBSA is the size of the burn injury. Starting from the time of burn injury, half of the fluid is given in the first 8 hours and the remaining half is given over the next 16 hours. It is important to note that, while formulas are useful in establishing goals of initial therapy, all therapy should be guided by measured endpoints of resuscitation such as urine output with hour-to-hour changes in the rate of infused fluid made based on these endpoints.

**Answer: E**

Cancio, L. (2014) Initial assessment and fluid resuscitation of burn patients. *Surgical Clinics of North America*, **94**, 741–754.
Cancio, L., Salinas, J., and Kramer, G. (2016) Protocolized resuscitation of burn patients. *Critical Care Clinics of North America*, **32**, 599–610.
Pham, T., Cancio, L., and Gibran, N. (2008) American Burn Association practice guidelines: burn shock resuscitation. *Journal of Burn Care and Research*, **29**, 257–266.

5  *A 26 year-old man presents to your emergency room via ambulance after self-extricating from a burning vehicle. The patient has full-thickness and partial-thickness burns involving the entirety of his bilateral lower extremities circumferentially, the entire anterior surface of his right upper extremity, the entire posterior surface of his left upper extremity, and the anterior upper half of his chest. What is his calculated percentage total body surface area involved by this burn?*

   **A**  *45% TBSA*
   **B**  *49.5% TBSA*
   **C**  *54% TBSA*
   **D**  *58.5% TBSA*
   **E**  *63% TBSA*

The "rule of nines" is a general rule used to make a quick assessment of the amount of involved partial-thickness and full-thickness burned tissue to help guide initial resuscitation. It is calculated by determining which areas of the body are involved with the burn. First-degree burns are not used to calculate the total body surface area burned. From there, one can determine the total body surface area by adding the total amount of burned tissue in each area of the body based on the anatomic location of the burns. The percentage of each area is as follows:

Head = 9%
Anterior chest = 18%
Posterior chest = 18%
Right upper extremity = 9%
Left upper extremity = 9%
Anterior right lower extremity = 9%
Posterior right lower extremity = 9%
Anterior left lower extremity = 9%
Posterior left lower extremity = 9%
Perineum = 1%

Thus, in the scenario above, the patient had his bilateral lower extremities burned circumferentially (9 + 9 + 9 + 9), the anterior surface of his right upper extremity (4.5), the posterior surface of his left upper extremity (4.5), and the upper half of his anterior chest burned (9). Therefore, 9 + 9 + 9 + 9 + 4.5 + 4.5 + 9 = 54%.

**Answer: C**

Hartford, E.C. (2012) Chapter 6: Care of outpatient burns, in *Total Burn Care*, 4th edn (ed. D. Herndon), Chicago, Elsevier, pp. 81–92.

6  *Which of the following is the most reliable method of monitoring resuscitation of burn injured patients?*
   **A**  *Urine output*
   **B**  *Lactate normalization*
   **C**  *Abdominal compartment pressure monitoring*
   **D**  *Response of measured cardiac index to fluid bolus*
   **E**  *Direct tissue oxygen measurements*

Urine output, although the least technologically advanced of the described measures, remains the best validated method of guiding resuscitation. Abnormal admission arterial lactate and base excess values have been shown to correlate with the magnitude of injury and their failure to correct over time predicts mortality, but there remain no prospective studies to support the use of these parameters to guide fluid resuscitation. Abdominal compartment pressure monitoring can assist in the detection of abdominal compartment syndrome—a possible complication of overresuscitation—but does not provide a measure of adequate resuscitative efforts. Although several preliminary studies documented successful increases in preload and cardiac index with aggressive fluid resuscitation after burns, a prospective randomized control trial failed to confirm these benefits. Direct tissue oxygen measurements have also been investigated in preliminary studies but require additional study and are compromised by the edema that is associated with burn injury.

**Answer: A**

Caruso, D. and Matthews, M. (2016) Monitoring end points of burn resuscitation. *Critical Care Clinics of North America*, **32**, 525–537.

7   *A 70-kg patient with 40% TBSA burn has transferred to your facility after receiving >250 mL/kg of crystalloid for the 16 hours prior to transfer. On arrival, his abdomen is tense, his heart rate is 118 beats/min and his blood pressure is 94/42 mm Hg. He has an elevated CVP, and a bladder pressure measurement reveals a pressure of 40 mm Hg. The next appropriate step should be:*

   A *Diuresis with furosemide*
   B *500 mL of 5% albumin bolus over 5 minutes*
   C *Attempt at percutaneous catheter decompression of the abdomen*
   D *Emergent decompressive laparotomy in the emergency department*
   E *Allow the patient to auto-diuresis the excess fluid*

Bladder pressure monitoring should be initiated as part of the burn fluid resuscitation protocol of every patient with >30% TBSA burn. Patients who receive >250 mL/kg of crystalloid in the first 24 hours will likely require abdominal decompression. Percutaneous decompression is a minimally invasive procedure that should be attempted prior to resorting to laparotomy. The International Conference of Experts on Intra-Abdominal Hypertension and Abdominal Compartment Syndrome recommends that if less invasive maneuvers fail, decompressive laparotomy should be performed in patients with ACS that is refractory to other treatment options. The reported mortality rates for decompressive laparotomy for ACS can be as high as 88% to 100%.

**Answer: C**

Cheatam, M.L., Malbrain, M.L., Kirkpatrick, A., *et al.* (2007) Results from the International Conference on Experts on Intra-abdominal Hypertension and Abdominal Compartment Syndrome, II: recommendations. *Intensive Care Medicine*, **33**, 951–962.

Ivy, M.E., Atweh, N.A., Palmer, J., *et al.* (2000) Intra-abdominal hypertension and abdominal compartment syndrome in burn patients. *Journal of Trauma*, **49** (3), 387–391.

Latenser, B.A., Kowal-Vern, A., Kimball, D., *et al.* (2002) A pilot study comparing percutaneous decompression with decompressive laparotomy for acute abdominal compartment syndrome in thermal injury. *Journal of Burn Care Rehabilitation*, **23**, 190–195.

8   *A patient has suffered a 45% TBSA burn, which includes circumferential burns to his bilateral lower extremities, after falling into an open flame while camping. The patient is now 8 hours into his initial resuscitation. He is complaining of bilateral lower extremity pain that has steadily increased since his admission. He has received a total of 9 L of lactated Ringer's solution for resuscitation per the Parkland Formula. On examination, the patient has nonpalpable dorsalis pedis pulses bilaterally, weak Doppler signals appreciated on Doppler examination, and he has significant pain with passive dorsiflexion of his bilateral feet. What is the next best step in management of this patient?*

   A *Increase intravenous fluid resuscitation by 250 mL/ hr due to poor perfusion as evidenced by his abnormal peripheral vascular examination*
   B *Perform bilateral lower extremity fasciotomies*
   C *Give the patient 40 mg of furosemide to decrease anasarca*
   D *Perform bilateral lower extremity escharotomies*
   E *Perform ankle-brachial index measurements of the patient's bilateral lower extremities every 4 hours and continue to monitor*

The diagnosis of compartment syndrome is largely a clinical diagnosis, and in this patient the diagnosis is clear. Compartment syndrome should be expected when any of the six Ps are seen (poikilothermia, paresthesias, pallor, pain, pulselessness, and paralysis). In this patient, multiple findings in the stem point to a diagnosis of compartment syndrome. First, he has circumferential burns. Circumferential burns place patients at risk for developing a compartment syndrome as the overlying eschar acts as a restrictive band that does not allow the tissues to expand with the resuscitation often required in large burns. Next, the patient has received a significant amount of fluid in the first 8 hours of his resuscitation. This increases his risk of compartment syndrome as above. Lastly, his exam is very concerning in that he has pain out-of-proportion to his exam with passive motion of his extremities and pulselessness on physical exam with weak signals noted on Doppler examination. With these physical exam findings, a clinical diagnosis of compartment syndrome is readily made.

With regards to next steps in management, increasing resuscitation will only worsen the compartment syndrome by driving more fluid into the surround tissues making Answer A incorrect. Diuresis in the acute resuscitative phase is not indicated; moreover, diuresis would not address the ongoing compartment syndrome caused by the fluid already in the interstitial space making Answer C incorrect. While ankle-brachial index measurements and intracompartment pressure measurements can assist when the diagnosis is in question, further monitoring while likely lead to permanent neurologic deficits – if not frank limb loss – making Answer E incorrect. While multiple pathologic states can cause a compartment syndrome requiring a fasciotomy, circumferential burns rarely require fasciotomies; rather, simply releasing the burned tissue of the eschar down through the burn into the subcutaneous tissues will often allow immediate release of the compartment syndrome. Bleeding and pain are not encountered with escharotomies. As such, Answer D is correct in that escharotomies are the best treatment at this time, and Answer B is incorrect in that there is no sign that the fascia needs to be opened at this stage. An example of an escharotomy is shown in Figure 43.1.

**Answer: D**

Micak, R.P., Buffalo, C., and Jimenez, C.J. (2012) Pre-hospital management, transportation, and emergency care, in *Total Burn Care*, 4th edn (ed. D. Herndon), Chicago, Elsevier, pp. 93–102.

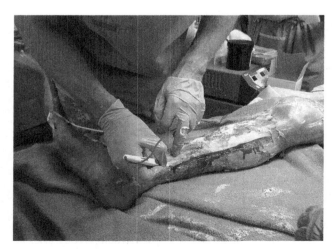

**Figure 43.1** An escharotomy.

9 *Reliable signs of infections among severely burned patients include:*
   A *Fever*
   B *Tachycardia*
   C *Tachypnea*
   D *Leukocytosis*
   E *None of the above*

Current definitions for sepsis and infection have many criteria routinely found in patients with extensive burns without infection or sepsis (i.e. fever, tachycardia, tachypnea, leukocytosis). The inflammatory and hyperdynamic responses associated with burns may result in fever, tachycardia, tachypnea, and even leukocytosis—all in the absence of infection. Useful clues of infection may, however, manifest in the form of increased fluid requirements, decreasing platelet counts >3 days after injury, altered mental status, worsening pulmonary status, and impaired renal function.

**Answer: E**

Latenser, B. (2009) Critical care of the burn patient: the first 48 hours. *Critical Care Medicine*, **37**, 2819–2826.

10 *Central line catheters are commonly required for severe burn victims. Given the risk of central line-associated blood-stream infections, these lines require special care. Reasonable approaches to minimize the risk and sequelae of infection from these lines include all of the following except:*
   A *Meticulous sterile technique with placement*
   B *Preferential utilization of a subclavian site when possible*
   C *Avoiding line placement through burn eschar whenever possible*
   D *Prophylactic systemic antibiotics after line placement*
   E *Daily assessment of line need*

Any infection in a burn patient should be considered to be from the central venous catheter until proven otherwise. If no other source is clearly attributable, the line should be removed after new access has been established; always utilizing meticulous sterile technique for every line placement is paramount in preventing infection. According to the 2011 NIH consensus statement on central venous catheter utilization, the subclavian site is preferred over jugular or femoral sites to potentially reduce the infection risks associated with these sites. The same guidelines support the daily practice of routine evaluation of line need and subsequent removal when an indication for central venous catheterization is no longer necessary. It should also be remembered that in the setting of severe burns, many of the traditional markers of infection (fever and tachycardia, for example) may be present without actual infection. Therefore, routine removal of a central line in patients with tachycardia or low-grade fever in the setting of a severe burn response, particularly if vascular access options are limited, should be avoided. If infection is documented by Gram stain or culture, or if clinical suspicion is strong, then removal and change of a line is indicated. The correct Answer is D; prophylactic systemic antibiotics have not demonstrated a role in the routine care of thermal injury.

**Answer: D**

Weber, J.M., Sheridan, R.L., Fagan, S.P., *et al.* (2013) Incidence of catheter-associated bloodstream infection after introduction of minocycline and rifampin antimicrobial-coated catheters in a pediatric burn population. *Journal of Burn Care Resuscitation*, **33**, 539–543.

Greenhalgh, D.G., Saffle, J.R., Holmes, J.H., *et al.* (2007) American Burn Association Consensus Conference to define sepsis and infection in burns. *Journal of Burn Care Research*, **28**, 71–75.

O'Grady, N.P., Alexander, M., Burns, L.A., *et al.* (2011) Guidelines for the prevention of intravascular catheter-related infections. *Clinical Infectious Diseases*, **52** (9), e162–e193.

11  *Which of the following is false regarding nutrition among burn patients?*
    **A** *Patients with 20% TBSA burns are unlikely to meet their nutritional needs with native oral intake alone*
    **B** *Patients fed early after thermal injury have shorter hospital stays*
    **C** *Parenteral nutrition is the first-line of nutritional delivery in severe burns*
    **D** *Early feeding is associated with enhanced wound healing*
    **E** *The hypermetabolism associated with burn injury can lead to a doubling of normal resting energy expenditure and higher caloric requirements*

Hypermetabolism can double energy expenditure and significantly increase caloric requirements of burn patients. Enteral nutrition is the most desirable route and should be started for these patients as soon as resuscitation is underway. Patients with ≥20% TBSA are not likely to meet their nutritional requirements by mouth alone and should have a transpyloric feeding tube placed if possible. Patients fed early have significantly enhanced wound healing and shorter hospital stays.

**Answer: C**

Faga, S.P., Bilodeau, M., and Goverman, J. (2014) Burn intensive care. *Surgical Clinics of North America*, **94**, 765–779

12  *Which of the following has not proven potentially beneficial for burn patients?*
    **A** *Glucose control*
    **B** *Routine exogenous cortisol*
    **C** *Oxandralone*
    **D** *Propanolol*
    **E** *Topical antimicrobial agents*

Although absolute adrenal insufficiency occurs in up to 36% of patients with major burns, there has not been a correlation between response to corticotropin stimulation or cortisol and survival. Glucose control in burn patients has been shown to be associated with decreased infectious complications and mortality rates. Anabolic steroids, including oxandralone, have been shown to promote regain of weight and lean mass two to three times faster than nutrition alone after burn injury. Beta-blockers like propanolol have been shown to attenuate hypermetabolism and reverse muscle protein catabolism. Once a wound is clean, topical antimicrobial agents limit bacterial proliferation and fungal colonization in burn wounds.

**Answer: B**

Ferrando, A.A., Chinkes, D.L., Wolf, S.E., *et al.* (1999) A submaximal dose of insulin promotes skeletal muscle protein synthesis in patients with severe burns. *Annals of Surgery*, **229**, 11–18.

Herndon, D.N., Hart, D.W., Wolf, S.E., *et al.* (2001) Reversal of catabolism by beta blockers after severe burns. *New England Journal of Medicine*, **345**, 1223–1229.

Wolf, S.E., Edelman, L.S., Kemalyan, N., *et al.* (2006) Effects of oxandrolone on outcome measures in the severely burned: a multicenter prospective randomized double-blind trial. *Journal of Burn Care and Research*, **27** (2), 131–139.

13  *Mafenide acetate (sulfamylon acetate) is a topical antimicrobial frequently utilized in burn wound care. This medication is associated with characteristic side effects including:*
    **A** *Hyponatremia*
    **B** *Hypochloremia*
    **C** *Methemoglobinemia*
    **D** *Hyperchloremic acidosis*
    **E** *Leukopenia*

Mafenide acetate (sulfamylon acetate) has a broad antimicrobial spectrum of action and excellent eshcar penetration. Some side effects that are worrisome with the use of this topical antimicrobial (either 10% cream or 5% soaks) are burning sensation, allergic reactions, and hyperchloremic acidosis. Silver sulfadiazine is essentially a combination of two antimicrobials, silver and a sulfonamide. It has a more moderate eschar penetration ability than mafenide acetate. Complications of silver sulfadiazine include allergic reactions, methemoglobinemia, and leukopenia. Silver nitrate also has a broad antimicrobial spectrum of topical action and can be associated with the side effects of hyponatremia, methemoglobinemia, and hypochloremia.

**Answer: D**

Gallagher, J.J., Branski, L.K., Williams-Bouyer, N., *et al.* (2012) Treatment of infection in burns, in *Total Burn Care*, 4th edn (ed. D. Herndon), Chicago, Elsevier, pp. 137–156.

**14** *All of the following constitute clear criteria for transfer to a burn center except:*
A *>10% TBSA partial thickness burns*
B *Inhalational injury*
C *Electrical injury*
D *Serious chemical injury*
E *6% TBSA partial thickness burn to the back of a previously healthy adult man with a nonoperative scaphoid fracture*

The American Burn Association has established criteria for burn patients who should be acutely transferred to a burn center: >10% TBSA partial thickness burns, any size full thickness burn, burns to special areas of function or cosmesis, inhalational injury including lightning, burns with trauma where burns are the major problem, pediatric burns if the referring hospital has no special pediatric capabilities, and smaller burns in patients with multiple co-morbidities. Patient E meets none of these criteria.

**Answer: E**

American Burn Association (2016) *Burn Center Referral Criteria*, at: www.ameriburn.org/BurnCenterReferralCriteria.pdf (accessed October 23, 2016).

**15** *A 34-year-old man is brought to your emergency department after a house fire. He has a cough productive of carbonaceous sputum and has singed facial hairs and eyebrows. He complains of mild shortness of breath. All of the following have a potential role in the treatment of inhalational injury except:*

A *Early intubation for airway protection*
B *Treatment of bronchospasm with alpha agonists*
C *N-acteylcysteine nebulized treatments*
D *Inhaled steroids*
E *Nebulized heparin*

Inhalational injury can progress very rapidly and the identification of these injuries demands serious consideration of early intubation. Early bronchoscopy provides for diagnosis of inhalational injury, documentation of airway ulceration, and assessment of severity. Both nebulized heparin and *N*-acetylcysteine have been used to break down the casts that form following these injuries. Alpha-agonists are effective in the treatment of associated bronchospasm. Inhaled steroids have not been shown to be of benefit in inhalational injury and should not be given unless the patient is steroid-dependent before injury or has bronchospasm resistant to standard therapy.

**Answer: D**

Sheridan, R.L. (2016) Fire-related inhalation injury. *The New England Journal of Medicine*, **375**, 464–469.

**16** *A 24-year-old woman is struck by lightning during a golf outing. She has burns on her hands and a separate burn on her right thigh. Which of the following is not indicated:*
A *Initial ECG*
B *Fluid hydration to maintain urine output at 1.0 to 1.5 mL/kg/hr*
C *Vigilance for evidence of compartment syndrome*
D *Early detection of myoglobinuria*
E *Empiric use of bicarbonate infusions*

High-voltage injuries with electrical transmission from lightning strikes have serious potential sequelae that must be considered. Initial and delayed cardiac and neurogenic abnormalities are frequent manifestations. Compartment syndromes under areas of unaffected skin can complicate the course, particularly if not recognized early. Subsequent muscle injury from the transmission effects as well as compartment pressure elevations can lead to myoglobinuria and renal failure. Urine output should be maintained at 1.0 to 1.5 mL/kg/hr to minimize the renal effects of myoglobinuria. While bicarbonate and mannitol have been used in attempts at renal protection, hydration alone has proven sufficient in the treatment of myoglobinuria that accompanies the deep muscle necrosis and acidosis in these injuries.

**Answer: E**

Lee, R.C. (1997) Injury by electrical forces: pathophysiology, manifestations, and therapy. *Current Problems in Surgery*, **34** (9), 677–764.

Sheridan, R.L. and Greenhalgh, D. (2014) Special problems in burns. *Surgical Clinics of North America*, **94**, 781–791.

**17** *Central nervous system injury is common in lightning strike victims. These sequelae may be characterized by all of the following except:*
  **A** *Early symptoms followed by universal resolution within hours*
  **B** *Loss of consciousness*
  **C** *Hypoxic ischemic neuropathy*
  **D** *Epidural hematomas due to associated falls*
  **E** *Keraunoparalysis*

Neurologic effects of lightning injuries may be both temporary and permanent. These can be classified into four groups. Group 1 effects are immediate and transient, and are very common. These include loss of consciousness (75%), amnesia, paresthesias (80%), and keraunoparalysis. Keraunoparalysis (Charcot's paralysis) is a neurologic disorder specific to lightning victims which features transient paralysis, often predominantly affecting the lower extremities, and accompanied by loss of sensation; it lasts several hours and then resolves. Group 2 neurologic effects are immediate, prolonged, or permanent in nature. These include hypoxic ischemic neuropathies, intracranial hemorrhage, post-arrest cerebral infarctions, and cerebellar syndromes. Group 3 neurologic effects are possibly delayed syndromes, including motor neuron diseases and movement disorders. Finally, group 4 injuries such as subdural or epidural hematomas occur as a result of associated falls or blasts.

**Answer: A**

Cherington, M. (2003) Neurologic manifestations of lightning strikes. *Neurology*, **60** (2), 182–185.

**18** *The most common cause of death after lighting strikes is:*
  **A** *Flash pulmonary edema*
  **B** *Cardiopulmonary arrest and apnea*
  **C** *Multiorgan failure*
  **D** *Grand mal seizures*
  **E** *Myoglobinuria*

The most common causes of death from lighting injury are cardiopulmonary arrest and apnea. The interruption of normal cardiac conduction by the associated direct current results in asystole, but—like a defibrillator—spontaneous cardiac activity typically resumes shortly thereafter.

The apnea that results from the same direct current is caused by effects on the brain's respiratory center; however, it is longer lasting and—if left untreated—will result in hypoxia, arrhythmias, and secondary cardiac arrest.

**Answer: B**

Davis, C., Engeln, A., Johnson, E., *et al.* (2014) Wilderness medical society practice guidelines for the prevention and treatment of lightning injuries: 2014 update. *Wilderness and Environmental Medicine*, **25**, S86–S95.

**19** *Early burn wound excision and grafting of deep second- and third-degree burns is associated with:*
  **A** *Increased infection rates*
  **B** *Increased blood loss*
  **C** *Improved survival*
  **D** *Increased length of hospital stay*
  **E** *All of the above*

Deep second- and third-degree burns do not heal in a timely fashion without autografting. The persistence of these burned tissues serves as a nidus for inflammation and infection that can lead to sepsis and death. Early excision and grafting of these wounds is now practiced in most burn centers and has been associated with improved survival, decreased blood loss, and shorter hospitalizations.

**Answer: C**

Sheridan, R.L. and Chang, P. (2014) Acute burn procedures. *Surgical Clinics of North America*, **94**, 755–764.

**20** *For a patient with a localized burn to the ear and exposed cartilage, which topical agent is most likely to be beneficial in minimizing the risk of cartilaginous infection?*
  **A** *Silver sulfdiazene*
  **B** *Mafenide acetate*
  **C** *Bacitracin*
  **D** *Topical steroids*
  **E** *All of the above are just as likely to minimize risk*

Mafenide acetate is the best choice for this location, as it has the best eschar or cartilaginous penetration. Silver sulfdiazine, comparatively, has poorer penetration of these tissues. Bacitracin has even less effectiveness in this regard. Steroids are of no benefit in the avoidance of chondritis.

**Answer: B**

Skedros, D.G., Goldfarb, I.W., Slater, H., and Rocco, J. (1992) Chrondritis of the burned ear: a review. *Ear Nose and Throat Journal*, **71** (8), 359–362.

**21** *While working at an industrial site, a worker is sprayed with a strong alkali material on the leg. Which of the following is the best first step in treating this chemical burn?*

A *Application of dry gauze to the site of the chemical burn*

B *Copious irrigation of the wound with tap water*

C *Application of silver sulfadiazine to the site to prevent bacterial superinfection*

D *Immediate operative tangential excision and debridement of the effected tissues*

E *Application of a weak acid to neutralize the alkali*

Alkali compounds cause cellular damage through a variety of mechanisms: saponification of fats allow expeditious deep penetration of the wound, exothermic reaction potentiates the cellular damage due to thermal injury of the tissues, alkali compounds are hygroscopic by nature leading to desiccation of the tissues, and alkali compounds form chemical bonds with proteins (forming water soluble alkali proteinates), which cause liquefactive necrosis of the surrounding tissues as well. As such, limiting the time tissue is exposed to alkali substances is critical to limiting the amount of tissue damaged. Copious irrigation of exposed tissue is the first key step to treating alkali burns.

Application of dry gauze will trap the alkali material on the skin, thus potentiating the burn. Topical antimicrobials are not indicated in the acute phase of managing a chemical burn. Operative debridement of tissues may be indicated after removing the compound and resuscitating the patient; however, it should not be considered first-line therapy. Application of a neutralizing acid—while intuitive from a basic science context—is ill advised in treating alkali burns. Neutralization with acids causes an inherently exothermic reaction which potentiates thermal burns at the site of alkali exposure. Also, there are significant difficulties with titrating an appropriate amount of acid such that the alkali is neutralized but not causing an acidic environment at the site. Moreover, there are significant difficulties with applying the acid to only areas of the body that were exposed to the alkali compound. Application of acid to nonalkali exposed tissues will likely cause an area of an acid burn near the alkaliexposed tissues.

**Answer: B**

Greenwood, J.E., Tan, J.L., Ming, J.C.T., *et al.* (2015) Alkalis and skin. *The Journal of Burn Care and Research*, **37** (2), 135–141.

**22** *A 54-year-old taxidermist presents to the local burn emergency room after spilling a large amount of hydrofluoric acid on his bilateral upper extremities and chest while preparing hides for tanning. Beyond copiously irrigating the wound to remove the offending acid, what is the next step in management of this condition?*

A *Application of dry gauze to the site of the chemical burn*

B *Application of silver mafenide to the site of the burn*

C *Application of topical calcium gluconate gel at the site of the burn*

D *Application of a weak alkali to neutralize the hydrofluoric acid*

E *Immediate operative tangential excision and debridement of the effected tissues*

Acidic compounds cause localized cellular damage at the site of exposure via coagulative necrosis and cell death. Typically, there is less penetration of the acid into the subcutaneous tissues unlike in alkali burns. However, several acid compounds can have more systemic effects that require more intervention than simple irrigation of the tissue and local wound care.

Hydrofluoric acid is a common corrosive used in industrial settings and some trades, such as taxidermy and tanning. Beyond the local tissue damage caused by the acid, the fluoride ions can cause significant systemic pathology. Fluoride acts as a direct chelator of calcium and magnesium ions in the local tissues. This chelation causes local cells to efflux calcium stores thus causing osmotic shifts and cell death locally. Fluoride can also enter the systemic circulation and absorb calcium and magnesium on a systemic level leading to muscle contraction, cellular dysfunction, and ventricular fibrillation. Treatment of this particular acid requires local—and occasionally systemic—administration of calcium gluconate to help chelate the free fluoride ions. Typical administration of local therapy includes applying calcium gluconate gel to the site, injecting subcutaneous calcium gluconate in the effected tissues, and some providers advocate for intraarterial administration of calcium gluconate to effected extremities with extremity burns. Serial chemistry panels and continuous telemetry are necessary for large exposures. Occasionally, hemodialysis may be an adjunct required to clear the free fluoride ions as well.

**Answer: C**

Elija, I.E., Sanford, A.P., and Lee, J.O. (2012) Chemical burns, in *Total Burn Care*, 4th edn (ed. D. Herndon), Chicago, Elsevier, pp. 455–460.

# 44

# Gynecologic Surgery
*K. Aviva Bashan-Gilzenrat, MD*

1 *A 32-year-old woman with history of right ovarian cysts presents to the emergency department with the complaint of sudden onset of intense right-sided pelvic pain; she has never had this type of pain before. She denies fevers, but reports nausea and vomiting. She states that the pain radiates to the right lumbar area. Vital signs are normal. Her abdominal and pelvic exams reveal only focal tenderness in the right lower quadrant. β-human chorionic gonadotropin (HCG) is negative, the urinalysis is normal, and WBC is 8500/ microL. Regarding further evaluation, which of the following is true regarding adnexal torsion?*

A *The patient should undergo immediate laparoscopy*

B *Ultrasound can rule out adnexal torsion*

C *The absence of fever is consistent with the diagnosis*

D *Adnexal torsion rarely occurs on the right, and this diagnosis should not be pursued*

E *CT Scan and MRI provide no useful information with regards to the diagnosis*

Adnexal torsion may involve twisting of the ovary alone, the ovary and fallopian tube together, or the fallopian tube alone. This entity is rare in postmenopausal women. In children and adolescents, the cause is usually increased mobility of the pedicle, while in adult women a cyst is typically the precipitant. Torsion is more likely to occur on the right than the left, as the right-sided utero-ovarian ligament is longer. Some authors speculate that the presence of the sigmoid colon reduces space of the left pelvis, and decreases the likelihood of left sided torsion. Any condition that results in increased adnexal weight is a risk factor for torsion. These include ovarian cysts and tumors, corpus luteum cysts, tubal pregnancies, and hemo and hydrosalpinx. Patients undergoing ovarian stimulation for *in vitro* fertilization are at increased risk. The patients present with sudden onset of intense unilateral pelvic pain, which may radiate to the lumbar area. The pain episodes may be intermittent, if the adnexal structures spontaneously torse and detorse. Nausea and vomiting, but not fevers, are common. Physical examination may reveal the presence of a tender adnexal mass. In a patient with a negative β-HCG, adnexal torsion, pelvic inflammatory disease and even appendicitis remain in the differential. Ultrasound is the next best step, as it may identify pathologic adnexa, abscess, or appendicitis. However, it is specific but not sensitive for adnexal torsion, as pathologic adnexa may be undetected in up to 25% of cases. Doppler investigation of the presence or absence of venous or arterial flow is useful only when the flow is absent; the presence of flow does not rule out partial or intermittent torsion. A CT scan can be helpful in identifying abnormal ovaries and associated findings of loss of fat planes and ascites, but is less useful in determining ischemia. Contrast-enhanced MRI may identify non-enhancement of the ovary consistent with infarction, but this would not be helpful in early torsion. The diagnosis is definitively made with diagnostic laparoscopy. Detorsion is performed, and ischemic or necrotic appearing structures are resected. Oophoropexy is an option if the ovary appears viable.

**Answer: C**

Huchon, C. and Fauconnier, A. (2010) Adnexal torsion: a literature review. *European Journal of Obstetrics and Gynecology and Reproductive Biology*, **150**, 8–12.

McWilliams, G.D.E., Hill, M.J., and Dietrich, C.S. (2008) Gyneco-logic emergencies. *Surgical Clinics of North America*, **88**, 265–283.

Vandermeer, F.Q. and Wong-You-Cheong, J.J. (2009) Imaging of acute pelvic pain. *Clinical Obstetrics and Gynecology*, **52** (1), 2–20.

2 *A 22-year-old woman with past medical history remarkable only for previously treated sexually transmitted disease, presents with a complaint of acute onset of severe pelvic pain. She denies a history of trauma, and states that there is no possibility of pregnancy.*

*Surgical Critical Care and Emergency Surgery: Clinical Questions and Answers*, Second Edition.
Edited by Forrest "Dell" Moore, Peter Rhee, and Gerard J. Fulda.
© 2018 John Wiley & Sons Ltd. Published 2018 by John Wiley & Sons Ltd.
Companion website: www.wiley.com/go/moore/surgical_criticalcare_and_emergency_surgery

*She cannot recall the date of her last menses. On exam, she is mildly hypotensive; her abdomen is soft but moderately distended, and she has nonfocal pain to palpation, without peritoneal signs. Pelvic exam reveals exquisite tenderness to palpation at the left adnexa, but no cervical motion tenderness. Stat labs reveal a positive β-HCG, hemoglobin of 6 gm/dL, and normal urinalysis. Which of the following does not support the diagnosis of ruptured ectopic pregnancy as the cause of this patient's abdominal pain and anemia?*

**A** *Sonographic finding of complex adnexal mass*
**B** *Sonographic finding of echogenic free fluid*
**C** *History of irregular vaginal bleeding*
**D** *History of neck and shoulder pain*
**E** *Absence of intrauterine pregnancy by ultrasound, with quantitative β-HCG of 500 mIU/mL*

Patients with ectopic pregnancy typically present with history of abdominal pain and amenorrhea. Irregular vaginal bleeding may also occur. The presence of rupture is suggested by a history of severe, stabbing pelvic pain. Irritation of the diaphragm by hemoperitoneum may also result in complaint of neck or shoulder pain. Abdominal exam is typically remarkable for ipsilateral pelvic tenderness, and bimanual exam is painful. In a hemodynamically normal patient, the diagnosis is secured with a pregnancy test and transvaginal ultrasound. The first goal of sonography is to identify the presence or absence of an intrauterine pregnancy, and this should be possible if the quantitative β-HCG is 2000 mIU/mL. With levels of β-HCG greater than 1500 mIU/mL (and definitely 800 mIU/mL), an intrauterine gestational sac is typically detected with a normal pregnancy. Absence of an intrauterine pregnancy, along with findings of a complex adnexal mass and echogenic free fluid (blood) supports the diagnosis of ruptured ectopic pregnancy. In austere settings, culdocentesis can be used to make the diagnosis. In this procedure, the posterior lip of the cervix is retracted anteriorly, and a needle is passed parallel to the cervix through the posterior vaginal fornix in order to aspirate the posterior cul-de-sac; the presence of non-clotting blood is consistent with bleeding secondary to ruptured ectopic pregnancy. However, hypotensive patients with (+)β-HCG should be taken directly to the operating room. The decision for laparoscopy versus laparotomy rests on the comfort level of the surgeon. Either salpingostomy (opening of the salpinx), salpingotomy (opening of the salpinx followed by suture closure), or salpingectomy may be performed. Salpingectomy is indicated if needed for hemostasis, if the salpinx has had prior damage, or if the patient does not desire the option of future fertility. Risk factors for ectopic pregnancy include prior episodes of salpingitis, prior tubal surgeries, or history of assisted reproduction.

**Answer: E**

Cunningham, F.G., Leveno, K.J., Bloom, S.L., *et al.* (2005) Ectopic pregnancy, in *Williams Obstetrics*, 22nd edn (ed. F.G. Cunningham), McGraw-Hill, New York, pp. 253–272.

McWilliams, G.D.E., Hill, M.J., and Dietrich, C.S. (2008) Gyneco-logic emergencies. *Surgical Clinics of North America*, **88**, 265–283.

Vandermeer, F.Q. and Wong-You-Cheong, J.J. (2009) Imaging of acute pelvic pain. *Clinical Obstetrics and Gynecology*, **52** (1), 2–20.

**3** *Regarding pelvic inflammatory disease (PID), which of the following is correct?*

**A** *Even mild to moderate PID should be treated on an inpatient basis*
**B** *Transvaginal ultrasound has excellent specificity but poor sensitivity*
**C** *Laparotomy is the gold standard for diagnosis*
**D** *Tubo-ovarian abscess is an indication for immediate surgical intervention*
**E** *Surgery is indicated for tubo-ovarian abscess that fails to respond to medical therapy*

Pelvic inflammatory disease is a polymicrobial infection of the upper genital tract that typically occurs in young women of reproductive age, secondary to sexually transmitted organisms or lower genital tract flora. The symptoms may be gradual in onset, with pelvic pain and fevers being the most prominent complaints. Exam typically reveals an ill-appearing young woman, with abdominal tenderness to palpation, as well as cervical motion tenderness and bilateral adnexal tenderness on pelvic exam. Laboratories reveal leukocytosis. The diagnosis can be difficult, and requires the abdominal and pelvic exam findings, as well as one of the following secondary findings: T 38.3 °C, purulent cervical drainage, elevated erythrocyte sedimentation rate or C-reactive protein, *C. Trachomatis* or *N. Gonorrhoeae* cervical infection, or presence of adnexal mass on sonography. Transvaginal ultrasound has excellent specificity, and can distinguish uncomplicated PID from tubo-ovarian abscess. However, it has poor sensitivity. Oral and IV-contrasted CT scan is useful in the face of an unremarkable ultrasound. It may identify early inflammatory changes as well as delineate the architecture of the complex adnexal masses and fluid collections that comprise tubo-ovarian abscess. An MRI may be a useful alternative in the context of a pregnant patient. (β-HCG should be obtained, as early pregnancy and pelvic inflammatory disease co-exist in 3–4% of patients.)

Laparoscopy is regarded as the gold standard for diagnosis. Patients with mild to moderate disease may be treated as outpatients; coverage should include agents active against *C. trachomatis* and *N. gonorrhoeae*. With the exception of fluoroquinolones (to which there are a growing number of resistant *N. gonorrhoeae* isolates), there are many broad spectrum antibiotic regimens that are effective. One that has been studied extensively for outpatient use is a single intramuscular dose of cefoxitin plus a single dose of oral probenecid plus oral doxycycline for 14 days. Tubo-ovarian abscess is an indication for hospitalization. Patients who fail to respond to medical management may be considered for percutaneous drainage. Surgical intervention is reserved for patients with life-threatening infection, ruptured tubo-ovarian abscess, or symptomatic/recurrent adnexal masses.

**Answer: B**

Eckert, L.O. and Lentz, G.M. (2007) Infections of the upper genital tract, in *Comprehensive Gynecology*, 5th edn (ed. V. Katz), Mosby, Philadelphia PA, pp. 607–632.

Lareau, S.M. and Beigi, R.H. (2008) Pelvic inflammatory disease and tubo-ovarian abscess. *Infectious Disease Clinics of North America*, **22**, 693–708.

McWilliams, G.D.E., Hill, M.J., and Dietrich, C.S. (2008) Gynecologic emergencies. *Surgical Clinics of North America*, **88**, 265–83.

Ness, R.B., Soper, D.E., Holley, R.L., *et al.* (2002) Effectiveness of inpatient and outpatient treatment strategies for women with pelvic inflammatory disease: results from the Pelvic Inflammatory Disease Evaluation and Clinical Health (PEACH) randomized trial. *American Journal of Obstetrics and Gynecology*, **186** (5), 929.

Vandermeer, F.Q. and Wong-You-Cheong, J.J. (2009) Imaging of acute pelvic pain. *Clinical Obstetrics and Gynecology*, **52** (1), 2–20.

*The following vignette applies to questions 4–6:*
A 21-year-old G2P1001 woman at 32 weeks of pregnancy presents to the ER with a 1-day history of umbilical pain pain, moderate nausea and one episode of non-bloody, non-bilious emesis. Vital signs are as follows: temperature 38.4 °C, heart rate 105, blood pressure 100/60, respiratory rate of 16, $O_2$ saturation 99% on room air. Examination is significant for a gravid abdomen with right lower quadrant tenderness. The patient exhibits some guarding with deep palpation, but no rebound tenderness. Laboratory studies are significant for a WBC of 16 400 cells/microL with a left shift, a ß-HCG of 5400 mIU/ml and a normal urinalysis.

**4** *The most appropriate initial imaging study to establish the diagnosis is:*
   **A** *MRI abdomen and pelvis with gadolinium*
   **B** *CT abdomen and pelvis without IV contrast*
   **C** *Ultrasound with Doppler of bilateral ovaries*
   **D** *Ultrasound with graded compression*
   **E** *CT abdomen and pelvis with IV and PO contrast*

The patient's presentation is suggestive of acute appendicitis, which is the most common general surgery problem encountered during pregnancy. The clinical diagnosis should be strongly suspected in pregnant women with classic findings: abdominal pain that migrates to the right lower quadrant, right lower quadrant tenderness, nausea/vomiting, fever, and leukocytosis with left shift. The most appropriate initial imaging technique should be ultrasound with graded compression. Diagnosis of suspected appendicitis is supported by identification of a noncompressible blind-ended tubular structure in the right lower quadrant with a maximal diameter greater than 6 mm. For pregnant women whose ultrasound examination is inconclusive for appendicitis, magnetic resonance imaging (MRI) is the preferred next test as it avoids the ionizing radiation of computed tomography. When MRI is performed in pregnant women, gadolinium is not routinely administered because of theoretical fetal safety concerns, but may be used if essential.

CT scan has the highest fetal ionizing radiation exposure of the three imaging techniques. Modifications to the CT protocol can limit estimated fetal radiation exposure to less than 3 mGy, well below doses known to potentially cause adverse fetal effects (30 mGy for risk of carcinogenesis, 50 mGy for deterministic effects), and do not limit diagnostic performance. Standard abdominal CT scanning with an oral contrast preparation and intravenous contrast or a specialized appendiceal CT scanning protocol can also be used, but are associated with higher fetal radiation exposure (20–40 mGy).

**Answer: D**

Abbasi, N., Patenaude, V., and Abenhaim, H.A. (2014) Management and outcomes of acute appendicitis in pregnancy-population-based study of over 7000 cases. *BJOG: An International Journal of Obstetrics and Gynaecology*, **121** (12), 1509.

Williams, R. and Shaw, J. (2007) Ultrasound scanning in the diagnosis of acute appendicitis in pregnancy. *Emergency Medicine Journal*, **24** (5), 359–360.

**5** *The best treatment for acute unperforated appendicitis in an otherwise healthy woman in the third trimester of her pregnancy is:*

A *Laparoscopic appendectomy*

B *IV antibiotics 48 hours followed by 5 additional days of PO antibiotics alone*

C *IV antibiotics 48 hours followed by 5 additional days of PO antibiotics, followed by interval appendectomy after delivery*

D *Open appendectomy*

E *IV antibiotic therapy for 7 days followed by interval appendectomy after delivery*

The current standard treatment of acute appendicitis is appendectomy. Management with antibiotic therapy alone is currently not recommended because it is associated with both short-term and long-term failure, with minimal data in pregnant patients. Maternal morbidity following appendectomy is comparable to that in non-pregnant women and low, except in patients in whom the appendix has perforated. Importantly, the risk of fetal loss is increased when the appendix perforates (fetal loss 36% versus 1.5% without perforation) or when there is generalized peritonitis or a peritoneal abscess. Laparoscopy can be performed successfully during all trimesters and with few complications although it may be more difficult. Port positioning should take into account fundal height as well as the location of the appendix on imaging.

**Answer: A**

Abbasi, N., Patenaude, V., and Abenhaim, H.A. (2014) Management and outcomes of acute appendicitis in pregnancy-population-based study of over 7000 cases. *BJOG: An International Journal of Obstetrics and Gynaecology*, **121** (12),1509.

Guidelines Committee of the Society of American Gastrointestinal and Endoscopic Surgeons (2008) Guidelines for diagnosis, treatment, and use of laparoscopy for surgical problems during pregnancy. *Surgical Endoscopy*, **22** (4), 849–861.

Mourad, J., Elliott, J.P., Erickson, L., and Lisboa, L. (2000). Appendicitis in pregnancy: new information that contradicts long-held clinical beliefs. *American Journal of Obstetrics and Gynecology*, **182** (5), 1027.

6 *The most recent guidelines for laparoscopic appendectomy in pregnant patients includes which of the following:*

A *Continuous intraoperative fetal monitoring should be utilized*

B *CO₂ insufflation of 15 mm Hg can be safely used*

C *Prophylactic tocolytics should be given preoperatively*

D *Gravid patients should be placed in the right lateral decubitus position*

E *Safe initial abdominal access can only be accomplished with the Hasson technique*

As previously discussed, laparoscopic appendectomy is safe in all trimesters of pregnancy. As long as fundal height and previous incisions are taken into account, Hasson technique, Veress needle and optical trocar are all safe methods of initially accessing the abdomen. With regard to insufflation, pressures of 15 mm Hg have been used in pregnant patients without increasing adverse outcomes to the patient or her fetus. There has not been any literature in support of prophylactic tocolytics; they are appropriate for use in the case of threatened preterm labor. Gravid patients should be positioned in the left lateral decubitus position any time they will need to be supine for any period of time. This serves to decrease compression of the IVC. While intraoperative fetal heart monitoring was once thought to be the most accurate method to detect fetal distress, no intraoperative abnormalities have been reported in the literature. Therefore, the current recommendation for pre- and post-operative monitoring only.

**Answer: B**

Guidelines Committee of the Society of American Gastrointestinal and Endoscopic Surgeons (2008) Guidelines for diagnosis, treatment, and use of laparoscopy for surgical problems during pregnancy. *Surgical Endoscopy*, **22** (4), 849–861.

*The following vignette applies to questions 7–8.*

*A 27-year-old G1P1001 woman is immediately postpartum following caesarian section delivery after an uncomplicated full term pregnancy when she abruptly becomes hypoxic with an oxygen saturation of 67% on pulse oximetry. The patient becomes confused and then unresponsive. She is rapidly transferred to the SICU, intubated and shortly thereafter becomes hypotensive, requiring vasopressors. Transesophageal echocardiography shows elevated pulmonary arterial pressure, and right ventricular failure.*

7 *The established treatment for this clinical entity includes:*

A *High dose hydrocortisone*

B *Plasmapheresis*

C *IVIg administration*

D *Placement of an intra-aortic balloon pump*

E *Supportive therapy only*

There are numerous causes of hypotension, hypoxemia, and/or hemorrhage in women who are pregnant or postpartum. Amniotic fluid embolism syndrome (AFES) is a clinical diagnosis that is based upon the constellation of clinical findings, and it should be considered whenever shock and/or respiratory compromise develops during or immediately postpartum. There is no specific treatment other than supportive therapy. The goal of therapy is to correct hypoxemia and hypotension to avoid ischemic consequences (hypoxic brain injury, acute kidney injury, inadequate fetal oxygen delivery if woman has not yet delivered). There have been case reports of use of nitric oxide, right ventricular assist device with right heart failure, as well as use of extracorporeal membrane oxygenation (ECMO) and intraaortic balloon pump for severe left ventricular failure and hypoxemia.

**Answer: E**

Gist, R.S., Stafford, I.P., Leibowitz, A.B., and Beilin, Y. (2009) Amniotic fluid embolism. *Anesthesia and Analgesia*, **108** (5), 1599.

Knight, M., Tuffnell. D., Brocklehurst, P., *et al.* (2010). Incidence and risk factors for amniotic-fluid embolism. *Obstetrical and Gynecological Survey*, **115** (5), 910.

8 The coagulopathy most commonly associated with amniotic fluid embolism syndrome (AFES) will be demonstrated by:
   A normal PT, normal aPTT, normal platelet count, low plasma fibrinogen
   B prolonged PT, normal aPTT, normal platelet count, low plasma fibrinogen
   C normal PT, prolonged aPTT, normal platelet count, normal plasma fibrinogen
   D prolonged PT and aPTT, thrombocytopenia, low plasma fibrinogen
   E thrombocytopenia alone

As many as 80% of patients with AFES develop disseminated intravascular coagulation (DIC). It can begin as quickly as 10 to 30 minutes after the onset of cardiopulmonary symptoms and signs, or may be delayed by several days. Prolonged bleeding from sites of invasive interventions and bruising are the most common manifestations of DIC. Blood product transfusion, including the transfusion of recombinant factor VIIa, may be required for some patients with coagulopathy or bleeding due to DIC. Laboratory diagnosis of DIC is based on findings of coagulopathy and/or fibrinolysis. Findings such as thrombocytopenia, low fibrinogen, and elevated D-dimer are relatively sensitive for the diagnosis.

**Answer: D**

Gist, R.S., Stafford, I.P., Leibowitz, A.B., and Beilin, Y. (2009) Amniotic fluid embolism. *Anesthesia and Analgesia*, **108** (5), 1599.

*The following vignette applies to questions 9-10.*

*A 17-year-old G2P1001 woman at 39 weeks of pregnancy presents to the ER after being assaulted with fists to the face and abdomen, as well as a scald burn with hot water to the abdomen. Primary survey is intact, Glasgow Coma Scale is 15, and vital signs are only significant for a heart rate of 115 beats/minute. Secondary survey reveals right periorbital ecchymosis and a 6% TBSA superficial partial thickness burn to the patient's gravid abdomen.*

9 Which of the following regarding intimate partner violence (IPV) and pregnancy is true?
   A 2% of all pregnancies in the United States are complicated by physical abuse
   B Abused pregnant women have a threefold increased risk of being the victim of attempted or completed homicide
   C Acute UTI, but not pyelonephritis, occurs with higher likelihood in abused pregnant patients
   D IPV in pregnancy is associated with increased risk of macrosomia
   E Hypertension occurs with lower likelihood in abused pregnant patients

Intimate partner violence (IPV) often begins or escalates during pregnancy. Risk factors include being a young female, alcohol or drug use, being less educated, and family history or prior exposure to violence. A US national survey found that between 4 and 8% of pregnant women reported being abused at least once during the pregnancy, and abused pregnant women have a threefold higher risk of being victims of attempted/completed homicide. IPV is associated with a number of pregnancy complications: UTI, pyelonephritis, hypertension, vaginal bleeding, severe nausea and vomiting, and preterm labor. The fetus is at increased risk of preterm delivery, low birth weight, and requiring ICU care. Abruption, fetal fractures, premature labor, and perinatal death have also been associated with IPV.

**Answer: B**

Tjaden, P. and Thoennes, N. (2005) *Full report of the prevalence, incidence, and consequences of violence against women: findings from the National Violence Against Women Survey.* Publication no. NCJ-183781, US Department of Justice, Washington, DC.

Wallace, M.E., Hoyert, D., Williams, C., and Mendola, P. (2016) Pregnancy-associated homicide and suicide in 37 US states with enhanced pregnancy surveillance. *American Journal of Obstetrics and Gynecology*, **215** (3), 364.

**10** Which of the following treatments should not be used
   for the patient's scald burn?
   **A** Silver sulfadiazine
   **B** Silver nitrate
   **C** Bacitracin
   **D** Mafenide
   **E** Mupirocin

Given that the burn is superficial partial thickness in
nature, it will likely heal without tangential excision and
skin grafting. However, the patient will require dressing
changes with topical antimicrobial therapy to reduce
the incidence of infection. Although these medications
are applied topically, it is important to consider that
they may be absorbed and circulate systemically. These
topical antibiotics are all used in pregnancy with the
exception of silver sulfadiazine, which can cause hyper-
bilirubinemia and kernicterus. Silver sulfadiazine is
therefore contraindicated for use near-term, on premature infants, or on newborn infants during the first 2
months of life.

**Answer: A**

Wasiak, J., Cleland, H., and Campbell, F. (2008). Dressings
   for superficial and partial thickness burns. *Cochrane
   Database of Systematic Reviews*, **8** (4)

*The following vignette applies to questions 11-12.*

*An unknown age woman is brought emergently to the
trauma bay after involvement in a high speed motor vehicle collision. On arrival, primary survey is intact and
vital signs include a heart rate of 137 beats/min, a manual blood pressure of 84/43 mm Hg, a respiratory rate of
30 breaths/min and a pulse oximetry of 93%. Glasgow
coma scale is 14. The patient is complaining of severe
abdominal pain. Secondary survey reveals a 5 cm forehead laceration, left periorbital ecchymosis, a gravid
abdomen that is rigid with a fundal height about 8 cm
above the umbilicus, transverse lower abdominal ecchymosis in a lap belt pattern, and right calf deformity.*

**11** Which of the following is true regarding this patient's
   initial assessment and treatment?
   **A** Trauma patients should not be placed in the left lat-
      eral decubitus position due to risk of spinal injury
   **B** Blood transfusion should be deferred in favor of
      crystalloid resuscitation in pregnant patients
   **C** CT scans should be deferred in favor of MRI to
      limit radiation exposure to the fetus
   **D** Maternal oxygen saturation should be main-
      tained at > 95% for optimal fetal oxygen delivery
   **E** Tachycardia and hypotension develop after 10%
      total blood volume loss in pregnancy

Approach to evaluation and management of trauma in
pregnant women is dictated by its severity and influenced by the gestational age. Gestational age can be
estimated by location of the uterine fundus: if below the
umbilicus, gestation is likely less than 20 weeks, if
above, then it is likely greater than 20 weeks. If the
gestational age is greater than 20 weeks, the patient
should be placed in the left lateral decubitus position to
decrease compression of the vena cava. If spine precautions must be maintained, this can be accomplished
by placing a wedge to achieve a 30 degree tilt. If transfusion is indicated, transfusion protocols and targets
are similar to those in non-pregnant individuals, with
the exception of a target fibrinogen of >200 (pregnant
women have higher fibrinogen levels at baseline). Any
diagnostic test of treatment that is required to save the
mother's life should be undertaken, as in most cases
morbidity to the surviving fetus is related to the consequences of maternal trauma. When techniques involving
ionizing radiation are required, the information
obtained nearly always outweighs the radiation risk to
the fetus since fetal radiation exposure from diagnostic
studies is generally small. One of the physiologic changes
of pregnancy is hypervolemia, therefore substantial
changes in vital signs may not occur until 15–20% of
total blood volume loss.

**Answer: D**

Brown, H.L. (2009) Trauma in pregnancy. *Obstetrics and
   Gynecology*, **114** (1), 147–160.
Schiff, M.A. and Holt, V.L. (2005). Pregnancy outcomes
   following hospitalization for motor vehicle crashes in
   Washington State from 1989 to 2001. *American Journal
   of Epidemiology*, **161** (6), 503.

*Two large bore peripheral IVs are placed and fluid
resuscitation is initiated. Shortly thereafter, the patient's
oxygen saturation drops, she becomes bradycardic and
then asystolic. CPR is initiated immediately and epinephrine is given.*

**12** Which of the following is true regarding CPR and
   emergent caesarean section in this situation?
   **A** Emergent caesarean section has been shown to
      improve fetal, but not maternal, mortality
   **B** Optimal survival is obtained when the fetus is deliv-
      ered within 15 minutes of maternal cardiac arrest
   **C** Caesarean delivery should be initiated within 4
      minutes of maternal cardiac arrest
   **D** External chest compression efficacy is reduced due
      to increased chest compliance in pregnancy
   **E** Emergent caesarean section should not be under-
      taken if the fetus is at the limit of viability

CPR is more difficult during pregnancy for several reasons. There is reduced chest compliance, which makes external chest compressions more difficult and potentially less efficacious. In addition, there is significant aortocaval compression in the supine position by the uterus in late pregnancy, which significantly reduces cardiac output. Given these facts, delivery increases the effectiveness of CPR and can save a mother's life, even if the fetus will not benefit due to early gestational age. Optimal maternal and newborn survival is achieved when caesarean is initiated within 4 minutes of maternal cardiac arrest and the fetus is delivered within 5 minutes of unsuccessful CPR. Fetal survival falls to 5% after 15 minutes of unsuccessful CPR.

**Answer: C**

Katz, V., Balderston, K., and DeFreest, M. (2005) Perimortem cesarean delivery: were our assumptions correct? *American Journal of Obstetrics and Gynecology*, **192** (6), 1916.

# 45

## Cardiovascular and Thoracic Surgery
*Jonathan Nguyen, DO and Bryan C. Morse, MS, MD*

1 *A 63-year-old woman is admitted to the surgical intensive care unit with acute respiratory failure two days after total hip arthroplasty. On admission, the patient is intubated and sedated with a paO$_2$ of 180 mm Hg on 100% FiO$_2$. She requires infusions of dopamine (10 µg/kg/min) and norepinephrine (20 µg/min) to maintain adequate hemodynamics. A bedside echocardiogram reveals moderate-to-severe-right ventricular dysfunction, moderately depressed left ventricular function and no obvious intracardiac thrombus. In addition to anticoagulation, which of the following interventions would be appropriate for this patient?*
   A *Surgical or transvenous pulmonary embolectomy*
   B *Anticoagulation alone*
   C *Systemic intravenous thrombolytic therapy*
   D *Venovenous extracorporeal membrane oxygenation (ECMO)*
   E *Anticoagulation and IVC filter placement*

Immediate and aggressive anticoagulation with either intravenous unfractionated heparin or subcutaneous low-molecular-weight heparin is the mainstay of treatment for acute pulmonary embolism. By accelerating the action of circulating antithrombin III, heparin permits more rapid endogenous thrombolysis and retards the propagation of pulmonary arterial thrombus.

When associated with significant hemodynamic compromise, acute pulmonary embolism (PE) carries a mortality rate more than 50%. Accordingly, more aggressive treatment with thrombolytic therapy or surgical embolectomy should be considered for any patient with massive PE presenting in shock. There are no large-scale prospective studies demonstrating a mortality benefit for either of these modalities compared to anticoagulation alone. However, evidence from numerous case series and the high historical mortality in patients with acute PE and hypotension have led to a consensus that anticoagulation

alone is not the optimal treatment for this small subset of patients. The use of surgical embolectomy or thrombolytics for PE patients with right ventricular dysfunction in the absence of hemodynamic instability is not well established, although these modalities may improve outcome.

The choice between thrombolysis and surgical embolectomy is controversial and often driven by institutional resources and experience. However, systemic thrombolytics are contraindicated in the setting of recent major surgery or trauma and thrombolytics introduce a significant risk of intracranial hemorrhage or other bleeding complications even in the absence of a known contraindication. Patients receiving heparin plus systemic thrombolytics have been shown to have a higher risk of intracranial and non-intracranial bleeding when compared to heparin alone. More recently, catheter-based embolectomy has been reported for PE with encouraging results.

The current patient presents with a massive pulmonary embolism (Figure 45.1) and hemodynamic instability after adequate resuscitation. Her recent major orthopedic operation represents a contraindication to systemic thrombolytic treatment. If available, surgical embolectomy is indicated on an emergent basis. Percutaneous catheter-direct embolectomy would be a reasonable alternative treatment, although less well established. Importantly, surgical embolectomy is only appropriate for patients such as this with a large central thromboembolic burden. When not contraindicated, thrombolysis may have a relative advantage over embolectomy in patients with more distal or diffuse embolization.

Extracorporeal membrane oxygenation may be appropriate in select patients with massive PE and shock, with reports of its successful use as a temporary stabilizing measure to allow more definitive treatment or as a bridge to recovery by maintaining oxygenation and perfusion and unloading the right ventricle during the period of native thrombolysis. However, ECMO support for the present patient would require venoarterial rather

*Surgical Critical Care and Emergency Surgery: Clinical Questions and Answers*, Second Edition.
Edited by Forrest "Dell" Moore, Peter Rhee, and Gerard J. Fulda.
© 2018 John Wiley & Sons Ltd. Published 2018 by John Wiley & Sons Ltd.
Companion website: www.wiley.com/go/moore/surgical_criticalcare_and_emergency_surgery

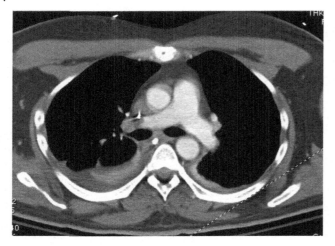

**Figure 45.1** Large right pulmonary embolus on CT scan.

than venovenous circuitry. Venovenous ECMO would allow for better oxygenation but would not address this patient's hemodynamic compromise.

**Answer: A**

Buller, H.R., Agnelli, G., Hull, R.D., *et al.* (2004) Antithrombotic therapy for venous thromboembolic disease: the seventh ACCP conference on antithrombotic and thrombolytic therapy. *Chest*, **126**, 401S–428S.

Kucher, N. (2007) Catheter embolectomy for acute pulmonary embolism. *Chest*, **132**, 657–663.

Meyer, E., Vicaut, E., Danays, T., et al. (2014) Fibrinolysis for patients with Intermediate Risk Pulmonary Embolism. *New England Journal of Medicine*, **370**, 1402–1411.

**2** *A 64-year-old diabetic, hypertensive man, was admitted to the hospital with an acute ST-elevation myocardial infarction (STEMI) after emergent angioplasty and stent placement. He is being treated with aspirin, clopidogrel, and subcutaneous low-molecular-weight heparin. On the third hospital day, the patient develops sudden hypotension associated with acute pulmonary edema and respiratory failure. Physical examination reveals distended neck veins, pulmonary rales, and a previously undetected prominent systolic murmur. Which of the following is/are a likely explanation for this patient's sudden hemodynamic compromise?*

**A** *Ventricular free wall rupture with cardiac tamponade*
**B** *Atrial septal rupture*
**C** *Papillary muscle rupture with acute mitral regurgitation*
**D** *Acute stent thrombosis*
**E** *Stent migration*

Mechanical complications after acute myocardial infarction include papillary muscle rupture, ventricular septal rupture, and ventricular free wall rupture. The majority of patients with post-infarct mechanical complications present within two weeks of an ST-elevation myocardial infarction in the setting of anatomically limited coronary artery disease with inadequate collateral blood flow. All of these complications must be considered in any post-infarct patient presenting with new hypotension or shock, as all three mandate urgent surgical correction.

Ventricular free-wall rupture is the most common mechanical complication of acute myocardial infarction and typically results in immediate death. In some cases, a controlled state of tamponade may ensue allowing time for emergent surgical repair. Although a patient with contained ventricular rupture and cardiac tamponade could certainly present with new hypotension and distended neck veins, pulmonary rales and a prominent systolic murmur are not typical features of patients with tamponade.

Papillary muscle rupture typically occurs in association with an inferior myocardial infarction. Because of its acute nature, the severe mitral regurgitation seen after papillary muscle rupture is generally associated with fulminant heart failure and pulmonary edema. As opposed to atrial septal rupture, which does not occur in this setting, ventricular septal rupture after myocardial infarction results in an acute left-to-right intracardiac shunt with associated pulmonary vascular congestion and a variable degree of systemic hypoperfusion. It is associated with a new pansystolic murmur in the majority of cases.

Although acute thrombosis is a known complication of coronary stent placement and could manifest as sudden, severe left ventricular dysfunction, this would be a highly unlikely event within the first several days of stenting, particularly in a fully anticoagulated patient.

**Answer: C**

Reeder, S. (1995) Identification and treatment of complications of myocardial infarction. *Mayo Clinic Proceedings*, **70**, 880–884.

**3** *A 74-year-old man was admitted to the intensive care unit for unstable angina and left main coronary artery stenosis. He is presently pain-free and hemodynamically stable with an intra-aortic balloon pump (IABP) in place via a right femoral arterial sheath. The patient is awaiting planned coronary artery bypass. After the patient complains of new pain in his right foot, your physical examination reveals absent right pedal pulses with an otherwise stable neurovascular examination. Appropriate intervention(s) at this point would include which of the following?*

**A** *Reduction from 1:1 to 1:2 IABP pulsation*
**B** *IABP removal and replacement in the left leg*
**C** *Downsizing of IABP*
**D** *Leave IABP in place and schedule emergent coronary artery bypass*
**E** *IABP removal and immediate four-compartment fasciotomy*

Limb ischemia is the most common complication of IABP counterpulsation and is associated with significant morbidity and mortality. Other less common complications of IABP use include bleeding, paraplegia, and arterial dissection.

All patients undergoing IABP treatment must be assessed with frequent neurovascular examinations. Any significant distal pulse deficit necessitates immediate balloon pump removal. If IABP removal does not restore adequate distal perfusion, emergent bidirectional thromboembolectomy or even bypass is indicated. Concomitant arterial bypass and/or limb fasciotomy may be indicated in selected cases.

Reducing the rate of IABP counterpulsation would have no effect on distal limb ischemia and is not indicated in this case. In the above clinical scenario, immediate IABP removal is indicated. If continued IABP therapy is absolutely required, the balloon pump may be placed via the contralateral femoral artery. Fasciotomy is not indicated in the absence of clinical evidence of lower extremity compartment syndrome. Emergent coronary bypass in this stable patient would be inappropriate without first addressing his acute limb ischemia.

**Answer: B**

Arafa, O.E., Pedersen, T.H., Svennevig, J.L., *et al.* (1999) Vascular complications of the intraaortic balloon pump in patients undergoing open heart operations: a 15-year experience. *Annals of Thoracic Surgery*, **67** (3), 645–651.

Severi, L., Vaccaro, P., Covotta, M., *et al.* (2012) Severe intra-aortic balloon pump complications: a single center 12 year experience. *Journal of Cardiothoracic and Vascular Anesthesia*, **26** (4), 604–607.

4 *A 64-year-old man underwent right pneumonectomy for non-small cell lung carcinoma five days earlier suddenly develops respiratory distress associated with severe tachypnea and copious frothy pink respiratory secretions. Which of the following interventions represent(s) appropriate initial treatment?*
  **A** *Placement of a large-bore right tube thoracostomy to 20 cm $H_2O$ suction*
  **B** *Tracheostomy*

**C** *Immediate reoperation*
**D** *Immediate CT scan of the chest*
**E** *Placement of a large-bore right tube thoracostomy to water seal*

The above description is the classic presentation for acute bronchopleural fistula (BPF) after lung resection, which occurs most frequently after right pneumonectomy. BPF after pneumonectomy indicates a loss of bronchial stump integrity. Although this is an uncommon complication, it carries a mortality more than 30% and demands immediate recognition and treatment.

The greatest immediate risk in a patient with early BPF after pneumonectomy is soilage of the remaining lung and subsequent aspiration pneumonia or acute lung injury. Initial treatment is therefore predicated upon immediate drainage of the affected pleural space and protection of the contralateral lung by way of either postural maneuvers or endotracheal intubation (ideally with the cuff distal to the affected bronchial stump). A tube thoracostomy after pneumonectomy should not be placed to suction until the mediastinum has stabilized (typically at about two weeks). The use of suction before mediastinal stabilization may result in mediastinal herniation and acute hemodynamic compromise. Immediate tube thoracostomy is indicated in the patient above, but the tube should be placed to water seal rather than suction.

After these initial measures and the initiation of broad-spectrum antibiotic therapy, bronchoscopy is performed to evaluate the degree of bronchial stump disruption and to plan appropriate treatment. In some instances, fibrin glue may now be used endoscopically to seal the defect. Although CT scan may be a useful diagnostic adjunct in these patients after initial evaluation and treatment, it has no role in the acute setting. Reoperation with reinforced closure of the fistula is likely the treatment of choice for early BPF after pneumonectomy, but should not be performed until the immediate risk of aspiration has been addressed, and the patient adequately stabilized.

**Answer: E**

Darling, G.E., Abdurahman, A., Yi, Q-L., *et al.* (2005) Risk of a right pneumonectomy: role of bronchopleural fistula. *Annals of Thoracic Surgery*, **79**, 433–437.

Fuso L, *et al.* (2016). Incidence and management of post lobectomy and pneumonectomy bronchopleural fistula. *Lung*, **194** (2), 299–305.

Puskas, J.D., Mathisen, D.J., Grillo, H.C., *et al.* (1995) Treatment strategies for bronchopleural fistula. *Journal of Thoracic Cardiovascular Surgery*, **109**, 989–995.

**5** *A 44-year-old man with longstanding hypertension presents to the ED with acute chest pain. CXR reveals a markedly widened mediastinum and CT scan of the chest reveals an acute aortic dissection. The cardiac surgical team is en route for planned emergent operative repair. The patient presently has a heart rate of 96 beats/min with a systolic blood pressure of 86 mm Hg. Plausible explanations for this patient's hypotension include all of the following except:*

**A** *Cardiac tamponade*

**B** *Acute coronary occlusion*

**C** *Free thoracic aortic rupture*

**D** *Acute aortic valve insufficiency*

**E** *Proximal propagation of aortic dissection*

As patients with acute aortic dissection typically present with hypertension and tachycardia, the finding of hypotension in a patient with known aortic dissection is highly suggestive of a secondary complication. Proximal propagation of an aortic dissection may lead to hemopericardium with cardiac tamponade, coronary ostial disruption with myocardial ischemia, or aortic annular dilatation with valvular insufficiency and associated malperfusion. All three of these scenarios are plausible explanations for hypotension in the above patient. Free thoracic aortic rupture would normally lead to immediate exsanguination and death.

**Answer: C**

Nienaber, C.A. and Eagle, K.A. (2003) Aortic dissection: new frontiers in diagnosis and management; part II: therapeutic management and follow-up. *Circulation*, **108**, 772–778.

Reece, T.B., Green, G.R., and Kron, I.L. (2008) Aortic dissection, in *Cardiac Surgery in the Adult*, 3rd edn (ed. L. Cohn), McGraw-Hill, New York, pp. 1195–222.

**6** *A 60-year-old woman is admitted to the intensive care unit with an acute dissection limited to the descending thoracic aorta. Her admission blood pressure is 185/110 mm Hg with a heart rate of 110 beats/min. There is no evidence of end-organ malperfusion. Which of the following would constitute appropriate management?*

**A** *Immediate operative repair*

**B** *Initial blood pressure control with intravenous sodium nitroprusside infusion alone*

**C** *Initial blood pressure control with intravenous esmolol infusion alone*

**D** *Heart rate control with intravenous infusions of amiodarone*

**E** *Initial blood pressure control with nitroglycerine*

Patients with acute aortic dissection limited to the descending thoracic aorta ("Stanford" Type B, "DeBakey" Type III) are treated non-surgically in the absence of rupture, malperfusion, or refractory pain. The mainstay of medical treatment for these patients is strict control of blood pressure and heart rate to reduce aortic sheer forces and minimize the risk of propagation or rupture. Beta-blockers or calcium channel blockers are the appropriate initial therapy (in addition to intravenous narcotics), with the addition of vasodilatory agents such as sodium nitroprusside for patients with persistent hypertension. The use of a pure vasodilator alone in patients with acute aortic dissection may lead to an increase in the rate of rise of aortic pressure with a concomitant increase in aortic shear stress. An infusion of nitroprusside alone would therefore not be an appropriate therapy in this patient.

**Answer: C**

Nienaber, C.A. and Eagle, K.A. (2003) Aortic dissection: new frontiers in diagnosis and management; part II: therapeutic management and follow-up. *Circulation*, **108**, 772–778.

Reece, T.B., Green, G.R., and Kron, I.L. (2008) Aortic dissection, in *Cardiac Surgery in the Adult*, 3rd edn (ed. L. Cohn), McGraw-Hill, New York, pp. 1195–1222.

**7** *A 48-year-old woman develops new relative hypotension, oliguria and dyspnea two days after aortic valve replacement with a mechanical valve. Bedside echocardiography reveals a large pericardial effusion. Which of the following measures would constitute appropriate treatment?*

**A** *Urgent bedside subxiphoid pericardial window*

**B** *Image-guided catheter drainage of the pericardium*

**C** *Urgent reoperation*

**D** *Aggressive diuresis*

**E** *NSAIDs*

Cardiac tamponade must be an immediate consideration in any patient with malperfusion after cardiac surgery. The risk of tamponade is increased in patients on anticoagulant medications. Her echocardiogram depicts a large pericardial effusion, confirming this diagnosis. When diagnosed and treated promptly, postoperative cardiac tamponade should not significantly affect mortality.

Early tamponade (within the first several days of surgery) is generally indicative of a surgical source of bleeding and is best addressed with an urgent reoperation. Bedside drainage would be ill-advised in a patient with early postoperative tamponade as drainage of the effusion in such patients often leads to profound hemodynamic derangement and one must be prepared to address immediately the source of bleeding. In patients with profound hemodynamic collapse or if an operating theater is not immediately available, a bedside reoperation is a treatment option. However, this operation would be approached by reopening the patient's sternotomy rather than via a subxiphoid incision.

Image-guided catheter drainage is likely the treatment of choice for patients with delayed pericardial effusion after cardiac surgery but is not indicated for early postoperative tamponade. Diuretics have no role in the treatment of patients with postoperative tamponade.

**Answer: C**

Kuvin, J.T., Harati, N.A., Pandian, N.G., *et al.* (2002) Postoperative cardiac tamponade in the modern surgical era. *Annals of Thoracic Surgery*, **74**, 1148–1153.

Mangi, A.A., Palacios, I.F., and Torchiana, D.F. (2002) Catheter pericardiocentesis for delayed tamponade after cardiac valve operation. *Annals of Thoracic Surgery*, **73** (5), 1479–1483.

**8** *A 22-year-old otherwise healthy man is admitted to the intensive care unit with chest pain, dyspnea, and a CT scan that reveals a large anterior mediastinal mass with >50% tracheal compression. After a non-diagnostic CT-guided core biopsy, a surgical biopsy is planned. Which of the following would be appropriate anesthetic strategies for this operation?*

**A** *Conventional general anesthesia with the use of inhaled agent and intravenous neuromuscular blockade*

**B** *Local anesthesia with intravenous sedation*

**C** *Anesthesia with neuromuscular blockers and intravenous sedation*

**D** *Definitive resection using adjunctive cardiopulmonary bypass*

**E** *Definitive resection using left-heart bypass*

In patients with anterior mediastinal masses, a tissue diagnosis is essential before resection, as lymphoma and most germ-cell tumors are not optimally treated with primary resection. Pre-treatment of patients with massive anterior mediastinal masses with steroids, empiric radiotherapy or chemotherapy may alleviate airway obstruction but may also adversely affect the accuracy of subsequent tissue diagnosis. The risks of anesthesia in patients with anterior mediastinal masses can be estimated based on the presence of symptoms such as stridor, dyspnea at rest, or dyspnea in the recumbent position. Airway compression of greater than 50% on CT imaging also indicated an increased risk of airway obstruction during general anesthesia.

Muscular relaxation causes loss of chest wall tone and reduces the external support of narrowed airways. Therefore, most advocate the maintenance of spontaneous respiration and the avoidance of muscular relaxation during general anesthesia in patients with large anterior mediastinal masses. Conventional general anesthesia in the upright position followed by rigid bronchoscopy to maintain airway patency has also been advocated for these patients, although this is probably a more appropriate approach in patients for whom definitive resection rather than biopsy is planned.

Wherever possible, biopsy for large anterior mediastinal masses should be attempted under local anesthetic with intravenous sedation. Anterior mediastinotomy and biopsy for the patient above could likely be performed in this manner. If general anesthesia was felt to be required, it would optimally be performed under spontaneous ventilation without the use of paralytics. Cardiopulmonary bypass may be indicated for extreme cases in patients with massive anterior mediastinal masses, but resection of this mass without prior tissue diagnosis would not be an appropriate therapeutic strategy.

**Answer: B**

Goh, M.H. and Goh, Y.S. (1999) Anterior mediastinal masses: an anaesthetic challenge. *Anaesthesia*, **54**, 670–672.

Gothard, J.W.W. (2008) Anesthetic considerations for patients with anterior mediastinal masses. *Anesthesiology Clinics*, **26**, 305–314.

**9** *A 44-year-old man with known metastatic small-cell lung cancer is admitted to the intensive care unit with worsening hemoptysis. He has expectorated approximately 400 mL of blood over the past six hours. He was mildly hypotensive on presentation but stabilized with intravenous resuscitation. Which of the following would constitute appropriate therapeutic considerations at this time?*

**A** *Emergent rigid and flexible bronchoscopy in the operating room*

**B** *Emergent bronchial artery embolization (BAE)*

**C** *Immediate tracheostomy*

**D** *Immediate bedside flexible bronchoscopy*

**E** *Thoracotomy for lung resection*

The definition of "massive" hemoptysis varies in the literature, but hemoptysis of greater than 600 mL in 24 hours is a widely accepted criterion. Certainly, any patient presenting with hemoptysis and associated hypotension meets the criteria of massive hemoptysis, which is associated with a mortality rate of 25–50%.

Patients with massive hemoptysis typically die of asphyxiation rather than exsanguination. Airway control is therefore of paramount importance, and endotracheal intubation would be appropriate in the case above. If the source of hemoptysis is known a double-lumen endotracheal tube or bronchial blocker may be useful for temporary isolation of the bleeding source.

Bronchoscopy is indicated in all patients with hemoptysis to localize the source of bleeding and for local control. In all but the most unstable patients, bronchoscopy should be preceded by chest imaging to aid in the identification of a bleeding source. For patients with massive hemoptysis, rigid bronchoscopy is the initial procedure of choice as it allows greater suctioning ability and maintenance of airway patency compared to flexible bronchoscopy. After placement of a rigid bronchoscope (through which ventilation may be maintained), the flexible scope can be introduced to assess the more distal airways as needed. Bedside flexible bronchoscopy is not an appropriate initial procedure for a patient with massive hemoptysis. After a bleeding source is localized by rigid bronchoscopy, bleeding can often be controlled with a combination of mechanical tamponade or dilute epinephrine injection.

Bronchial artery embolization (BAE) is highly effective in the initial management of hemoptysis with control rates consistently greater than 80%. It is not indicated or effective when the source of bleeding is not from the bronchial circulation. For patients with massive hemoptysis with a known resectable source and suitable reserve, surgical resection is likely the treatment of choice, although surgery may optimally be delayed until the patient has been stabilized and airway patency ensured. Surgery would not be appropriate in a patient with a known terminal malignancy unless all available nonsurgical means for control had been exhausted.

**Answer: A**

Ayed, A. (2003) Pulmonary resection for massive hemoptysis of benign etiology. *European Journal of Thoracic Surgery*, **24**, 689–693.

Endo, S., Otani, S., Saito, N., *et al.* (2003) Management of massive hemoptysis in a thoracic surgical unit. *European Journal of Thoracic Surgery*, **23** (4), 467–472.

Jean-Baptiste, E. (2000) Clinical assessment and management of massive hemoptysis. *Critical Care Medicine*, **28**, 1642–1647.

Shigemura, N., Wan, I.Y., Yu, S.C.H., *et al.* (2008) Multidisciplinary management of life-threatening massive hemoptysis: a 10-year experience. *Annals of Thoracic Surgery*, **87**, 849–853.

**10** *A 19-year-old man is brought to the trauma bay after sustaining a gunshot wound to the right chest just lateral to the sternal border. Chest radiograph shows a large right hemothorax. A thoracostomy tube is placed on the right with the return of 1600 mL of blood. The patient is taken to the operating room, and a right lateral thoracotomy is performed. A through-and-through injury is noted in the right upper lobe with continued hemorrhage from both wounds. Which of the following is the next best step to control the pulmonary hemorrhage?*

**A** *Close each lung wound with absorbable sutures*

**B** *Right pneumonectomy*

**C** *Right upper lobectomy*

**D** *Right pulmonary tractotomy and ligation of bleeding vessels*

**E** *Gain venous access for cardiopulmonary bypass*

Damage control strategies have been demonstrated to improve survival by stemming the untoward effects of the lethal triad. Several operative techniques have been described for damage control thoracotomy to control hemorrhage and decrease operative time and transfusion requirements, as well as improving survival. Stapled pneumonectomy in trauma is indicated when there is an irreparable main bronchus injury with significant intraoperative hemodynamic instability. Although trauma pneumonectomy is a last-resort procedure, simultaneously stapled pneumonectomy may potentially improve outcomes. Lobectomy can be performed if there is a destructive injury isolated to one lobe. Pulmonary tractotomy (pulmonotomy) is the most commonly utilized damage control technique in the chest. Indications for lung-sparing pulmonary tractotomy are penetrating or blunt through-and-through pulmonary parenchymal injury that does not involve the hilar structures. Cardiopulmonary bypass is rarely necessary for management of lung injury and is not indicated in this case.

**Answer: D**

Roberts, D.J., Bobrovitz, N., Zygun, D.A., *et al.* (2015). Indications for use of thoracic, abdominal, pelvic, and vascular damage control interventions in trauma patients: A content analysis and expert appropriateness rating study. *Journal of Trauma and Acute Care Surgery*, **79** (4), 568–579.

Garcia, A., Martinez, J., Rodriguez., J, *et al.* (2015). Damage-control techniques in the management of severe lung trauma. *Journal of Trauma and Acute Care Surgery*, **78** (1), 45–51.

**11** *A 35-year-old woman with metastatic renal cell cancer presents with worsening dyspnea and CXR* *with complete opacification of the left chest. A left tube thoracostomy is placed with the immediate drainage of two liters of straw-colored pleural fluid. During preparations to replace the patient's full pleural drainage chamber for continued chest tube output, the patient develops a refractory cough, worsening tachypnea and the expectoration of copious frothy white sputum. Which of the following constitute appropriate maneuvers at this time?*

**A** *Immediately clamping the patient's chest tube*
**B** *Placement of a second left chest tube*
**C** *Replacement of the patient's pleural drainage chamber and continued suction evacuation*
**D** *Intravenous fluid challenge*
**E** *None of the above*

Re-expansion pulmonary edema (RPE) is a rare complication from drainage of a large pleural effusion but is associated with mortality as high as 20%. It may occur with lung re-expansion after pneumothorax in addition to after the drainage of a large pleural effusion, and patients with a longstanding effusion are likely at higher risk. Although expert consensus suggests limiting drainage in one setting to 1L to avoid this complication or the monitoring of pleural pressures during drainage, there is little scientific evidence to support the efficacy of these practices in reducing the risks of RPE.

Patients with RPE may experience dyspnea, pain, cough with or without pink/foamy sputum or cyanosis. Symptoms typically occur within the first two hours of lung expansion but may be delayed by as many as 24–48 hours.

The mainstay of therapy for RPE is mainly supportive and short lived. Treatment includes supplemental oxygen, a low threshold for mechanical ventilation with positive end-expiratory pressure, diuresis, and hemodynamic support as needed. For this patient with RPE, drainage of her pleural effusion should be immediately halted with the institution of supplemental oxygen, intravenous diuretic therapy, and airway/hemodynamic support as needed. Placing an additional chest tube would have no effect on this complication.

**Answer: A**

Feller-Kopman, D., Berkowitz, D., Boiselle, P., and Ernst, A. (2007) Large-volume thoracentesis and the risk of reexpansion pulmonary edema. *Annals of Thoracic Surgery*, **84**, 1656–1662.
Mahfood, S., Hix, W.R., Aaroon, B.L., *et al.* (1997) Reexpansion pulmonary edema. *Annals of Thoracic Surgery*, **63**, 1206–1027.

**12** *A 22-year-old man with multi-organ injury and paraplegia due to a high-speed motor vehicle accident underwent tracheostomy ten days ago. You are called to the bedside because of a report of bright red blood from the tracheostomy site and tube but are unable to detect any bleeding on your assessment. Appropriate diagnostic maneuvers would include which of the following?*

**A** *Rigid bronchoscopy after tracheostomy removal in the operating room*
**B** *Urgent angiography*
**C** *Bedside examination during bag-mask ventilation after tracheostomy removal*
**D** *CT Scan of the neck and chest*
**E** *Flexible bronchoscopy at the bedside*

Any patient with bleeding from a tracheostomy tube after the first 48 hours of placement must be suspected of having a tracheo-innominate fistula (TIF), an uncommon but highly lethal complication of open or percutaneous tracheostomy.

An episode of transient, low-volume minor bleeding ("herald" or "sentinel" bleed), as described above, is a common feature in patients with TIF and must be addressed immediately. The diagnostic procedure of choice is flexible and/or rigid bronchoscopy in the operating room, allowing immediate subsequent repair if needed.

Angiography and CT imaging have no role in the diagnosis of TIF. Bedside tracheostomy removal without definitive airway control and preparations for an immediate operation would be contraindicated.

**Answer: A**

Ailawadi, G. (2009) Technique for managing tracheoinnominate arterial fistula. *Operative Techniques in Thoracic and Cardiovascular Surgery*, **2**, 66–72.
Thorp, A., Hurt, T.L., Kim, T.Y., and Brown, L. (2005) Tracheoinnominate artery fistula. A rare and often fatal complication of indwelling tracheostomy tubes. *Pediatric Emergency Care*, **21**, 763–766.

**13** *A 64-year-old woman presents with ongoing bright red hemorrhage from her tracheostomy tube site 14 days after percutaneous tracheostomy. Which of the following would constitute appropriate initial management?*

**A** *Urgent angiography and embolization*
**B** *Deflation of the tracheostomy cuff*
**C** *Endotracheal intubation, tracheostomy removal and digital compression*
**D** *Immediate, flexible bronchoscopy*
**E** *Urgent cervical exploration*

Massive bleeding from a tracheostomy site must be assumed to be associated with a tracheo-innominate fistula (TIF). The immediate goals in treating such patients involve airway protection and temporary control of active bleeding. After these initial measures, the patient should be resuscitated, blood products made available, and the patient taken to the operating room to investigate for TIF and perform a definitive repair if identified. Overinflation of the tracheostomy cuff is successful in temporarily arresting bleeding in 85% of cases. If this is unsuccessful, the innominate artery may be digitally compressed against the sternum after tracheostomy removal and endotracheal intubation. Flexible bronchoscopy before the use of these initial measures and transport to the operating room is not advised as it often fails to visualize the area of concern and may exacerbate bleeding by destabilizing the clot.

Definitive repair after initial stabilization is approached via upper hemi-sternotomy or more often complete sternotomy. Cervical exploration is never indicated as it does not allow vascular control of the innominate artery before encountering the fistula site. Angiographic embolization is not an appropriate treatment for TIF.

**Answer: C**

Ailawadi, G. (2009) Technique for managing tracheoinnominate arterial fistula. *Operative Techniques in Thoracic and Cardiovascular Surgery*, **2**, 66–72.

Thorp, A., Hurt, T.L., Kim, T.Y., and Brown, L. (2005) Tracheoinnominate artery fistula. A rare and often fatal complication of indwelling tracheostomy tubes. *Pediatric Emergency Care*, **21**, 763–766.

14 *A 48-year-old man is treated at a trauma center after a motorcycle collision. The patient complains of right side chest wall pain and blood pressure = 135/60 mm Hg, heart rate = 85 beats/min, oxygen saturation = 94% on 3 liters nasal cannula. Chest x-ray demonstrates a right side hemothorax and a right tube thoracostomy is placed with the return of 500 mL dark blood. As part of the evaluation for injuries, CT chest shows a retained hemothorax of 450 mL. What is the next appropriate step in the management of retained hemothorax?*

 A *Early VATS evacuation of hemothorax*
 B *Placement of second right tube thoracostomy*
 C *Plan delayed thoracotomy*
 D *Instillation of streptokinase into chest tube to degrade hemothorax*
 E *Observation alone*

Post-traumatic retained hemothorax (RH) represents a clinical challenge due to the high rates of fibrothorax and empyema and management. A number of therapies and procedures have been developed to address RH including observation, image-guided drainage, additional thoracostomy, VATS, intrapleural fibrinolytics, and thoracotomy. Image-guided drainage and placing an additional thoracostomy may evacuate hemothorax but have a high rate of needing additional procedures to resolve RH completely. The role of fibrinolytics in RH is controversial as it may cause uncontrolled bleeding and also has a high rate of additional procedures and is not indicated in this patient. Thoracotomy will afford excellent exposure for evacuation of RH; however, it also carries the highest operative risk and is usually performed with patients for volume of RH > 900 mL. VATS evacuation of RH has been associated with reduced ICU, and hospital stays compared to other techniques especially when performed early < 72 hours from injury. While observation may be an option in RH management, small RH (300 mL) is an independent predictor of successful outcome. Based on this, observation is not a good choice in this case.

**Answer: A**

DuBose, J., Inaba, K., Demetriades, D., *et al.* (2012) Management of post-traumatic retained hemothorax: a prospective, observational, multicenter AAST study. *Journal of Trauma and Acute Care Surgery*, **72** (1), 11–22, 22–24.

15 *A 36-year-old woman with recently diagnosed non-Hodgkin's lymphoma is awaiting planned initiation of systemic chemotherapy. In the interim, she is transferred to the intensive care unit for worsening facial and upper extremity edema, mild dyspnea and CT scan revealing a large anterior mediastinal mass. Which of the following modalities are appropriate for immediate management?*

 A *Immediate institution of chemotherapy*
 B *Immediate angiographic stent placement*
 C *Urgent surgical bypass between the innominate vein and the right atrium*
 D *Vigorous intravenous hydration*
 E *No management necessary due to collateral circulation*

Superior vena cava (SVC) syndrome is characterized by SVC obstruction due to either external compression or internal thrombus. Patients may present with edema of the head, neck, and arms, with cyanosis or plethora, respiratory symptoms, or in extreme cases with signs of cerebral edema. Although this condition may present in a clinically dramatic fashion, mortality from

SVC obstruction alone is extremely rare, and most patients have developed significant collateral venous flow by the time of presentation.

Malignancy is the most common contemporary etiology of SVC syndrome, most often bronchogenic carcinoma or lymphoma. Benign etiologies include SVC thrombosis, mediastinal fibrosis, and complications of intravascular devices and catheters.

In the absence of hemodynamic compromise or evidence of cerebral edema, most cases of SVC syndrome associated with intrathoracic malignancy are best managed by the immediate institution of specific cancer treatment. In the case presented above, this patient's planned chemotherapy should be instituted immediately and will likely ameliorate her SVC syndrome in short order. Although of unproven benefit, steroids and diuretics are generally instituted for the initial treatment of patients with SVC syndrome.

For the rare patient with SVC syndrome presenting in extremis, endovascular therapy is very effective for treatment. Endovascular treatment is also indicated for patients with malignant SVC syndrome due to malignancy without available effective medical therapies. For the stable patient presented above, immediate invasive treatment is not indicated. Surgical bypass of the SVC is a treatment option for cases not amenable to medical or percutaneous therapies or in particular for SVC syndrome of benign etiology, for whom a durable modality is needed.

**Answer: A**

Cheng, S. (2009) Superior vena cava syndrome. A contemporary review of a historic disease. *Cardiology in Review*, **17**, 16–22.

Yu, J.B., Wilson, L.D., Detterbeck, F.C. (2008) Superior vena cava syndrome: a proposed classification system and algorithm for management. *Journal of Thoracic Oncology*, **3**, 811–814.

16 *A 50-year-old man is transferred to the intensive care unit for new dyspnea and pleuritic right chest pain after an attempted right internal jugular venous catheter placement. On physical examination, his respirations are rapid and labored. Right-sided breath sounds are absent. His heart rate is 126 beats/min, and his blood pressure is 88/60 mm Hg. Which of the following measures constitute appropriate immediate therapy?*

   A *Two liters warm lactated ringers*
   B *Endotracheal intubation*
   C *Portable chest radiography (CXR)*
   D *Placement of a right tube thoracostomy*
   E *Initiation of vasoactive support*

This patient's presentation is consistent with a pneumothorax related to attempted central venous line placement. The presence of tachycardia and hypotension in this setting is indicative of tension pneumothorax, a life-threatening condition requiring immediate treatment. Tension pneumothorax is a clinical diagnosis. There is no indication for a CXR before treatment as this would introduce an unnecessary delay in therapy.

Tension pneumothorax may be treated by needle thoracostomy with a needle or cannulae of at least 4.5 cm length (followed by tube thoracostomy) or by immediate tube thoracostomy. The patient's hypotension and respiratory distress will likely be immediately resolved by treatment of his pneumothorax. Intubation or vasoactive support would not be indicated unless the patient manifested persistent cardiopulmonary compromise after appropriate treatment of his mechanical complication.

**Answer: D**

Hoyt, D.B., Coimbra, R., and Acosta, J. (2007) Management of acute trauma, in *Sabiston Textbook of Surgery*, 18th edn (ed. C.M. Townsend), WB Saunders, Philadelphia, PA, pp. 477–520.

Zenergink, I., Brink, P.R., Laupland, K.B., *et al.* (2008) Needle thoracostomy in the treatment of a tension pneumothorax in trauma patients: what size needle? *Journal of Trauma*, **64**, 111–114.

17 *A 54-year-old diabetic man without prior cardiac disease presented to the hospital four days ago with fevers and new left arm weakness. A non-contrast CT scan of the head reveals an acute right thalamic hemorrhage. Echocardiography revealed multiple 3–5 mm vegetations on the mitral valve and severe mitral valve regurgitation. His admission blood cultures grew out Streptococcus viridans. The patient has manifested a steady hemodynamic and respiratory decline since admission. As of this morning, he required intubation and is requiring infusions of vasopressin (0.04 units/min), milrinone (0.5 μg/kg/min), and escalating doses of epinephrine (currently 12 μg/min) to maintain acceptable hemodynamics. Which of the following is an appropriate course of action at this point?*

   A *Urgent mitral valve repair*
   B *Urgent mitral valve replacement with prosthetic valve*
   C *Urgent mitral valve repair with biologic valve*
   D *Continuation of intravenous antibiotics and respiratory/hemodynamic support*
   E *Mitral valve debridement only*

Approximately 50% of patients with bacterial endocarditis will require surgical treatment. Indications for surgery in endocarditis include refractory bacteremia or sepsis, recurrent embolic phenomena, congestive heart failure, and myocardial extension. Congestive heart failure from endocarditis that is severe and refractory to medical treatment is the most common indication for surgery for endocarditis, and early surgical intervention has the potential to substantially reduce mortality in this group of patients.

The patient above has evidence of cardiogenic shock due to acute severe mitral valve regurgitation from his endocarditis. This is a clear surgical indication. Mitral valve repair or replacement may be performed, although repair is preferred whenever this can be achieved in concert with the complete eradication of all infected tissues. Unfortunately, this patient's acute hemorrhagic cerebrovascular accident (CVA) presents an absolute contraindication to mitral valve surgery at this time. The requirement for high-dose anticoagulation during cardiopulmonary bypass would present prohibitive risk and would likely be associated with a dismal neurological outcome.

This patient's prognosis is extremely poor, but there is no role for surgery at this time. He should be treated with continued antibiotic therapy and respiratory/hemodynamic support. Given his requirement for escalating doses of inotropic and vasopressor support, IABP placement would be a reasonable adjunct (although not optimal in a patient with recent bacteremia). If he survives, surgical intervention could be contemplated after an interval of four weeks from his hemorrhagic event.

**Answer: D**

Feringa, H.H.H., Shaw, L.J., Poldermans, D., *et al.* (2007) Mitral valve repair and replacement in endocarditis: a systematic review of literature. *Annals of Thoracic Surgery*, **83**, 564–571.

Lester, S.J. and Wilansky, S. (2007) Endocarditis and associated complications. *Critical Care Medicine*, **35**, S384–S391.

Prendergast, B.D. and Tornos, P. (2010) Surgery for infective endocarditis. Who and when? *Circulation*, **121**, 1141–1152.

**18** *A 68-year-old man developed a leak with sepsis and multi-organ dysfunction after sigmoid colectomy for diverticulitis. He has been ventilator-dependent for 14 days and is receiving enteral nutrition via a nasogastric (NG) tube. Over the past two days, he has developed increasing pulmonary secretions, progressive abdominal distension, and loss of ventilatory volumes. Panendoscopy confirms a moderate-size tracheoesophageal fistula (TEF). Which of the following would represent appropriate management at this time?*

A *Immediate repair by fistula division and repair of trachea and esophagus*

B *Decompressing gastrostomy, feeding jejunostomy, placement of endotracheal tube cuff distal to fistula*

C *Immediate esophageal exclusion/diversion*

D *Esophagectomy and spit fistula*

E *Observation*

Cuff-related tracheal injury due to prolonged intubation is the most common cause of acquired nonmalignant TEF. In general, this complication may be prevented by scrutiny of the endotracheal tube (ETT) and tracheostomy cuff pressures and avoiding the use of stiff, indwelling NG tubes in ventilated patients. Spontaneous fistula closure is rare.

The optimal management for most patients with acquired nonmalignant TEF is fistula division with primary repair of the trachea and esophagus and the interposition of viable tissue. In the case of more extensive TEF, tracheal resection, and end-to-end anastomosis may be indicated.

However, TEF repair should only be applied in patients who can be immediately extubated after repair, as there is otherwise a prohibitive risk of recurrence or failure of repair.

Until patients with TEF can be weaned from mechanical ventilation, this complication should be treated conservatively, with the placement of the ETT or tracheostomy cuff distal to the fistula site, NG tube removal, a decompressive gastrostomy, and feeding jejunostomy tube placement. Antibiotics are also appropriate. Single-stage repair is performed after the patient is weaned from mechanical ventilation.

For patients with a fistula near the carina in whom effective distal ventilation cannot be achieved, cervical esophageal exclusion may be applied. Esophageal stenting may be an option for the management of patients with TEF, but is probably not the treatment of choice for most patients.

**Answer: B**

Landreneau, R.J., Hazelrigg, S.R., Boley, T.M., *et al.* (1991) Management of an extensive tracheoesophageal fistula by cervical esophageal exclusion. *Chest*, **99**, 777–780.

Mathisen, D.J., Grillo, H.C., Wain, J.C., and Hilgenberg, A.D. (1991) Management of acquired nonmalignant tracheoesophageal fistula. *Annals of Thoracic Surgery*, **52**, 759–765.

Yeh, C.-M. and Chou, C.-M. (2008) Early repair of acquired tracheoesophageal fistula. *Asian Cardiovascular and Thoracic Annals*, **16**, 318–320.

**19** *A 35-year-old man with a traumatic brain injury and dysphagia undergoes a difficult esophagogastroduodenoscopy (EGD) for placement of a percutaneous endoscopic gastrostomy (PEG) tube. Several hours after the procedure the patient develops fever, tachycardia, and crepitance in the neck. The best next steps in management include:*

**A** *IV antibiotics, fluid resuscitation, contrast swallow, attempted nonoperative management*

**B** *IV antibiotics, fluid resuscitation, and immediate cervical exploration*

**C** *IV antibiotics, fluid resuscitation, and left thoracotomy*

**D** *IV antibiotics, fluid resuscitation, and right thoracotomy*

**E** *IV antibiotics, fluid resuscitation, and laparotomy*

This patient sustained a perforation of the cervical esophagus as a complication of his upper endoscopy. Esophageal perforation can result from iatrogenesis, trauma, malignancy, inflammatory process, or infection. Iatrogenic injury is the most common cause of esophageal perforation, usually as a result of an upper endoscopy. The diagnosis of esophageal perforation is suspected with a history of prior esophageal instrumentation or trauma, but the diagnosis is usually confirmed with a contrast swallow (Figure 45.2).

General management of esophageal perforation includes broad-spectrum intravenous antibiotics and fluid resuscitation. The decision for operative versus nonoperative management depends on several factors including location of perforation, the cause of perforation, time since perforation occurred, whether or not the leak is contained, and the overall status of the patient. In general, patients with a localized perforation (particularly of the cervical esophagus after instrumentation), who have the leak identified in a timely fashion and are clinically stable, are potential candidates for nonoperative management. If operative management is required the surgical approach depends on the location of perforation, and may require a cervical incision, left or right thoracotomy, or laparotomy.

**Answer: A**

Altorjay, A., Kiss, J., and Bohak, A. (1997) Nonoperative management of esophageal perforations. Is it justified? *Annals of Surgery*, **225**, 415–421.

DeMeester, S.R. (2008) Esophageal perforation, in *Current Surgical Therapy*, 9th edn, (ed. J.L. Cameron), Mosby, Philadelphia, PA, pp. 16–20.

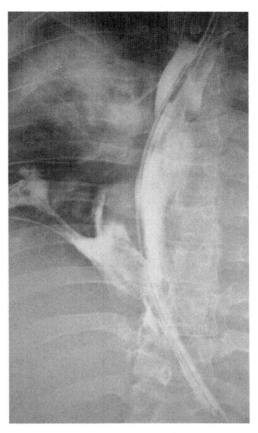

**Figure 45.2** Free esophageal perforation into the right pleural cavity.

**20** *A 17-year-old girl who ingests laundry bleach in a suicide attempt presents to the emergency department with oropharyngeal pain, difficulty swallowing, and excessive drooling. Management priorities include which of the following:*

**A** *Placement of a nasogastric tube for activated charcoal administration.*

**B** *Airway evaluation.*

**C** *Ingestion of agents to neutralize or dilute the acid.*

**D** *Upper endoscopy within 1–2 weeks to evaluate the extent of the injury.*

**E** *Neck x-rays to rule out perforation*

Caustic injuries of the esophagus usually result from an accidental ingestion in children or a suicide attempt in adults. The severity of injury to the esophagus depends on the type of agent ingested and the amount and concentration of the agent. Most common ingestions involve acid or alkaline substances, with an alkali ingestion leading to more extensive injury and associated mortality. Acids have a low viscosity leading to rapid transit time through the esophagus and cause a coagulation necrosis that causes a more superficial injury to the esophagus.

In contrast, ingested alkalis cause a liquefactive necrosis and deep esophageal injury. Furthermore, alkali substances have higher viscosity, slowing transit time and prolonging exposure to the esophagus.

Clinical presentation after caustic ingestion typically includes oropharyngeal pain, dysphagia, salivation, and may include chest or abdominal pain. However, presenting symptoms are poor predictors for the extent of the injury. Essential in evaluation and treatment of a patient with a caustic ingestion includes early identification of the ingested agent and the amount ingested. Initial evaluation should focus on the airway by physical exam for direct visualization with laryngoscopy or fiber optic Naso pharyngoscopy, and with any suspicion of airway compromise the patient should be endotracheally intubated. Further evaluation with chest or abdominal x-rays may indicate evidence of full thickness perforation. The mainstay of diagnosis and evaluation of the extent of the injury is early endoscopic evaluation within 12–24 hours.

Treatment for mild injury seen by endoscopy includes antibiotics, acid suppression therapy, and nutritional support if needed. Patients with moderate to severe injury seen on endoscopy require the same therapy as those with mild injury, but the physician must maintain a high index of suspicion for progression of injury during the next 24–48 hours. Patients initially managed nonoperatively need a gastrograffin swallow or upper endoscopy several weeks after the injury to evaluate for stricture formation. Patients with evidence of perforation require emergent surgery via thoracotomy, laparotomy, or both. Blind passage of nasogastric tubes or any attempt to neutralize or dilute the offending agent should be avoided.

**Answer: B**

Fischer, A.C. (2008) Chemical esophageal injuries, in *Current Surgical Therapy*, 9th edn, (ed. J.L. Cameron), Mosby, Philadelphia, PA, pp. 49–52.
Hugh, T.B. and Kelly, M.D. (1999) Corrosive ingestion and the surgeon. *Journal of the American College of Surgeons*, **189**, 508–522.

21 *A 68-year-old man has just undergone an Ivor Lewis esophagectomy with a thoracic anastomosis. Postoperative day 1 his white count is 12 000, and he was intermittently hypotensive requiring resuscitation and norepinephrine infusion. Two days later, his white count is now 19 000; vital signs: blood pressure = 88/46 mmHg, heart rate = 126 beats/min, and temperature = 101.9 F. What is the next best step in management?*

   **A** *Antibiotics, increase pressors and resuscitate*
   **B** *Antibiotics, CT scan of the chest, resuscitate*

   **C** *Emergent re-exploration of the chest*
   **D** *Emergent re-exploration of the abdomen*

Given the segmental nature of the blood supply to the esophagus and the arteries that are sacrificed to mobilize the stomach, there is some risk for the anastomotic leak. In addition, the patient has been hypotensive throughout the first 24 hours after his surgery and required pressors to maintain his blood pressure. These factors together should raise the suspicion that the patient has a leak at his esophagogastric anastomosis. The next best step is broad spectrum antibiotics, resuscitation, and imaging which will confirm the diagnosis. Gastrografin ingestion or via an NGT that is usually left near the anastomosis can also be helpful in confirming the diagnosis. Once the diagnosis is confirmed, operative intervention can be pursued if needed. In some instances, small leaks can be managed non-operatively with simple percutaneous drainage of a local abscess.

**Answer: B**

Atkins, B.Z., Shah, A.S. and Hutcheson, K.A. *et al.* (2004) Reducing hospital morbidity and mortality following esophagectomy. *Annals of Thoracic Surgery*, **78**, 1170–1176.
Law, S.K and Long, J. (2007) Esophagogastrectomy for carcinoma of the esophagus and gastric cardia, and the esophageal anastomosis, in *Mastery of Surgery*, 5th ed. (eds. A.C. Fischer, K. Bland, and M. Callery), Wolters Kluwer Health/Lippincott Williams & Wilkins, Philadelphia, PA, pp. 752–771.

22 *A 36-year-old man was admitted to the floor at a trauma center where he is being treated for flail chest with incentive spirometer and intravenous morphine for pain. After admission, the patient's pain is not controlled. He can only pull 400 mL on bedside spirometry and complains of worsening dyspnea. Temperature = 37.0 °C, saturation = 93% on 5 liters nasal cannula $O_2$. Arterial blood gas: pH = 7.35, $pCO_2$ = 48 mm Hg, $pO_2$ = 62 mm Hg. What is the next best step in management?*

   **A** *Start intravenous ceftriaxone for community-acquired pneumonia*
   **B** *Increase dosage of morphine and change to PCA delivery.*
   **C** *Intubate patient immediately*
   **D** *Surgical stabilization of flail rib fractures*
   **E** *Start hyperbaric oxygen*

Fractures of the ribs after trauma are a common and potentially debilitating injury. Flail chest results when three consecutive ribs are fractured in two or more places.

Patients with flail chest are at risk for prolonged respiratory failure and pneumonia. Historically, these fractures were managed with pneumatic stabilization of the chest wall with mechanical ventilation due to poorly engineered stabilization hardware. However, new devices are available to fit over the rib. Several studies have demonstrated improvement in respiratory failure and tracheostomy rates as well as a reduction in days of mechanical ventilation, ICU length of stay and hospital length of stay. In this case, where a patient has an impending respiratory failure due to pain from rib fractures, operative stabilization is an appropriate choice.

There is no clinical evidence of pneumonia so starting antibiotics would not be appropriate. This patient does not meet criteria for emergent intubation. While it is important to optimize pain control, the patient already has an elevated $pCO_2$ which may worsen the acidosis with increasing dosage of narcotics. There is, however, level I evidence to support early use of epidural analgesia in patients with rib fractures. Hyperbaric oxygen is not indicated for this patient.

**Answer: D**

Nickerson, T.P., Thiels, C.A., Kim, B.D., *et al.* (2016) Outcomes of complete versus partial surgical stabilization of flail chest. *World Journal of Surgery,* **40** (1), 236–241.

Pieracci, F.M., Lin, Y., Rodil, M., *et al.* (2016) A prospective, controlled clinical evaluation of surgical stabilization of severe rib fractures. *Journal of Trauma and Acute Care Surgery,* **80** (2), 187–194.

# 46

# Pediatric Surgery

*Matthew Martin, MD, Aaron Cunningham, MD and Mubeen Jafri, MD*

1 *A 3-year-old child is struck by a car and has a GCS of 5 on arrival to the trauma center. The trauma surgeon determines that immediate endotracheal intubation is indicated. Which of the following is an important consideration when managing the airway of pediatric trauma patients?*

   A *The length of the trachea in children results in more left main stem intubations than in adults*

   B *The vocal cords are the narrowest portion of the pediatric airway and are commonly the site of obstruction*

   C *Cricothyroidotomy in children has a similar risk of complications as in adults*

   D *The larynx in children sits higher and more anterior than in adults*

   E *Children have an increased functional residual capacity as compared to adults, giving them increased reserve during respiratory compromise*

Management of the pediatric airway can represent a unique set of challenges. The airway diameter in younger children is typically smaller, the larynx is higher and more anterior, the tongue is proportionally larger, and the trachea is shorter than in adults. Children's airways are relatively narrower than those of adults, leading to an increased resistance that makes them more prone to respiratory failure. The narrowest portion of the airway is at the cricoid ring as opposed to the vocal cords in adults, making this a common location for obstruction. The shortened trachea predisposes to possible airway problems that must be always considered. This includes the risk of right mainstem intubation that is often poorly tolerated in these patients, as well as the risk of inadvertent extubation with even relatively small degrees of tube movement. Typically, children >8 years have an airway similar to adults. Many of the same principles in airway management are similar in children, including supplemental oxygenation, suctioning, and use of oral and nasal airway adjuncts. These are, however, tailored to the pediatric airway. Infants preferentially are nasal breathers and nasal suctioning can be of great benefit. Care must be exercised in using nasal airways due to the acute angle between the nasopharynx and oropharynx, and in general nasal airways in children should be avoided if at all possible. Emergent surgical airways in children carry a higher risk of complications compared with adults. These include injury to the airway, tube misplacement or dislodgment, and longer-term risks of subglottic stenosis. In particular, cricothyroidotomy should be avoided in children, particularly smaller children (<12 years old), as this is the narrowest part of the airway and is also immediately adjacent to the vocal cords. Tracheostomy should be the preferred urgent surgical airway, and urgent temporary oxygenation can be obtained using a needle cricothyroidotomy. Children have significantly less functional residual capacity than adults, and thus have less reserve and shorter time to desaturate when not being ventilated.

**Answer: D**

Gaines, B.A., Scheidler, M.G., Lynch, J.M., and Ford, H.R. (2008) Pediatric trauma, in *The Trauma Manual: Trauma and Acute Care Surgery*, 3rd edn (eds A.B. Peitzman, M. Rhodes, C.W. Schwab, *et al.*), Lippencott Williams & Wilkins, Philadelphia, PA, pp. 499–514.

Santillanes, G. and Gausche-Hill, M. (2008) Pediatric airway management. *Emergency Medical Clinics of North America*, **26**, 961–675.

2 *Which of the following statements about emergent endotracheal intubation in the pediatric patient is correct?*

   A *Bag-valve-mask ventilation is frequently ineffective in children*

   B *All pediatric patients should be intubated with an appropriately sized UNCUFFED endotracheal tube*

*Surgical Critical Care and Emergency Surgery: Clinical Questions and Answers*, Second Edition.
Edited by Forrest "Dell" Moore, Peter Rhee, and Gerard J. Fulda.
© 2018 John Wiley & Sons Ltd. Published 2018 by John Wiley & Sons Ltd.
Companion website: www.wiley.com/go/moore/surgical_criticalcare_and_emergency_surgery

C Bradycardia can occur during rapid sequence intubation, and can be treated with atropine administration

D The presence of bilateral breath sounds is the "gold standard" for confirming appropriate endotracheal tube placement

E A laryngeal mask airway (LMA) is considered an acceptable alternative definitive airway in pediatric trauma patients

One of the more common errors during emergency intubation of children, particularly by less-experienced providers, is to perform inadequate initial basic airway management and fully preoxygenate prior to intubation attempts. Bag-valve-mask (BVM) ventilation by hand should be possible in almost all children, barring an actual mechanical obstruction in the airway. An oral airway should be inserted if there is inadequate BVM ventilation due to a large tongue. Although previous recommendations were for uncuffed tubes in pediatric patients, current guidelines support the use of cuffed tubes for emergent intubation in children. Pediatric patients can develop significant bradycardia during rapid sequence intubation, and thus should either be premedicated with atropine, or atropine should be standing by for immediate use. The gold standard for confirming correct tube placement is visualization of the tube passing through the vocal cords, and confirmation with capnography demonstrating end-tidal $CO_2$. A cuffed tube in the trachea is the only "definitive" airway, although temporary airway devices such as the LMA or combined esophageal/tracheal tubes (such as Combitube, King airway) can provide initial airway control and oxygenation/ventilation until a definitive airway can be established.

**Answer: C**

Bano, S., Akhtar, S., Zia, N., *et al.* (2012) Pediatric endotracheal intubations for airway management in the emergency department. *Pediatric Emergency Care*, **28** (11), 1129–1131.

Castilla, D.M., Dinh, C.T., and Younis, R. (2012) Pediatric airway management in craniofacial trauma. *Juornal of Craniofacial Surgery*, **22** (4), 1175–1178.

Sagarin, M.J., Chiang, V., Sakles, J.C., *et al.* (2002) Rapid sequence intubation for pediatric emergency airway management. *Pediatric Emergency Care*, **18** (6), 417–423.

3 Spinal cord injury without radiographic abnormality (SCIWORA) is characterized by which of the following?

A SCIWORA injuries typically show no abnormalities on magnetic resonance imaging (MRI), which is of no benefit in predicting the prognosis of the injury

B SCIWORA lesions in younger children (<9 years) often occur at higher cervical level and are more severe than SCIWORA injuries in older children (9–16 years)

C A SCIWORA injury does not require further immobilization since there is lack of fracture or ligamentous damage

D SCIWORA is a more common injury in older children aged 9–16 years, due to decreased elasticity of the spinal cord

E Pseudosubluxation on cervical spine imaging is a diagnostic hallmark of SCIWORA

SCIWORA is an injury that occurs primarily in children, and is most common in those younger than 9 years. It is characterized by physical examination evidence of a spinal cord injury in the setting of normal x-ray and computed tomography imaging. However, an MRI will typically demonstrate signs of ligamentous and/or spinal cord injury in these patients. Patients with SCIWORA who have a normal MRI, minor hemorrhage, or edema only, have an improved prognosis compared to that predicted by the initial neurological examination. It is thought to occur through hyperextension, flexion, distraction, and spinal cord ischemia. The hypermobility of the juvenile spinal column allows for the spinal cord to stretch beyond its ability to withstand injury, and to create a significant injury without associated bony fracture of the vertebral column. Pooled data from multiple studies estimates that 63% of children with spinal cord injury (SCI) age 0–9 have SCIWORA whereas 20% of children with SCI age 10–17 have SCIWORA. In children age 0–9, 78% of these injuries were classified as severe, whereas only 13% of injuries were severe in those 10–17 years old. Younger children also have a higher incidence of higher level cervical spine injuries (C1–C4 level). Although in some cases no radiographic spinal column injury is identified, recurrent injury has been documented up to 10 weeks after the initial presentation prompting recommendations for up to 3 months of spinal immobilization. Pseudosubluxation of the cervical spine is a common radiographic finding in the pediatric population, and is characterized by anterior subluxation with normal alignment of the posterior vertebral bodies and spinous processes. No immobilization or further workup is required for this isolated radiographic finding in the absence of any symptoms of spinal column or cord injury.

**Answer: B**

Liao, C.C., Lui, T.N., Chen, L.R., *et al.* (2005) Spinal cord injury without radiological abnormality in preschool-aged children: correlation of magnetic resonance imaging findings with neurological outcomes. *Journal of Neurosurgery (Pediatrics 1)*, **103**, 17–23.

Pang, D. (2004) Spinal cord injury without radiographic abnormality in children, 2 decades later. *Neurosurgery*, **55**, 1325–1343.

Shaw, M., Burnett, H., Wilson, A., and Chan, O. (1999) Pseudosubluxation of C2 on C3 in polytraumatized children–prevalence and significance. *Clinical Radiology*, **54** (6), 377–380.

**4** *A 6-year-old, 22 kg boy who was a restrained passenger in the back seat of a car involved in a motor vehicle collision has a grade III splenic laceration. He arrives with a systolic blood pressure of 70 mm Hg and a heart rate of 140 beats/min. Which of the following would be an appropriate initial fluid bolus for crystalloid and packed red blood cells (pRBCs)?*

**A** *660 mL normal saline, 220 mL pRBCs*
**B** *440 mL lactated Ringers, 440 mL pRBCs*
**C** *660 mL lactated Ringers, 440 mL pRBCs*
**D** *440 mL lactated Ringers, 220 mL pRBCs*
**E** *1000 mL normal saline, 1 unit pRBCs*

The Advanced Trauma Life Support guidelines for initial adult resuscitation begins with 2L of crystalloid (either normal saline or lactated Ringers) followed by pRBC if there is no response or a transient response to crystalloid, or obvious signs of ongoing hemorrhage. In contrast to adults, fluid and blood product resuscitation in children is based on weight. Often an exact weight is unknown and can be best estimated using the Breslow Pediatric Emergency Tape. Initial boluses of warm, isotonic crystalloid are given in 20 mL/kg volumes. After one or two boluses, packed red blood cells should be considered based on the child's response to the initial fluid volume and anticipation of ongoing bleeding. Packed red cells are given in 10 mL/kg boluses. For a 22 kg male, 22 kg × 20 mL/kg = 440 mL bolus of crystalloid plus 22 kg × 10mL/kg = 220 mL pRBCs are recommended by ATLS guidelines as the initial transfusion. Guidelines for massive transfusion in pediatric patients are much less well defined than for adults, although similar overall principals should be followed.

**Answer: D**

American College of Surgeons (ed.) (2012) Pediatric trauma, in *Advanced Trauma Life Support*, 9th edn, Elsevier, Chicago, IL, pp. 246–271.

Dehmer, J.J. and Adamson, W.T. (2010) Massive transfusion and blood product use in the pediatric trauma patient. *Seminars in Pediatric Surgery*, **19**, 286–291.

**5** *The patient in question 4 receives the initial boluses of lactated Ringer's solution and pRBCs, but remains persistently hypotensive and tachycardic. He is taken emergently to the operating room and found to have large-volume hemoperitoneum with a grade 5 splenic injury and grade 3 liver injury and ongoing hemorrhage. He is hypothermic and has an arterial pH of 7.21. Which of the following would be the optimal approach to resuscitation in this patient?*

**A** *He does not yet meet criteria to activate a "massive transfusion" protocol*
**B** *A stat prothrombin time/INR should be sent, and fresh frozen plasma administered for an INR above 1.3*
**C** *There is a proven survival benefit of resuscitating with a 1:1:1 ratio of pRBC to plasma to platelets in the pediatric trauma population*
**D** *Recombinant activated factor VII (rFVIIa) should be administered immediately*
**E** *Immediate fresh frozen plasma should be administered along with each pRBC bolus until hemorrhage control is obtained*

This patient has clear evidence of ongoing hemorrhage and physiologic shock, as evidenced by persistent hypotension, tachycardia, hypothermia, and systemic acidosis. The presence of proven or suspected large-volume bleeding and the above risk factors are all well-accepted criteria to initiate large-volume blood-product resuscitation. This is best done through a pre-existing "massive transfusion protocol" that can be rapidly activated, and then deactivated when no longer required. Although exact features of a pediatric massive transfusion protocol will vary between centers, there are universal basic principles that should be followed. This includes the early administration of plasma along with pRBCs rather than waiting for laboratory evidence of coagulopathy. Although there is evidence of benefit of a 1:1:1 ratio in adult patients, there is no similar benefit yet demonstrated in pediatric trauma patients. The question of the optimal exact ratio of blood products in pediatric patients remains poorly characterized, although most current protocols utilize ratios of 1:1 or 1:2 for FFP:pRBC. There is no evidence of benefit for rFVIIa administration, particularly in pediatric patients, and the trauma community has largely abandoned this agent. There is currently no standardized accepted definition for "massive transfusion" in the pediatric population, although the best available data supports a blood loss of 40 cc/kg (approximately half of the pediatric circulating blood volume) as a reasonable and valid definition for massive transfusion.

**Answer: E**

Edwards, M.J., Lustik, M.B., Clark, M.E., *et al.* (2015) The effects of balanced blood component resuscitation and crystalloid administration in pediatric trauma patients requiring transfusion in Afghanistan and Iraq 2002 to 2012. *Journal of Trauma and Acute Care Surgery*, **78** (2), 330–335.

Neff, L.P., Cannon, J.W., Morrison, J.J., *et al.* (2015). Clearly defining pediatric massive transfusion: cutting through the fog and friction with combat data. *Journal of Trauma and Acute Care Surgery*, **78** (1), 22–29.

Smith, S.A., Livingston, M.H., and Merritt, N.H. (2016) Early coagulopathy and metabolic acidosis predict transfusion of packed red blood cells in pediatric trauma patients. *Journal of Pediatric Surgery*, **51** (5), 848–852.

6 The mechanism of injury responsible for the most pediatric trauma deaths is which of the following?
   A Motor vehicle crash
   B All-terrain vehicle accident
   C Non-accidental trauma
   D Burn-related injury
   E Falls

Blunt injury mechanisms are much more common than penetrating injury in pediatric patients overall and in all age subgroups, making up approximately 86% of all injuries. However, the relative incidence of penetrating trauma rises sharply with age, particularly among teenage males. The most common presenting mechanism for pediatric trauma is falls, but these rarely result in major morbidity or mortality. Motor-vehicle accidents are the leading cause of pediatric deaths, followed by drownings, house fires, homicides, and falls. Similar to adults, males comprise approximately 60% of all pediatric trauma admissions. Burn-related injuries are much less common, but are a cause of significant morbidity and often lifelong disability. Nonaccidental trauma is also less common, but is significantly underrecognized and underreported. Routine screening of all pediatric trauma patients for nonaccidental trauma has been shown to significantly improve the recognition, early treatment, and outcomes associated with nonaccidental trauma.

**Answer: A**

American College of Surgeons (ed.) (2012) Pediatric trauma, in *Advanced Trauma Life Support*, 9th edn, Elsevier, Chicago, IL, pp. 246–271.

Cooper, A., Barlow, B., DiScala, C., and String, D. (1994) Mortality and truncal injury: the pediatric perspective. *Journal of Pediatric Surgery*, **29** (1), 33–38.

Guice, K.S., Cassidy, L.D., and Oldham, K.T. (2007) Traumatic injury and children: a national assessment. *Journal of Trauma*, **63**, S68–S80.

Roaten, J.B., Partrick, D.A., Nydam, T.L., *et al.* (2006) Nonaccidental trauma is a major cause of morbidity and mortality among patients at a regional level 1 pediatric trauma center. *Journal of Pediatric Surgery*, **41** (12), 2013–2015.

7 Which child below would be considered both hypotensive and tachycardic based on the admission vital signs?
   A 4-year-old boy with HR 148 beats/minute, SBP 69 mm Hg
   B 8-month-old girl with HR 156 beats/minute, SBP 63 mm Hg
   C 2-year-old girl with HR 149 beats/minute, SBP 73 mm Hg
   D 10-year-old boy with HR 115 beats/minute, SBP 85 mm Hg
   E 7-year-old girl with HR 116 beats/minute, SBP 84 mm Hg

When caring for pediatric trauma patients, it is important to know the ranges for normal vital signs at a given age, and also the characteristic hemodynamic response of children to injury and hemorrhage (Table 46.1). Of note, tachycardia is the most important early indicator of hypovolemic shock in the pediatric patient. Systolic

**Table 46.1** Pediatric vital sign normal ranges.

| Age Group | Respiratory Rate | Heart Rate | Systolic Blood Pressure | Weight in kilos | Weight in pounds |
| --- | --- | --- | --- | --- | --- |
| Newborn | 30–50 | 120–160 | 50–70 | 2–3 | 4.5–7 |
| Infant (1–12 months) | 20–30 | 80–140 | 70–100 | 4–10 | 9–22 |
| Toddler (1–3 yrs.) | 20–30 | 80–130 | 80–110 | 10–14 | 22–31 |
| Preschooler (3–5 yrs.) | 20–30 | 80–120 | 80–110 | 14–18 | 31–40 |
| School Age (6–12 yrs.) | 20–30 | 70–110 | 80–120 | 20–42 | 41–92 |
| Adolescent (13+ yrs.) | 12–20 | 55–105 | 110–120 | >50 | >110 |

blood pressure can give a false sense of security and may not be significantly low until almost 50% of the blood volume is lost. A 4-year-old boy should have a HR less than 140 beats/min and a SBP >75 mm Hg. The characteristic response to ongoing hemorrhage in children includes progressively worsening tachycardia with relatively sustained blood pressure until class 4 shock is reached. They will then exhibit a rapid and precipitous decline manifested by hypotension and then bradycardia before progressing to complete cardiopulmonary arrest. A change from tachycardia to bradycardia is an ominous sign that indicates impending arrest, and should prompt rapid and immediate interventions as well as resuscitation.

**Answer: A**

American College of Surgeons (ed.) (2012) Pediatric trauma, in *Advanced Trauma Life Support*, 9th edn, Elsevier, Chicago, IL, pp. 246–271.

Gaines, B.A., Scheidler, M.G., Lynch, J.M., and Ford, H.R. (2008) Pediatric trauma in *The Trauma Manual: Trauma and Acute Care Surgery*, 3rd edn (eds A.B. Peitzman, M. Rhodes, C.W. Schwab, *et al.*), Lippencott Williams & Wilkins, Philadelphia, PA, pp. 499–514.

**8** *A 5-year-old, 22 kg boy presents after falling 10 feet off a deck. He was immobilized on a spine board before transport by medics. His workup reveals a fractured left radius. The AP cervical spine film is normal and his lateral cervical spine film reveals mild anterior displacement (1 mm) of C2 on C3. His cranial nerves are intact and he has no peripheral weakness or sensory deficits. He denies pain in his neck with palpation. What is the next appropriate step in management?*

**A** *Flexion and extension c-spine x-rays*
**B** *CT scan to evaluate for a missed c-spine fracture*
**C** *MRI to evaluate for cervical spinal cord injury*
**D** *Cervical collar immobilization and repeat x-rays in 4–6 weeks*
**E** *Observation*

An appreciation of the normal variation of c-spine anatomy is important in caring for children. Pseudosubluxation of C2 on C3 is a common variant. Reviews of normal, uninjured children reveal that this variation occurs in 22–46% of children <8 years old. A true dislocation of C2 on C3 can be differentiated from pseuodosubluxation by drawing Swischuk's line. Swischuk's line is drawn along the anterior aspect of the spinous processes of C1 and C3. If the line is more than 2 mm anterior to the anterior process of C2, then it suggests a true dislocation. Because the patient has no neurological symptoms or neck pain,

further x-rays or immobilization are not necessary. Routine CT in pediatric patients following trauma is not recommended unless x-ray studies are inadequate, show suspicious findings, or are abnormal. MRI would be recommended if neurological symptoms were present, x-rays were abnormal, or the c-collar could not be cleared due to neck pain or instability.

**Answer: E**

Easter, J.S., Barkin, R., Rosen, C.L., and Ban, K. (2010) Cervical spine injuries in children, part II: management and special considerations. *Journal of Emergency Medicine*, **41** (2), 142–150.

Shaw, M., Burnett, H., Wilson, A., and Chan, O. (1999) Pseudosubluxation of C2 on C3 in polytraumatized children—prevalence and significance. *Clinical Radiology*, **54** (6), 377–380.

**9** *A 6-year-old, 25 kg girl who was a back seat passenger involved in a motor vehicle crash is diagnosed with a severe splenic laceration. Which of the following would mandate surgical exploration and splenectomy?*

**A** *Tachycardia and hypotension prior to resuscitation*
**B** *Transfusion requirement of 1 unit of pRBCs within the first 8 hours*
**C** *Transfusion requirement of 1L of pRBCs within the first 24 hours*
**D** *Grade IV or V splenic laceration on CT scan*
**E** *Grade IV or V splenic laceration with blush on CT scan*

Splenic preservation has become the standard of care for management of blunt splenic injuries. Nonoperative management avoids complications associated with laparotomy as well as overwhelming postsplenectomy infection. This is most important in children less than five years of age who have a serious infection rate of greater than 10%. The risk for postsplenectomy sepsis in adults is around 1% or less. Nonoperative management of blunt splenic injury is successful in greater than 90% of all children, and is influenced by the grade of injury. Grade III injury and above has been shown to be an independent risk factor for splenectomy. Despite this, a study by Potoka *et al.* found splenic preservation to be as high as 82% for grade IV and 52% for grade V splenic injury at pediatric trauma centers. Hemodynamic instability is an absolute indication for splenectomy, but splenectomy is also indicated when blood transfusion of greater than half the blood volume (40 mL/kg) is anticipated or when other significant intraabdominal injuries are present. A 25 kg child has an approximate blood volume of 80 mL/kg × 25 or 2 L. A transfusion requirement of 1 L of pRBCs would be a significant enough transfusion requirement to mandate splenectomy. For hemodynamically normal patients with grade IV or V splenic injuries with blush identified on CT scan, angioembolization is warranted.

**Answer: C**

Jim, J., Leonardi, M.J., Cryer, H.G., *et al.* (2008) Management of high-grade splenic injury in children. *American Journal of Surgery*, **74** (10), 988–992.

Mooney, D.P., Downard, C., Johnson, S., *et al.* (2005) Physiology after pediatric splenic injury. *Journal of Trauma*, **58**, 108–111.

Potoka, D.A., Schall, L.C., and Ford, H.R. (2002) Risk factors for splenectomy in children with blunt splenic trauma. *Journal of Pediatric Surgery*, **37**, 294–299.

10  *A 2-year-old boy apparently fell down the stairs a few days previously. Areas of bruising of varying age are suspicious of nonaccidental trauma. Which of the following actions should be taken?*

   **A** *Notify child protection services*

   **B** *Obtain a skeletal survey, CT head, and ophthalmological exam, and notify child protection services only if additional injuries are found*

   **C** *Consult the hospital ethics committee to advise*

   **D** *Notify child protection services only if the child has a history of prior visits for trauma*

   **E** *Defer to the child's own pediatrician who knows his full history*

Health professionals caring for pediatric trauma patients should remain on alert for potential signs of child abuse. Laws in all 50 states require the examining physician to report all suspicious cases of child abuse to child protective services for review. Red flags include an inconsistent history, inconsistent mechanism, repeated ED visits, significant delay between injury and presentation, bruises or fractures in different stages of healing, long bone fractures in children <3 years, and multiple subdural hematomas. The workup includes an admission to the hospital, CT scan of the head, skeletal survey for patients under 2 years, ophthalmologic exam for those under 3 years, and any additional studies tailored to specific clinical concern. Child protective services should be notified for all cases of suspected nonaccidental trauma. An ethics consult or a consultation with the child's pediatrician is not necessary.

**Answer: A**

Adamsbaum, C., Mejean, N., Merzoug, V., and Rey-Salmon, C. (2010) How to explore and report children with suspected non-accidental trauma. *Pediatric Radiolology*, **40**, 932–938.

Tuggle, D.W. and Garza, J. (2008) Pediatric trauma. In Feliciano DV, Mattox KL, Moore EE (eds) *Trauma*, 6th edn, McGraw-Hill, New York, pp. 987–1002.

11  *An 8-year-old, 28 kg boy was shot with a stray bullet in the right chest while riding his bike. En route to the hospital he was transiently hypotensive, but responded to infusion of 1 L normal and 250 mL pRBCs. His workup in the ED has revealed a right-sided hemopneumothorax for which a right-sided chest tube was placed. Approximately 600 mL of blood was evacuated from the right chest. Which of the following is the most appropriate treatment course?*

   **A** *Obtain a CT of the chest to further evaluate the intrathoracic injury*

   **B** *Transfer directly to the OR for thoracic exploration*

   **C** *Transfer to the ICU for close evaluation and take to the OR if bloody output exceeds 3 mL/kg over the next 4 h*

   **D** *Transfer to the ICU for close evaluation and take to the OR if requires more than 40 mL/kg of pRBCs within 24 hours*

   **E** *Transfer to the ICU. Operative management would only be necessary if the child becomes hemodynamically unstable*

Penetrating thoracic trauma in the pediatric patient is a relatively infrequent occurrence. A single institutional study found the incidence to be around 1–2%. Of these, 54% ($n = 7$) required operative intervention. As with any penetrating trauma, low threshold for operative intervention should be maintained. Hemodynamic instability unresponsive to resuscitation or a significant bloody chest tube output (>15 mL/kg initially) or 2–3 mL/kg over the next 4 hours would mandate operative intervention. For the above patient, greater than $28 \times 15$ mL/kg or 420 mL of blood would be significant enough to justify operative intervention. A CT scan of the chest in this situation would delay intervention and put the patient at risk for decompensating during the scan. If the patient had minimal chest tube output initially and was hemodynamically normal, then a CT of the chest and close observation of chest tube output, oxygenation, and hemodynamics in the ICU would be reasonable.

**Answer: B**

Peterson, R.J., Tiwary, A.D., Kissoon, N., *et al.* (1994) Pediatric penetrating thoracic trauma: a five-year experience. *Pediatric Emergency Care*, **10** (3), 129–131.

Tuggle, D.W. and Garza, J. (2008) Pediatric trauma. In *Trauma*, 6th edn (eds D.V. Feliciano, K.L. Mattox, and E.E. Moore), McGraw-Hill, New York, pp. 987–1002.

**12** Which of the following statements regarding comparing adult and pediatric nutrition is true?
  **A** Pediatric patients have a similar overall energy expenditure compared to adults
  **B** Pediatric patients have a greater energy reserve due to proportionally larger fat stores
  **C** Unlike adults, pediatric patients do not increase total energy expenditure after traumatic injury
  **D** Children are at minimal risk for gut mucosal atrophy and bacterial translocation and therefore TPN is a good alternative to enteral feeding
  **E** Pediatric patients have a lower daily protein requirement per kilogram than adults

As with adults, optimal nutrition is an important component of treatment for pediatric trauma patients. While many of the aspects of nutritional support are similar with adults and children, some important distinctions exist. One of the main distinguishing characteristics in pediatric nutrition is that children do not increase their overall energy consumption after trauma as seen in adults. Instead, they shift their energy from growth support to the hypermetabolic response. Children also have higher baseline energy expenditure per kilogram and a higher protein requirement per kilogram compared to adults. Protein support becomes vital in children because they have a higher requirement, decreased stores, and decreased ability to tolerate protein deficiency without complications of infection, respiratory failure, and wound healing. Most recommend supplemental enteral or parenteral feedings to commence if more than three days without a diet is anticipated. As with adults, enteral feeding is recommended if it can be tolerated due to risk of central venous catheter complications, infection, and bacterial translocation from gut mucosal atrophy. It is recommended that children fed enterally have a 10% increase in calorie content due to obligate intestinal malabsorption.

**Answer: C**

Cook, R.C. and Blinman, T.A. (2010) Nutritional support of the pediatric trauma patient. *Seminars in Pediatric Surgery*, **19**, 242–251.
Jaksic, T. (2002) Effective and efficient nutritional support for the injured child. *Surgical Clinics of North America*, **82**, 379–391.

**13** An 8-year-old boy is admitted to the PICU with sepsis and respiratory failure. He is intubated and sedated. All of the following are supported as early endpoints of resuscitation except?
  **A** Normalization of blood pressure for age
  **B** Capillary refill </= 2 seconds
  **C** Normal pulse exam with no differential between peripheral and central pulses
  **D** Urine output > 1cc/kg/hr
  **E** Hemoglobin levels > 12 mg/dl

Pediatric sepsis resuscitation generally follows similar guidelines to adults, with several "special considerations" that take into account the unique pediatric physiology and response to overwhelming infection. The Surviving Sepsis Guidelines emphasize the importance of minimizing the time to recognition and initiation of critical therapies for pediatric sepsis. These include administration of broad-spectrum antibiotics (preferably after cultures have been obtained), fluid resuscitation, and source control. Initial endpoints of resuscitation for septic shock include capillary refill </= 2 seconds, normal blood pressure for age, normal pulse exam with no differential between peripheral and central pulses, normal urine output, warm extremities, and normal mental status. Later endpoints after initial resuscitation include a central venous $O_2$ saturation ($ScvO_2$) >/= 70% and cardiac index between 3.3 and 6 L/min/m$^2$. It should be noted however that several recent trials have questioned the value of using $ScvO_2$ as an endpoint, and alternative endpoints such as lactate or dynamic ultrasound assessment may be substituted. Similar hemoglobin targets to adults are recommended in pediatric patients, and a hemoglobin target of > 7g/dL is appropriate after initial resuscitation and stabilization. There is clearly no benefit of transfusing pediatric patients to hemoglobin of greater than 7–10 g/dL

**Answer: E**

Dellinger, R.P., Levy, M.M., Rhodes, A., *et al.* (2013) Surviving sepsis campaign: international guidelines for management of severe sepsis and septic shock: 2012. *Critical Care Medicine*, **41** (2), 580–637.
Surviving Sepsis Campaign (2013) Recommendations: special considerations in pediatrics, at: http://www.survivingsepsis.org/Guidelines/Documents/Pediatric%20table.pdf (accessed November 12, 2017).

**14** A 10-year-old girl is admitted to the PICU with progressive hypoxic respiratory failure following emergent surgery. She is intubated and placed on mechanical ventilation. Her pulse oximeter $O_2$ saturation is 90% on an $FiO_2$ of 0.8, and her mean airway pressure is 20 mm Hg. An arterial blood gas is obtained with pH 7.25, $pCO_2$ 65, and $pO_2$ 80. She has bilateral diffuse interstitial infiltrates on x-ray and no clinical evidence of cardiogenic edema. Which of the following statements is correct?

A *This patient does not meet diagnostic criteria for acute respiratory distress syndrome (ARDS), but meets criteria for acute lung injury (ALI)*

B *The P/F ratio in this patient is > 200*

C *Minute ventilation should be increased to correct the respiratory acidosis*

D *The Oxygenation Index is 20, indicating severe ARDS.*

E *The diagnosis and categorization of pediatric ARDS requires the measurement of the PaO$_2$ from an arterial blood gas*

This patient has significant hypoxemic respiratory failure in the postoperative setting consistent with acute respiratory distress syndrome, and meets all currently accepted criteria for a diagnosis of ARDS. Similar management principles to adults should be utilized, including low tidal volume ventilation and tolerance of permissive hypercapnia and mild to moderate respiratory acidosis (pH > 7.20). The previous ARDS classification system that included the diagnosis of "acute lung injury" has been abandoned in favor of the "Berlin Criteria." This categorizes the severity of ARDS based on the P/F ratio as mild (</=100), moderate (101–200), or severe (201–300). The P/F ratio in this patient is 100, consistent with severe ARDS. However, these criteria were developed for adult patients, and did not take into account unique features of pediatric disease, as well as alternative measures of oxygenation used in pediatric critical care. In 2015 the Pediatric Acute Lung Injury Consensus Conference Group published

their pediatric-specific consensus diagnostic criteria and treatment guidelines for pediatric ARDS (see Table 46.2). This includes the use of the alternative indices of oxygenation index (OI) or oxygen saturation index (OSI). The OI has the advantage of including information about mean airway pressures, while the OSI has the advantage of requiring only a pulse oximetry reading instead of an arterial blood gas. Table 46.2 shows the OI and OSI cutoffs for determining the severity of ARDS in pediatric patients. In this patient, the OI is 20, and the OSI is 17.8, both of which result in a categorization of severe ARDS. These measures have also been shown to be useful for predicting mortality, as well as serving as criteria for consideration of ECMO in patients with an OI > 40.

The OI is calculated as OI = (FiO$_2$ × Mean Airway Pressure × 100)/PaO$_2$

The OSI is calculated as OSI = (FiO$_2$ × Mean Airway Pressure × 100)/SpO$_2$

**Answer: D**

Khemani, R.G., Smith, L.S., Zimmerman, J.J., *et al.* (2015) Pediatric acute respiratory distress syndrome: definition, incidence, and epidemiology: proceedings from the Pediatric Acute Lung Injury Consensus Conference. *Pediatric Critical Care Medicine*, **16** (5 Suppl 1), S23–40.

Rimensberger, P.C., Cheifetz, I.M., and Pediatric Acute Lung Injury Consensus Conference G. (2015) Ventilatory support in children with pediatric acute respiratory distress syndrome: proceedings from the

**Table 46.2** The OI and OSI cutoffs for determining the severity of ARDS in pediatric patients.

| Age | Exclude patients with peri-natal related lung disease | | | |
|---|---|---|---|---|
| **Timing** | Within 7 days of known clinical insult | | | |
| **Origin of Edema** | Respiratory failure not fully explained by cardiac failure or fluid overload | | | |
| **Chest Imaging** | Chest imaging findings of new infiltrate(s) consistent with acute pulmonary parenchymal disease | | | |
| **Oxygenation** | **Non Invasive mechanical ventilation** | **Invasive mechanical ventilation** | | |
| | PARDS (No severity stratification) | Mild | Moderate | Severe |
| | Full face-mask bi-level ventilation or CPAP ≥ 5 cm H$_2$O[2] PF ratios ≤ 300 SF ratio ≤ 264[1] | 4 ≤ OI < 8 5 ≤ OSI < 7.5[1] | 8 < OI < 16 7.5 ≤ OSI < 12.3[1] | OI ≥ 16 OSI ≥ 12.3[1] |
| | **Special Populations** | | | |
| **Cyanotic Heart Disease** | Standard Criteria above for age, timing, origin of edema and chest imaging with an acute deterioration in oxygenation not explained by underlying cardiac disease.[3] | | | |
| **Chronic Lung Disease** | Standard Criteria above for age, timing, and origin of edema with chest imaging consistent with new infiltrate and acute deterioration in oxygenation from baseline which meet oxygenation criteria above.[3] | | | |
| **Left Ventricular dysfunction** | Standard Criteria for age, timing and origin of edema with chest imaging changes consistent with new infiltrate and acute deterioration in oxygenation which meet criteria above not explained by left ventricular dysfunction. | | | |

*Source*: Reprinted with permission from: Pediatric Acute Lung Injury Consensus Conference Group (2015) *Pediatric Critical Care Medicine*, **16** (5), 428–439

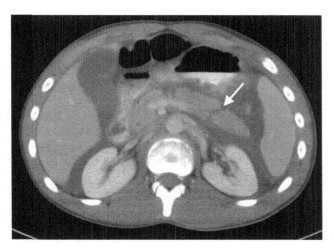

**Figure 46.1**

Pediatric Acute Lung Injury Consensus Conference. *Pediatric Critical Care Medicine*, **16** (5 Suppl 1), S51–60.

Tamburro, R.F., Kneyber, M.C., and Pediatric Acute Lung Injury Consensus Conference G. (2015) Pulmonary specific ancillary treatment for pediatric acute respiratory distress syndrome: proceedings from the Pediatric Acute Lung Injury Consensus Conference. *Pediatric Critical Care Medicine*, **16** (5 Suppl 1), S61–72.

**15** *A 12-year-old boy crashes while riding his bicycle and strikes his abdomen on the handlebars. He has epigastric pain and tenderness, but normal labs and a negative FAST exam. He is admitted for observation and serial exams. On hospital day 2 he develops an acute increase in epigastric pain, fevers, nausea, and emesis. A serum lipase is 1750. He has a stat CT scan of his abdomen performed, as shown in Figure 46.1. What is the optimal management strategy for this injury?*

**A** *Operative exploration and distal pancreatectomy*

**B** *NPO, start parenteral nutrition and continued observation*

**C** *Continue regular diet and serial exams, and repeat CT scan in 48 hours*

**D** *Operative exploration without pancreatic resection, placement of closed-suction drains at site of injury*

**E** *Gastroenterology consultation for ERCP and placement of pancreatic duct stent*

The described mechanism of a sharp blow to the epigastrium from a bicycle crash is frequently associated with several specific injuries. These include a pancreatic injury or an injury to the duodenum. This patient has a classic presentation for a pancreatic injury, including a somewhat delayed presentation of clear clinical manifestations of

**Table 46.3** The American Association for the Surgery of Trauma Organ Injury Scale (AAST-OIS) for pancreatic injuries. Reproduced with permission from Moore *et al.* (1990) *Journal of Trauma*, **30**, 1427–1429.

| Grade* | Type of Injury | Description of Injury |
|---|---|---|
| I | Hematoma | Minor contusion without duct injury |
| | Laceration | Superficial laceration without duct injury |
| II | Hematoma | Major contusion without duct injury or tissue loss |
| | Laceration | Major laceration without duct injury or tissue loss |
| III | Laceration | Distal transection or parenchymal injury with duct injury |
| IV | Laceration | Proximal[?] transection or parenchymal injury involving ampulla |
| V | Laceration | Massive disruption of pancreatic head |

*Advance one grade for multiple injuries up to grade III.

worsening abdominal pain, fevers, nausea/emesis, and an elevated lipase. The CT scan confirms an injury to the distal pancreas. The two most important factors in determining both prognosis and optimal management are 1) the location of the injury and 2) the integrity of the main pancreatic duct. This is reflected in the AAST Organ Injury Scale for pancreatic injuries (see Table 46.3). Injuries that have a better prognosis and that are most amenable to nonoperative management are injuries to the body/tail that do not involve the main pancreatic duct (PD). Injuries that involve the main PD typically require some type of immediate intervention to resolve or control the leakage of pancreatic enzymes into the lesser sac and abdominal cavity. This patient has an injury to the distal pancreas (arrow in Figure 46.1) that is a complete transection and thus clearly involves the main PD. Although there is some debate about operative versus nonoperative management, for pediatric patients with a distal injury and a transected PD, several series have demonstrated consistently superior outcomes with surgical intervention rather than attempts at nonoperative management. This injury is best managed with a distal pancreatectomy, and with splenic preservation if possible. Managing a pancreatic injury with drains only would be most appropriate for a grade I or II injury that involves parenchyma and not the main PD, or injuries to the pancreatic head.

**Answer: A**

Beres, A.L., Wales, P.W., Christison-Lagay, E.R., *et al.* (2013) Non-operative management of high-grade pancreatic trauma: is it worth the wait? *Journal of Pediatric Surgery*, **48** (5), 1060–1064.

Iqbal, C.W., St Peter, S.D., Tsao, K., *et al.* (2014) Operative vs nonoperative management for blunt pancreatic transection in children: multi-institutional outcomes. *Journal of the American College of Surgeons*, **218** (2), 157–162.

16  *A 6-year-old male presents to the emergency department via emergency medical services following a low-speed 30 mph MVC where he was a restrained passenger. Emesis and abdominal pain reported at the scene and concurrently in the ED. He is hemodynamically normal upon arrival and during resuscitation, reports diffuse abdominal pain but is nontender on exam. CBC, LFTs, lipase, and UA are all within normal limits. What is the most appropriate next step?*

   A  *Observation overnight, with serial abdominal exams*
   B  *Urgent CT of the abdomen and pelvis*
   C  *Abdominal ultrasound exam (FAST)*
   D  *Proceed to the operating room for urgent laparotomy*
   E  *Trial oral diet in the ED and discharge to home*

As the operative management of blunt abdominal trauma becomes more selective with the increasing specificity and availability of CT imaging, considerations regarding radiation exposure in the pediatric patient have come into question and prediction rules have been developed to guide the use of CT in pediatric trauma. Holmes *et al.* have developed a prediction rule to identify children at very low risk for intraabdominal injury (IAI) following trauma, identifying patients with whom CT scan could be avoided. Absence of abdominal wall trauma/seat belt sign, GCS > 13, absence of abdominal pain/tenderness or thoracic wall trauma, no decreased breath sounds and no vomiting had a NPV of 99.9% and a sensitivity of 97% for predicting absence IAI. Per their findings, the above patient with only abdominal pain but no objective findings on exam has a 0.7% chance of IAI. Routine laboratory screening for IAI with LFTs, lipase, CBC, and UA is routine and has shown to be predictive in the identification of abdominal injury. While FAST is excellent at predicting the need for laparotomy in the hypotensive *adult* patient, that sensitivity has not translated to the pediatric population. Abdominal ultrasonography in children is limited due to 1) the proportional decrease in intraabdominal fluid despite clinically significant injury and conversely, 2) the prevalence, among children, of clinically significant injury without hemoperitoneum (26–34% of abdominal injuries). Conversely, observation with serial abdominal exams in a hemodynamically stable patient without laboratory findings of intraabdominal injury has been shown to be effective at detecting low likelihood abdominal injuries without added morbidity.

**Answer: A**

Holmes, J.F., Gladman, A., and Chang, C.H. (2007) Performance of abdominal ultrasonography in pediatric blunt trauma patients: a meta-analysis. *Journal of Pediatric Surgery*, **42** (9), 1588–1594.

Holmes, J.F., Lillis, K., Monroe, D., *et al.* (2013). Identifying children at very low risk of clinically important blunt abdominal injuries. *Annals of Emergency Medicine*, **62** (2), 107–116.

Holmes, J.F., Sokolove, P.E., Brant, W.E., *et al.* (2002) Identification of children with intra-abdominal injuries after blunt trauma. *Annals of Emergency Medicine*, **39** (5), 500–509.

17  *Which of the following is TRUE regarding the management of burn injuries in the pediatric patient?*

   A  *The modified rule of nines inaccurately estimates total body surface area (TBSA) in children by overestimating the surface area of the head and neck and underestimating the surface area of the lower extremities*
   B  *Children under the age of two should be resuscitated with lactated ringer's solution alone during the first 24 hours after injury*
   C  *The Parkland formula, and other weight-based fluid resuscitation formulas, grossly overestimate resuscitation in severely burned children*
   D  *Children are less vulnerable to protein-calorie malnutrition following burn injury because of their proportionally increased body fat and large muscle mass as compared to adults*
   E  *Growth hormone and IGF-1 are up-regulated following burn injury*

Extensive burn injury creates an impressive stress on the body initiating a diffuse catabolic state with excessive protein loss and requiring large volume fluid resuscitation. Early management focuses on removing the source of injury, fluid resuscitation, wound management, addressing increased nutritional needs due to hypermetabolic state, and analgesia. While much of the principles of burn management are identical between children and adults there are a few notable differences. Since children have a greater body surface area (BSA) in relation to weight as compared to adults, weight-based fluid resuscitation guidelines often underestimate resuscitation volumes in small burns and overestimate it in severe burns. The most accurate measurement of BSA is with the modified rule of nines with proportionally larger percentage of BSA attributed to the head and neck in children. Children under the age of two should be resuscitated with dextrose-containing isotonic fluid because of the limited glycogen stores in that age group. Children are classically more susceptible to protein-calorie malnutrition because of their decreased fat and muscle stores. Extensive burn injuries create a diffuse catabolic state where growth hormone and IGF-1 are classically down-regulated.

**Answer: C**

Chung, D.H., Colon, N.C., Herndon, D.N. (2012) Burns, in *Pediatric Surgery*, 7th edn (eds A.G. Coran, N.S. Adzick, and A.A. Caldamore), Elsevier, Philadelphia, PA, pp. 369–384.

Graves, T.A., Captain, M.C., Cioffi, W.G., *et al.* (1988) Fluid resuscitation of infants and children with massive thermal injury. *Journal of Trauma and Acute Care Surgery*, **28** (12), 1656–1659

**18** *Which of the following patients should receive venous thromboembolism (VTE) prophylaxis in the ICU?*

  A *12-year-old girl with grade 3 splenic laceration following a motor vehicle collision*

  B *5-year-old girl with bilateral femur fractures following fall from third-story window*

  C *8-year-old girl with left femur fracture, GCS 11, currently, intubated, sedated*

  D *14-year-old boy with pelvic fracture, GCS 8, currently receiving total parenteral nutrition*

  E *3-year-old boy intubated, sedated with known IPH*

While venous thromboembolic disease has been shown to be a large source of morbidity in the adult trauma patient, this risk has not directly translated to the pediatric cohort. Large retrospective studies have shown exceedingly low rates of unprovoked VTE in trauma patients < 13 years old (Azu *et al.* report 0/1192 DVTs over 10 years). However, the risk for VTE appears to increase with age from exceedingly low in children to near adult rates in late adolescents. Risk factors for VTE in the pediatric population are parenteral nutrition supplementation, central venous catheter, deep sedation, and neuromuscular blockade. Sepsis, long bone fracture and spinal cord injury were not associated with increased risk.

**Answer: D**

Azu, M.C., McCormack, J.E., Scriven, R.J., *et al.* (2005) Venous thromboembolic events in pediatric trauma patients: is prophylaxis necessary? *Journal of Trauma and Acute Care Surgery*, **59** (6), 1345–1349.

Hanson, S.J., Punzalan, R.C., Greenup, R.A., *et al.* (2010) Incidence and risk factors for venous thromboembolism in critically ill children after trauma. *Journal of Trauma and Acute Care Surgery*, **68** (1), 52–56

**19** *Which of the following regarding pediatric solid organ injuries is not true?*

  A *They are the most common injury modality following blunt abdominal trauma*

  B *Conservative management fails in approximately 23% of cases*

  C *When managed by adult trauma surgeons, pediatric patients have significantly higher rates of laparotomy*

  D *Solid organ injury is associated with additional intraabdominal injury in approximately 18% of cases*

  E *Delayed hemorrhage after blunt splenic or liver injury is rare*

Solid organ injury is the most common injury modality in blunt abdominal trauma and treatment continues to evolve towards progressive nonoperative management with >90% success rate. Despite this success, management practices differ depending on treatment setting and the training of the surgeon with significantly higher rates of laparotomy amongst nonlevel 1 trauma facilities, rural hospitals, and nonpediatric surgeons. Solid organ injury is associated with a low rate (18%) of other intraabdominal injury and delayed solid organ hemorrhage is exceedingly rare (0.33% as noted by Davies et al.)

**Answer: B**

Davies, D.A., Fecteau, A., Himidan, S., *et al.* (2009) What's the incidence of delayed splenic bleeding in children after blunt trauma? An institutional experience and review of the literature. *Journal of Trauma and Acute Care Surgery*, **67** (3), 573–577

Morse, M.A. and Garcia, V.F. (1994) Selective nonoperative management of pediatric blunt splenic trauma: Risk for missed associated injuries. *Journal of Pediatric Surgery*, **29** (1), 23–27

Sims, C.A., Wiebe, D.J., and Nance, M.L. (2008) Blunt solid organ injury: do adult and pediatric surgeons treat children differently? *Journal of Trauma and Acute Care Surgery*, **65** (3), 698–703

**20** *Which of the following patients with head trauma has the strongest indication for performing a head CT scan?*

  A *2-year-old girl who fell while running in playground, no LOC, 5 cm frontal scalp hematoma but no palpable skull fracture, alert, interactive, and appropriate per teacher*

  B *11-month-old girl who fell from highchair. Reportedly loss consciousness for 5 seconds before crying, no scalp hematoma on exam, now acting appropriately per parents*

C *10-year-old girl tripped while running up stair, hitting her head. She has a 3 cm frontal scalp hematoma, denies loss of consciousness or headache, GCS 15*

D *4-year-old boy who fell from monkey bars, 10 sec LOC, no palpable skull fracture, GCS 14*

E *18-month-old boy who fell from ottoman with 3-4 sec LOC, no external signs of trauma, now acting normally per parents*

Identifying clinically important traumatic brain injury has become paramount in the trauma assessment and has markedly improved as CT imaging evolves. However, over utilization of ionizing radiation can increase the risk of malignancy significantly in the pediatric population. Clinical prediction rules have been developed with a NPV of 99.9–100% to identify patients in a low-risk group for TBI. Per Kuppermann et al. normal mental status, absence of scalp hematoma except frontal, LOC < 5 seconds, nonsevere injury mechanism, absence palpable skull fracture, and normal affect per parents predicts low-risk for clinically significant TBI in patients < 2 years. Similar rules apply to the rest of the pediatric population with the exception that those > 2 years old, any LOC raises the suspicion of possible TBI.

**Answer: D**

Kuppermann, N., Holmes, J.F., Dayan, P.S., *et al.* (2009) Identification of children at very low risk of clinically-important brain injuries after head trauma: a prospective cohort study. *Lancet*, **374** (9696), 1160–1170.

Osmond, M.H., Klassen, T.P., Wells, G.A., *et al.* (2010) CATCH: a clinical decision rule for the use of computed tomography in children with minor head injury. *Canadian Medical Association Journal*, **182** (4), 341–348.

21 *A pediatric trauma patient requires computed tomography imaging of the brain, abdomen, and pelvis. Which of the following will significantly reduce the total dose of radiation the patient receives from the CT scan?*

A *Decreasing the slice thickness to 2mm from 5mm*

B *Using an older 16-slice CT scanner versus a newer 64-slice machine*

C *Keeping the arms at the patient's side during the abdominal CT scan*

D *Decreasing the beam energy and CT tube current*

E *Performing the Head CT and the abdomen/pelvis CT at different times*

Although CT scanning has become the default imaging strategy for most adult trauma patients, it should be used much more sparingly in pediatric trauma patients. This is due to the increased appreciation of the longer-term risks of radiation exposure, including an increased lifetime risk of cancers. This risk appears to correlate with total radiation exposure, which can accumulate rapidly with the liberal use of x-rays and CT scans for routine diagnostic imaging. This has led to the widespread adoption of the principle of ALARA (as low are reasonably achievable) when it comes to pediatric radiation exposure. The most important factor to reduce total radiation dose is to limit unnecessary imaging, or to use modalities such as ultrasound and MRI that do not carry the same risks of exposure. For the pediatric patient who does require imaging, particularly with computed tomography, there are multiple adjustments that can be made to decrease the radiation exposure and received dose. These include using thicker image cuts (avoiding "fine cut" imaging), using the latest generation of CT scanners, raising the arms above the head for body imaging, and decreasing the CT beam energy and the tube current (correct answer to above question). Performing the studies concurrently or at different times will not have an appreciable effect on the total dose of radiation received.

**Answer: D**

Brinkman, A.S., Gill, K.G., Leys, C.M., and Gosain, A. (2015) Computed tomography–related radiation exposure in children transferred to a Level I pediatric trauma center. *Journal of Trauma and Acute Care Surgery*, **78** (6), 1134–1137.

Eeg, K.R., Khoury, A.E., Halachmi, S., *et al.* (2009) Single center experience with application of the ALARA concept to serial imaging studies after blunt renal trauma in children–is ultrasound enough? *Journal of Urology*, **181** (4), 1834–1840.

Zacharias, C., Alessio, A.M., Otto, R.K., *et al.* (2013) Pediatric CT, strategies to lower radiation dose. *American Journal of Roentology*, **200** (5), 950–956.

# 47

# Geriatrics

*K. Aviva Bashan-Gilzenrat, MD and Bryan Morse, MS, MD*

The *following vignette applies to questions 1– 4. A 76-year-old woman is admitted to the intensive care unit following a fall down some stairs. Her injuries include a 6 mm subdural hematoma, a type II odontoid fracture, and fractures of left ribs 3–9 with moderate hemopneumothorax. On presentation, she has a blood pressure of 160/96 mm Hg, heart rate of 70 beats/min, and oxygen saturation of 91% on 6 L of oxygen by nasal cannula. Her GCS is 14. Her medical history is significant for the use of warfarin for paroxysmal atrial fibrillation, with a presenting international normalized ratio (INR) of 3.1.*

1 *Which of the following statements is true:*
   A *Chronic amyloid deposits in the myocardium increase cardiac contractility*
   B *Ventricular filling is improved by cardiac myocyte hypertrophy creating a vacuum effect during diastole*
   C *Diastolic compliance is reduced and diastolic filling delayed*
   D *"Silent" or unrecognized myocardial infarction is uncommon in geriatric patients*
   E *The volume of crystalloid, blood, and blood products should be minimized to avoid congestive heart failure in the elderly patient*

There are numerous age-related changes in the heart. The replacement of normal elastin fibers and the deposition of calcium contribute to progressive loss of elasticity in the arterial tree. Arteriosclerosis leads to systolic hypertension, impaired impedance matching, and myocardial hypertrophy. Similarly, the heart itself becomes increasingly stiff due to amyloid deposits in the myocardium with as much as a 30% increase in ventricular wall thickness. The combination of myocyte hypertrophy and increased left ventricular afterload prolongs myocardial contraction. This extended contraction leads to a delay in diastolic filling by 50% due to reduced diastolic compliance of the left ventricle. This renders the left ventricle dependent on

atrial filling pressures to maintain end-diastolic volume and preserve ejection fraction in elderly patients. Furthermore, chronic amyloid deposits in the myocardium can also be a cause of conduction abnormalities and decrease cardiac function.

The Framingham heart study found that more than 40% of subjects over the age of 75 years had silent or unrecognized ischemia. All of these factors contribute to the elderly heart being much more reliant on preload, rather than heart rate, to maintain adequate cardiac output. For this reason careful attention must be paid to adequately restoring circulating volume and maintaining sinus rhythm to maximize diastolic filling and cardiac output making E incorrect

**Answer: C**

Alvis, B.D. and Hughes, C.G. (2015) Physiology considerations in geriatric patients. *Anesthesiology Clinics*, **33** (3), 447–456.

Kannel, W.B., Bannenberg, A.L., and Abbott, R.D. (1985) Unrecognized myocardial infarction and hypertension: The Framingham Study. *American Heart Journal*, **109**, 581–585.

Oxenham, H. and Sharpe, N. (2003) Cardiovascular aging and heart failure. *European Journal of Heart Failure*, **5**, 427–434.

2 *Because of the patient's rib fractures and intracranial hemorrhage she is admitted to the ICU for close observation and treatment. A small-bore pigtail chest tube has been placed on the left and drained 200 ml of blood. She is requiring 6 L oxygen by nasal cannula to maintain her oxygen saturation above 90%. Multiple rib fractures in an elderly patient:*
   A *Result in the same risk for mortality as seen in younger patients*
   B *Lead to pneumonia twice as often as in younger patients with similar injury and occurs 33% of the time.*

C *Usually result in mortality in the first 72 hours after injury*

D *Result in complications with the same frequency whether epidural analgesia or opioids are used for pain control*

E *Require significant mechanism of injury to occur*

In the geriatric population, rib fractures and other chest trauma are frequent, and can occur in two-thirds of blunt injured trauma patients, and up to 35% of these may have pulmonary complications. Mechanism of injury is frequently misleading. Elderly patients with same level falls had much higher injury severity than younger patients with the same mechanism of injury, and the injury from falls is much more likely to result in death. The mortality rate in the elderly is much higher than in younger patients. Death from isolated chest trauma occurs late; in one study, an average of 23 days after trauma. The mortality is late and not early in the hospitalization. Pneumonia is frequent in the elderly after rib fractures, occurring in nearly one-third of patients, a rate much higher than younger patients. Epidural and other regional anesthesia offers significant benefit for patients and has been shown to both reduce the number of ventilator days and the rate of pneumonia. The elderly can break multiple ribs as they are calcified and have less compliance. The younger patient can absorb tremendous kinetic energy, enough to cause significant pulmonary contusions without breaking ribs. However, the elderly can break many ribs with lesser amounts of kinetic energy. How they respond to the fractured ribs is also different to the younger patient.

**Answer: B**

Bergeron, E., Lavoie, A., Clas, D., *et al.* (2003) Elderly trauma patients with rib fractures are at greater risk of death and pneumonia. *Journal of Trauma*, **54**, 478–485.

Bulger, E.M., Arneson, M.A., Mock, C.N., and Jurkovich, G.J. (2000) Rib fractures in the elderly. *Journal of Trauma*, **48** (6), 1040–1046.

Bulger, E.M., Edwards, T., Klotz, P., and Jurkovich, G.J. (2004) Epidural analgesia improves outcome after multiple rib fractures. *Surgery*, **136** (2), 426–430.

3 *Despite aggressive pulmonary hygiene measures and adequate pain control she eventually progresses to respiratory failure, is intubated, and placed on mechanical ventilation. When managing mechanical ventilation in the elderly, which of the following is the most true:*

A *Position will have little effect, as the work of breathing will be the same in the supine and upright positions*

B *Chest wall compliance will be increased due to weakening of connective tissue and loss of muscle strength*

C *The use of positive end-expiratory pressure (PEEP) is important to overcome the greater tendency of the lungs to collapse at higher volumes*

D *Higher tidal volumes should be used in order to overcome the loss of elasticity in the alveoli*

E *Standard weaning parameters for extubation show the same predictive power as in younger patients*

The elderly patient has numerous changes in pulmonary physiology. Declines in vital capacity, forced expiratory volume in one second, arterial oxygen tension, and maximal oxygen consumption are all clinically relevant. Upright positioning has been shown to decrease oxygen consumption compared to the sitting position and thus A is not correct. Chest wall compliance is also decreased in the elderly due to calcification of the ribs and spine and thus Answer B is not correct. PEEP is helpful in elderly patients, as the loss of elasticity in the airways results in closure of the lung at much higher volumes and is thus the correct answer. The tendency of the airways to close, and the use of high tidal volumes, results in over aeration of the healthy lung and begins a cycle of progressive lung injury and decline. This causes barotrauma and thus Answer D is not correct. Standard weaning parameters have been shown to be less accurate in predicting successful weaning from mechanical ventilation in geriatric patients.

**Answer: C**

Brandi, L.S., Bertoline, R., Janni, A., *et al.* (1996) Energy metabolism of thoracic surgical patients in the early postoperative period. *Effect of posture. Chest*, **109**, 630–637.

Gee, M.H., Gottlieb, J.E., Albertine, K.H., *et al.* (1990) Physiology of aging related to outcome in the adult respiratory distress syndrome. *Journal of Applied Physiology*, **69**, 822–829.

Krieger, B.P., Ershowsky, P.F., Becker, D.A., Gazeroglu, H.B. (1989) Evaluation of conventional criteria for predicting successful weaning from mechanical ventilatory support in elderly patients. *Critical Care Medicine*, **17**, 858–861.

4 *The patient has a subdural hematoma in the setting of warfarin use with an INR of 3.1. Which statement is most accurate for trauma patients on preinjury warfarin?*

A *All trauma patients on warfarin have a greater incidence of death and disability than patients with no history of warfarin use*

**B** *Presenting INR and Glasgow Coma Score can be used to accurately identify patients with intracranial hemorrhage in trauma*

**C** *Warfarin use is present in less than 5% of geriatric trauma patients*

**D** *Reversal of anticoagulation with prothrombin complex concentrate (PCC) is more rapid than vitamin K and fresh frozen plasma*

**E** *Elderly trauma patients on warfarin with no CT evidence of intracranial hemorrhage can safely be discharged from the emergency department*

Despite this, multiple studies have seen no change in mortality in the absence of traumatic intracranial hemorrhage. Intracranial hemorrhage is only reliably detected in these patients by liberal use of CT scans. Warfarin use in elderly patients is quite common, and may be present in as many as 9% of patients presenting after trauma. In geriatric patients, rapid reversal of anticoagulation with prothrombin complex concentrate (PCC) is quicker than vitamin K and plasma with a reduced rate of intracranial hemorrhage expansion. The rate of significant bleeding may approach 7–14% with absent or minimal symptoms. In addition, decompensation after minor injury is common, and patients require monitoring as an inpatient for at least 24 hours, although the INR does not need to be corrected unless intracranial hemorrhage is present.

**Answer: D**

Edavettal, M., Rogers, A., Rogers, F., *et al.* (2014) Prothrombin complex concentrate accelerates international normalized ratio reversal and diminishes the extension of intracranial hemorrhage in geriatric trauma patients. *American Surgeon*, **80**, 372–376.

Ivascu, F.A., Howells, G.A., Junn, F.S., *et al.* (2005) Rapid warfarin reversal in anticoagulated patients with traumatic intracranial hemorrhage reduces hemorrhage progression and mortality. *Journal of Trauma*, **59**, 1131–1139.

Mina, A.A., Bair, H.A., Howells, G.A., and Bendick, P.J. (2003) Complications of preinjury warfarin use in the trauma patient. *Journal of Trauma*, **54**, 842–847.

*The following vignette applies to questions 5 and 6. An 84-year-old patient with a history of mild Alzheimer's disease was admitted to the ICU after undergoing emergent colectomy for complications of diverticular disease. He was successfully weaned from mechanical ventilation on postoperative day 2. Since extubation he has been intermittently confused and at times agitated, usually at night.*

**5** *Delirium in the ICU:*

**A** *Is easily identified and diagnosed in the critically ill patients*

**B** *Is unavoidable due to required sedation and analgesia*

**C** *Is minimized by use of constant infusions of sedatives to prevent the detrimental cognitive effects of sleep loss*

**D** *Is best managed by restraints and immobilization to prevent injury during exacerbations*

**E** *Can be reduced by the use of gamma-aminobutyric acid (GABA) receptor sparing agents such as opioids and dexmedetomidine instead of benzodiazepines*

**Answer: E**

**6** *Which of the following medications should be avoided in the elderly, delirious patient?*

**A** *Haldol*

**B** *Risperidone*

**C** *Benadryl*

**D** *Fentanyl*

**E** *Quetiapine*

Delirium in the ICU is frequent and is often under recognized by the treatment team. The classic presentation of agitation and confusion at night makes up less than half of the patients with delirium. Daily screening measures should be employed such as the Confusion Assessment Method for the ICU (CAM-ICU) assessment. Sedation and analgesia are, of course, required in the mechanically ventilated patient, but techniques are available to avoid delirium. Intermittent, rather than continuous infusions can result in less delirium, and the duration of the first episode may be shorter. Daily sedation interruptions are an essential part of critical care. Sleep disturbance is almost uniform in the ICU, with the average patient getting only 2 hours of sleep over 24 hours. In addition the time spent in rapid eye movement (REM) sleep is reduced. Restraints are a last resort, and should only be employed when medically needed to protect the patient and medically necessary devices. The immobilization actually contributes to delirium. Newer GABA-sparing agents such as dexmedetomidine have less incidence of delirium than benzodiazepines.

Benzodiazepines in the elderly are often a source of itatrogenic problems as they typically have very long half-life and active metabolites. After trying to orient the patient, if the benzodiazepines are administered, the patient will be amnestic as that is one of the major effects of benzodiazepines. Thus this could add to the problem of confusion and delirium. In the setting of traumatic brain injury or intracranial hemorrhage the administration of benzodiazepines can be difficult to separate whether the confusion, and altered mental status is due to delirium, dementia, worsening traumatic brain injury or due to the benzodiazepines. Current recommendations are to avoid benzodiazepines in the elderly for delirium and, if they are to be used for possible alcohol withdrawal, that it is used in intermittent doses and not to be used as continuous effusions. Drugs with long half-lives with active metabolites should not be used as infusions in general in the SICU.

After ruling out metabolic sources of delirium, pharmacologic treatment of delirium is employed. Haldol is the recommended drug of choice for the treatment of ICU delirium by Society of Critical Care Medicine. Use of other newer antipsychotics, such as risperidone, ziprasidone, and quetiapine, can be useful in the treatment of delirium, but are not as useful for treatment of acute exacerbations. Anticholinergic drugs such as benadryl should be avoided in elderly patients. Atypical reactions are common and can exacerbate alterations in mental status. Opiates, like fentanyl, remifentanil, morphine and hydromorphone, are often used in the ICU as sedative-analgesics, especially in cases of agitation caused by pain. Abnormal pharmacokinetic modifying variables, like age and renal function, can magnify differences among the agents and can potentially worsen delirium.

**Answer: C**

Girard, T.D., Pandharipande, P.P., and Ely, E.W. (2008) Delirium in the intensive care unit. *Critical Care*, **12** (suppl. 3), S3.

Jacobi, J., Fraser, G.L., Coursin, D.B., *et al.* (2002) Clinical practice guidelines for the sustained use of sedatives and analgesics in the critically ill adult. *Critical Care Medicine*, **30** (1), 119–141.

Ouimet, S., Kavanagh, B.P., Gottfried, S.B., and Skrobik, Y. (2007) Incidence, risk factors and consequences of ICU delirium. *Intensive Care Medicine*, **33**, 66–73.

*The following vignette applies to questions 7 and 8. A 65-year-old woman has been transferred to the ICU from the surgical floor for respiratory insufficiency. She underwent repair of pelvic fractures two days ago and had been recovering well until this morning, when she became hypoxic, tachycardic, and tachypneic. A presumptive diagnosis of pulmonary embolism is made, and a CT pulmonary angiogram has been ordered. She has a baseline creatinine of 1.1 mg/dL.*

**7** To prevent contrast-induced nephropathy in this patient:

  **A** *Normal creatinine levels indicate that renal function is preserved and no measures are needed*

  **B** *Dopamine should be administered to vasodilate the renal bed and promote renal function*

  **C** *Fluid use should be minimized prior to CT scan to prevent volume overload*

  **D** *Statin administration along with IV hydration prior to contrast administration should be utilized*

  **E** *The use of antioxidants such as ascorbic acid is indicated*

**Answer: D**

**8** *Following the CT scan the patient is noted to have renal dysfunction, which eventually progresses to anuria. In an elderly patient with acute kidney injury (AKI) in the ICU:*

  **A** *There is little chance of return to normal renal function if renal replacement therapy is required*

  **B** *Is most commonly due to prerenal factors*

  **C** *Furosemide should be administered to convert anuric renal failure to oliguric renal failure*

  **D** *Protein administration should be limited to prevent further damage to the kidney*

  **E** *Renal replacement therapy will be required in up to 85% of patients with oliguric renal failure, and should follow the same medical indications as younger patients*

The risk of contrast-induced nephropathy (CIN) is relatively low overall but the risk factors for renal dysfunction are much more prevalent in the geriatric patient, and efforts should be made to avoid this adverse effect. Creatinine should be assessed in all patients prior to administration of contrast. Normal creatinine is not always indicative of normal glomerular filtration rate and age is a determinant. Typically it takes loss of 75% of the nephrons before creatinine rises in general. Older patients have decreased number of nephrons compared to the younger population despite the normal creatinine levels. Optimization of fluids and the avoidance of dehydration remain important. Although the contrast is a direct nephrotoxic agent, it is especially nephrotoxic in the setting of prerenal dehydration.

A recent large meta-analysis found an important protective effect of statins with IV fluids compared to IV fluid. The role of prophylaxis with sodium bicarbonate and N-acetylcysteine remain unclear although it was originally suggestive of being protective. Vasodilators such as dopamine and fenoldopam, and antioxidants have not proven to be beneficial in preventing renal dysfunction in clinical studies.

In the elderly, prerenal ARF is the predominant type seen in hospitalized patients, usually secondary to dehydration. Acute tubular necrosis, however, is the most frequent cause of intrinsic ARF, and accounts for up to 76% of ARF in the in intensive care unit. Furosemide is frequently administered in an effort to increase urine output. Although urine output may be increased this does not translate into any improvement in clinical outcome or mortality, and is not recommended. High doses of furosemide are nephrotoxic, especially in the prerenal setting. The initiation of renal replacement is a complex decision, but the medical indications are the same as in younger patients, and the decision should be made according to the patient's directives. Many elderly patients, up to 57%, have complete return of renal function to baseline. The elderly are frequently malnourished and hypermetabolic in the setting of critical illness. Adequate nutrition is important to overall care and protein should not be withheld.

**Answer: E**

Cheung, C.M., Ponnusamy, A., and Anderton, J.G. (2008) Management of acute renal failure in the elderly patient. *Drugs and Aging*, **25** (6), 455–476.

Subramanian, R.M., Wilson, R.F., Turban, S., *et al.* (2016) Contrast-*Induced Nephropathy: Comparative Effectiveness of Preventive Measures. Comparative Effectiveness Review No. 156*. (Prepared by the Johns Hopkins University Evidence-based Practice Center under Contract No. 290-2012-00007-I.) AHRQ Publication No. 15(16)-EHC023-EF. Agency for Healthcare Research and Quality, Rockville, MD.

Pannu, N., Weibe, N., Tonelli, M., *et al.* (2006) Prophylaxis strategies for contrast-induced nephropathy. *Journal of the American Medical Association* Surgery, **295** (23), 2765–2779.

*The following vignette applies to questions 9–11. An 88-year-old man was transported by helicopter to a level I trauma center from the scene where he was struck by a car while crossing the street. In the trauma bay, his Glasgow Coma Score = 13 and he is noted to have the following vital signs: blood pressure 88/46 mm Hg and heart rate = 66 beats/ min and oxygen saturation = 95% on 2L nasal cannula $O_2$. He relates that he is on blood pressure medication, statin, insulin, and herbal supplements at home.*

9 *Which of the following is true regarding the patient's cardiac physiology:*

**A** *Chronic arteriosclerosis reduces systemic vascular resistance*

**B** *Tachycardia in response to hemorrhage can be blunted by β-adrenergic blocking medications*

**C** *For chronically hypertensive patients, a "normal" blood pressure improves end-organ perfusion*

**D** *Cardiac afterload in decreased due to decreased elastin in large arteries*

**E** *Systolic blood pressure significantly decreases with age, while diastolic blood pressure increases to a lesser extent, leading to decrease in pulse pressure*

Many structural and physiologic changes occur in the cardiovascular system in the natural aging process. Significant cardiac changes include progressive arteriosclerosis, which can lead to elevated systemic vascular resistance resulting in chronic hypertension. It is important to keep in mind that, for elderly patients with chronic hypertension, a "normal" blood pressure may produce relative hypotension with end-organ ischemia. Pulse pressure *increases* with age as systolic blood pressure significantly rises but diastolic blood pressure rises to a lesser extent. Cardiac output also decreases in geriatric patients. While basal heart rate remains relatively unchanged, the aging heart is less sensitive to sympathetic stimulation and cannot compensate for an increased need of cardiac output by significantly increasing the heart rate. Medications, especially β-blockers, may further blunt tachycardia in response to shock states. Afterload increases as a result of decreased elastin in the aorta and major vessels, and, essentially, the heart becomes preload dependent making the cardiovascular system sensitive to minor changes in volume status. In elderly patients with bradycardia, it should be initially assumed that the patient is on *β-adrenergic blocking medications*.

**Answer: B**

Nagappan, R. and Parkin, G. (2003). Geriatric critical care. *Critical Care Clinics*, **19**, 253–270

Menaker, J. and Scalea, T.M. (2010). Geriatric care in the surgical intensive care unit. *Critical Care Medicine*, **38** (9), S452–S459

*After resuscitation with two units of packed red blood cells and intravenous fluids, his blood pressure is 130/75 mm Hg and GCS = 15. CT scan head is negative, but CT abdomen/pelvis shows moderate amount of blood in LUQ and pelvis with no solid organ injury. You are preparing for transport to the operating room for exploration when the patient tells you he does not want an operation because he has end-stage lung cancer and does not want to be on a ventilator. He states he understands when told that not operating could be fatal. There is no family available.*

10 *Next step in management should be?*

**A** *Proceed to exploratory laparotomy after documenting medical necessity in chart*

**B** *Request ethics committee and psychiatry consults*

**C** *Admit to ICU and continue resuscitation and allow patient to consider operation*

**D** *Discharge patient home because he does not comply with surgical plan*

**E** *Have case manager call other family members to give consent*

Informed consent plays a significant role in the development of the relationship between the surgeon and patient. Legal statutes have determined that informed consent involves meeting the needs of the "reasonable patient" including providing the patient general information in nontechnical terms regarding an operation. Refusal of an operative intervention after an adequate informed consent process usually results from a state of indecision related to ambivalence to alternatives or fear of surgery. It is important that the surgeon not express disappointment or threaten the patient when this occurs especially given that this does not preclude future surgical intervention. However, the surgeon should explain, especially in emergent situations, that the risks and benefit and outcomes of operation may change and are time dependent. Refusal of surgery is not necessarily an indication of lack of competency. In these cases, the surgeon should review the patient's comprehension of the procedure as well as understanding other external patient concerns and acknowledge any value differences with the patient. Nonoperative management may be a useful alternative supported by a patient's values and allow the patient time to reconsider other strategies. It should be remembered that most patients are not aware of the risks and benefits, and it is important for the physician to assess the social scenario as much as possible and make the proper recommendation rather than just giving a patient a choice when they do not fully understand the consequences. However in the scenario where the patient is cognitive of the situation and is capable, surgery against their will can be interpreted as physical battery.

In many states, there are laws to allow surrogates, usually family or designated by advance directives, to make decisions for family members with diminished competence. The primary objective is to establish goals based on the patient's desires. However, in 70% of important medical decisions, surrogate care inaccurately reflects the patient's wishes. In cases of disputes, courts can be petitioned to select a surrogate.

**Answer: C**

Hare, J. Pratt, C., and Nelson C. (1992) Agreement between patients and their self-selected surrogates on difficult medical decisions. *Archives of Internal Medicine*, **152**. 1049–1054.

Jones, J.W., McCullough, L.B., and Richman, B.W. (2003) The surgeon's obligations to the noncompliant patient. *Journal of Vascular Surgery*, **38**, 626–627.

Jones, J.W. and McCullough, L.B., (2002) Refusal of life-saving treatment in the aged. *Journal of Vascular Surgery*, **35**, 1067.

Shalowitz, D.I., Garrett-Mayer, E., and Wendler, D. (2006) The accuracy of surrogate decision makers: a systematic review. *Archives of Internal Medicine*, **166** (5), 493–497.

11 *A 68-year-old man presents to the emergency department with 2 week history of "gnawing" abdominal pain which is better after eating but has been gradually worsening. His only medication is ibuprofen for chronic back pain. Surgery is consulted for abdominal pain. Which of the following is true regarding peptic ulcer disease (PUD) in the elderly?*

A *Compared to younger patients, elderly patients present with initial complaint of abdominal pain*

B *Compared to younger patients, elderly patients with peptic ulcer disease have lower incidence of Helicobacter pylori*

C *Absence of free air on abdominal plain x-rays excludes perforation*

D *Gastric outlet obstruction is the most common complication of PUD in elderly patients*

E *The most common presenting sign of PUD in elderly patients is melena*

Peptic ulcer disease (PUD) is a common and often undiagnosed disease among elderly patients. The diagnosis is challenging because, for patients with endoscopically proven PUD, elderly patients (65%) are less likely to present with abdominal pain compared to younger patients (92%). The most common presenting sign is melena, but approximately half of elderly patients with PUD initially present with a perforation followed by other complications include hemorrhage, gastric outlet obstruction, and erosion. Diagnosis of these complications can be challenging as vital signs may be normal and free air is appreciated on only about 40% of plain radiographs. Indications for operation are similar to that of the general population.

Worldwide, there is increasing prevalence of *H. pylori* infection with age, reaching 40–60% in asymptomatic elderly individuals and >70% in elderly patients with gastroduodenal disease. The prevalence is particularly high amongst institutionalized elderly patients, with a range of 70–85%.

**Answer: E**

Leuthauser, A. and McVane, B. (2016) Abdominal pain in the geriatric patient. *Emergency Medicine Clinics of North America*, **34** (2), 363–375.

Pilotto, A. and Franceschi, M. (2014) *Helicobacter pylori* infection in older people. *World Journal of Gastroenterology*, **20** (21), 6364–6367.

12 *A 72-year-old woman presents to the emergency department from a nursing home with 1 day history of vague periumbilical abdominal pain which is now localized to the right lower quadrant. According to a report from the nursing home she is refusing to eat.*

*She has a history of stroke, hypertension, and coronary artery disease. On exam, she has rebound tenderness in right lower quadrant. Surgery is consulted for abdominal pain.*

*Which of the following is true regarding appendicitis in elderly patients?*

A *Initial treatment in geriatric patients with appendicitis should be with antibiotics alone*

B *In general, open appendectomy has a higher overall rate of complications compared to laparoscopic appendectomy*

C *Due to advances in CT technology, misdiagnosis of appendicitis in geriatric patients is negligible*

D *Appendicitis is the most common indication for emergent abdominal surgery in geriatric patients*

E *In elderly patients, physical exam is the superior method for diagnosis because classically described symptoms and signs are usually present*

As life expectancy increases in the elderly patients, the incidence of appendicitis increases in this population. Currently, appendectomy is not the most common but the third most common indication for abdominal surgery in elderly patients. Although the overall incidence is lower in the elderly population compared with the general population, the mortality rate is four to eight times higher due to delay in diagnosis and frequent misdiagnosis in approximately 50% of cases. Classic symptoms of fever, anorexia, and leukocytosis are present in less than one-third of patients. Less than one-third of patients have fever, anorexia, right lower quadrant pain, or leukocytosis on presentation. Laparoscopic appendectomy is the primary operation for appendicitis. For patients who present with RLQ abscess, the ideal therapy would be drainage and antibiotics as open or laparoscopic surgery would be difficult. Although there is a growing body of evidence to support antibiotic use alone in treatment of appendicitis, it is not currently recommended as first-line therapy for appendicitis in elderly patients unless there are absolute contraindications to operation.

**Answer: B**

Kot, A., Kenig, J., and Wałęga, P. (2016) Treatment of acute appendicitis in geriatric patients – literature review. *Polski przeglad chirurgiczny*, **88** (3), 136–141

Omari, A.H., Khammash, M.R., Qasaimeh, G.R., *et al.* (2014) Acute appendicitis in the elderly: risk factors for perforation. *World Journal of Emergency Surgery*, **9**, 6.

Storm-Dickerson, T.L. and Horratas, M.C. (2003). What have we learned over the past 20 years about appendicitis in the elderly? *American Journal of Surgery*, **185**, 198–201.

13 *An 85-year-old woman is evaluated in the trauma bay for after being found in her bedroom beside a bottle of pills and multiple superficial lacerations to her wrist in an apparent suicide attempt. She was intubated in the field for Glasgow Coma Score = 7 and remainder of primary survey is normal. Secondary survey only demonstrates prehospital intubation and superficial lacerations which are bandaged. Current vital signs temperature = 38.1 °C, blood pressure = 100/60 and heart rate = 92 beats/ min. Electrocardiogram shows QRS duration of 130 ms with sinus tachycardia. Urine toxicology screen is positive for tricyclic antidepressants. In addition to ICU admission and ventilator support, what is the most appropriate next step in management?*

A *Administer intravenous flumazenil*

B *Administer amiodarone intravenous bolus*

C *Sodium bicarbonate infusion*

D *Administer intravenous naloxone*

E *Administer procainamide intravenous*

Elderly patients have the highest rate of suicide of any age group (19 deaths/100,000 persons). Late-life depression, a leading risk for suicide, is frequently treated with tricyclic antidepressants (TCAs). Death from TCA overdose is most frequently due to cardiovascular collapse and lethal arrhythmias. Sodium bicarbonate infusion raises serum pH minimizing binding of the drug to sodium channels as well as serum sodium levels decreasing the risk of arrhythmic potentials in the myocardium. QRS normalization should be monitored with serial electrocardiograms. Procainamide, which inhibits cardiac sodium channels similarly to TCAs, is contraindicated. Amiodarone may prolong the QRS interval and exacerbate arrhythmias. Naloxone and flumazenil are not indicated as there is no evidence of benefit from narcotic or benzodiazepine use.

**Answer: C**

Body, R., Bartram, T., Azam, F., and Mackway-Jones, K. (2011) Guidelines in Emergency Medicine Network (GEMNet): guideline for the management of tricyclic antidepressant overdose. *Emergency Medicine Journal*, **28** (4), 347–368

Uncapher, H. and Areán, P.A. (2000). Physicians are less willing to treat suicidal ideation in older patients. *Journal of the American Geriatrics Society*, **48** (2), 188–192.

*The following vignette applies to questions 14 and 15. An 81-year-old man was admitted to the surgical intensive care unit 6 days ago after segmental sigmoid colectomy and colostomy for septic shock related to perforated diverticulitis with massive contamination. He is mechanically ventilated. He has started to have stool from the colostomy.*

**14** *Which of the following is the most appropriate next step in management of this patient's nutritional support?*

   **A** *Place a central venous line and start parenteral nutrition*

   **B** *Start a hypertonic (2 kcal/mL) preparation to prevent volume overload via nasogastric route*

   **C** *Start an isotonic (1 kcal/mL) preparation via nasogastric route alone*

   **D** *Start isotonic (1 kcal/mL) preparation via nasogastric tube with intravenous lipid supplementation*

   **E** *Start isotonic enteral feeding enhanced with L-arginine via nasogastric route*

The goal of nutritional support in critically ill patients include diminishing the untoward effects of malnutrition especially in the high risk geriatric population. The enteral route is generally well-tolerated with low complication rates. Parenteral nutrition is associated with a higher number of complications especially when including mechanical complications. While it has not been shown to be superior to the enteral route, indications for parenteral nutrition include intolerance of intestinal feeding or contraindication to enteral nutrition for a prolonged period (usually > 7 days). Immuno-modulating enteral tube feeds enhanced with L-arginine or other nutrients while initially thought to be beneficial is currently controversial and not indicated at this time. The currently accepted guidelines are that no nutrition is associated with poor outcome, excessive nutrition is associated with poor outcome and that permissive underfeeding (75%) is associated with the best outcome.

**Answer: C**

McClave, S.A., Martindale, R.G., Vanek, V.W., *et al.* (2009). Guidelines for the provision and assessment of nutrition support therapy in the adult critically ill patient: Society of Critical Care Medicine (SCCM) and American Society for Parenteral and Enteral Nutrition (A.S.P.E.N.). *Journal of Parenteral and Enteral Nutrition*, **33** (3), 277–316

**15** *Which of the following is true regarding the effects of aging on nutrition and metabolism?*

   **A** *Decreased oral food intake is the primary factor in decreased resting metabolic rate*

   **B** *Weight loss in elderly patients predominantly related to decrease in physical activity*

   **C** *Lean body mass increases due to a decrease in fat mass*

   **D** *Changes in total energy expenditure are related to increases in ATPase and triiodothyronine*

   **E** *Body mass index peaks at age 70 years*

Advanced age is characterized by a number of physiologic changes including reduction in lean body mass, predominantly skeletal muscle (decreases ~40% from 20 to 70 years of age), an increase in fat mass (maximal fat mass is reached at ~70 years of age), and a redistribution of fat from the periphery to central locations. Furthermore, total energy expenditure decreases with age due to, not only a decline in physical activity, but also by a decreased resting metabolic rate. Decrease in resting metabolic rate in geriatric patients is multifactorial and is related to a decline in Na + K+ adenosine triphosphatase (ATPase) activity, a decline in triiodothyronine, a decrease in the postreceptor effect of norepinephrine, and a decrease in food intake. Weight loss is not predominantly due to decrease in physical activity and has to do with metabolism and hormones as well. Lean body mass may increase but is not solely due to decrease in fat mass. Mean body weight and BMI increase most of adult life and reach peak values at 50–59 years of age in both men and women. After age 60, mean body weight and BMI tend to decrease.

**Answer: A**

Morley, J.E. and Thomas, D.R. (1999) Anorexia and aging: pathophysiology. *Nutrition*, **15** (6), 499–503.

Reid, M.B. and Allard-Gould, P. (2004) Malnutrition and the critically ill elderly patient. *Critical Care Nursing Clinics of North America*, **16** (4), 531–536.

*This vignette applies to questions 16 and 17. A 75 year-old woman is evaluated in the trauma bay for fall from standing at home. She notes palpitations and dizziness that began shortly before the fall. She has a history of hypothyroidism, hypertension, and heart failure with preserved ejection fraction. Blood pressure = 85/45 mm Hg, heart rate = 145 beats/min, and oxygen saturation = 92% on 4 L via nasal cannula. Secondary survey reveals an irregularly irregular rhythm with tachycardia along with bruising on the right side of her face. Her Glasgow Coma Score = 15. FAST and chest and pelvis x-rays are negative. Electrocardiogram reveals atrial fibrillation with rapid ventricular rate.*

**16** *Which of the following is the most appropriate next step in acute management?*

   **A** *Diltiazem intravenous push*

   **B** *Diltiazem intravenous drip*

C *Amiodarone bolus followed by intravenous drip*
D *Metoprolol intravenous push*
E *Cardioversion*

Atrial fibrillation is the most common cardiac arrhythmia in elderly patients and prevalence increases with age. Patients with atrial fibrillation who are hemodynamically unstable should undergo immediate cardioversion although there is a risk of an embolic event. Cardioversion is very successful (approximately 90%) in restoring a normal sinus rhythm. While diltiazem and metoprolol are useful for rate control, these medications could exacerbate the hypotension, and with the history of heart failure, they may induce pulmonary edema. Amiodarone may be useful to convert atrial fibrillation in hemodynamically stable patients and can be utilized as an oral agent for atrial fibrillation prevention.

**Answer: E**

Riley, A.B. and Manning, W.J. (2011) Atrial fibrillation: an epidemic in the elderly. *Expert Reviews of Cardiovascular Therapy*, **9**, 1081–1090.
Zimetbaum, P. (2010) In the clinic. Atrial fibrillation. *Annals of Internal Medicine*, **153** (11), ITC6 -1–ITC6-16

**17** Which of the following is the most true regarding syncope in elderly adults?
   A Orthostatic hypotension is the most common cause of syncope
   B Initial evaluation of syncope should include routine echocardiography
   C Syncopal episodes in elderly patients rarely result in injury
   D Provocative tests such as postural vital signs are not recommended for evaluation syncope because they lack sensitivity
   E Carotid sinus syndrome and vasovagal events are neurally-mediated causes of syncope

Syncope is a transient loss of consciousness related to cerebral hypoperfusion. The prevalence of syncope increases with age and is associated with an estimated 2-year mortality rate of over 25%. Furthermore, syncope is strongly associated with falls and over one-third of events result in injury.

There are three etiologies of syncope related to pathophysiology. Neurally-mediated etiologies such as vasovagal syncope and carotid sinus syndrome are the most common cause of syncope in older adults. Orthostatic hypotension is another common cause with a prevalence reported as high as 30% among those aged > 75 years. In neurally-mediated syncope, autonomic reflexes are hyperactive whereas orthostatic hypotension occurs as a result of impaired autonomic reflexes. Cardiac syncope occurs in the setting of heart disease and portends a worse prognosis.

The initial workup for syncope should include a history, physical examination, and 12-lead electrocardiogram, which may obviate the need for echocardiogram in the absence of suggestive cardiac findings. Other provocative tests such as postural vital signs are cost-effective in the initial evaluation of syncope.

**Answer: E**

Goyal, P. and Maurer, M.S. (2016) Syncope in older adults. *Journal of Geriatric Cardiology*, **13** (5), 380–386.

**18** A 71-year-old man is brought to the hospital after sustaining 32% deep partial and full thickness burns to bilateral lower extremities after attempting to burn trash in his yard. He is admitted to the burn ICU, started on resuscitative IV fluids, a foley catheter is placed, and escharotomies are performed on bilateral lower extremities.
   Which of the following is the most true regarding burns in the elderly population?
   A The mortality for lower extremity burns in the elderly is the same as that of younger adults
   B Resuscitative fluids should be reduced by half in elderly burn patients to avoid fluid overload
   C Transfer to a dedicated burn center is only necessary for greater than 30% TBSA burns in the elderly
   D The mortality rate for a 15% TBSA burn in an 85 year old is the same as the mortality rate for a 90% TBSA in a 20 year old
   E The elderly only experience increased mortality rates with the addition of inhalation injury

The elderly have significantly higher mortality for any size burn, in any location, than younger adults. The latest data would suggest that there is a 50% mortality rate for a healthy adult with a 90% TBSA burn, based on advances in resuscitation, infection control and support of hypermetabolism. For patients aged 60–70 years, the 50% mortality rate occurred at 43.1% TBSA, for those aged 70 to 80 it was 25.9% TBSA, and for those 80 and older it was only 13.1% TBSA.

Elderly burn patients, although unable to tolerate volume overload as well as a younger patient, still do need significant resuscitation and care must be taken not to underresuscitate as this would increase patient likelihood of death. Instead, resuscitation must be guided by clinical response. The need for careful intervention, especially in geriatric patients, dictates that they should be transferred to a dedicated burn center with everything but minor burn injuries.

**Answer: D**

Klein, M., Goverman, J., Hayden, D., *et al.* (2014). Benchmark for the care of the critically ill burn patient. *Annals of Surgery,* **259**, 833–841.

Wibbenmeyer, L.A., Amelon, M.J., Morgan, L.J., *et al.* (2001) Predicting survival in an elderly burn patient population. *Burns,* **27** (6), 583–590.

**19** *After a fall from standing, a 76-year-old woman with a medical history of rheumatoid arthritis is brought to the emergency room for evaluation. Her GCS is 15, her vital signs are stable and she denies loss of consciousness. She is lucid and has no complaints. Physical exam is only notable for bilateral upper extremity grip strength of 4/5, with 5/5 strength in bilateral lower extremities. She has no midline spinal tenderness and no other injuries.*

*Which of the following is true regarding cervical spine clearance in geriatric patients?*

**A** *Based on NEXUS criteria, the patient does not require cervical spine imaging and can be cleared clinically*

**B** *The Canadian Cervical Spine Rule specifically lays out criteria for imaging after trauma in the elderly*

**C** *This patient's age places her at increased risk for central cord syndrome secondary to hyperextension injury*

**D** *This patient's history of rheumatoid arthritis places her at increased risk for central cord syndrome secondary to hyperflexion injury*

**E** *Elderly patients have an increased incidence of low cervical spine injuries from seemingly minor mechanisms*

The incidence of cervical spine injury is greater in elderly patients, and evaluation can be more difficult. Therefore, NEXUS and the Canadian Cervical Spine Rule studies specifically excluded elderly patients. The fact that the patient also is not neurologically normal as her upper extremities are not normal excludes her from clinical clearance. High cervical fractures, particularly type II odontoid fractures, can occur with relatively minor seeming mechanisms. Cervical stenosis, osteoarthritis, and rheumatoid arthritis can make the spine more vulnerable as well. Central cord syndrome occurs more frequently in the elderly trauma patient. It is most frequently the result of a hyperextension injury (not hyperextension injury, making D incorrect), and is characterized by

greater motor impairment in upper extremities, bladder dysfunction and a variable amount of sensory loss.

**Answer: C**

Hoffman, J.R., Mower, W.R., Wolfson, A.B., *et al.* (2000) Validity of a set of clinical criteria to rule out injury to the cervical spine in patients with blunt trauma. National Emergency X-Radiography Utilization Study Group. *New England Journal of Medicine,* **343** (2), 94–99.

Stiell I.G., Wells G.A., Vandemheen K.L., *et al.* (2001) The Canadian C-spine rule for radiography in alert and stable trauma patients. *Journal of the American Medical Association* Surgery, **286** (15), 1841–1848.

Reinhold, M., Bellabarba, C., Bransford, R., *et al.* (2011) Radiographic analysis of type II odontoid fractures in a geriatric patient population: description and pathomechanism of the "Geier"-deformity. *European Spine Journal,* **20** (11), 1929–1939.

**20** *A consult is called to the Acute Care Surgery team regarding a patient admitted to the MICU for a CHF exacerbation. The patient is a 78-year-old male with an EF of 20%, admitted with severe dyspnea, orthopnea, and worsening peripheral edema. He also complained of epigastric pain which started a few hours prior to presentation. His medical problems included dilated cardiomyopathy, type 2 diabetes mellitus, hypertension, hyperlipidemia, and polysubstance abuse. Blood urea nitrogen and creatinine were 59 mg/dL and 1.9 mg/dL respectively. The patient is started on treatment for exacerbation of congestive heart failure, which includes several doses of diuretics. Two days later, he develops crampy, moderately severe abdominal pain. A noncontrast CT scan of the abdomen showed mildly thickened and distended small bowel, but no evidence of perforation. CBC reveals a WBC of 12,000 and a lactate mildly elevated at 2.5 mmol/L. What should be the next step in management?*

**A** *Emergent exploratory laparotomy*

**B** *Diagnostic laparoscopy*

**C** *Placement of invasive monitoring and resuscitation to restore intravascular volume*

**D** *Continue diuretic therapy to optimize the patient from a pulmonary standpoint*

**E** *CT abdomen pelvis with PO and IV contrast*

The majority of cases of nonocclusive mesenteric ischemia (NOMI) involve spasm of branches of the superior mesenteric artery supplying the small intestine and proximal colon. Pathogenesis is related to a homeostatic mechanism that maintains cardiac and cerebral blood flow at the expense of the splanchnic and peripheral circulation. Spasm may also be triggered by vasoactive and cardiotonic drugs. These patients are typically critically ill, often with severe cardiovascular disease, and have life-threatening complications such as sepsis, myocardial infarction, or congestive heart failure.

The goal of treatment of patients with nonocclusive mesenteric ischemia is to restore intestinal blood flow as rapidly as possible which is accomplished by the removal inciting factors, treating underlying causes (i.e. heart failure), hemodynamic support and monitoring, and, less commonly, intraarterial infusion of vasodilators. There is no evidence of perforation, and therefore surgery is not strictly indicated at this time, thus A and B are incorrect. Continuation of diuretic therapy may cause worsening hypovolemia, causing even worse splanchnic flow, and therefore D is incorrect as well. The patient does need imaging, but with an elevated creatinine, there is significant risk of renal failure with an IV contrast bolus, thus making Answer E incorrect.

**Answer: C**

Oliva, I.B., Davarpanah, A.H., Rybicki, F.J., and Desjardins, B. (2013) ACR appropriateness criteria imaging of mesenteric ischemia. *Abdominal Imaging*, **38** (4), 714.

Park, W.M., Gloviczki, P., Cherry, K.J., *et al.* (2002) Contemporary management of acute mesenteric ischemia: Factors associated with survival. *Journal of Vascular Surgery*, **35** (3), 445–452.

Ward, D., Vernava, A.M., Kaminski, D.L., *et al.* (1995) Improved outcome by identification of high-risk nonocclusive mesenteric ischemia, aggressive reexploration, and delayed anastomosis. *American Journal of Surgery*, **170** (6), 577.

**48**

# Telemedicine and Telepresence for Surgery and Trauma

*Kalterina Latifi, MS and Rifat Latifi, MD*

1 *Telemedicine and telepresence can be performed through:*
   A *Local Area Network (LAN) and Wide Area Network (WAN) or Virtual Private Network (VPN)*
   B *Wireless Networks (3G or 4G)*
   C *Private network, closed or restricted network such as a corporate network*
   D *Wired network, network transmissions via fiber or copper cabling*
   E *All of the above*

Telemedicine requires electronic data communications networks to facilitate the exchange of patient information between two or more parties. Each network technology has its own unique features that distinguish it from other technologies. These should be carefully considered in accordance with the needs and future plans of any telemedicine program. What type of network is needed will depend on the specific needs for the telemedicine service, but bandwidth, security, and mobility requirements, the initial and recurring costs of the network, and in some cases, the distances between networked locations, are important factors. There are numerous networks that make possible completion of telemedicine programs.

**Answer: E**

Hadeed, H.G., Holcomb, M., and Latifi, R. (2010) Communication technologies – an overview of telemedicine connectivity, in *Telemedicine for Trauma, Emergency and Disaster Management* (ed. R. Latifi), Artech House, London, pp. 37–52.

SNMPTools.net (2010) *Network Basics: LAN, WAN, VPN*, at: ccessed February, 2010. http://www.snmptools.net/netbasics/lanwan/(accessed November 15, 2017).

Qiang, C.Z., Yamamichi, M., Hausman, V., and Altman, D. (2011) *Mobile Applications for the Health Sector*, The World Bank, ICT Sector Unit, Washington, DC.

2 *Telesurgery has evolved to an important field of telemedicine as we know it today, and involves surgical telementoring, teleproctoring, and other education activities as well as actual performance of the operation at the distance. Which of the following statements is not true?*
   A *Several studies have demonstrated the practicality, effectiveness and safety of surgical telementoring*
   B *Two- and three-dimensional video-based laparoscopic procedures are an ideal platform for real-time transmission and development of telesurgery*
   C *Experienced surgeons at a remote site can be safely guided and supervised by an expert*
   D *When comparing the traditional presence of the mentor with "telepresence" of the mentor from a distance, there are no significant differences in the performances of the operating surgeons or in outcomes of the operations*
   E *Laparoscopic training cannot be done via distance*

Real-time interactive long-distance teaching of surgical techniques was performed many decades ago but it was not until the late 1990s that telesurgical mentoring was reported as feasible, useful, and an acceptable teaching technique and practice. As advances in technologies and communications progressed, telesurgery was popularized by "live demonstrations" at many of the various annual surgical societies meetings, supported by industry and commercially available surgical systems. Now, we are at the point where telesurgery has expanded and one can see in the literature reports from educational and clinical telesurgical programs around the world. This is remarkable progress in surgery and medicine overall, but we have still a long road ahead of us before we can declare telesurgery a common practice in our professional lives. This is despite that fact that numerous studies have demonstrated that an inexperienced surgeon at a remote site can be safely guided and supervised by an

*Surgical Critical Care and Emergency Surgery: Clinical Questions and Answers*, Second Edition.
Edited by Forrest "Dell" Moore, Peter Rhee, and Gerard J. Fulda.
© 2018 John Wiley & Sons Ltd. Published 2018 by John Wiley & Sons Ltd.
Companion website: www.wiley.com/go/moore/surgical_criticalcare_and_emergency_surgery

expert, and when comparing the traditional presence of the mentor with "telepresence" of the mentor from a distance there are no significant differences in the performances of the operating surgeons or in outcomes of the operations. Furthermore, the safety and potentially cost effectiveness of advanced training in laparoscopic procedures from the distance was demonstrated. An experienced surgeon can guide a less experienced surgeon to perform advanced laparoscopic procedures using simple technologies such as plain old telephone with a band of 12 kbps [9] even from extreme conditions. While the real long-term value of application of telementoring is not established, this represents a new means of educating surgeons throughout the world in the latest surgical practices and technology. Accordingly, these and other studies have led to establishment of clinical telesurgical programs for real rural world. A recent survey of 159 rural surgeons practicing in communities smaller than 50,000 people, 78.6 % felt that telementoring would be useful to their practice, and 69.8 % thought it would benefit their hospitals. There was no correlation between years of practice and perceived usefulness of surgical telementoring. When asked the single most useful, or primary, application of surgical telementoring there was a split between learning new techniques (46.5 %) and intraoperative assistance with unexpected findings (39.0 %). When asked to select all applications in which they would be interested in using telementoring from a list of possible uses, surgeons most frequently selected: intraoperative consultation for unexpected findings (67.7 %), trauma consultation (32.9 %), and laparoscopic colectomy (32.9 %). Future applications of video technology are being developed, including possible integration into accreditation and board certification.

**Answer: E**

Anvari, M., McKinley, C., and Stein, H. (2005) Establishment of world's first telerobotic surgical service: for provision of advanced laparoscopic surgery in a rural community. *Annals of Surgery*, **241**, 460–464.

Bauer, J.J., Lee, B.R., Bishoff, J.T., *et al.* (2000) International surgical telementoring using a robotic arm: our experience. *Telemedicine Journal*, **6**, 25–31.

Cubano, M., Poulose, B., Talamini, M., *et al.* (1999) Long distance telementoring: A novel tool for laparoscopy aboard the USS Abraham Lincoln. *Surgical Endoscopy*, **13**, 673–678.

Glenn, I.C., Bruns, N.E., Hayek, D. *et al.* (2016) Rural surgeons would embrace surgical telementoring for help with difficult cases and acquisition of new skills. *Surgical Endoscopy*, **31** (3), 1264–1268.

Ibrahim, A.M., Varban, O.A., and Dimick, J.B. (2016) Novel uses of video to accelerate the surgical learning curve.

*Journal of Laparoendoscopic & Advanced Surgical Techniques*, **26** (4), 240–242.

Janetschek, G., Bartsch, G., and Kavoussi, L.R. (1998) Transcontinental interactive laparoscopic telesurgery between the United States and Europe. *Journal of Urology*, **160**, 1413.

Lee, B.R., Bishoff, J.T., Janetschek, G., *et al.* (1998) A novel method of surgical instruction: international telementoring. *Journal of Urology*, **16**, 367–370.

Lee, B.R., Png, D.J., Liew, L., *et al.* (2000) Laparoscopic telesurgery between the United States and Singapore. *Annals/Academy of Medicine, Singapore*, **29**, 665–668.

Marescaux, J., Leroy, J., Rubino, F., *et al.* (2002) Transcontinental robot-assisted remote telesurgery; feasibility and potential applications. *Annals of Surgery*, **235**, 487–492.

Rosser, J., Gabriel, N., Herman, B., *et al.* (2001) Telementoring and teleproctoring. *World Journal of Surgery*, **25**, 1438–1448.

Rosser, J., Bell, R., Harnett, B., et al. (1999) Use of mobile low-bandwidth telemedical techniques for extreme telemedicine applications. *Journal of the American College of Surgeons*, **189**, 397–404.

3  Which of the following is true regarding virtual intensive care?
   A  The critical specialist is confined to the intensive care unit of the hospital
   B  There is no need for nursing staff
   C  There is better compliance with evidence-based medicine and guideline compliance using telemedicine and e-health tools
   D  It is not expensive and has become very common practice already
   E  Most common technology is "open source"

Telemedicine application in the intensive care units has become a reality in many institutions in the United States. There are multiple reports suggesting better compliance with evidence-based medical guidelines and protocols when a centralized telemedicine process is in place. In one study, a remote care program used intensivists and physician extenders to provide supplemental monitoring and management of ICU patients for 19 hrs/day (noon to 7 a.m.) from a centralized, off-site facility (eICU). Supporting software, including electronic data display, physician note- and order-writing applications, and a computer-based decision-support tool, were available both in the ICU and at the remote site. They reported lower hospital mortality for ICU patients and ICU length of stay. In another study, lower variable costs per case and higher hospital revenues (from increased case volumes) generated financial benefits in excess of program costs were reported. A meta-analysis of 11 observational studies showed that telemedicine, compared to standard care, is associated with lower ICU mortality and overall hospital mortality. The cost savings were associated with a lower incidence of complications. More recently, other studies by Thomas *et al.* and Morrison *et al.* did not demonstrate mortality benefit. Virtual intensive care unit is most commonly done through a proprietary technology and not an open source. The installation and running costs are still expensive.

**Answer: C**

Breslow, M.J., Rosenfeld, B.A., Doerfler, M., *et al.* (2004) Effect of a multiple-site intensive care unit telemedicine program on clinical and economic outcomes: An alternative paradigm for intensivists staffing. *Critical Care Medicine*, **32**, 31–38.

Morrison, J.L., Cai, Q., Davis, N., *et al.* (2010) Clinical and economic outcomes of the electronic intensive care unit: Results from two community hospitals. *Critical Care Medicine*, **38**, 2–8.

Rosenfeld, B.A., Dorman, T., Breslow, M.J., *et al.* (2000) Intensive care unit telemedicine: alternate paradigm for providing continuous intensivists care. *Critical Care Medicine*, **28** (12), 3925–3931.

Thomas, E.J., Lucke, J.F., Wueste, L., *et al.* (2009) Association of Telemedicine for Remote Monitoring of Intensive Care Patients With Mortality, Complications, and Length of *Stay Journal of the American Medical Association*, **302** (24), 2671–2678.

Wilcox, M.E. and Adhikari, N.K.J. (2012) The effect of telemedicine in critically ill patients: systematic review and meta-analysis. *Critical Care*, **16**, R127.

4 *Which of the following about telemedicine for trauma and emergency management is true?*
   A *It is performed on a secured virtual private network under HIPAA regulations*
   B *Should be used only amongst small hospitals in order that they can help each other*
   C *When it comes to teletrauma, HIPAA regulations do not apply*
   D *You need to complete a fellowship in telemedicine in order to be able to get privileges for telemedicine*
   E *The best technology is an open source*

Technologies used for teletrauma and telepresence vary, in a way, each of them is in a constant experimental phase. Some systems may be more feature packed than others. One element, however, is important for all such technologies: the network connectivity is the backbone. Dedicated telemedicine networks use dedicated lines for its connectivity while others rely on a combination of technologies. In the past some programs use Integrated Services Digital Network (ISDN), however lately Digital Subscriber Lines (DSL) or Cable in the home is more common. Yet others prefer satellite, since it provides a mobile and reliable source for connectivity during times of uncertainty. What is important is for reliable technology to be in place, for policies and procedures to be well-rehearsed, and for all personnel to be well-versed in the use of the technology. It should be "online" 24/7 and can be used for any other conditions. HIPPA regulations apply as in any other patient relationship and care. There is no extra fellowship, but training should be taken before the teletrauma is practiced. Most programs do not use an open source currently. A secured network is a must.

**Answer: A**

Hadeed, H.G., Holcomb, M., and Latifi, R. (2010) Communication technologies – an overview of telemedicine connectivity, in *Telemedicine for Trauma, Emergency and Disaster Management* (ed. R. Latifi), Artech House, London, pp. 37–52.

5 *Which of the following best describes teletrauma?*
   A *Trauma surgeons cannot provide care in rural hospitals through telepresence*
   B *During teletrauma sessions, experts cannot identify knowledge gaps of provider in remote areas*
   C *The acceptance of teletrauma by trauma surgeons, referring physicians, nurses, and other providers, as well as by patients, has been reported*
   D *As technology becomes friendlier and cheaper, the concepts of teletrauma, telepresence, and teleresuscitation will not be needed any more*

Recent advances in technology, coupled with the decreasing cost of equipment, have opened the door for wider adoption of teletrauma. Robust systems can now be implemented that bring the telepresence of trauma surgeons and other emergency specialists into any rural hospital emergency room, allowing definitive trauma care to begin almost immediately after a patient's arrival at a rural hospital. Trauma surgeons can now assist in the evaluation, resuscitation, and care of the patient – a process that is often difficult to accomplish over the telephone alone. The ability to completely visualize the patient in real time is invaluable, enabling firsthand assessment by the surgeon as well as constant monitoring of the patient while the emergency team is at work. Telepresence can help prevent departures from the standard of care and avoid errors experienced in low-volume rural emergency centers. The field of trauma and emergency care management is ripe with opportunities for using telemedicine as patient care is complex and time sensitive, whereas the ability of the healthcare providers of a small hospital to remain equipped with the capacity, knowledge, and ability to deliver the timely care is limited.

Teletrauma may be able to prevent numerous deaths. Often, intervention, even if minor, will have a significant impact on the outcome of the patient. Teletrauma can not only ensure that an injured patient will not die, but also prevent the complicated course, morbidity, and cost associated with suboptimal care (or with no care at all). The biggest promise of teletrauma is the transformation of the concept of intervention from the "golden hour" to the "golden minutes," during which the patient is stabilized through appropriate teleresuscitation and then safely transported, if need be, to a trauma center. The initial experiences with teletrauma in saving lives of trauma patients, and in reducing the overall cost of trauma care have been reported. The acceptance of teletrauma by trauma surgeons, referring physicians, nurses, and other providers, as well as by patients, has been excellent. The telepresence of trauma surgeons through the teletrauma system is providing the missing segment of care in rural hospitals. Furthermore, during teletrauma sessions, experts can often identify significant knowledge gaps and the need for instituting new outreach educational programs in such hospitals. As technology becomes more user-friendly and cheaper, the concepts of teletrauma, telepresence, and teleresuscitation continue to evolve and to become more integrated into the modern care of trauma and surgical patients.

**Answer: C**

Baker, S.P., Whitfield, R.A., and O'Neil, B. (1987) Geographic variation from mortality from vehicle crashes. *New England Journal of Medicine*, **316**, 1384–1387.

Flow, K.M., Cunningham, P.R.G., and Foil, M.B. (1995) Rural trauma. *Annals of Surgery*, **27**, 29–39.

Latifi, R., Hadeed, G.J., Rhee, P., *et al.* (2009) Initial experiences and outcomes of telepresence in the management of trauma and emergency surgical patients. *American Journal of Surgery*, **198** (6), 905–910.

Ricci, M.A., Caputo, M., Amour, J., *et al.* (2003) Telemedicine reduces discrepancies in rural trauma care. *Telemedicine and e-Health*, **9**, 3–11.

Rogers, F., Ricci, M., Shackford, S., *et al.* (2001) The use of telemedicine for real-time video consultation between trauma center and community hospital in a rural setting improves early trauma care. Preliminary results. *Journal of Trauma*, **51** (6), 1037–1041.

**6** *Which of the following is true about real-time trauma resuscitation?*

  **A** *Reduces the unnecessary transport of trauma patients and may prevent preventable deaths*

  **B** *Does not helps with resuscitation when there is no trauma surgeon present in the remote site*

  **C** *Has never proved to be useful in the rural setting*

  **D** *You do not need privileges in a remote hospital to practice telemedicine since you are not there physically*

  **E** *There is high rate of malpractice law suits in teletrauma*

The first attempt to simulate the use of telemedicine in real-time trauma resuscitation was in 1978 by Dr R. Adams Cowley, who staged a disaster exercise at Friendship Airport in Baltimore, in an aged DC-6 aircraft, using old cumbersome satellite technology. Rogers et al. reported their use of a teletrauma service in rural Vermont; 68% of that state's population lives in rural areas. Their initial experience with 41 teletrauma consultations was very encouraging. Of 41 patients seen via the teletrauma system, 31 were transferred to a tertiary care center. For 59% of the patients, transfer was recommended immediately, because of their critical condition; 41% of transfers were accomplished by helicopter. In three patients, teletrauma consultation was considered lifesaving. The most common recommendations from the teletrauma consultant concerned patient disposition; for example, for 15% of the patients, the consultant recommended keeping them at the referring facility. Other recommendations included suggestions for diagnostics (such as obtaining or foregoing a computed tomography scan) and for additional therapeutics (such as placement of a nasogastric tube, placement of a chest tube, or transfusion of blood). Other investigators have described various applications of teletrauma in rural settings, such as the management of orthopedic injuries, including the evaluation and treatment of extremity and pelvic injuries. In one study, 68 of 100 patients referred for teletrauma were able to remain in the rural community hospital with pelvic fractures. That outcome certainly has major cost implications, minimizing the number of costly transfers to major medical centers, increasing the use of local healthcare facilities, and avoiding the array of social and financial issues involved with treating patients away from their families. The clinical accuracy of teletrauma has also been affirmed. Of our own first 59 patients evaluated, 35 (59%) were treated for trauma and 24 (41%) for general surgery. Of the 35 trauma patients, 32 (91%) suffered blunt injuries and three (9%), penetrating injuries. Policies and procedures need to be in place in order to practice telemedicine for trauma. Privileges, usually limited ones, must be obtained in each of the hospitals that one practices telemedicine. Today there is no report of malpractice involving telemedicine for trauma. Most commonly, telemedicine for trauma is practiced between the rural hospital and urban trauma center.

**Answer: A**

Aucar, J., Granchi, T., Liscum, K., (2000) Is regionalization of trauma care using telemedicine feasible and desirable. *American Journal of Surgery*, **180**, 535–539.

Duchesne, J.C., Kyle, A., Simmons, J., *et al.* (2008) Injury, infection, and critical care: impact of telemedicine upon rural trauma care, *Journal of Trauma*, **64** 1, 92–98.

Latifi, R. (2008) The do's and don'ts when you establish telemedicine and e-health (not only) in developing countries. *Studies in Health Technology and Informatics*, 39–44.

Latifi, R., Peck, K., Porter, J.M., *et al.* (2004) Telepresence and telementoring in trauma and emergency care management, in *Establishing Telemedicine in Developing Countries: From Inception to Implementation* (ed. R. Latifi), IOS Press, Amsterdam, pp. 193–199.

Latifi, R., Weinstein, R.S., Porter, J.M. *et al.* (2007) Telemedicine and telepresence for trauma and emergency care management. *Scandinavian Journal of Surgery*, **96** (4), 281–219.

Maull, K. (2002) The Friendship Airport disaster exercise: pioneering effort in trauma telemedicine. *European Journal of Medical Research*, 7 (Suppl), 48.

Rogers, F.B., Shackford, S.R., Osler, T.M., *et al.* (1999) Rural trauma: the challenge for the next decade. *Journal of Trauma*, **47**, 801–821.

**7** *What are the proven benefits of implementing telemedicine in critical care units?*

 **A** *Technology is leveraged given shortage of intensivists' populations to meet the demands of ICU care across the country.*

 **B** *Demand for ICU staff and expertise will continue to increase in the coming years.*

 **C** *It could address health disparity and inequality issues at a local level.*

 **D** *Reduce hospital and ICU length of stays.*

 **E** *All of the above*

One of the fundamental core concepts of telemedicine is bring expertise to a resource limited facility/department. By bringing intensivists to ICUs that lack appropriate staff the system is able to utilize technology to bridge the connection between areas of advanced technology and staffing models to areas of limited resources and staff. The technology itself allows optimal physician/patient ratios that can also be leveraged across multiple institutions and regardless of location. The lack of intensivists is against the backdrop of an increasingly aging population. It is estimated that the US elderly population will increase 50% by 2020 and will double by 2030. Patients older than 64 years use the ICU at 3.5 times the rate of the population younger than 64 years of age. Health disparities and inequality are of particular concern for health organizations across the United States. For critically ill patients across certain parts of the country, access to an ICU and a critical care specialist would mean improved outcomes and fewer complications. Telemedicine offers an ideal solution for resource limited areas, lack of staffing, increased volume of patients and improved outcomes.

**Answer: E**

Angus, D.C., Kelley, M.A., Schmitz, R.J., *et al.* (2000) Caring for the critically ill patient: current and projected workforce requirements for care of the critically ill and patients with pulmonary disease Can we meet the requirements of an aging population? *Journal of the American Medical Association Surgery*, **284**, 2762–2770.

Angus, D.C., Shorr, A.F., White, A., *et al.* (2006) Critical care delivery in the United States: distribution of services and compliance with Leapfrog recommendations. *Critical Care Medicine*, **34**, 1016–1024.

Lilly, C.M., Cody, S., Zhao, H., *et al.* (2011) Hospital mortality, length of stay, and preventable complications among critically ill patients before and after tele-ICU reengineering of critical care processes. *Journal of the American Medical Association Surgery*, **305** (21), 2175–2183.

Martin, G.S. (2006) Healthcare disparities in critically ill patients, in *Yearbook of Intensive Care and Emergency Medicine* (ed. J.L. Vincent), New York, Springer, pp. 778–785.

US Department of Health and Human Services, Health Resources and Services Administration (2003) *Report to Congress: The Critical Care Workforce; A Study of the Supply and Demand for Critical Care Physicians*. US Department of Health and Human Services, Washington, DC.

# 49

## Statistics

*Alan Cook, MD*

**1** *Cohort studies follow a group of subjects over a period of time. Each of the following is false regarding cohort studies, except:*
  **A** *They are not vulnerable to patient loss to follow up*
  **B** *They are a valid way of studying risk factors for a disease*
  **C** *They do not take very long to complete*
  **D** *They are synonymous to randomized, controlled trials because both studies follow subjects over time*
  **E** *They are generally resource efficient*

Cohort studies follow a group of study subjects, cohort, including both exposed and unexposed subjects over a period of time to compare the incidence or outcomes of a disease (see Table 49.1). The length of time required for the completion of cohort studies is determined by the problem studied. If a disease requires a lengthy period of exposure or there is a prolonged latency period, the study may require a substantial length of time to finish. Due to their longitudinal nature, cohort studies are vulnerable to patient drop out or loss to follow up. The most important difference between cohort studies and randomized, controlled trials is that some exposures are considered or known to be harmful so subjects cannot be randomized for such exposure. Thus, cohort studies are ideal for studying potentially harmful risk factors. Due to the followup time required, cohort studies tend to be resource intensive. Prospective (longitudinal) cohort studies between exposure and disease strongly aid in studying causal associations, though distinguishing true causality usually requires further corroboration from further experimental trials.

**Answer: B**

**2** *Cross-sectional studies analyze data from a group of subjects collected at a single point in time. The following are true of cross-sectional studies, except:*
  **A** *They are the design of choice to study the incidence of a disease*

**Table 49.1** Design of a cohort study.

| | Disease develops | Disease does not develop |
| --- | --- | --- |
| Exposure | *a* | *B* |
| No exposure | *c* | *D* |

  **B** *They are vulnerable to temporal bias*
  **C** *It is a type of observational study*
  **D** *Surveys are a type of cross-sectional study*
  **E** *They are often unable to include data on confounding factors*

Cross-sectional studies analyze data gathered at a single point in time, for example, a survey or poll. Due to the "snapshot-in-time" nature of this study design, we can only make inferences regarding the exposure (present or absent) and disease state (present or absent) at the same point in time. We cannot say which came first. When erroneous inferences about the proper temporal sequence of cause and effect are made, this is known as temporal bias. This study design cannot produce disease incidence rate data. We can only study disease prevalence in a cross-sectional study. Cross-sectional studies using data originally collected for other purposes often lack data pertaining to confounding factors.

**Answer: A**

**3** *An academic surgeon is planning to study the theoretical health and therapeutic effects of nutritional supplementation with vinegar extract in critically ill trauma patients. A randomized, placebo-controlled, blind trial is proposed with hyperglycemia as the primary endpoint. The hypothesized treatment effect of vinegar supplementation will be a 21% decrease in the proportion of hyperglycemic patients compared to the control group. Which of the following choices are true regarding sample size?*

*Surgical Critical Care and Emergency Surgery: Clinical Questions and Answers,* Second Edition.
Edited by Forrest "Dell" Moore, Peter Rhee, and Gerard J. Fulda.
© 2018 John Wiley & Sons Ltd. Published 2018 by John Wiley & Sons Ltd.
Companion website: www.wiley.com/go/moore/surgical_criticalcare_and_emergency_surgery

**A** *As the sample size decreases, the power to detect an actual difference increases.*

**B** *Studies with dichotomous predictors require fewer subjects to reject the null hypothesis*

**C** *The power of a sample (1-β) is the ability to detect a true significant difference between groups*

**D** *Statements of sample size calculation only need to be reported in studies that report significant differences between groups, (positive studies).*

**E** *Doubling the effect size increases the sample size by half.*

The size of a study sample is known as power and is expressed mathematically as $1-\beta$, where $\beta$ is the probability of a Type II error. The estimation of sample size is of paramount importance when planning any study, especially studies testing an intervention. In prospective trials, the cost of the study is proportional to the number of subjects in the study, as is the ability to detect a true (significant) difference between groups. Thus, the accurate estimation of the number of study subjects is a matter of scientific and economic necessity.

Dichotomizing continuous predictors, or dividing a continuous predictor variable into two mutually exclusive categories results in a substantial loss of power to detect real relationships. As such, more subjects are needed to compensate for the loss of power.

Sample size calculation should be stated in research manuscripts, especially in studies that report no difference between groups, the so called negative study. The reader needs to know if the null result is simply a matter of an insufficient sample size, a Type II error. Doubling the effect size reduces the sample size by factor of 4.

**Answer: C**

**4** *The first step in data analysis is describing characteristics of the study cohort in terms of basic differences between exposed and unexposed groups. The following are true about descriptive analyses, except:*

**A** *Tests for descriptive analyses include chi-square, t-test, Wilcoxon Rank Sum test*

**B** *They are usually found on Table 1*

**C** *Very often the variables are described with means and standard deviations (SD) or 95% confidence intervals (95% CI), medians with interquartile range (IQR)*

**D** *Multivariable logistic regression is a type of a descriptive test*

**E** *Categorizing continuous data can be useful for summarizing results, but not for statistical analysis*

Describing the characteristics of the study cohort is an important first step in the analysis of research data. Usually this is found in Table 1 and formatted to compare basic differences in the exposed and unexposed groups. The tests like those listed in answer A serve to identify any differences between groups. The measures listed in answer C describe the central tendency of the continuous data. Central tendency includes measures of the shape of the distribution of a variable. These describe the symmetry around the mean or if the distribution is skewed in one direction or another. Mean and SD suggest symmetry about the distribution of the variable. On the other hand, median and IQR are usually used when the data lack symmetry. The most common symmetric distribution is the normal or parametric distribution. Asymmetric distributions can be referred as skewed or nonparametric (Figure 49.1). Multivariable analyses are not considered descriptive tests, per se. Such analyses allow us to appraise the effect size of a predictor in the context of other predictors and confounders in the data. Categorizing a continuous variable reduces the amount of information available, though may make clinical decision making easier, (think if a value is in the "normal" range or not).

**Answer: D**

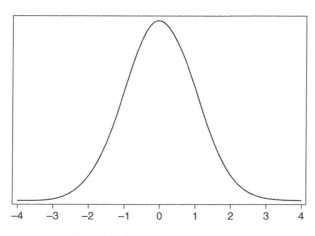 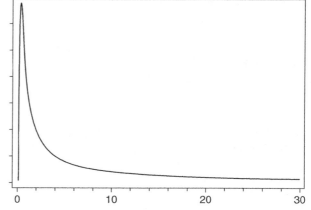

**Figure 49.1** Normal and asymmetric distributions.

**5** *In the previous question, the distinction between parametric and nonparametric data distributions was mentioned. Each distribution type requires unique tests of significance. The following tests are paired with the terms parametric or non-parametric. Which of the following are incorrectly paired?*
**A** *Parametric: Student's t-test*
**B** *Non-parametric: Wilcoxon rank sum*
**C** *Parametric: Kruskal-Wallis test*
**D** *Parametric: ANOVA*
**E** *Unpaired data: McNemar's test*

Statistical tests are each based on underlying assumptions. When the continuous data do not conform to those assumptions, inferences based on those results will be erroneous. As discussed above, the distinction of parametric versus non-parametric distribution is fundamental. Among the tests with the underlying assumption of normal or parametric distribution of continuous data are the Student's t-test and ANOVA. The Student's t-test compares the means of a continuous variable between two groups of subjects, for example, exposed and unexposed, from paired or independent samples. The ANOVA tests if a significant difference exists between means of a parametric, continuous variable among three or more groups of subjects on one or more factors. The tests appropriate for nonparametric variables include the Kruskal-Wallis and Wilcoxon rank sum. The Wilcoxon rank sum tests the null hypothesis that medians of two populations are equal and does not require the underlying populations to be normally distributed. However, the Wilcoxon rank sum does assume the distributions have the same general shape. Finally, the Kruskal-Wallis test is a nonparametric alternative to the one-way ANOVA and is used when a test of the means among more than two samples is needed or the analysis involves ordinal data. The McNemar's test takes the form of a $r \times c$ contingency table, (usually 2 x 2) for paired data.

**Answer: C**

**6** *The p-value gives us information about the results of a test. Which of the following is true regarding p-values?*
**A** *The importance of a finding is determined solely on the basis of a p-value less than 0.05*
**B** *P-values less than 0.05 indicate there is a less than 5% chance that a difference as big or bigger that the one observed will be the product of random chance*
**C** *Under ideal circumstances, all p-values in a study would be significant, $(p < 0.05)$*
**D** *A two-sided p-value tests only if the measure of interest for sample group A is greater than that for group B*

**E** *The p-value is said to be powerful to the extent that its distribution shifts toward 1 and away from 0 when the test hypothesis is false*

The p-value in statistical analyses is a measure of the probability of obtaining a result as large or larger than that observed if the null hypothesis is true. That is, the probability of incorrectly rejecting a true null hypothesis by random chance alone. When a study involves a sufficiently large cohort of subjects, even extremely small differences, including clinically or practically insignificant ones will have p-values less than 0.05. There are times when results with p-values greater than 0.05 are preferred. One example is testing the results of randomizations when groups are intended to be identical. Two-sided p-values are used in tests where the difference between A and B can be greater or lesser than 0. When the test hypothesis is true, the distribution of the p-value shifts toward 0.

**Answer: B**

**7** *In a randomized comparison of two different methods of chest tube insertion in blunt trauma patients, a new trocar device versus the conventional blunt dissection method, the investigator observes a difference in the mean insertion time. The alpha was set at $p < 0.05$. The manuscript reports the new trocar device was associated with a mean of 150 seconds (95% confidence interval (95%CI) 140–160 seconds). The mean of the conventional method was 160 seconds (95% CI 145–175). The p-value was 0.07. The result is reported as a real (significant) difference. What type of error was committed in this manuscript?*
**A** *Type I error*
**B** *Type II error*
**C** *Beta error*
**D** *No error has occurred. The authors correctly rejected the null hypothesis*
**E** *Gamma error*

The authors set the alpha, or level of significance at $p < 0.05$. The study results were associated with a p-value of 0.07. When the p-value of the result is greater than the alpha value, the null hypothesis is correct in that no real difference is present. When the null hypothesis is incorrectly rejected, a type I error has occurred. Type I error is also referred to as alpha error because it occurs at the frequency of alpha. When the null hypothesis is incorrectly retained, a type II error has occurred. Type II error is also referred to as beta error because it occurs at the frequency of beta (usually 0.8). Type II errors are frequently due to very small effect size for the predictor variable as well as small sample sizes. Also note that the 95% CIs overlap substantially. This is also an indication that the two groups differ insufficiently for a statistical significance.

**Answer: A**

8 Which of the following statements is true of p-values and 95% CIs?
  A P-values and 95% CIs are redundant measures of significance because the two add to 100
  B P-values less than 0.05 indicate there is a less than 5% chance that a difference as big or bigger than the one observed will be the product of random chance
  C The 95% CI indicates 95% of all of the data values in the population fall within the interval
  D The 95% CI indicates that if the population were randomly sampled repeatedly and 95% CIs were calculated for each sample, 95% of those CIs would contain the true population mean
  E C and E

The p-value and 95% CI are often the subjects of misinterpretation. To be valid and meaningful the results of statistical tests must take into account the uncertainty of the measure and the variability within the population of the measure in question, for example the time required to place a chest tube for each method studied. The most common measures of such requirements are the p-value and 95% CI. The p-value is discussed above. The 95% CI is a method of accounting for the variability of the phenomenon of interest (time of chest tube placement) in the target population (blunt trauma patients). The equation for the 95% CI includes terms for the sample mean $\mu$, the standard deviation $\sigma$ which measures the variability of chest tube placement in the cohort and the cohort size $n$. For the sake of completeness, the equation for the upper and lower bounds of the confidence interval is given below:

$$95\% CI = \mu \pm 1.96 \times \frac{\sigma}{\sqrt{n}}$$

**Answer: E**

9 In 2001, the rate of first-time diagnoses of pancreatitis in California was 44 per 100,000. At the same time, the prevalence of chronic pancreatitis was approximately 6 per 100,000. Which of the following is true about incidence and prevalence?
  A Incidence reflects the number of people in the target population exposed to a risk factor and might develop a disease during a specified period of time

  B Prevalence is the number of people in the population who have been successfully been treated for the disease and are now disease free during a specified period of time. They "prevailed" over the disease
  C Incidence reflects the number of people in the population who are newly diagnosed with the disease in the target population, here Californians, during a specific time period
  D Prevalence defines the number of existing cases of a disease within a population for a defined period of time
  E A and B

Incidence and prevalence are epidemiologic terms found throughout the medical literature. Incidence refers to the number of new cases in a population for a given time period. Prevalence is defined as the number of existing cases in a population for a given time period. Both incidence and prevalence are expressed as X per 100,000 (usually) population per time, usually year. There are some vital statistics expressed as X per 1,000 per year, such as infant mortality.

**Answer: A**

10 Which of the following is true regarding case-control studies:
  A Case-control studies are most useful for studying common diseases
  B Case-control studies are generally bias-free because they rely on patient recall
  C Like a cohort study, a case-control study follows groups of subjects exposed to a possible risk factor for the disease of interest
  D Case-control studies can explore associations between several exposures and the disease under study
  E The subjects in randomized, controlled trials are appropriately described as cases and controls

The characteristic of the case-control design is the first step of the study where subjects with the disease (cases) are selected then disease-free subjects with similar characteristics to the cases (controls) are selected to explore possible exposure associations. This method is valuable for studying rare diseases. Additionally, the evaluation of several exposures for association with the disease is possible. The matching of controls to the cases can be done by several methods to make the controls as similar to the cases to ensure confounders are similarly distributed between the two groups. The matching can be done at the group level to make proportions of certain characteristics, say socioeconomic status, equivalent between cases and controls. Alternatively, individual matching can be the method of choice when hospital controls are used. The major threat to the validity of case-control studies is known as recall bias. This occurs when the case subjects over report exposures in the past to explain the occurrence of the disease. Finally, a notable example of an early case-control design is that by Sir Richard Doll and A. Bradford Hill from 1950 that improved the evidence regarding the association between tobacco smoking and lung carcinoma. Subjects in randomized, controlled trials are not accurately described as cases and controls.

**Answer: D**

11  *Confounding can seriously compromise the results of a study. Which of the following is true?*

   **A** *The confounder also known as the confounding variable, is a result of the exposure*

   **B** *No known method exists for minimizing the effect of confounding in observational studies*

   **C** *Confounding biases the results of a study toward the null hypothesis*

   **D** *Confounding occurs when all or part of the observed association between exposure and outcome is partially or completely due to a variable(s) related to the outcome but not affected by the exposure*

   **E** *With the appropriate test or model, confounding can be completely controlled*

Confounding occurs when the following conditions are met: a variable is a known risk factor for the disease, and the variable is associated with the exposure, but is not a result of the exposure. Confounding in observational studies can be minimized in both the design and conduct of the study, as well as the analysis of the data. In the design phase, the cases can be matched to controls on the basis of the possible confounder. In the analysis stage, the problem of confounding can be handled by stratification of the cohort based on the confounder. Additionally, the analysis can be stratified on the confounder and by comparing the results across the strata. Another method for controlling confounding in the analysis is including the confounding variable(s) in a multivariable mode. This is adjustment or adjusting for the confounder(s). Confounding can bias the results either increasing or decreasing the effect size of the association. Confounding can persist after adjustment of the putatively measured confounders is known as residual confounding.

**Answer: D**

12  *An investigator wishes to study the association of endotracheal tubes with subglottic secretion suction compared to conventional endotracheal tubes on the*  *incidence of ventilator-associated pneumonia (VAP, yes/no) at any point in the patient's ICU stay. The other risk factors for VAP include patient age, gender, injury severity, GCS on ED arrival, days of mechanical ventilation, traumatic brain injury (yes/no), face fractures (yes/no), chlorhexidine oral hygiene, and so on. Since the incidence of VAP can be confounded by the presence or absence other factors, several variables must be controlled for simultaneously to estimate a patient's odds of VAP. The proper test for this analysis is:*

   **A** *Paired Student's t-test*

   **B** *Multivariable logistic regression*

   **C** *Multivariable linear regression*

   **D** *Cox proportional hazard ratio*

   **E** *The Mann-Whitney U test*

In the previous question, we discussed the phenomenon of confounding. The method of adjusting for one or more confounders in the analysis phase of a study is to control for them in a multivariable model. Here the outcome of interest is binary, VAP (yes/no). Therefore the paired Student's t-test, which compares the means of a variable for a group of individuals measured before and after an intervention like subjects' weight before and after a diet change is not appropriate. The Mann-Whitney U test is another name for the Wilcoxon Rank Sum test where one can compare the means of a variable between two independent groups of subjects when the distribution of the variable is nonparametric (See question 4). Again, this is a bivariate test and cannot accommodate the nine variables we list in the question. The Cox proportional hazard ratio is a multivariable model that incorporates a time-to-event component. The study in question is simply interested in whether or not VAP develops, not how long it takes to develop. Therefore, the required temporal component is absent. The Cox proportional hazard ratio is applied in survival analysis, for example. The multivariable linear regression would be an appropriate multivariable model if the outcome of interest is continuous and linear, like body temperature. The multivariable logistic regression is the model of choice for the analysis at hand. The logistic regression model is used to describe the relationship between a binary outcome variable, VAP, and a set of independent predictor variables whether they are continuous, categorical or binary. The results are reported as odds ratios with 95% CIs and p-values for the predictors.

**Answer: B**

13  *All of the following can be computed from a $2 \times 2$ contingency table, except:*

   **A** *Risk ratio, a.k.a. relative risk*

   **B** *Odds ratio*

C *Attributable risk*
D *Pearson's $X^2$*
E *Pearson's correlation coefficient*

The $2 \times 2$ contingency table is a fundamental construct in biostatistics. It can represent a test result (positive or negative) and the disease state (present or absent), a risk factor and the disease, and so on, see Table 49.1. All of the options listed in answers A–D can be calculated from the $2 \times 2$ table as follows:

$$\text{Risk ratio} = \frac{a/(a+b)}{c/(c+d)}$$ or the ratio of risk of an outcome in the exposed to that in the unexposed. The odds ratio $= \dfrac{ad}{bc}$ is the ratio of odds of an outcome in the exposed to the odds in the unexposed. Attributable risk $= a/(a+b) - c/(c+d)$ is the proportion of cases attributable to the exposure in relation to all cases. Then Pearson's $X^2$ is a test of significance for row x column tables, here $2 \times 2$, tables. The $X^2$ statistic calculation depends on the expected value ($E$) of each cell in the table $\left( \dfrac{(a+b)(a+c)}{a+b+c+d} \right)$ then the expression $(O_a - E_a)^2 / E_a$ is summed for all cells, where O is the observed value in the cell. Finally, Pearson's correlation coefficient is a measure of how well the relationship between two variables can be described using a linear function

**Answer: E**

14 *The following are true regarding randomization of subjects in a randomized trial, except:*
   A *The variation in outcome between treatment and control groups is either treatment effect or random variation*
   B *The best way to deal with concerns about confounding from unmeasured variables*
   C *The subject decides their group assignment*
   D *Requires informed consent*
   E *Can be stratified*

The concept of randomization, or random allocation of subjects as a basis for experimental design was developed in the early twentieth century by R. A. Fisher and colleagues. Randomization accounts for variability across groups in an experimental study. When a study cohort is properly randomized, the assignment of the next subject enrolled is nonpredictable. This ensures the personal judgements and ambitions of the investigators and subjects do not bias the allocation to the treatment or control group. Given the random allocation of subjects, variation in outcome across treatment groups that is unrelated to the treatment effect can be justifiably be

called random variation. Treatment assignment should be designed to minimize the bias of confounding. One approach to address this concern is stratified randomization. As an example, consider a disease that has a worse prognosis in older people. To ensure the equitable distribution of age in both groups of the study, subjects are first grouped by age (strata), then the subjects are randomized to treatment groups within each strata. Since the subjects do not select which group they will belong to, informed consent is critical to this study design. This informed consent requires the subject be informed: 1) that they are voluntarily participating in a research study for a specified period of time; 2) that the procedures or treatments in the study are experimental; 3) since their participation is voluntary, they can withdraw at any time; and 4) of the potential risks and benefits of their participation.

**Answer: C**

15 *Once again a group of academic clinician/investigators fixes their interest on ventilator-associated pneumonia (VAP). The group has hospital administrative data from the trauma and medical intensive care units. They hypothesize the difference in patient populations (trauma vs. medical) is associated with the observed difference in rates of VAP. One aspect of their study is a comparison of each group's time to the diagnosis of VAP in terms of days of mechanical ventilation. Their results are illustrated in the Figure 49.2. Which of the following is true?*
   A *The incidence of VAP is equivalent between the trauma ICU and medical ICU*
   B *The rate of VAP is constant over time*
   C *The line drops down when someone develops VAP or is extubated or dies*
   D *Medical patients are intubated longer than trauma patients*
   E *None of the above*

The graph depicts a Kaplan-Meier survival curve which can be thought of as a time-to-event analysis. Here the event is the diagnosis of VAP but the event could be patient death or some other discrete event. The distribution of survival times is characterized by the survival function. The survival function is the probability a patient will remain event-free beyond a point in time. When an event occurs, the line drops down at which point the survival function changes. In this fashion, the Kaplan-Meier estimator accommodates the variation of incidence rates over time. Next, this model allows subjects to leave the group at risk, or in this example be liberated from the ventilator, develop VAP or die. This is known as censoring. The inclusion of censored data

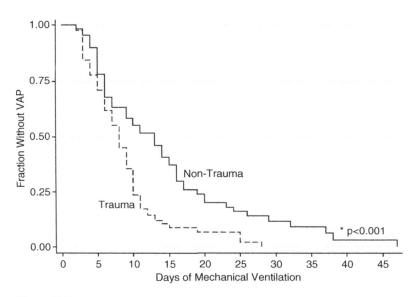

**Figure 49.2**

distinguishes survival analysis from other types of analysis. In contrast to the life-table method, the Kaplan-Meier uses the exact time-to-event for each patient instead of grouping events into specified time intervals. Here we see a greater incidence of VAP in the trauma patients beginning at approximately ventilator day 7 as the proportion of mechanically ventilated trauma patients without VAP decreases markedly compared to the medical ICU patients mechanically ventilated for an equal amount of time. We can also see the rate of VAP diagnoses decreases at about day 15 for the trauma patients and day 20 for the patients in the medical ICU. The investigators cannot infer if the trauma patients or medical patients remain intubated longer. What the graph does tell us is that after around 27 days, no intubated trauma patients remained VAP-free. Similarly no patient in the medical ICU was intubated and VAP-free beyond day 47.

**Answer: C**

Gordis, L. (2009) *Epidemiology*, 4th edn, Saunders, Philadelphia, PA.

Porta, M. (2014) *A Dictionary of Epidemiology*, 6th edn, Oxford University Press, New York.

Rosner, B. (2010) *Fundamentals of biostatistics*, 7th edn, Duxbury Press, New York.

Rothman, K.J., Greenland, S., and Lash, T.L. (eds) (2008) *Modern Epidemiology*, 3rd edn, Philadelphia, PA, Lippincott Williams & Wilkins.

# 50

## Ethics, End-of-Life, and Organ Retrieval
*Allyson Cook, MD and Lewis J. Kaplan, MD*

1 *An elderly woman is brought to the emergency department from her nursing home with obvious septic shock. She is intubated, fluid resuscitated and placed on a norepinephrine infusion. Her husband is dead and her sole surviving relative is her daughter. When the daughter arrives, she indicates that her mother would not want all of the care she is currently receiving and would wish to pursue comfort care. Which of the following principles is the care team using in pursuing the daughter's statement of her mother's wishes for comfort care?*
   A *Substituted judgment*
   B *Distributive justice*
   C *Ethical parity*
   D *Nonmalfeasance*
   E *Respect*

Since the patient is intubated, and cannot state her desires if she knew all of the information that the care team knows, one must obtain outside input. Using a family member who is more likely to understand the patient's desires is appropriate. Accepting that family member's input is termed substituted judgment. Distributive justice is the principle that applies the concept of justice across several individuals or groups of individuals instead of a single person. Ethical parity implies the equally appropriate application of ethical principles across different cultures and circumstances. Nonmalfeasance indicates a lack of wrongdoing by a public official, often in a financial undertaking. Respect is linked with the concept of autonomy, but does not address accepting another's representation of what individuals' wishes would be if they were only able to share them.

### Answer: A

Thompson, I.E. (1987) Fundamental ethical principles in healthcare. *British Medical Journal*, **295**, 1461–1465.

2 *A 67-year-old man has a potentially resectable colon cancer and has a tumor type that is thought to be favorably responsive to chemotherapy administration. After a lengthy discussion with you, his surgeon, he declines operative therapy as well as chemotherapy. What principle is being utilized in his decision to decline indicated and potentially life-saving therapy?*
   A *Nonrational thinking*
   B *Deontology*
   C *Autonomy*
   D *Munificence*
   E *Principlis*

This question addresses the role of patient autonomy in medical decision making. Autonomy is a key principle in Western medical ethics, which preserves a patient's ability to engage in self-determination with regard to goals of therapy, as well as diagnostic or therapeutic undertakings. If the physician believes that the patient has appropriate decisional capacity and understands the implications of the decisions being made, then respecting their informed and autonomous decision to decline medically indicated therapy is appropriate. Nonrational thinking is decision making based on obedience, imitation, feeling, desire, intuition, or habit. Deontology is rules-based decision-making. Munificence is generosity in giving and does not apply here. Principlism, generally a Western approach, embraces beneficence, nonmaleficence, and autonomy as well as justice, and as such is too broad an answer.

### Answer: C

Limentani, A.E. (1999) The role of ethical principles in health care and the implications for ethical codes. *Journal of Medical Ethics*, **25**, 394–398.
Thompson, I.E. (1987) Fundamental ethical principles in healthcare. *British Medical Journal*, **295**, 1461–1465.

*Surgical Critical Care and Emergency Surgery: Clinical Questions and Answers*, Second Edition.
Edited by Forrest "Dell" Moore, Peter Rhee, and Gerard J. Fulda.
© 2018 John Wiley & Sons Ltd. Published 2018 by John Wiley & Sons Ltd.
Companion website: www.wiley.com/go/moore/surgical_criticalcare_and_emergency_surgery

**3** *A 24-year-old male motorcyclist arrives with a severe traumatic brain injury (TBI) and within 48 hours has an examination and supportive investigations consistent with brain death. Which of the following strategies is associated with the greatest likelihood that his family's legally authorized representative will consent to organ donation on his behalf?*
   A *A structured interview with an organ donation recipient and family*
   B *Approach and consent obtained by the physician and nurse care team*
   C *Approach and consent by the organ procurement surgeon*
   D *Combined approach by the care team and organ procurement network team*
   E *Combined approach by nursing, social service, and chaplaincy representatives*

One of the challenges in organ procurement has been obtaining consent from the legally authorized representative of a potential donor patient. Components cited as contributing to failure in obtaining consent are: lack of consistent message between clinicians, lack of an appropriately constructed message based on what would render donation process easily understood, lack of understanding of organ donation in general, concerns regarding costs of organ donation, concerns regarding mutilation as well as religious concerns. Perhaps the most readily addressable set of concerns are those that discuss communication. A prefamily meeting "huddle" consisting of physicians, nurses, and representatives of the organ procurement organization to discuss the best approach for a given family has been demonstrated to significantly improve consent rates. Other members of the care team may also participate in the "huddle" as needed or appropriate. Engaging a donor recipient and family is appropriate for recipients and families but not the donor family. The organ procurement surgeon is ethically constrained from participating in the consent process due to a conflict of interest.

**Answer: D**

Rady, M.Y., Verheijde, J.L., and McGregor, J.L. (2010) Scientific, legal and ethical challenges of end-of-life organ procurement in emergency medicine. *Resuscitation*, **81** (9), 1061–1062.

**4** *The ethical and humane treatment of prisoners of war (POW) by physicians is specifically addressed by which of the following:*
   A *Hastings Center report*
   B *Nuremberg proceedings*
   C *North Atlantic Treaty Organization*
   D *World Health Organization*
   E *Geneva Conventions*

The ethical treatment of POWs is laid out in detail within the Geneva Conventions. The tenets are embraced and further articulated within a variety of military field manuals as well. Physicians are specifically constrained from being active combatants but are expected to be able to defend themselves and the patients for whom they are providing care. The Geneva Convention also prohibits the deliberate attack of medical care providers, and torture of prisoners. Provision of nourishment, medical and surgical care, and humane holding conditions are also explicitly required within the document. The Hastings Center mission is to address fundamental ethical issues in the areas of health, medicine, and the environment as they affect individuals, communities, and societies. This center focuses ethical issues centered about end-of-life, public health issues, and new and emerging technology. Periodic reports are generated on these topics, but not treatment of POWs. The Nuremberg Proceedings addressed war crimes. NATO is a collection of allied countries with similar aims and who have signed mutual aid and intent treaties. The WHO is an organization that addresses world health issues. NATO and the WHO both endorse the Geneva Convention.

**Answer: E**

Carter, B.S. (1994) Ethical concerns for physicians deployed to Operation Desert Storm. *Military Medicine*, **159** (1), 55–59.

**5** *If one argues that principles and moral rules are not absolutely binding, but are instead prima facie, this means that the principles and moral rules are:*
   A *Self-evident and are context independent when rendering moral judgment*
   B *Duties that are binding unless in conflict with an equal or stronger duty*
   C *Unable to be equally applied across the same circumstance in different cultures*
   D *Only able to be understood within the context of virtue ethics and behavior*
   E *Rooted in Western culture and interwoven within the rules for social behavior*

*Prima facie* means that principles and moral rules are duties that are binding unless in conflict with an equal or stronger duty. In this way, *prima facie* recognizes that principles may come into conflict with one another and there is a context-sensitive nature to principles that may not translate from one culture to another. Therefore, *prima facie* allows one to allow contextual influences to help shape a moral judgment, instead of strictly adhering to a single set of rules. Thus, a need for overall balance is embedded in the concept of *prima facie*. Virtue ethics asserts that decision-maker characteristics are reflected in their behavior and ethics may be interpolated from a behavior set. This type of ethics implies that virtuous behavior is a type of moral excellence.

**Answer: B**

Limentani, A.E. (1999) The role of ethical principles in health care and the implications for ethical codes. *Journal of Medical Ethics*, **25**, 394–398.

**6** *Which of the following ethical principles may be used as a justification for performing scientific and medical research?*
   **A** *Nonmaleficence*
   **B** *Distributed justice*
   **C** *Beneficence*
   **D** *Autonomy*
   **E** *Pluralism*

Beneficence is acting for the greater good, and implies a sense of moral and ethical correctness in the assignation of good to a particular behavior or activity. Research may be justified using this concept in that the discovery of new knowledge may be applied to others with similar conditions to enable recovery, survival, or mitigate consequences of that particular, and other related, illnesses. Nonmaleficence is different in that it constrains one from willfully doing harm. Distributed justice implies equality in a particular element in either equal share, or in proportion to need, effort, contribution, or merit. Autonomy relates to an individual's right to self-determination. Pluralism is the philosophy that it is desirable and beneficial to have several distinct ethnic, religious, or cultural groups thrive within a single society. Pluralism also holds that no single explanatory or belief system may reliably and definitively account for all the phenomena of life. In this way pluralism supports many different ethical viewpoints and contextually specific moral judgments.

**Answer: C**

Beauchamp, T.L. and Childress, J.F. (eds) (2009) *Principles of Biomedical Ethics*, 6th edn, Oxford University Press, New York.
Limentani, A.E. (1999) The role of ethical principles in health care and the implications for ethical codes. *Journal of Medical Ethics*, **25**, 394–398.

**7** *A patient with metastatic colorectal cancer, with symptomatic bony and brain metastases, is critically ill in the ICU with severe sepsis and impending acute respiratory failure. As the intensivist, you have a discussion with the patient regarding his goals of therapy. He states that although he is aware that he has only a limited time to live based on his malignancy, he wishes to receive intubation, mechanical ventilation, and CPR if he has a pulmonary or cardiac arrest. His wife is on her way to the ICU but has not yet arrived. As the intensivist, you do not believe that those therapies are reasonable to pursue for this patient. The next most appropriate course of action is to:*
   **A** *Accept the patient's decisions to respect his autonomy*
   **B** *Enter a DNR/DNI order to respect your autonomy*
   **C** *Contact the hospital legal/risk management department*
   **D** *Discuss with the wife and accept her substituted judgment*
   **E** *Convene an ethics committee consultative visit*

This patient is critically ill and has brain metastasis. Therefore, his judgment may be compromised and he may not be able to appropriately interpret the consequences of his decisions. Moreover, as it is an emergency situation, asking a patient to articulate goals of therapy may be viewed as coercive. Furthermore, since you do not believe that intubation will help the patient achieve a reasonable goal it is appropriate to discuss goals of therapy with an individual who is not in severe sepsis and with impending respiratory failure. The next most appropriate individual is his wife. Were she not alive, then an adult child would be the next most appropriate individual. Others may have a legally authorized representative empowered by a durable healthcare power of attorney designation. Still others have a court appointed conservator when there is no kin to help make healthcare decisions—or when those who are present are unwilling or incapable of making such decisions. Accepting the goals as articulated by the most appropriate individual as those of the patient is known as substituted judgment. Substituted judgment relies on the perspective that the goals being related are those that the patient would most likely share with the care team if they were able to do so. The clinician must be careful to ensure that the goals do not instead reflect what the individual stating the goals wants for the patient, but rather what the patient would want for his or herself. Respecting autonomy also implies that the patient is competent to render a decision. Entering a DNR/DNI order to respect your autonomy is inappropriate and violates the patient's right to self-determination—either autonomously or via substituted judgment. Hospital agencies generally act to slowly to render a rapid decision regarding care, but are very helpful when there is the luxury of time to have an outside agency (not the primary healthcare team) review the case and share input regarding difficult ethical decisions.

**Answer: D**

Mazur, D.J. (2006) How successful are we at protecting preferences? Consent, informed consent, advance directives and substituted judgment. *Medical Decision Making*, **26** (2), 106–109.

Seckler, A.B., Meier, D.E., Mulvihill, M., and Paris, B.E. (1991) Substituted judgment: how accurate are proxy predictors? *Annals of Internal Medicine*, **115** (2), 92–98.

8   While on call at night in the ICU, one of the surgeon's brings up a patient from the OR after performing an adhesiolysis and small bowel resection for a small-bowel obstruction. The operation went smoothly and appears to have been performed in the usual fashion without complication. As the surgeon is discussing the patient with you in the ICU, it is clear to you that the surgeon's breath smells of alcohol and the surgeon appears to be intoxicated. You most appropriate course of action is to:
   A   Have a private conversation with the surgeon once sober
   B   Do nothing as you do not have laboratory evidence of intoxication
   C   Immediately contact your Chairman with your concerns
   D   Disenfranchise the surgeon from the patient's care due to incompetence
   E   Discuss your observations with the patient's family to provide full disclosure

Using the principle of nonmaleficence (do no harm), one is compelled to act in order to preserve patient safety. Operating while under the influence of alcohol is clearly unsafe, unethical, and morally unsupportable. The most appropriate action is to engage the hierarchical power structure that can directly intervene to protect patient's from harm. From the standpoint of beneficence (doing good), one must also act in the surgeon's best interest as if the surgeon is operating while intoxicated, it is a powerful marker of a personal health issue. While "blowing the whistle" may be superficially construed as damaging it is the most appropriate action to undertake from any perspective. A private conversation will not support patient safety, and nor will taking no action. One cannot unilaterally disenfranchise a surgeon from their patient's care. Providing disclosure without evidence that supports your suspicion of intoxication is also not appropriate at this time, especially if there is no direct evidence of harm.

**Answer: C**

Beauchamp, T.L. and Childress, J.F. (eds) (2009) *Principles of Biomedical Ethics*, 6th edn, Oxford University Press, New York.

9   A 36-year-old woman was involved in a motorcycle crash two days ago. She has severe TBI and the neurosurgeon believes it to be a nonsurvivable injury. She has a physical examination that describes the absence of brain stem reflexes by two physicians, and has a transcranial Doppler assessment through an ocular insonation window that demonstrates no optic flow. Her temperature is 32.8C, HR 102 beats/min, BP 96/42 mm Hg (MAP = 60 mm Hg), SaO$_2$ 98% on AC/VCV and FIO$_2$ 0.40 on fentanyl at 0.5 μg/kg/hour and midazolam at 2 mg/hour. She breathes only with the ventilator. The next most appropriate action is to:
   A   Start a norepinephrine infusion to raise her MAP
   B   Perform an apnea test to assess CO$_2$ responsivity
   C   Disconnect her from the ventilator as she is brain dead
   D   Obtain a radionuclide cerebral blood flow scan
   E   Change to fentanyl and propofol to minimize sedation

This patient may have a nonsurvivable brain injury in the neurosurgeon's opinion, but she does not meet criteria for the declaration of brain death. The absence of brain-stem reflexes is supportive, but she is still on sedating agents that need to be discontinued to render the examination valid. Transcranial Doppler examination is similarly insufficient to determine cerebral blood flow as a universally agreed upon standard. Universal standards include four-vessel cerebral angiography and cerebral radionuclide scanning. There remains controversy regarding cerebral computed tomogram angiography for the declaration of brain death. One does need to be warm as well to be declared brain dead. Given the low temperature and the analgesic and sedative agents, a radionuclide scan is the most appropriate method of supporting the determination of brain death of the choices offered as it is temperature and sedative independent, unlike an apnea test—which may be significantly influenced by sedative agents. Raising the MAP will also not help address whether or not she is brain dead, and MAP manipulation is best done in conjunction with determining cerebral perfusion pressure (MAP–ICP) and there is no ICP monitor in this patient.

**Answer: D**

Greer, D.M., Straczyk, D., and Schwamm, L.H. (2009) False positive CT angiography in brain death. *Neurocritical Care*, **11** (2), 272–275.

Tibbalis, J. (2010) A critique of the apneic oxygenation test for the diagnosis of "brain death." *Pediatric Critical Care Medicine,* **11** (4), 475–478.

Zuckier, L.S. and Kolano, J. (2008) Radionuclide studies in the determination of brain death: criteria, concepts and controversies. *Seminars in Nuclear Medicine,* **38** (4), 262–273.

**10** *A patient is declared brain dead and you have shared the news with the family. It is Wednesday evening and they request that you do not remove their father from the ventilator until Saturday as they want family to arrive from across the country. However, Friday is their father's wedding anniversary and their mother died only eight months ago. Which of the following paradigms best described the basis for the family members' thought process in requesting the three-day delay?*

**A** *Consequentialism*
**B** *Principlism*
**C** *Nonrationalism*
**D** *Virtue ethics*
**E** *Deontologism*

This patient's family is making an unsupportable request. It is superficially logical to the family but is inconsistent with appropriate medical care and legal rulings. Once one is declared brain dead then one is legally dead and may be disconnected from life support devices. The family has articulated a desire to delay disconnection, which is a nonrational request as they apparently understand that he is medically and legally dead. Nonrationalism identifies that decision and requests stem from feelings, desires, intuition, habit, obedience, or imitation. Consequentialism renders decisions based on the downstream effects of each individual decision. Principlism frames decisions within autonomy, beneficence, nonmaleficence, justice, and respect. Virtue ethics derives ethical values from the behavior of an individual who is believed to be virtuous as a kind of moral excellence. Deontologism renders ethical decisions based adherence to predefined and accepted rules.

**Answer: C**

Limentani, A.E. (1999) The role of ethical principles in health care and the implications for ethical codes. *Journal of Medical Ethics,* **25,** 394–398.

Thompson, I.E. (1987) Fundamental ethical principles in healthcare. *British Medical Journal,* **295,** 1461–1465.

**11** *A 72-year-old man is admitted to the surgical service after undergoing a left inguinal hernia as he had hypoxemia in the PACU and is now oxygen requiring.*

*He has underlying COPD, CAD, DM, and CRI (baseline creatinine 2.4); he is DNR but not DNI. You are called at 02:00 as part of your hospital's rapid response team for severe hypoxemia. When you arrive, the patient has a HR of 126 beats/min, RR of 36 breaths/min, A BP of 98/52 mm Hg (baseline 142/82 mm Hg), and a SaO$_2$ of 90% on 100% O$_2$ by nonrebreather while sitting bolt upright. Before proceeding with intubation, the anesthesiologist wants to obtain consent from the patient. Which of the following is the most appropriate course of action?*

**A** *Engage in a discussion of intubation to obtain an informed consent*
**B** *Obtain a CXR to look for treatable causes of hypoxemia*
**C** *Administer furosemide 80 mg IVP as well as nebulized albuterol*
**D** *Establish phone contact with a family member to obtain consent*
**E** *Proceed with intubation as consent in this situation is coercive*

The concept of informed consent embraces a plethora of issues including the clarity and scope of the discussion, the patient's ability to comprehend the discussion, the ability of the clinician to explain the procedure, and the ability of the patient to understand the consequences of agreeing or disagreeing to the intended procedure. Truly informed consent must allow for adequate time for questions, answers, discussion, and perhaps reflection as well. Emergency situations such as the one described preclude that process in large part with the patient as well as with family members. It also underscores the importance of having discussions that impact goals of therapy prior to elective hospitalization and early within the course of unplanned admission. Diagnostic or therapeutic undertakings that do not immediately address impending respiratory arrest are inappropriate compared with rapid airway and work of breathing control.

**Answer: E**

Brendel, R.W., Wei, M.H., Schouten, R., and Edersheim, J.G. (2010) An approach to selected legal issues: confidentiality, mandatory reporting, abuse and neglect, informed consent, capacity decisions, boundary issues, and malpractice claims. *Medical Clinics of North America,* **94** (6), 1229–1240.

**12** *You are caring for an injured patient who is being nonoperatively managed for a grade II liver injury and a grade III splenic injury but who also has a right femur fracture. The orthopedic surgeon on call, and who is ready to operate on the patient, is one* *whom you believe is less technically and cognitively competent than any of the other surgeons who take orthopedic trauma panel call. The patient's family asks you for your opinion of the orthopedic surgeon who is intending to operate on their mother. Your most appropriate course of action is to:*

A *Reassure the family that they should feel comfortable with the surgeon*

B *State the since you are not an orthopedist, you cannot comment*

C *Suggest that the family might want to obtain a second opinion*

D *Find a reason to delay the OR until a better surgeon is responsible*

E *Offer that it is their comfort with the surgeon that is important*

This question addresses both patient autonomy (the right to choose therapy and who will deliver it) and surgeon autonomy (the right to practice in an unrestricted fashion) in the setting of medical professionalism (professional conduct in patient care). Reassuring the family that "all is well" if one does not believe it to be so is patently lying and not to be condoned as appropriate behavior. Declining to comment about the surgeon since you have expertise in different aspects of the field is similarly untruthful and deceitful. Suggesting a second opinion may also infringe the orthopedist's practice and autonomy. Delaying an indicated operation on the basis of personal bias is medically inappropriate and morally incorrect. Therefore, the only appropriate answer is to identify that it is not your opinion that matters, but rather the family's comfort and confidence in the surgeon that is paramount. If you truly believe that the orthopedist is practicing below an acceptable standard of care, then there are performance-improvement data-driven mechanisms that one may engage to evaluate performance. Engaging your hospital's peer-review process is the professional and appropriate means to address your concerns regarding the orthopedist's skill set and professional judgment.

**Answer: E**

Lantos, J., Matlock, A.M., and Wendler, D. (2011) Clinical integrity and limits to patient autonomy. *Journal of the American Medical Association*, **305** (5), 495–499.

13 *A 14-year-old boy is struck by a vehicle at high speed and brought into the emergency department. On evaluation, the child has a GCS of 4, no pupillary responses, and a palpable open, depressed skull fracture. While the trauma team does not feel that there is a reasonable hope of survival, the patient is* intubated and resuscitated in the hopes that he could be an organ donor. Which of the following is true?

A *Providing futile care to the child is unethical, and all efforts should be halted*

B *Resuscitative efforts should be provided to give the family a chance to come to terms with the prognosis and decide on organ donation*

C *The local organ procurement organization (OPO) should be immediately called for consultation*

D *Resuscitation should proceed with set limits to give the appearance to the family that every effort was made*

E *The parents should be informed that their son will die and the decision left to them as to how to proceed*

The appropriateness of continuation of care is predicated on the determination of futility in further care of this patient and the intent of the actions behind those actions. Given the lack of certainty in the patient's prognosis in the acute setting, discontinuation of care would be premature at this stage. Similarly, contacting the OPO at this stage is premature as one is still engaged in actively providing care for a patient in whom the outcome is uncertain. Such contact may be construed as a conflict of interest in certain circumstances. When prognosis is definitively established, nonbeneficial procedures such as CPR may be considered in limited circumstances as a compassionate act for the benefit of the family, providing comfort and reassurance that everything possible was done for their child. For patients in whom organ transplantation is considered, the United States Uniform Anatomic Gift Act was revised in 2006 to permit the use of life-support systems at or near death in order to maximize the potential for organ procurement. The revised act presumes donation intent and the use of life support systems, overriding expressed intent, but has not yet been universally adopted in all states.

**Answer: B**

Sachdeva, R., Jefferson, L., Coss-Bu, J., *et al.* (1996) Resource consumption and extent of futile care among patients in a pediatric intensive care unit setting. *Journal of Pediatrics*, **128** (6), 742–747.

Truog, R.D. (2010) Is it always wrong to perform futile CPR? *New England Journal of Medicine*, **362**, 477–947.

Verheijde, J.L., Rady, M.Y., McGregor, J.L. (2007) The United States Revised Uniform Anatomical Gift Act (2006): new challenges to balancing patient rights and physician responsibilities. *Philosophy, Ethics, and Humanities in Medicine*, **2**, 19.

14 *During a routine preoperative chest x-ray in a 68-year-old woman, a suspicious nodule is found. The*

*reviewing physician feels that a CT scan is war-ranted, and she refers her to a radiology center that physician's husband owns and manages. Which of the following is true?*

**A** *The patient can be referred so long as the physician's financial ties are disclosed to the patient*

**B** *There is no violation of conflict of interest since the physician herself has no direct financial ties to the center*

**C** *The patient can referred since the center is an external facility, and regulations against self-referral only apply to internal facilities*

**D** *Referring to this center is a violation of Stark laws unless no other nearby facilities exist*

**E** *The physician cannot make the referral herself, but can have her physician's assistant fill out the referral*

Physician self-referral occurs when physicians refer patients to medical facilities in which they have a financial interest. Such arrangements are ethically questionable due to the potential for over-utilization of medical resources and subsequently, increased healthcare costs for society. The Stark laws, enacted in 1992, state that a physician cannot refer a Medicare or Medicaid patient to a facility in which he or she (or an immediate family member) has a financial relationship. An exception to this rule exists for rural settings in which no other facility is conveniently available. A mid-level practitioner operates under the supervision of the physician within the practice and therefore is not exempt.

**Answer: D**

Department of Health and Human Services, Centers for Medicare and Medicaid Services (2007) *42 CFR Parts 409, 410, et al. Medicare Program; Proposed Revisions to Payment Policies Under the Physician Fee Schedule, and Other Part B Payment Policies for CY 2008.* Department of Health and Human Services, Washington, DC.

Manchikanti, L., and McMahon, E.B. (2007) Physician refer thyself: is Stark II, phase III the final voyage? *Pain Physician*, **10** (6), 725–741.

**15** *A 45-year-old man suffers a massive intracranial hemorrhage from a previously undiagnosed aneurysm and despite aggressive medical and surgical management, is deemed unsalvageable. The surgical critical care fellow has been taking care of this patient and is very involved in the discussions with the family. The family eventually decides to withdraw care and consents to organ donation. At the time of organ harvest, the transplant surgeon invites the fellow to join them in the operating room since* *this is a good "teaching opportunity." The fellow should do which of the following?*

**A** *Accepting this could be seen as a conflict of interest, and he should therefore decline*

**B** *Accept this because as a trainee, there is no conflict of interest, and this would be an educational opportunity*

**C** *Accept this but as an observer only since he is a critical care fellow and not a transplant fellow*

**D** *Accept but go to the operating room only with the written consent of the family*

**E** *Accept and participate in the procedure since it is educational, but without informing the family*

Perceived conflict of interest can occur when there is overlap or confusion between the treating team and the transplantation team. Indeed, consent rates have been shown to be up to three times greater when an optimal request pattern was pursued, including clear separation between the treatment team and the donation requester. The surgical critical care fellow is a member of the treatment care team and, although he may not be involved in the discussion of organ donation and obtaining consent for transplantation, is at risk of appearing to have conflicting motivations.

**Answer: A**

Siminoff, L.A., Arnold, R.M., and Hewlett, J. (2001) The process of organ donation and its effect on consent. *Clinical Transplantation*, **15**, 39–47.

**16** *A surgery resident places an enteral access catheter to provide nutritional support in an elderly, debilitated patient in the ICU. On a followup chest X-ray, the catheter is found to have gone down the right mainstem bronchus and to be in the right pleural space with a large pneumothorax. The family is informed, the catheter is removed, and a chest tube is placed. The patient remains stable throughout, and the chest tube is removed five days later without complications. The family is irate and threatens to sue. Which is the best course of action?*

**A** *Conduct further discussions only in the presence of the Legal department*

**B** *Request the input of the hospital Ethics committee to determine the best course of action and to counsel the family*

**C** *Say as little as possible since the resident was unsupervised at the time*

**D** *Ignore the family's threat, since there is no medical liability due to the fact that no harm was done*

**E** *Schedule a family meeting to ensure that the family is fully informed and to discuss their concerns*

Mistakes are common in medicine. Full disclosure of medical errors can be difficult due to embarrassment and concerns over legal liability and erosion of the patient–physician relationship. However, studies have shown that when a policy of full disclosure is followed, no clear increases in lawsuits or healthcare costs occur. Moreover, the provider–patient relationship is strengthened with a policy of openness and honesty. Models for medical error compensation have been proposed and may lead to decreases in overall healthcare costs.

**Answer: E**

Hebert, P.C. (2001) Disclosure of adverse events and errors in healthcare: An ethical perspective. *Drug Safety*, **24** (15), 1095–1104.

Kachalia, A., Kaufman, S.R., Boothman, R., *et al.* (2010) Liability claims and costs before and after implementation of a medical error disclosure program. *Annals of Internal Medicine*, **153** (4), 213–221.

O'Connor, E., Coates, H.M., Yardley, I.E., *et al.* (2010) Disclosure of patient safety incidents: a comprehensive review. *International Journal for Quality in Health Care*, **22** (5), 371–379.

**17** *During the hernia repair of a patient with a history of IV drug use, the surgeon accidentally sticks himself with a 2-0 suture needle and breaks the skin. Which of the following is true?*

  **A** *Consent for HIV testing is not required, and the patient can be tested confidentially based on medical necessity*

  **B** *The patient may refuse to consent to testing and consent is required for HIV testing*

  **C** *If the patient refuses to be tested for HIV, the patient can be legally mandated to submit to testing*

  **D** *Nothing needs to be done since the risk of HIV transmission from nonhollow bore needlesticks is negligible*

  **E** *Testing of the patient without consent is allowable so long as test results are confidential and anonymous*

Testing for HIV without the patient's consent or knowledge is a violation of the patient's rights to privacy, self-determination, and autonomy. Patients must have the freedom and capacity to make an informed decision regarding testing and dealing with the emotional, personal, and structural consequences of an HIV-positive diagnosis. While there are no reported cases of HIV transmission from suture-related needlestick injuries, clinicians need to assess the severity of exposure and characterize the risk of HIV transmission to determine the appropriateness of antiretroviral prophylaxis. If testing of the source patient cannot be performed, then prophylactic treatment should be initiated and serial testing of the exposed surgeon performed. It should be noted that some states may authorize blood testing without patient consent in certain circumstances. Additionally, some institutions will accept verbal agreement and not require written consent for HIV testing.

**Answer: B**

Centers for Disease Control and Prevention (1995) Case-control study of HIV sero-conversion in health care workers after exposure to HIV infected blood—France, United Kingdom, and United States, January 1988–August 1994. *Morbidity and Mortality Weekly Report*, **44**, 929–933.

Cowan, E. and Macklin, R. (2012) Unconsented HIV testing in cases of occupational exposure: ethics, law, and policy. *Academic emergency medicine: official journal of the Society for Academic Emergency Medicine*, **19** (10), 1181–1187.

Hanssens, C. (2007) Legal and ethical implications of opt-out HIV testing. *Clinical Infectious Diseases*, **45** (suppl 4), S232–S239.

**18** *At the end of a routine orthopedic procedure, a patient is accidently given a large dose of a benzodiazepine instead of the narcotic she was supposed to receive for pain. As a consequence, she was unable to be extubated at the end of the case, and was left intubated overnight. She was subsequently extubated the next morning and went home without incident. What is the best course of action?*

  **A** *Nothing, since prolonged recovery from anesthesia is a known complication and covered in the initial consent*

  **B** *The anesthesia team should fully disclose to the patient what occurred and admit that a mistake was made*

  **C** *Tell the family that this is a known risk of anesthesia, and that it is not uncommon after operation*

  **D** *It is unnecessary to inform the family, but the hospital legal department needs to be informed of the incident*

  **E** *The family should be told about the details of the case without admission of fault*

While the patient suffered no long-term effects from her prolonged intubation, increased length of stay and risks of sedation cannot be dismissed as expected consequences of her procedure, and can be considered harmful. Often patients and families perceive adverse effects in a more broad sense than clinicians. Full disclosure of unexpected events and medical errors fosters communication and trust in the physician–patient relationship.

**Answer: B**

Gallagher, T.H., Waterman, A.D., Ebers, A.G., *et al.* (2003) Patients' and physicians' attitudes regarding the disclosure of medical errors. *Journal of the American Medical Association*, **289**, 1001–1007.

Institute of Medicine (2000) *To Err Is Human: Building A Safer Health System*, National Academy Press, Washington, DC.

O'Connor, E., Coates, H., Yardley, I., *et al.* (2010) Disclosure of patient safety incidents: a comprehensive review. *International Journal of Quality in Health Care*, **22** (5), 371–379.

**19** *A 12-year-old girl falls onto a glass table with a deep laceration to her thigh and loses a significant volume of blood before being found. She is brought into the emergency department tachycardic, hypotensive, and profoundly anemic. Her parents, who are Jehovah's Witnesses, refuse to consent to blood transfusion based on their religious beliefs. What is the most appropriate course of action?*

**A** *Try to obtain the patient's consent to transfusion*
**B** *Respect the wishes of the parents since the patient is a minor*
**C** *Transfuse the patient, since her condition is life-threatening*
**D** *Obtain a court order to override the wishes of the parents*
**E** *Contact the congregation elder to negotiate with the family*

The Jehovah's Witness Society is notable for their religious stance against transfusion of blood, even in the face of life-threatening anemia. In the competent adult patient, adherence to the patient's wishes is in accordance with *respect for persons* and the patient's right to self-determination. However, in the case of the child, the patient is incapable of formulating a rational, informed choice and expressing those views, therefore transfusion is justified by our societal obligation to the child's best interests, based on the principle of *beneficence*.

**Answer: C**

Gillon, R. (1994) Medical ethics: four principles plus attention to scope. *British Medical Journal*, **309**, 184–188.

Gillon, R. (2003) Four scenarios. *Journal of Medical Ethics*, **29** (5), 267–268.

Woolley, S. (2005) Children of Jehovah's Witnesses and adolescent Jehovah's Witnesses: what are their rights? *Archives of Disease in Childhood*, **90** (7), 715–719.

Woolley, S. (2005) Jehovah's Witnesses in the emergency department: what are their rights? *Emergency Medicine Journal*, **22** (12), 869–871.

**20** *On review of his monthly billings, a physician notices that he billed for the incorrect procedure on a patient. The claim had already been accepted and paid out by the insurance company. What is the appropriate course of action?*

**A** *Nothing, since the RVUs between the two procedures is similar*
**B** *If the claim amount is less than $10 000, no correction is necessary*
**C** *Report the error, refund the monies, and resubmit with justification*
**D** *Report the error to the insurance company and refund the claim*
**E** *Nothing can be done since the claim is already paid to the physician*

Policies differ between insurance carriers and Medicare/Medicaid in terms of correction of incorrect claims. Review and understanding of these agreements is important in minimizing your exposure to liability and prosecution. In general, failure to report errors in billing is subject to repayment of claims and imposed fines. Reporting, refunding, and resubmitting an honest error with justification will cover all of the requirements for full disclosure and accuracy in correcting incorrect billing claims. This strategy may not ensure that there is not an associated fine, but is consistent with the concept of distributed justice across the healthcare system, and is internally consistent with the concept of virtuous behavior. The worst course of action is to do nothing and hope that the incorrect billing is not noticed.

**Answer: C**

Vogel, R.L. (2010) The False Claims Act and its impact on medical practices. *Journal of Medical Practice Management*, **26** (1), 21–24.

# Index

Note: Page numbers in *italic* indicate Figures and those in **bold** indicate Tables.

2×2 contingency table  487–488
95% confidence intervals (CIs) and
    p-values  486

## a

A-a gradient calculation  10
abdominal compartment syndrome
    assessment for  81
    causes and prognosis in neonates
        and infants  236
    definition and risk factors  314–315
    in resuscitated burn patients  425
abdominal injury  307–315
abdominal paracentesis, performance
    in the ICU  259–260
AC/VCV ventilation
    auto-PEEP waveform and
        intervention to correct  87, *87*
    high peak airway pressures in a
        postoperative patient  83–84
    intervention to improve
        oxygenation  82
    waveform analysis  88, *88*
acetaminophen
    clinical manifestations of acute
        intoxication  175
    features of hepatotoxicity
        174–175
    mortality in the United States  240
    NAC antidote administration  240
    prevention of hepatotoxicity in
        overdose  240
    treatment of acetaminophen
        poisoning  175
acetylcholine, role in development of
    delirium  129
acid-base balance  135–144

acid-base disorders
    caused by vomiting  136
    diabetic ketoacidosis  141
    diagnosis of metabolic
        acidosis  137
    non-anion gap type metabolic
        acidosis  140
    *see also* metabolic acidosis;
        metabolic alkalosis
acid burns, treatment  430
acidosis, "lethal triad" of
    coagulopathy, acidosis, and
    hypothermia  117
*Acinetobacter* species, beta-lactamase
    production  105
activity scales  75
acute adrenal dysfunction, signs and
    symptoms  146–147
acute carpal tunnel syndrome,
    management  324–325
acute coronary syndrome with DAPT,
    timing of future surgery
    33–34
acute coronary syndromes  33–50
acute decompensated heart failure
    (ADHF)  8, 9
acute fatty liver of pregnancy (AFLP),
    diagnosis and
    treatment  219–220
acute head injury, initial
    management  277–279
acute kidney injury (AKI)  159–167
    advantages of renal replacement
        therapy  165–166
    criteria for stage 3 AKI
        159–160, **160**
    definition  159, **160**

determining the cause using FENa
    and FEUrea  166–167
diagnosis of intrinsic and prerenal
    causes  163–164
diagnosis of prerenal
    disorders  166
distinguishing intrinsic and
    prerenal causes  164
distinguishing renal and prerenal
    disorders  166–167
drugs associated with 165
effects of dopamine  165
effects of furosemide  164–165
etiologies  76
FENa calculation  166
indications for acute dialysis
    162–163
indications for dialysis  161–162
initial workup for postoperative
    oliguria  160–161
KDOGO criteria stages of AKI
    159–160, **160**
nutritional management  167
potential perioperative causes  161
prevention of contrast-induced
    nephropathy (CIN)  163
risk factors in pediatric ICU
    patients  233
risk in elderly trauma patients
    468–469
signs and symptoms of
    hyperkalemia due to
    stage 3 AKI  163
treatment of traumatic
    rhabdomyolosis  162
acute liver failure, clinical features
    and mortality risk  173–174

*Surgical Critical Care and Emergency Surgery: Clinical Questions and Answers*, Second Edition.
Edited by Forrest "Dell" Moore, Peter Rhee, and Gerard J. Fulda.
© 2018 John Wiley & Sons Ltd. Published 2018 by John Wiley & Sons Ltd.
Companion website: www.wiley.com/go/moore/surgical_criticalcare_and_emergency_surgery

acute lung injury (ALI)
  associated with transfusion (TRALI) 110
  pulmonary edema 14
acute pericarditis 39–40, *39, 40*
acute phase proteins (APP)
  functions of negative APPs 178–179
  mediators involved in production of 177–178
  response to severe injury 177
acute phase response (APR) 177
acute respiratory distress syndrome (ARDS)
  additional therapies to decrease mortality 86–87
  diagnosis in children 459–461, **460**
  differences between pediatric and adult ARDS 229, *229*
  ECMO for ARDS 30
  effect of PEEP in a severely hypoxic patients 6
  immunonutrition recommendations 183–184
  location of optimal PEEP on a volume-pressure curve 13
  pediatric patient *see* pediatric acute respiratory distress syndrome (PARDS)
  positional therapy for severe ARDS 29–30
  pulmonary edema 14
  transmembrane fluid flux 14
acute respiratory failure and mechanical ventilation 79–88
acute stent thrombosis, diagnosis and treatment 440
acute tubular necrosis, diagnostic criteria 160
Addisonian crisis, signs and symptoms 146–147
adnexal torsion, diagnosis and treatment 431
adrenal insufficiency, after traumatic brain injury 148
Advanced Trauma Life Support (ATLS) protocol, control of active bleeding 328–329
*Aeromonas* species, diagnosis of NSTI caused by 412
age-related changes *see* elderly patients
air leaks, sources in trauma patients 300–301

airway management 69–78
  emergency airway in pediatric patients 297
  pediatric trauma patients 453
  pregnant trauma patient 355
  tracheal injury 297
airway pressure release ventilation (APRV), effects on oxygenation 82–83
albumin
  effect on anion-gap type metabolic acidosis 143
  use in pediatric burn patients 227–228
alcohol dependence
  risk of critical illness 133
  risk of hospital mortality 133
alcohol withdrawal pathophysiology 132–134
  neurotransmitters responsible for 132
  treatment 132–133, **133**
alkali burns, initial treatment 430
alpha error 485
alvimopan (Entereg), prescribing limitations 98–99, **98**
American Academy of Orthopedic Surgery (AAOS), guidelines for PE and bleeding prophylaxis 205–206, **206**
American College of Chest Physicians (ACCP), VTE prevention and treatment guidelines 205, 206
American Heart Association (AHA)
  guidelines for CPR 15
  recommendations for sudden cardiac arrest 17
American Pediatric Surgical Association (APSA), guidelines for pediatric blunt trauma injury 234–235, *234*
American Society of Anesthesiologists (ASA), classification of physical status 71
American Society of Regional Anesthesia and Pain Medicine (ASRA), guidelines on LMWHs and epidurals 204
amino acids
  administration of branched-chain amino acids in critically-ill patients 183
  functions of arginine 180
  functions of glutamine 178

functions of glutamine 180
  requirements of critically-ill and injured patients 179
amiodarone 15–16
amniotic fluid embolism, diagnosis and treatment 221
amniotic fluid embolism syndrome (AFES)
  coagulopathy associated with 435
  development of disseminated intravascular coagulation (DIC) 435
  diagnosis and management 434–435
amphetamine intoxication, symptoms and treatment 246–247
amphotericin B, advantages of lipid formulations 102
amphotericin B deoxycholate, renal toxicity 102
amputation, risk in combined skeletal and arterial injuries 333–334, *334*
analgesia 121–128
  delirium prevention strategies 130
  postoperative pain in a patient with kidney disease 122
anesthesia 121–128
  causes of continued paralysis 70–71
  indicators of malignant hyperthermia 126
  malignant hyperthermia (MH) 77–78
  postdural puncture headache 125–126
anesthetic agents
  for patients with liver disease 124
  for patients with previous gastrectomy 124
  for patients with vitamin B12 deficiency 124
  potential hepatotoxicity 124
  respiratory depression side effect 128
angiotensin receptor blockers (ARB) 147
ANOVA 485
anterior mediastinal mass, anesthetic considerations 443
antibiotic resistance
  avoiding misuse and overuse of antibiotics 103–104

extended-spectrum beta-lactamase (ESBL) microorganisms 95–96
  mechanisms related to beta-lactamase production 105–106
  risk factors for MDR pneumonia 96
antibiotics 100–108
  black box warnings 108
  choice based on risk of MDR VAP 104–105, **104**
  duration of antibiotic therapy 90
  effect on outcomes of sepsis 56
  for ESBL organisms 105
  for necrotizing soft tissue infection 95, 106–107
  indications for combination therapy 92–93
  interactions between NMBAs and aminoglycoside antibiotics 70–71
  polyene antibiotic family 102
  principles of antibiotic therapy 103–104
  prophylactic antibiotics in critically-ill patients 93
  treatment of extended-spectrum beta-lactamase-producing organisms 53
anticoagulants 99–100
anticoagulated trauma patients
  management for surgery 33–34, **34**
  management of intracranial hemorrhage following TBI 285–286
  management of patients with HIT 100–101
  patients with cirrhosis 210–211
  rapid reversal of anticoagulation 118–119, **118**
  rapid reversal of coagulopathy 114
antidepressant overdose, clinical presentation of TCA toxicity 239–240
antidiuretic hormone (ADH)
  deficiency following traumatic brain injury 145
  lack of ADH release in central diabetes insipidus 135
antifungals, treatment for cryptococcal meningitis 53–54
antiemetics, choice for critically-ill patients 99

antioxidants, supplementation in critically-ill patients 182–183
antiphospholipid syndrome (APS), diagnosis and management 207
antiplatelet therapy, perioperative management 116–117
antithrombin III deficiency 26
antithymocyte antibodies, side effects when used as induction agents 216–217
aortic dissection
  management of limited dissection 442
  presentation 442
  secondary complications 442
aortic injury
  CXR findings 272
  diagnosis following blunt trauma 304
  diagnosis of traumatic aortic injury 305
  treatment for traumatic aortic injury 305
APACHE II prognostic model, applications 169
APACHE III prognostic model, applications 169
apixaban, rapid reversal in trauma patients 118–119, **118**
appendicitis
  diagnosis 376
  guidelines for laparoscopic appendectomy in pregnant patients 434
  management options 376–377
  presentation and diagnosis in pregnancy 433
  treatment in elderly patients 470–471
  treatment of acute appendicitis in pregnancy 433–434
appendix 371–383
  carcinoid tumor 373
  pseudomyxoma peritonei symptoms and treatment 373
ARDS *see* acute respiratory distress syndrome
arginine, requirements in trauma and critical care patients 180
arrhythmias 33–50
  multifocal atrial tachycardia (MAT) 80

arterial catheterization
  complications 254
  indications for 254
arterial line catheters, effects of increasing distance from the heart 61
ascites, treatment for intractable ascites in cirrhosis 173
asthma attack, respiratory failure and cardiomyopathy 36
asymmetric (skewed, non-parametric) distribution 484, *484*
atelectasis, signs of 80
atracurium
  Hofmann elimination 97, **98**
  reversal drugs 107
atracuronium, mechanism of action 123
atrial fibrillation, management in elderly patients 472–473
atrial flutter 42–44, *43*
atrial thrombus 43
attributable risk 487–488
autonomy principle 491, 493
  competence to make decisions 493–494
  right to choose therapy and who will deliver it 495–496
auto-PEEP, waveform and intervention to correct 87, *87*
Avalon Elite BiCaval Dual Lumen catheter, complications 28–29

**b**

bacterial endocarditis, diagnosis and treatment 447–448
barbiturate therapy, use in management of traumatic brain injury 194–195
bariatric surgery 415–422
  causes of early mortality 420
  recommendation for obesity 415
beneficence principle 491, 493, 499
benzamides, antiemetic action 99
benzocaine, methemoglobinemia associated with 140
benzodiazepines
  mechanism of action 101–102
  treatment of overdose 101–102
  use in the ICU for sedation 101–102

beta blockers
  overdose symptoms and
      management   247
  role in postoperative myocardial
      infarction prevention   73
beta error   485
beta-lactam antibiotics   95–96
beta-lactamase inhibitors   105–106
beta-lactamases, microorganisms
      that produce   105–106
Bezold–Jarisch reflex   48
bile duct injury
  factors in successful
      reconstruction   385
  iatrogenic injury   385
bile duct stones, MRCP imaging
      266–267
biliary anatomy   388
biliary infection, empiric treatment
      regimen for specific patient
      populations   387
bladder injury
  associated with pelvic fractures
      318, *318*
  extraperitoneal injury
      management   338
  management of penetrating
      injury   337, *338*
bleeding risk, prophylaxis for total
      knee or hip replacement
      205–206, **206**
blood component therapy for
      transfusion   109
blood glucose control, multiply-
      injured trauma patient   146
blunt abdominal trauma
  APSA guidelines for pediatric solid
      organ injury   234–235, *234*
  CT scan evaluation   263
  hepatic or splenic blush on CT
      scan in pediatric
      patients   231
  management of injuries in
      pediatric patients   235, 462
  management of pediatric blunt
      kidney trauma   235
  management of pediatric liver or
      spleen injury   234–235, *234*
  non-accidental trauma in young
      children   235
  small bowel mesenteric injury
      379–380, *379*
blunt cardiac injury (BCI), screening
      tools   304

blunt cerebrovascular injury (BCVI)
      288–289, *289*, **289**
  diagnosis and management
      277, *278*
  diagnostic imaging   268
  indications for BCVI
      screening   290
  indications for endovascular
      interventions   290–291, **290**
  injury scale   290–291, **290**
blunt neck trauma   287–297
blunt trauma, splenic artery
      embolization caused
      by   263–264
blunt vertebral artery injury,
      diagnosis and management
      277, *278*
body mass index (BMI)
  calculation   415
  changes related to aging   472
  classification   415, **416**
Boerhaave's syndrome, diagnosis and
      treatment   359–360
Bowel Injury Prediction Score
      (BIPS)   379–380
bowel obstruction
  gallstone ileus   388–389
  Meckel's diverticulum   377, *377*
bowel perforation, symptoms in
      steroid-treated patients   149
brachial artery injury
  evaluation and management   330
  presentation   330
brain death
  criteria for declaration
      494–495
  nonrational requests from the
      family   495
brain injury *see* traumatic brain
      injury
Brain Injury Guidelines (BIG)
      284–285, **285**
brain oxygenation monitoring
      techniques   195
Brain Trauma Foundation, Guidelines
      for the management of severe
      traumatic brain injury   198
branched-chain amino acids
      (BCCAs), administration in
      critically-ill patients   183
broken heart syndrome   36
bronchopleural fistula (BPF),
      complication of lung
      resection   441

bronchoscopy
  for diagnosis of ventilator-
      associated pneumonia   258
  for Zone II penetrating neck
      trauma   294
Brugada syndrome   35–36, *35*
bupivacaine (Marcaine), mechanism
      of action   72
burn shock pathophysiology   423
burns   423–430
  abdominal compartment syndrome
      monitoring and
      treatment   425
  albumin use in pediatric patients
      227–228
  area assessment   424
  bladder pressure monitoring   425
  burn center transfer criteria   428
  burn shock pathophysiology   423
  compartment syndrome
      diagnosis   425–426
  compartment syndrome
      management   425–426, *426*
  compartment syndrome risk in
      circumferential burns
      425–426
  compromised chest wall movement
      and ventilation   85
  deep second- and third-degree
      burns   429
  elderly patients   473–474
  escharotomy for compartment
      syndrome   425–426, *426*
  fluid resuscitation of burn
      patients   423
  full-thickness circumferential
      burns of the torso   85
  hyperkalemia risk   122
  infection risk from central line
      catheters   426–427
  inhalational injury treatment   428
  initial resuscitation of burn
      victims   423
  neuromuscular blocker choice for
      intubation   122
  nutritional requirements of burn
      patients   427
  nutritional therapy for burn
      patients   188
  parenteral nutrition in severe burn
      patients   427
  pediatric patients   462–463
  percentage total body surface area
      involved   424

potentially beneficial additional treatments 427
resuscitation monitoring 424–425
"rule of nines" used in area assessment 424
scald burn treatment in a pregnant patient 436
sequelae of initial burn injury 423
side effects of topical antimicrobials 427–428
signs of infection 426
thoracic escharotomy 85
topical agent for burned ear with exposed cartilage 429
topical antimicrobials 429
butyrophenones, antiemetic action 99

**C**
C1 fracture, Jefferson fracture 295, *295*
C2 fracture, association with vertebral artery injury 295–296, *295*
caffeine, mechanism of action 250–251
calcineurin inhibitors
    adverse effects 210, 215
    mechanisms of action 214–215
calcineurin toxicity, caused by drug-drug interactions 209–210, **210**
*Candida glabrata*, antibiotic resistance 96
*Candida* species
    association with CRBSI 63
    intravascular infection risk factors and treatment 56
candidemia in critically ill patients, treatment 56
candidiasis
    invasive, empiric antifungal therapy 106
    postoperative, antibiotic prophylaxis 93
    risk factors in critically-ill patients 106
candiduria in critically ill patients, treatment 56
"cannot intubate, cannot oxygenate" (CICO) scenario 293–294
CaO$_2$ (oxygen content) of blood, calculation 18

carbapenem-resistant microorganisms 95–96
carbapenems, action against ESBL organisms 105
carbon monoxide (CO) poisoning
    mechanism 242
    symptoms, treatment, and outcomes 242
carcinoid tumor of the appendix 373
cardiac allograft vasculopathy (CAV)
    distinction for coronary artery disease (CAD) 213
    medications to decrease CAV 213–214
cardiac arrest
    AHA recommendations for sudden cardiac arrest 17
    AHA treatment guidelines 15
    positive predictors of survival 15
    suspected cardiac etiology 17–18
    underlying causes of PEA arrest 16
    unstable patient requiring pressor support 17–18
    ventricular fibrillation following MI 49–50, *49*
    ventricular fibrillation treatment in the field 15–16
cardiac arrhythmias, management in elderly patients 472–473
cardiac cycle events 7–8, *7*
cardiac injury
    mitral valve tenea corda disruption 301
    posttraumatic signs of internal cardiac injuries 301
    prognostic indicators for penetrating injury 303
    repair of cardiac laceration 303–304
    screening for blunt cardiac injury (BCI) 304
cardiac pacing, temporary transvenous cardiac pacemaker 255
cardiac pressure-volume loops, physiologic processes represented 4, *4*
cardiac surgery, postoperative cardiac tamponade 442–443
cardiac tamponade
    diagnosis following penetrating injury 299–300
    following cardiac surgery 442–443

cardiac transplantation
    cardiac allograft vasculopathy (CAV) diagnosis 213
    medications to decrease CAV 213–214
cardiogenic shock
    features and etiology 20
    role of endothelin-1 58
cardiopulmonary resuscitation *see* CPR
cardiothoracic injury 299–306
cardiovascular collapse, indications for ED thoracotomy (EDT) 304–305
cardiovascular physiology 3–14
cardiovascular surgery 439–451
cardiovascular system, age-related changes 469
cardioversion, medications given after 41–42, *41–42*
carotid cavernous fistula
    diagnosis 275, *276*
    initial treatment and management 275
carpal tunnel symptoms, related to distal radius fracture 324–325
case-control studies 486–487
catheter-associated urinary tract infection (CAUTI), risk factors 93–94
catheter-directed thrombolytics (CDT) for DVT 201
catheter-related bloodstream infections (CRBSI)
    common causative organisms 63
    guidelines for prevention 62
    prevention practices 94
    treatment 53
catheterized critically-ill patients, *Candida* infection risk and treatment 56
caustic substance ingestion
    esophageal injuries 449–450
    evaluation of injuries 365
    initial assessment and management 365–366
cecal volvulus, diagnosis and management 378, *378*
cefepime, antimicrobial action 104, 105
ceftazidime, antimicrobial action 105
cell biology 209–217

central cord syndrome, association with falls in the elderly 193
central diabetes insipidus
after traumatic brain injury 145–146
free water deficit 135
pathophysiology and treatment 135
central line catheters, managing infection risk in burn patients 426–427
central nervous system infections, antifungal treatment 53–54
central pontine myelinolysis 139
central venous catheter (CVC), timing of intravascular pressure measurement 66–67
central venous catheter (CVC) placement
best practice guidelines 62
prevention of central line-associated bloodstream infection (CLABSI) 253
ultrasound guidance 270–271
ultrasound guidance versus the landmark technique 253–254
central venous pressure (CVP)
cause of acute rapid rise 66
definition 66
cerebral artery aneurysm
rupture causing subarachnoid hemorrhage 192
vasospasm following surgical or endovascular management 192
cerebral blood flow, zone of normal cerebral autoregulation 196
cerebral perfusion pressure (CPP), optimizing in traumatic brain injury 196, 283–284
cerebral salt wasting syndrome (CSW) 139
cerebrospinal fluid (CSF), penetration by antifungals 53–54
cerebrospinal fluid (CSF) rhinorrhea, tests to detect 276
cervical esophageal injury
evaluation 361–362
operative repair 362
cervical necrotizing fasciitis, causes and treatment 413–414

cervical spinal cord injury
initial management of blunt injuries 195
pulmonary function testing 288
cervical spine, normal anatomical variation in children 457
cervical spine clearance
in elderly patients 474
timing of 296–297
cervical spine injury, diagnosis in children 457
Cesarean section
in trauma patient undergoing CPR 436–437
prophylactic antibiotics 225
CHA$_2$DS$_2$-VASc score 33, **34**
CHADS$_2$ score 33
chemical burns
initial treatment of strong alkali burns 430
treatment of acid burns 430
chemical esophageal injuries 449–450
chemotherapy
neutropenia complication 54
neutropenic enterocolitis complication 375
chest compartment syndrome, signs and treatment 84–85
chest trauma
indications for urgent/emergent thoracotomy 303
retained hemothorax 306
widened mediastinum following blunt trauma 304
chest tube, sources of air leaks in trauma patients 300–301
child abuse, signs of non-accidental trauma 458
child protection services, notification of suspected child abuse 458
Child–Turcotte–Pugh (CTP) prognostic model 169
chi-square test 484
cholecystectomy
indications for prophylactic procedure 385–386
laparoscopic method 385
choledocholithiasis
management in pregnancy 389
treatment in Roux-en-Y gastric bypass patient 417–418
Chvostek's sign 145
ciprofloxacin, use in VAP 104–105

cisatracurium
Hofmann elimination 97, **98**
mechanism of action 122
metabolism and elimination 72
reversal drugs 107
use for patients with liver or renal disease 122–123
*Citrobacter* species, beta-lactamase production 105
clindamycin, interaction with neuromuscular blocking agents 70–71
Clinical Institute Withdrawal Assessment for Alcohol Scale (CIWA-Ar) 133
Clinical Pulmonary Infection Score (CPIS) 90
clopidogrel 44
*Clostridium difficile*, postoperative infection
management 89–90
*Clostridium difficile* colitis
management 372
treatment of refractory infection 100
coagulation 109–119
diagnosis and treatment of disseminated intravascular coagulation (DIC) 114
etiology of excessive bleeding after trauma or surgery 115
rapid reversal of anticoagulation in trauma patients 114, 118–119, **118**
coagulation system, role in the sepsis-induced inflammatory cascade 57
coagulopathy
bleeding in uremic patients 116
"lethal triad" of coagulopathy, acidosis, and hypothermia 117
cocaine
intoxication symptoms and treatment 246–247
mechanism of action 250–251
cocaine-associated chest pain (CACP), evaluation and management 246–247
cohort studies 483, **483**
colon 371–383
management of *Clostridium difficile* colitis 372

postoperative complications of destructive colon injuries   311

treatment of intraperitoneal gunshot wounds   375

colon tumor

chemotherapy for metastases   376

symptoms and management   376

colonic pseudo-obstruction, treatment   374

communication failures, risk factor for wrong-site surgical procedures   73

compartment syndrome

indication for a therapeutic decompressive fasciotomy   333

indications in closed tibia and fibula fracture   321

length of fasciotomy incision for the leg   322, *322*,

management in burn patients   425–426, *426*

medical malpractice liability issues   321–322

of the chest   84–85

pressure threshold for decompression   322

risk in burn patients   425–426

*see also* abdominal compartment syndrome

compensatory anti-inflammatory response syndrome (CARS) 178–179

complicated skin and soft tissue infections (cSSTIs)

antibiotic choice   410–411

management   409

types of   409

component separation technique, for hernia repair   405

computed tomography *see* CT

confidence intervals (CI) in statistics   484

confounding in studies   487, 488

Confusion Assessment Management (CAM) tool   130, **131**

consequentialism   495

continuous renal replacement therapy, for volume status management   340

contrast-induced nephropathy (CIN)   76

prevention in elderly trauma patients   468

prevention strategies   163

CO-oximetry

blood constituents measured by   60

measurement of oxygen saturation ($SpO_2$)   59–60

COPD exacerbations, use of NIPPV   86

core body temperature, at levels of hypothermia   154

coronary artery bypass grafting (CABG), for acute coronary syndrome   44

coronary artery disease (CAD)

distinction from cardiac allograft vasculopathy (CAV)   213

smoking risk factor   49

corticosteroids, indications for use in septic shock   52

Cox proportional hazard ratio   487

CPR (cardiopulmonary resuscitation)   15–21

American Heart Association guidelines   15

percentage of myocardial and cerebral blood flow provided by   16–17

CRBSI *see* catheter-related bloodstream infections

cricothyrotomy

predictors of difficult cricothyrotomy   69

SMART assessment tool   69

critical oxygen delivery   13–14

critically-ill patients

*Candida* intravascular infection risk and treatment   56

factors in successful fluid resuscitation   65–66

nutritional support   77

optimizing oxygen delivery ($DO_2$)   65

pharmacokinetic and pharmacodynamic principles   102–103

refeeding syndrome (RFS)   77

role of lactate clearance in successful fluid resuscitation   65–66

cross-sectional studies   483

cryptococcal meningitis, antifungal treatment   53–54

CT (computed tomography)

evaluation of blunt abdominal trauma   263

reducing radiation dose in children   464

CT angiography

blunt vertebral artery injury 277, *278*

diagnostic evaluation of penetrating neck trauma   265

CT arteriography, use in penetrating peripheral vascular trauma   265–266

Cushing's syndrome   147

CXR, findings in traumatic aortic injury   272

cyanide toxicity

associated with nitroprusside treatment   247–248

symptoms and treatment 247–248

cyclizine, antiemetic action   99

cyclosporine

immunosuppression in transplant patients   210

mechanism of action 214–215

side effects   215

cystoprostatectomy, postoperative complications   339, *339*

cytokine release syndrome, management in transplant patients   216–217

cytomegalovirus (CMV) infection

opportunistic infection in immunosuppressed patients   93

treatment in transplant patients 215–216

**d**

D-dimer, diagnostic use in DVT and PE   203–204

dabigatran, rapid reversal in trauma patients   118–119, **118**

dalteparin, prophylactic use   203

damage-control laparotomy (DCL), concept and indications   312

damage-control surgery (DCS), aim of the second phase   313

data analysis, descriptive analyses 484, *484*

decompressive craniectomy, in traumatic brain injury 283–284

decompressive craniotomy, for traumatic intracranial hypertension   197–198

DECRA trial (2011) findings 197–198

deep vein thrombosis *see* DVT
delirium   129–134
   causes and risk factors   129
   Confusion Assessment
      Management (CAM) tool
      130, **131**
   DSM-V diagnostic criteria   129
   effects of medications   131
   incidence in hospital and the
      ICU   129
   long-term risks associated with
      131–132
   medications to avoid   467–468
   prevention strategies in the ICU
      130, 467
   primary evaluation and
      management   130, 131
delirium tremens
   RASS evaluation   **133**, 133
   signs and symptoms   132
   treatment of alcohol withdrawal
      132–133, **133**
Denver screening criteria for blunt
      cerebrovascular injury (BCVI)
      288–289, *289*, **289**
deontology   491, 495
depression in elderly people, suicide
      risk of tricyclic
      antidepressants (TCAs)   471
descriptive analyses, features of
      484, *484*
desflurane, metabolism   124
desomorphine (Krokodil), effects of
      use as alternative to heroin
      248–250
dexmedetomidine, mechanism of
      action   102, 121–122, 128
diabetes insipidus (DI), after traumatic
      brain injury   145–146
diabetic foot infections
   predominant pathogens associated
      with   413
   presentation of severe SSTIs   413
diabetic ketoacidosis
   presentation and assessment   141
   treatment in addition to
      insulin   150
diagnostic imaging   261–272
dialysis, indications for acute dialysis
      162–163
diaphragmatic injury, detection
      following penetrating
      trauma   301
diazepam, mechanism of action   128

Dieulafoy's lesion, diagnosis and
      management   368
diffuse axonal injury, diagnosis   282
digitalis toxicity, association with
      electrolyte abnormalities
      138, *138*
dilaudid, mechanism of action   122
diltiazem, drug-drug interactions
      209–210, **210**
diphenhydramine, antiemetic
      action   99
disseminated intravascular
      coagulation (DIC)
   associated with amniotic fluid
      embolism syndrome
      (AFES)   435
   diagnosis and treatment   114
distributive justice   491, 493
diverticulitis, management according
      to the Hinchey staging
      system   371
$DO_2$ (oxygen delivery)
      calculation   18
dobutamine, mechanism of action of
      vasodilatory effects   62
domperidone, antiemetic action   99
dopamine, effects in acute kidney
      injury (AKI)   165
droperidol, antiemetic action and side
      effects   99
drug-drug interactions
   in transplant patients
      209–210, **210**
   neuromuscular blocking agents
      and aminoglycoside
      antibiotics   70–71
drugs associated with acute kidney
      injury (AKI)   165
Duke Activity Status Index
      (DASI)   75
duodenum   359–369
   management of obstructive
      duodenal hematoma   366–367
   management of penetrating
      injury   367
   symptoms and treatment of a
      perforated duodenal
      ulcer   363–364
duplex ultrasound, evaluation of
      peripheral vascular
      trauma   328
DVT (deep vein thrombosis)
   catheter-directed thrombolytics
      (CDT)   201

   diagnostic use of D-dimer
      203–204
   incidence and management
      202–203
   inferior vena cava (IVC) filter
      placement   255–256
   post-thrombotic syndrome
      (PTS)   200
DVT prophylaxis
   effectiveness of IPC devices and
      GCSs   199–200
   protocols for pelvic fracture
      318–319

***e***
ECG, multifocal atrial tachycardia
      (MAT)   80
echocardiography, surgeon-
      performed in the ICU
      271–272
ECMO (extracorporeal membrane
      oxygenation)   23–31
   bleeding from a previously
      non-draining chest
      tube   27–28
   causes of acute change   31
   choice between VA ECMO and VV
      ECMO   30
   coagulopathy associated with   26
   correcting acid-base abnormality
      26–27
   criteria for use in respiratory
      failure   29–30
   distance between cannulas in VV
      ECMO   30
   factors affecting patient
      survival   24–26, *25*
   Harlequin Syndrome   23–24, 29
   in ARDS with sepsis   30
   indicator of time to trial off
      ECMO   27
   management of bleeding   27–28
   patient selection   24–26, *25*
   pediatric patient
      consequences of malpositioned
         veno-venous cannula
         237–238, *238*
      management of massive
         hemothorax   236–237, *237*
      verification of correct placement
         of a veno-venous cannula
         237–238, *238*
   rate of sweep gas in the ECMO
      circuit   26–27

recognising adequate support   24
relative contraindications   23
RESP score   25–26, **25**
role in respiratory failure
    management   87
signs and causes of recirculation   30
use in acute hypoxic respiratory
    failure in trauma patients   26
veno-arterial ECMO   23–24
veno-venous ECMO   23–24
ectopic pregnancy
    presentation and diagnosis of
        ruptured ectopic pregnancy
        431–432
    risk factors   431–432
    treatment of ruptured ectopic
        pregnancy   431-2
edema, resuscitation fluids which
        promote edema   143–144
edrophonium, cholinesterase
        inhibitor   107, 108
eFAST (extended focused assessment
        sonography for trauma),
        injuries detected by   262–263
EKG
    left axis deviation   37–38
    measuring SR elevation   39–40,
        *39, 40*
    ST segment elevation and PR
        segment elevation
        39–40, *39, 40*
elderly patients
    age-related cardiovascular changes
        465, 469
    age-related changes in nutrition
        and metabolism   472
    appendicitis   470–471
    cardiac arrhythmias   472–473
    decision-making by surrogates
        469–470
    nutritional support in critical
        illness   471–472
    presentation of peptic ulcer
        disease   470
    prevalence and etiologies of
        syncope   473
    prevalence of *H. pylori*
        infection   470
    suicide rates   471
    TCA overdose   471
elderly trauma patients
    avoiding delirium in the ICU
        467–468
    burn injuries   473–474

cervical spine clearance   474
effects of use of warfarin   466–467
incidence and consequences of rib
        fractures   465–466
loss of upper extremity motor
        function after a fall   193
mechanical ventilation   466
patient refusal of surgery   469–470
rapid reversal of anticoagulation
        466–467
renal dysfunction   468–469
electrolyte abnormalities
    associated with digitalis toxicity
        138, *138*
    associated with massive
        transfusion   113–114
    caused by vomiting   136
    diagnosis of hyponatremia   176
electrolytes   135–144
Eliquis *see* apixaban
emergency department thoracotomy
        (EDT), indications for
        304–305
end-diastolic volume   4, *4*
end-of-life care   491–499
    patient who may have impaired
        judgment   493–494
    substituted judgment   491,
        493–494
end-organ profusion, ways to
        promote   4–5
endocarditis, diagnosis and
        treatment   447–448
endocrinopathies   145–151
endoscopy, considerations before
        performing in the ICU
        258–259
endothelin-1, role in cardiogenic
        shock   58
endotracheal intubation
    emergent intubation in pediatric
        patients   453–454
    techniques for successful
        intubation   256
enoxaparin
    administration for pulmonary
        embolism   99–100
    VTE prophylactic dosing and
        monitoring   207
enteral nutrition (EN)
    biochemical derangement in
        refeeding syndrome
        (RFS)   77
    delivery in the ICU   186

in the critically-ill patient   77
monitoring in the ICU   186
tolerance in pediatric critical care
        patients   232
Entereg (alvimopan), prescribing
        limitations   98–99, **98**
*Enterobacter* species
    antibiotic to treat extended-
        spectrum beta-lactamase-
        producing strains   53
    association with CRBSI   63
    association with VAP   55, 96
    beta-lactamase production   105
*Enterococcus* species, association with
        CRBSI   63
envenomations   239–251
epidural analgesia, and
        LMWHs   204
epidural hematoma
    diagnosis   281
    surgical management of acute
        hematoma   281
epigastric blunt injury, management
        of multiple injuries in children
        461–462, *461*, **461**
epinephrine   15
error types in statistics   485–486
ESBL *see* extended-spectrum
        beta-lactamase
escharotomy, for compartment
        syndrome in burn patients
        425–426, *426*
*Escherichia coli*, antibiotic regimen
        for ESBL *E. coli*   95–96
esophageal balloon catheter values,
        interpretation   11
esophageal injury
    caustic substance ingestion
        449–450
    cervical esophageal injury
        repair   362
    esophageal laceration repair   292
    evaluation of cervical esophageal
        injury   361–362
    gunshot wounds   364–365
    management approaches
        292–293
esophageal perforation
    antibiotic regimen   360–361
    Boerhaave's syndrome diagnosis
        and treatment   359–360
    causes   449, *449*
    iatrogenic   360, 449, *449*
    morbidity and mortality rates   360

esophageal varices, prevention of variceal bleeding 172
esophagogastric anastomosis, diagnosis of anastomotic leak 450
esophagoscopy, for Zone II penetrating neck trauma 294
esophagus 359–369
  anatomy 359
  blood supply 359
ethical parity 491
ethical principles 491
ethics 491–499
ethylene glycol ingestion, toxicity and treatment 243
etomidate
  influence on postoperative outcome 150
  inhibition of adrenal steroid production 124–125
  risk of adrenal insufficiency 150
extended-spectrum beta-lactamase (ESBL) organisms
  antibiotic regimen for ESBL *Escherichia coli* 95–96
  antibiotics to treat 53
  choice of antimicrobial treatment 105
extracorporeal membrane oxygenation *see* ECMO
extraperitoneal penetrating trauma management 382
extraperitoneal rectal injuries, recommended treatment 313–314
extubation
  determinants for safe extubation 85–86
  negative pressure pulmonary edema 79–80
  use of the rapid shallow breathing index (RSBI) 85–86

*f*
Factor V Leiden mutation, perioperative risk 205
falling, history of 36–37, *37*
falls in the elderly, central cord syndrome 193
family of deceased, nonrational requests from 495
fasciotomy
  length of incision to decompress the leg compartments 322, *322*
  predictors of the need for 333

FAST exam (Focused Assessment with Sonography for Trauma), sensitivity and specificity 269, *270*
femoral hernia
  borders that define the femoral ring 404
  comparison with inguinal hernia 404
  repair 404
  repair options for incarcerated hernia 406–407
femoral vein injury, options for repair 332
fentanyl
  mechanism of action 122
  postoperative pain management 98
fingers, replantation of traumatic amputations 323
flail chest
  cause and management 300
  causes of hypoxia related to 300
  risk factors and management 450–451
flexible bronchoscopy, diagnostic and therapeutic indications 258
fluconazole, use in central nervous system infections 53–54
fluid and electrolytes 135–144
fluid movement across capillary membranes 14
fluid resuscitation, role of lactate clearance in the critically-ill patient 65–66
flumazenil, mechanism of action 101–102
fondaparinux, use in DVT prophylaxis 202–203
Fournier's gangrene, management 341
Frank–Starling law of the heart 4
free air in the chest and abdomen, cause in steroid-treated trauma patient 149
fulminant liver failure
  clinical features and mortality risk 173–174
  treatment of acetaminophen poisoning 175
functional capacity, pre-surgery assessment 75

fungal infection in transplant patients, antifungal treatment 211
furosemide, effects in acute kidney injury (AKI) 164–165
futile care, issues related to continuation 496

*g*
gallbladder 385–392
  cancer diagnosis and management 390
gallbladder polyps, classification and management 389–390
gallstone disease, management during pregnancy 389
gallstone ileus, clinical presentation and management 388–389
gallstones
  management of asymptomatic gallstones 385–386
  risk factors for developing 387
gamma-aminobutyric acid (GABA), role in alcohol withdrawal pathophysiology 132
gastric band patient
  cause of poor PO tolerance 419
  removal of band fluid 419
  signs and symptoms of gastric band erosion 418
  treatment of gastric band erosion 418–419
gastric band port site infection, cause of 418
gastric bypass
  anastomotic leak detection and treatment 368–369
  *see also* Roux-en-Y gastric bypass
gastric decontamination procedure for drug overdose 241
gastric Dieulafoy's lesion, diagnosis and management 368
gastric dysmotility, effects in pediatric critical care patients 232
gastric outlet obstruction, management of malignant obstruction 364
Geneva Conventions 492
Geneva Score (revised) for PE diagnosis 204
gentamicin, interaction with neuromuscular blocking agents 70–71

geriatrics 465–475
Glasgow Coma Score
  determination for all injured
    patients 276–277, **277**
  prediction of poor outcome in
    penetrating brain injury
    191–192
glutamate, role in alcohol withdrawal
    pathophysiology 132
glutamine
  requirements in trauma and critical
    care patients 180
  role in nutritional support for
    critically-ill patients 178
goal-directed echocardiography
    (GDE) examination, standard
    views 261–262
graduated compression stockings
    (GCSs), effectiveness for
    DVT prophylaxis
    199–200
granisetron, antiemetic action 99
Graves' disease, postoperative thyroid
    storm 148
Greenfield filter, long-term follow-up
    of patients 207–208
groin hernia, surgical evaluation for
    repair 403
Guillain–Barré syndrome, diagnosis
    and therapy 197
gunshot wounds
  brain injury 191–192
  control of pulmonary
    hemorrhage 444
  detection and treatment of ureteral
    injury 341–342, **342**
  factors which help limb
    salvage 335, *335*
  indications of underlying vascular
    injury 327
  management of esophageal injuries
    364–365
  management of major vascular and
    musculoskeletal injuries
    335, *335*
  management of multiple
    penetrating injuries and
    bleeding 338–339, *339*
  pediatric penetrating thoracic
    trauma 458
  predictor of poor outcome in brain
    injury 191–192
  revascularization of injuries
    335, *335*

treatment of intraperitoneal colon
    injury 375
type of vascular injuries from
    shotgun wounds 334–335
use of intravascular shunting
    335, *335*
gynecologic surgery 431–437

**h**
*Haemophilus influenzae*, association
    with VAP 96
Hagen-Poiseuille equation 3
haloperidol, side-effects 131
halothane, potential side effects 124
hand trauma 317–325
hanging (non-lethal), common
    presenting injuries 291
head trauma, indications for CT scan
    in pediatric patients 463–464
heart, age-related changes 465
heat exchange, types of 153
heat exhaustion, definition 154–155
heat loss from the body,
    mechanisms 153
heat-related illness, medications
    which increase the risk of
    156–157
heat stroke, definition 154–155
*Helicobacter pylori* infection
  increasing prevalence with age 470
  methods of testing for 367–368
HELLP syndrome, distinction from
    acute fatty liver of pregnancy
    (AFLP)
hemodynamic monitoring 59–67
hemolytic uremic syndrome (HUS),
    pregnant patient 222–223
hemoperitoneum, diagnosis and
    treatment 118
hemophilia, excessive bleeding after
    trauma or surgery 115
hemoptysis, management of massive
    hemoptysis 443–444
hemorrhage
  activation of massive transfusion
    protocol 329, 455–456
  indications for REBOA 314
  management of pulsatile
    hemorrhage from deep stab
    wounds 329
  pediatric trauma patients requiring
    massive transfusion 455–456
  use of tourniquet to control
    328–329

hemorrhagic shock, diagnosis and
    treatment 21
hemorrhoids
  conditions referred to as
    381–382
  diagnosis and management
    381–382
hemostasis 109–119
  "lethal triad" of coagulopathy,
    acidosis, and
    hypothermia 117
  hemoperitoneum diagnosis and
    treatment 118
  use of rapid thromboelastography
    (TEG) in trauma patients
    112, *112*
  use of tranexamic acid (TXA) in
    trauma patients 110–111
hemothorax, post-traumatic retained
    hemothorax 446
heparin anticoagulation 99–100
heparin-induced thrombocytopenia
    (HIT)
  diagnosis and management
    100–101, 115–116
  treatment when platelet count
    normalizes 101
hepatic artery thrombosis (HAT),
    diagnosis in liver transplant
    patients 217
hepatic blush on CT, pediatric blunt
    abdominal trauma
    patients 231
hepatic dysfunction, choice of
    neuromuscular blocking
    agent 97, **98**
hepatic encephalopathy,
    pathophysiology and
    treatment 171–172
hepaticojejunostomy 385
hepatolithiasis, diagnosis and
    management 390
hepatopulmonary syndrome,
    diagnosis 175–176
hepatorenal syndrome
  distinction from prerenal
    azotemia 209
  pathogenesis 170–171
hepatotoxicity, features of acute
    acetaminophen intoxication
    174–175
hernias 403–407
  repair using the component
    separation technique 405

heroin users, effects of use of Krokodil alternative to heroin 248–250

hiatal hernia
  symptoms and management 366
  types of 366

high-frequency oscillation ventilation, parenchymal-pleural fistula (PPF) management 82

hip dislocation, diagnosis and management 324

HIV
  testing of patients 498
  transmission risk for healthcare workers 498

HIV/AIDS patients, opportunistic infections 93

Hofmann elimination process 97, **98**

hospital-acquired infections, catheter-related bloodstream infections (CRBSI) 62, 63

hospital antibiograms, use in choice of antibiotic therapy for VAP 104

hydatid disease of the liver, cause and treatment 394

hydromorphone, postoperative pain management 97–98

hyperacute rejection, symptoms and management 213–214

hyperbaric oxygen (HBO) therapy, use as adjunctive treatment for NSTIs 413

hypercalcemia
  definition and etiologies 140
  symptoms and treatment 140

hyperglycemic hyperosmolar state (HHS), diagnosis and treatment 150–151

hyperkalemia
  diagnosis and treatment 139
  etiologies 139
  indications for dialysis 161–162
  prevention of malignant ventricular arrhythmias 164
  risk associated with succinylcholine 137
  signs and symptoms of stage 3 AKI 163

hypertension
  appropriate choice of medication 147
  preoperative medications to control 147–148
  treatment during pregnancy 38 221–222

hypertensive emergencies 33–50

hyperthermia 153–157
  effect of fever in brain injury 156
  risk related to age 153

hypoalbuminemia, anion gap in ICU patients 143

hypocalcemia
  presentation 141
  risk after parathyroidectomy 145
  with hypomagnesemia 141

hypocortisolism, signs and symptoms 146–147

hypoglycemia, from overdose of a hypoglycemic agent 244–245

hypomagnesemia
  association with digitalis toxicity 138, *138*
  symptoms 16
  with hypocalcemia 141

hyponatremia
  causes and treatment 136
  diagnosis and pathophysiology in cirrhosis 176
  management of acute hyponatremia 139
  symptoms of acute hyponatremia 139
  treatment in edematous patients 136–137

hypophosphatemia, pathophysiology in critically-ill patients 141–142

hypotension in trauma patients
  causes in intubated sedated patient 124–125
  causes in trauma patients 293
  indications for REBOA 314
  intervention to maximize oxygen delivery ($DO_2$) 6
  treatment for persistent hypotension in the ICU patient 137

hypothalamic-pituitary-adrenal (HPA) axis 148

hypothermia 153–157
  cardiovascular and hemodynamic effects 156
  changes in core body temperature 154
  "lethal triad" of coagulopathy, acidosis, and hypothermia 117
  metabolic consequences 157
  perioperative risk and consequences 155–156
  rewarming method and rate 154
  role in mortality of trauma patients 117
  role in perioperative complications 126
  signs and symptoms 154
  therapeutic 155, 157

hypotonic hyponatremia, causes and treatment 136

hypovolemic shock
  diagnosis and treatment 21
  hypotension caused by 293
  oxygen extraction ($O_2ER$) calculation 19
  ways to promote end-organ profusion 4–5

hypoxemia, etiologies 10–11

*i*

ICU, common procedures 253–260

idarucizumab, reversal agent for dabigatran 118–119, **118**

ideal body weight (IBW) calculation 416

idiopathic thrombocytopenic purpura (ITP), management 398–399

iliac vein injuries, factors affecting mortality and morbidity 310–311

imaging in pediatric patients, ways to reduce the total dose of radiation 464

immune-enhancing formulas
  effects in critically-ill patients 184, 185
  role of nucleotides 185

immune-suppressed patients, combination antibiotic therapy 92–93

immunology 209–217

immunonutrition
  effects in critically-ill patients 185
  recommendations for ARDS patients 183–184

immunosuppression in transplant patients 209–210, **210**

incarcerated hernias 403–407
  para-colostomy hernia small bowel obstruction 406, *406*
  repair options for femoral hernia 406–407
  umbilical hernia in patient with cirrhosis 381
incidence, definition 486
incisional hernia, principles for repair 405
infectious disease 89–96
Infectious Disease Society of America (IDSA), guidelines for management of VAP 104–105, **104**
inferior vena cava (IVC) filter
  indications for 255–256
  management of a damaged filter 207–208
  potential complications 255–256
inflammatory response to injury 51–58
informed consent
  for participation in research studies 488
  in emergency situations 495
  issues in end-of-life care 495
  patient refusal of treatment 469–470
inguinal hernia, comparison with femoral hernia 404
inhalational burn injury, treatment 428
injury and stress, phases of response to 177
inotropic support, mechanism of action of dobutamine 62
insulin therapy, multiply-injured trauma patient 146
insurance companies, correction of incorrect claims 499
intermittent pneumatic compression devices (IPCs), effectiveness for DVT prophylaxis 199–200
interquartile range (IQR) 484
interventional radiology 261–272
intimate partner violence (IPV), risk factors and consequences in pregnancy 435
intra-abdominal HTN, assessment for 81
intra-abdominal hypertension, definition and risk factors 314–315

intra-abdominal insufflation, physiologic changes caused by 76
intra-abdominal pressure measurement, using bladder pressure 81
intra-aortic balloon pump (IABP)
  complications 440–441
  indications, placement, and physiology 11–12
intracranial hemorrhage, in anticoagulated elderly patients 466–467
intracranial hypertension, common causes 189
intracranial pressure (ICP)
  decompressive craniotomy 197–198
  DECRA trial (2011) findings 197–198
  decreasing ICP without lowering BP 284
  management of elevated ICP 190
  management of elevated ICP in pediatric trauma patients 196–197
  optimizing in traumatic brain injury 283–284
  RESCUEicp trial (2016) findings 197–198
  surgical management of uncontrollable elevation 197–198
  therapy for increased ICP in traumatic brain injury 280–281
  use of mannitol for osmotic therapy to reduce 190–191
intracranial pressure (ICP) monitoring
  devices used for 193–194
  objective in traumatic brain injury 189–190
  severe traumatic brain injury patients 279
intraparenchymal cerebral hematoma, indications for immediate surgery 190
intravascular catheter-related infection, prevention practices 94
intravascular volume status, indications from stroke volume variability (SVV) 60

intravenous immunoglobulin (IVIG)
  treatment of NSTIs 412
  treatment of refractory *C. difficile* infection 100
intubation
  identifying unrecognised misplaced intubation (UMI) 64–65
  Mallampati classification 69, *70*, **70**
  modalities to improve success rate in Mallampati IV airway 69–70
  prediction of difficult intubation 69, *70*, **70**
invasive candidiasis
  empiric antifungal therapy 106
  risk factors for 106
invasive zygomycosis, initial treatment 414
ischemia reperfusion lung injury (IRLI), following lung transplant 215
ischemic colitis diagnosis and management 380–381
isoflurane, metabolism 124

*j*
Jefferson fracture 295, *295*
Jehovah's Witness patient, management of splenic injury 401
Jehovah's Witnesses, refusal of blood transfusion for a child 499

*k*
Kaplan-Meier survival curve 488–489, *489*
Kcentra (PCC), use for rapid reversal of anticoagulation 114
ketamine
  amnestic and analgesic effects 127–128
  dissociative anesthetic 127–128
  use in rapid-sequence intubation 72–73
ketorolac, mechanism of action 122
*Klebsiella* species
  antibiotic resistance in *K. pneumoniae* 95–96
  association with CRBSI 63
  association with VAP 96

knee dislocation
  management of high-energy
    dislocation   322–323
  management of low-energy
    dislocation   323
  popliteal artery injury associated
    with   331–332
Krokodil (Crocodile, Krok, Croc),
    effects of use as alternative to
    heroin   248–250
Kruskal-Wallis test   485

## l

laboratory risk indicator for
    necrotizing fasciitis (LRINEC)
    score   341, 411, **411**
lactic acid, role of lactate clearance in
    successful fluid
    resuscitation   65–66
laparoscopic cholecystectomy   385
  early versus delayed
    procedure   386
laparoscopy, physiologic changes
    caused by intra-abdominal
    insufflation   76
Law of LaPlace   5
left anterior fascicular block (LAFB),
    EKG deviation   37–38
left ventricular pseudoaneurysm
    38–39, *38*
*Legionella pneumophila*
    infection   55
lidocaine   15–16
  effects of addition of
    epinephrine   72
  mechanism of action   72
life-saving therapy, patient refusal
    of   491
lightning strike victims
  initial concerns and management
    428–429
  most common cause of
    death   429
  neurologic sequelae   429
linezolid, use in VAP   104–105
lipid administration in critically-ill
    patients   182
lisinopril, mechanism of action   147
lithium overdose, toxic effects and
    treatment   242–243
liver   393–398
  anatomy   396–397, *396*
liver abscess, pyogenic and amebic
    types   393

liver cirrhosis
  diagnosis of hepatopulmonary
    syndrome   175–176
  effect on morbidity and mortality
    in trauma patients   395–396
  fluid leakage from umbilical
    hernia   404–405
  hyponatremia diagnosis and
    pathophysiology   176
  management of esophageal
    varices   170
  management of hepatic
    encephalopathy   171–172
  management of intractable
    ascites   173
  management of persistent
    bleeding   173
  management of pulmonary
    embolism   210–211
  management of upper
    gastrointestinal bleeding   170
  prognostic models for surgical
    patients   169, **170**
  risk of increased morbidity and
    mortality after surgery
    397–398, **397**
  symptoms and treatment of *Vibrio
    vulnificus* infection   211–212
liver cirrhosis and ascites,
    incarcerated/strangulated
    umbilical hernia   381
liver disease, pathogenesis of
    hepatorenal syndrome
    170–171
liver failure   169–176
  clinical features and mortality
    risk   173–174
  distinction between prerenal
    azotemia and hepatorenal
    syndrome   209
  nutritional therapy   187
  treatment of acetaminophen
    poisoning   175
liver injury
  abdominal computed tomography
    (CT)   393–394, *394*
  APSA guidelines for pediatric blunt
    trauma   234–235, *234*
  bile leak following laparotomy and
    hepatorraphy   309
  blush on CT scan   308
  criteria for nonoperative
    management   307
  delayed complications   395

indications for angiography and
    possible embolization   308
  nonoperative management
    393–394, *394*
  post-injury biloma
    complication   394–395
  post-injury hemobilia   395
liver transplantation
  diagnosis of hepatic artery
    thrombosis (HAT)   217
  indications and
    contraindications   214
  indications and outcomes
    173–174
  use of calcineurin inhibitors   210
liver trauma
  management of blunt trauma   393
  nonoperative management   393
liver tumors
  classification as benign or
    malignant   **397**, 397
  types of   **397**, 397
local anesthesics
  amino ester and amino amide
    types   126
  early clinical signs of central
    nervous system toxicity   125
  ester and amide types   72
  mechanism of action   71–72
lorazepam, mechanism of action
    101–102
low-molecular-weight heparin
    (LMWH) anticoagulation
    99–100
  epidural analgesia and   204
  prophylactic use   203
lower extremity ulceration, illicit drug
    likely to cause   248–250
lower gastrointestinal bleeding,
    management   375–376
LRINEC score   341, 411, **411**
lumbar puncture
  complications   260
  use in the ICU   260
lung resection, acute bronchopleural
    fistula (BPF)
    complication   441
lung transplantation
  causes of postoperative
    pneumonia   216
  etiology of respiratory failure   215
  risk of ischemia reperfusion lung
    injury (IRLI)   215
lungs, West lung zones   12

## m

mafenide acetate antimicrobial, side effects   427–428

magnesium sulfate   15

malignant gastric outlet obstruction, management   364

malignant hyperthermia (MH)
  causes, symptoms, and treatment   77–78
  indicators of   126

malignant ventricular arrhythmias, prevention in severe hyperkalemia   164

Mallampati classification   69, *70*, **70**

Mallory-Weiss tear, definition and management   361

mannitol, use in osmotic therapy to reduce intracranial pressure   190–191

Mann-Whitney U test   487

massive transfusion
  blood component therapy   109
  definition   111–112
  electrolyte abnormalities associated with   113–114
  hypocalcemia associated with   113–114
  plasma for patient of unknown blood type   112–113
  ratio and type of platelets   113

massive transfusion protocol (MTP)   329
  activation criteria   111–112
  for pediatric patients   455–456

McNemar's test   485

MDMA (Ecstasy/Bath salts), mechanism of action   250–251

mean (measure of central tendency)   484

mechanical ventilation *see* ventilator support

Meckel's diverticulum, diagnosis and management   377, *377*

median (measure of central tendency)   484

mediastinitis, postoperative
  initial management   89
  microorganism associated with   89

medical errors, disclosure and liability   497–498

medical insurance, correction of incorrect claims   499

medical malpractice, liability issues in compartment syndrome   321–322

medical professionalism   495–496

medical research, justification for performing   493

medications, effect on risk of heat-related illness   156–157

melena, presenting sign of PUD in elderly patients   470

meperidine
  mechanism of action   122
  postoperative pain management   98

meropenem, antimicrobial action   105

mesenteric ischemia (NOMI), identification and management   474–475

mesenteric venous ischemia associated with thrombosis   380, *380*

metabolic acidosis
  anion gap type   141, 143
  effect of albumin on anion-gap type   143
  diagnosis and assessment   137
  indications for use of sodium bicarbonate   167
  non-anion gap type   140, 141

metabolic alkalosis, causes   136

metabolic equivalents (METS) measure of functional capacity   75

metabolic illness   145–151

metabolism, effects of aging   472

methanol ingestion, toxicity and treatment   243

methemoglobinemia
  diagnosis and treatment   139–140
  drugs associated with   140
  etiologies and treatment   123–124

methicillin-resistant *Staphylococcus aureus* (MRSA) *see* MRSA

methicillin-susceptible *Staphylococcus aureus* (MSSA)   89, 96

metoclopramide, antiemetic action   99

metoprolol overdose, symptoms and management   247

metronidazole, use in VAP   104–105

micronutrients, supplementation in critically-ill patients   182–183

midazolam
  hemodynamic side effects   72–73
  mechanism of action   101–102, 128

Model for End-stage Liver Disease (MELD) risk scoring system   169, **170**

moral judgment, *prima facie* concept   492–493

*Moraxella* species, association with VAP   96

morphine
  mechanism of action   122
  postoperative pain management   97–98

motor bike accident trauma patient, evaluation and management   281–282

MRCP (magnetic resonance cholangiopancreatography), preoperative detection of common bile duct stones   266–267

MRSA (methicillin-resistant *Staphylococcus aureus*)
  association with VAP   55, 96
  risk factors for VAP   104–105, **104**

MRSA soft tissue infections, predictor of treatment failure and hospital mortality   410

MSSA (methicillin-susceptible *Staphylococcus aureus*)   89, 96

multidrug resistant (MDR) pathogens, risk factors in VAP   104–105, **104**

multidrug resistant (MDR) pneumonia, risk factors for   96

multifocal atrial tachycardia (MAT), ECG trace and treatment   80

multi-organ dysfunction syndrome (MODS), definition   51

multivariable analyses   484

multivariable linear regression   487

multivariable logistic regression   487

munificence   491

muscle protein catabolism in critically-ill and injured patients   179

*Mycoplasma* infection   55

myelinolysis   139

myocardial infarction (MI)
  complications   40–41, *40*
  complications after 48–49
  perioperative preventive
      medication   73
  right-sided ventricular infarction
      45–48, *46, 47*
  ventricular fibrillation following
      49–50, *49*
myocardial oxygen consumption
    (MVO$_2$), factors
    influencing   5
myonecrosis, most common cause
    411–412
myxedema coma, diagnosis and
    treatment   151

**n**
near infrared spectroscopy (NIRS)
  monitoring of pediatric critical
      care patients   228
  tissue oxygenation assessment   228
neck
  vascular anatomy   287, *288*
  zones of the neck   287, *288*
neck trauma   287–297
  anterior Zone II stab wound
      289–290
  blunt cerebrovascular injury
      (BCVI)   288–289, *289*, **289**
  "clothesline" injury
      management   297
  indications for BCVI
      screening   290
  operative versus non-operative
      management   287, *288*
  repair of esophageal
      laceration   292
  repair of tracheal laceration   292
  seatbelt sign   288–289, *289*,
      **289**, 290
  tracheal injury   289–290
  Zone II penetrating trauma
      management   287–288, 294
necrotizing fasciitis
  cervical necrotizing fasciitis
      413–414
  choice of antibiotic   106–107
  laboratory risk indicator (LRNEC)
      score   411, **411**
  most common cause   411–412
necrotizing pancreatitis
  antibiotic prophylaxis   392
  diagnosis and treatment
      approaches   390–391

necrotizing soft tissue infections
    (NSTIs)   409–414
  antibiotic choice   106–107
  antibiotic regimen   95
  causative organisms   94–95
  classification   95, 412
  diagnosis   409–410, *410*
  diagnosis of *Vibrio* or *Aeromonas*
      infection   412
  hard signs   409, *410*
  hyperbaric oxygen (HBO)
      therapy   413
  IVIG therapy   412
  microbiologic etiologies   412
  negative-pressure wound therapy
      (NPWT)   412
  perineal region   341
  signs   94–95
negative pressure pulmonary edema,
    following extubation   79–80
negative-pressure wound therapy
    (NPWT), use in NSTI
    management   412
neostigmine, action as NMBA
    reversal agent   107, 108
nephrogenic diabetes insipidus,
    diagnosis   145
neurocritical care   189–198
neurogenic shock
  diagnosis, etiology and
      treatment   21
  hypotension caused by   293
neuromuscular blocking agents
    (NMBAs)
  causes of continued
      paralysis   70–71
  choice for burn victims   122
  choice in patients with hepatic
      and/or renal dysfunction
      97, **98**
  choice of appropriate agent   72
  effects of inadequate reversal   79
  for critically-ill patients with liver
      or renal disease   122–123
  interaction with aminoglycoside
      antibiotics   70–71
  methods of elimination   97, **98**
  patient with a contraindication to
      succinylcholine   123
  reversal agents   107
  risk factors for inadequate
      reversal   79
neurotrauma   275–286
neutropenia, treatment of
    infections   54

neutropenic enterocolitis,
    complication of chemotherapy
    374–375
Nimbex *see* cisatracurium
nitric oxide (NO), role in vasodilation
    57–58
nitroprusside, cyanide toxicity
    associated with   247–248
nitrous oxide, risks for patients with
    vitamin B12 deficiency   124
non-accidental trauma in children
  blunt abdominal trauma   235
  reporting suspicious cases   458
non-ethanol alcohols, toxicity and
    treatment   243
non-invasive positive pressure
    ventilation (NIPPV)
  contraindications   86
  method and uses   86
non-invasive ventilation (NIV),
    effects in the immediate
    postoperative setting   79
nonmaleficence   491, 493
nonmalfeasance   491
non-occlusive mesenteric ischemia
    (NOMI), identification and
    management   474–475
non-parametric (asymmetric,
    skewed) distribution
    484, *484*
non-parametric tests of
    significance   485
nonrational requests from patient's
    family   495
nonrational thinking   491
normal (parametric) distribution
    484, *484*
normal saline (0.9% NaCl solution),
    effect on plasma volume   144
nosocomial infections, common
    pathogens   105–106
nucleotides
  functions of   185
  role in immunonutrition   185
null hypothesis, criteria for
    rejection   485–486
nutrients, location of absorption
    within the GI tract   419–420
nutrition
  effects of ageing   472
  requirements of children compared
      to adults   459
nutritional support
  deficiencies after bariatric
      surgery   419, 420

for critically-ill elderly patients 471–472
in acute kidney injury (AKI) 167
in critically-ill patients 177–188
preferred routes 77
refeeding syndrome (RFS) 77
requirement of burn patients 427
nutritional therapy
burn patients 188
in hepatic failure 187
in pulmonary failure 186–187
obese critically-ill patients 188
severe pancreatitis 187–188

**o**
obese patients 415–422
body mass index (BMI) classification 415, **416**
effects of obesity on pulmonary physiology 415
increase in prevalence of obesity 415
nutritional therapy for critically-ill patients 188
recommendation for bariatric surgery 415
risks from obstructive sleep apnea (OSA) 416–417
tracheostomy complication rates 416
ventilator tidal volume setting 416
obstetric critical care 219–226
obstructive sleep apnea (OSA), risk in obese patients 416–417
odds ratio 487–488
Ogilvie's syndrome 374
ondansetron, antiemetic action 99
open fractures
choice of antibiotic prophylaxis 321
duration of intravenous cefazolin administration 320
infection risk 319–320, *319*
timing of debridement in trauma patients 320
organ donation
avoiding the appearance of conflict of interest 497
issue of continuation of futile care 496
obtaining consent for 492, 497
separation of the treatment and organ transplant teams 497
orthopedic trauma 317–325
ovary, pseudomyxoma peritonei symptoms and treatment 373
overdose patient
gastric decontamination procedure 241
use of whole bowel irrigation (WBI) to prevent drug absorption 239
overwhelming postsplenectomy infection (OPSI), risk of 401–402
oxycodone, postoperative pain management 98
oxygen content ($CaO_2$) of blood, calculation 18
oxygen delivery ($DO_2$) 15–21
calculation 18, 65
definition 65
intervention to maximize in refractory hypotension 6
optimizing in the critically-ill patient 65
oxygen delivery index ($DO_2I$), calculation 65
oxygen-dissociation curve, factors which shift the curve to the right or left 19
oxygen extraction ($O_2ER$) calculation 19
oxygen saturation ($SpO_2$), methods of measurement 59–60
oxygen uptake/consumption ($VO_2$) calculation 18

**p**
p-values 485
relationship to 95% confidence intervals (CIs) 486
packed red blood cell (PRBC) transfusion
effects of liberal transfusion 111
pediatric critically-ill patients 228–229
pain management, analgesics for postoperative pain 97–98
*see also* analgesia
paired Student's t-test 487
pancreas 385–392
pancreas transplantation, effects on complications of diabetes 217
pancreatic injuries
AAST classification 391
caused by blunt trauma 310
evaluation and management 391
management challenges 391–392
management of blunt trauma in children 461–462, *461*, **461**
pancreatitis
acute flare-up 141
antibiotic prophylaxis 392
optimal nutritional support 386–387
pancuronium
mechanism of action 122, 123
metabolism and elimination 72, 97, **98**
reversal drugs 107
papillary muscle rupture 40–41, *40*
para-colostomy hernia
incarcerated hernia with small bowel obstruction 406, *406*
incidence and risk factors 405–406
paraesophageal hernia
symptoms and management 366
types of 366
parametric (normal) distribution 484, *484*
parametric tests of significance 485
parastomal hernia, incidence and risk factors 405–406
parathyroidectomy, postoperative hypocalcemia risk 145
parenchymal-pleural fistula (PPF) management 82
parenteral nutrition, in severe burn patients 427
patient autonomy 491
PCP, mechanism of action 250–251
peak airway pressures
high pressures in a postoperative patient 83–84
pressure versus volume tracing assessment 83–84
significance of rising pressures 81
Pearson's correlation coefficient 487–488
Pearson's $X^2$ test 487–488
pediatric acute respiratory distress syndrome (PARDS)
ancillary treatment 230–231
definition 229, *229*
titration of mechanical ventilatory support 230
ventilation support recommendations 229–230

pediatric critical care   227–238
pediatric massive transfusion
        protocol   455–456
pediatric trauma patients
    airway management   453–454
    blood transfusion for children of
        Jehovah's Witnesses   499
    emergency airway   297
    emergent endotracheal
        intubation   453–454
    evaluation of injuries from caustic
        substance ingestion   365
    initial assessment following caustic
        ingestion   365–366
    management of elevated ICP in
        traumatic brain
        injury   196–197
    mechanisms of fatal injury   456
    non-accidental trauma   456, 458
    normal ranges for vital
        signs   456–457, **456**
    nutritional requirements   459
    reporting suspected non-accidental
        trauma   458
    surgery   453–464
PEEP *see* positive end-expiratory
        pressure
pelvic angiography
    possible complications   264–265
    use in pelvic fracture   264
pelvic fractures
    application of a pelvic binder or
        sheet   317, *318*
    causes of bleeding associated with
        317–318
    diagnostic use of pelvic X-ray   271
    DVT prophylaxis
        protocols   318–319
    indicators of urethral injury   308
    management of hypotension
        associated with   307–308
    types associated with bladder
        injury   318, *318*
pelvic inflammatory disease, causes,
        diagnosis, and treatment
        432–433
pelvic ring injuries, common
        symptoms and problems in
        women   319
penetrating neck trauma   287–297
    diagnostic evaluation with CT
        angiography   265
penetrating peripheral vascular trauma
    evaluation and management   266
    use of CT arteriography   265–266

penetrating torso trauma, use of
        triple contrast CT scans
        267–268
penicillin-allergic patient, antibiotic
        choices   414
peptic ulcer disease (PUD)
    causes   362–363
    presentation in elderly patients   470
    treatment of bleeding from
        ulcers   362–363
percutaneous coronary intervention
        (PCI), effect on subsequent
        non-cardiac surgery   75
percutaneous endoscopic
        gastrostomy (PEG) tube
    considerations for tube
        placement   259
    esophageal perforation   449, *449*
perianal hematoma, diagnosis and
        management   381–382
pericardial effusion, assessment via
        transthoracic echocardiography
        (TTE)   261
periclavicular gunshot wound,
        evaluation   302–303
perilunate dislocation, avoiding delay
        in diagnosis and
        management   325
perineum, management of penetrating
        traumatic injury   382
perioperative hypothermia
    definition, consequences, and
        prevention   155–156
    role in perioperative
        complications   126
perioperative management   69–78
peripartum cardiomyopathy,
        diagnosis and
        management   220
peripheral arterial injury
    management   329
    use of a temporary intravascular
        shunt (TIVS)   329–330
peripheral vascular injury
    benefits of completion angiography
        after repair   330–331, *331*
    factors affecting survival
        330–331, *331*
peripheral vascular resistance (PVR),
        calculation   67
peripheral vascular trauma   327–335
    diagnostic testing   328
    indication for a therapeutic
        decompressive
        fasciotomy   333

pharmacodynamics
    alterations in critically-ill patients
        102–103
    definition   103
pharmacokinetics
    alterations in critically-ill
        patients   102–103
    definition   103
pharmacology 97–108
phenothiazines, antiemetic action
        and side effects   99
pheochromocytoma, symptoms,
        incidence, and management
        147–148
phlebostatic axis, definition   66
physical status, American Society of
        Anesthesiologists (ASA)
        classification   71
physician incompetence, action
        required   494
physician self-referral, ethical and
        legal issues   496–497
piperacillin/tazobactam, antimicrobial
        activity   105–106
placental abruption, diagnosis and
        management   219
Plasma-Lyte resuscitation fluid,
        properties   142
platelet inhibitor therapy, perioperative
        management   116–117
Plavix   44
pluralism   493
pneumonectomy, acute
        bronchopleural fistula (BPF)
        complication   441
pneumonia
    causes in lung transplant
        patients   216
    risk factors in trauma patients   94
pneumothorax
    diagnosis and management   447
    signs of   80
poisonings   239–251
    AACT/EAPCCT guidelines for
        management   243
polyene antibiotic family, mechanism
        of action   102
polymorphic ventricular tachycardia
        41–42, *41–42*
popliteal artery injuries
    associated with knee dislocation
        331–332
    evaluation and management
        331–332
    rate of limb salvage   331–332

portal-systemic encephalopathy, pathophysiology and treatment 171–172

positive end-expiratory pressure (PEEP)
effect in a severely hypoxic patient with ARDS 6
effect in patients who have ARDS 9
optimal location on a volume-pressure curve 13

positive pressure ventilation, effects on cardiac function 5–6

postdural puncture headache, symptoms and treatment 125–126

postoperative acute respiratory failure, most likely cause 79

postoperative *Candida glabrata* infection, antifungal treatment 96

postoperative candidiasis, antibiotic prophylaxis 93

postoperative *Clostridium difficile* infection, management 89–90

postoperative mediastinitis
initial management 89
microorganism associated with 89

postoperative mortality, medications likely to decrease mortality risk 93

postoperative myocardial infarction, preventive medication 73

postoperative nausea and vomiting, antiemetics 99

postoperative oliguria, initial workup 160–161

postoperative pain management, choice of analgesic 97–98

postpartum patient
causes of hypotension, hypoxemia, and/or hemorrhage 434–435
endometriosis diagnosis and treatment 225
risk of VTE 201–202

postpartum septic pelvic thrombophlebitis, diagnosis and management 223–224

post-thrombotic syndrome (PTS), pathophysiology and management 200

power of a study sample 483–484

Pradaxa *see* dabigatran

prealbumin, function as a negative acute phase protein 178–179

Precedex *see* dexmedetomidine

pregnancy
cardiovascular changes during 11
management of choledocholithiasis 389
management of gallstone disease 389
respiratory and metabolic changes 221
risk of VTE 201–202
safe antihypertensive medications 38

pregnant patient 345–357
airway management 355
cardiotocographic monitoring after blunt trauma 345
causes of hypotension, hypoxemia, and/or hemorrhage 434–435
characteristics of VTE in pregnancy 223
CPR and emergent Cesarian section 436–437
diagnosis and treatment of pulmonary embolism 224–225
differential diagnosis for altered mental state (AMS) 352
fetal risk of critical care medications 222
fetal survival in maternal cardiac arrest 437
guidelines for laparoscopic appendectomy 434
hemolytic uremic syndrome (HUS) 222–223
hypercoagulability of pregnancy 349–350
imaging radiation exposure concerns 348–349
imaging risks and considerations 267
incidence and types of trauma in pregnancy 356
indications for emergency Cesarean section 349
initial assessment and treatment of trauma patients 436
management changes in initial evaluation and resuscitation 353
management of neurologic injury 348

mortality rate for trauma during pregnancy 356
normal laboratory studies in pregnancy 355–356
perimortem emergency C-section procedure 351–352
physiological changes associated with pregnancy 346–347
posterior reversible encephalopathy syndrome (PRES) 225
presentation and diagnosis of acute appendicitis 433
risk and consequences of intimate partner violence (IPV) 435
risk of intimate partner violence 351
risk of placental abruption and fetal demise 353–354
risk of thromboembolism in pregnancy 349–350
routine assessment of fetal well-being 354–355
seat belt use by pregnant women 350–351
thrombotic thrombocytopenic purpura (TTP) 222–223
tocolytic associated pulmonary edema 226
tocolytic medications to prevent premature labor 345–346
treatment of acute appendicitis 433–434
treatment of HELLP syndrome 352–353
treatment of scald burn injuries 436
use and interpretation of the Kleihauer-Betke test 347–348
uterine rupture caused by trauma 356–357

pre-renal azotemia
distinction from acute tubular necrosis 160
distinction from hepatorenal syndrome (HRS) 209

pressure-volume dysregulation, "bird's beak" phenomenon 88, *88*

preterm labor, tocolytic-associated pulmonary edema 226

prevalence, definition 486

prima facie nature of principles and moral rules 492–493

principlism 491, 495

prisoners of war (POWs), ethical and humane treatment by physicians 492

prochlorperazine, antiemetic action and side effects 99

professional conduct in patient care 495–496

progesterone, use in traumatic brain injury treatment 196

prognostic models, for surgical patient with liver cirrhosis 169, **170**

prolonged QT interval 42, 42

propofol
    common side effects 121
    hemodynamic side effects 72–73
    mechanism of action 121, 128
    metabolism 124

propofol infusion syndrome 125

protein synthesis
    in critically ill and injured patients 179
    process of mRNA translation 179–180
    sites of 179–180

prothrombin complex concentrate (PCC)
    for rapid reversal of anticoagulation 114, 118–119
    use to normalize INR 61–62

protocolized emergency department sepsis guideline 227

*Pseudomonas aeruginosa*
    antibiotic resistance 95–96
    association with VAP 55, 96
    beta-lactamase production 105–106
    choice of antimicrobial medication 105–106
    duration of antibiotic therapy for VAP 90
    risk factors for MDR *Pseudomonas* VAP 104–105, **104**
    use of combination antibiotic therapy 92–93

pseudomyxoma peritonei, symptoms and treatment 373

psychiatric disorders 129–134
    psychosis etiologies 134
    psychosis presentations and management 133–134

pulmonary artery catheter (PAC)
    false cardiac output measurement caused by cardiac abnormalities 62–63
    indications and contraindications for placement 63–64, 254–255
    information provided by 254–255
    pressure changes as the catheter is being placed 61–62
    thermodilution principle 62–63

pulmonary edema
    following myocardial infarction 40–41, *40*
    in ALI/ARDs 14
    re-expansion pulmonary edema 445
    tocolytic-associated pulmonary edema 226

pulmonary embolism (PE)
    AAOS recommendations for prophylaxis 205–206, **206**
    diagnosis and treatment in a pregnant patient 224–225
    diagnostic scoring systems 204
    diagnostic use of D-dimer 203–204
    enoxaparin administration 99–100
    following bariatric surgery 420
    following spleen injury 199
    incidence and management 202–203
    inferior vena cava (IVC) filter placement 255–256
    management in patients with cirrhosis 210–211
    prophylaxis for total knee or hip replacement 205–206, **206**
    treatment of acute PE 439–440, *440*

pulmonary failure, nutritional therapy 186–187

pulmonary physiology, effects of obesity 415

pulmonary trauma, control of pulmonary hemorrhage 444

pulse oximetry monitors, factors affecting the accuracy of readings 59–60

pulseless electrical activity (PEA) arrest 15, 16

*pulsus paradoxus*, definition and etiologies 20–21

**q**

quinupristin/dalfopristin, antimicrobial action 104

**r**

radiocontrast media, contrast-induced nephropathy (CIN) 76

radius, nerve injury in distal radius fractures 324–325

randomization of subjects in a study 488

rapid-sequence intubation
    choice of neuromuscular blocker 122
    drugs used for head-injured trauma patients 72–73

rapid shallow breathing index (RSBI) 64, 86

REBOA (resuscitative endovascular balloon occlusion of the aorta), indications and contraindications in trauma patients 306, 314

rectal bleeding
    colon tumor management 376
    ischemic colitis diagnosis and management 380–381

rectal foreign bodies, removal 383

rectal prolapse, assessment and management 378–379, *378*

rectum 371–383
    management of extraperitoneal penetrating trauma 382

re-expansion pulmonary edema, diagnosis and management 445
    following drainage of pulmonary effusion 445

refeeding syndrome (RFS), biochemical derangement in 77

relative risk 487–488

renal dysfunction
    choice of neuromuscular blocking agent 97, **98**
    risk in elderly trauma patients 468–469

renal injuries
    incidence and management in trauma patients 309–310
    pediatric blunt kidney trauma 235
    penetrating renal injury 342–343, *343*
    renal exploration for trauma 342–343, *343*

renal replacement therapy
 advantages over intermittent
   dialysis 165–166
 in elderly patients 468–469
renal transplant patients
 common causes of late
   deaths 212
 diagnosis of calcineurin toxicity
   209–210, **210**
 diagnosis of renal artery
   thrombosis 214
 drug-drug interactions
   209–210, **210**
 post-transplant
   complications 214
 side effects of thymoglobulin
   induction agent 216–217
 treatment for invasive fungal
   infection 211
renin-angiotensin-aldosterone
   system 147
RESCUEicp trial (2016) findings
   197–198
research, justification for
   performing 493
RESP score 25–26, **25**
respect (ethical principle) 491
respiratory acidosis
 adjustment of ventilator
   settings 84
 diagnosis and treatment 142–143
respiratory failure management, role
   of ECMO 87
respiratory monitoring 59–67
respiratory physiology 3–14
resuscitation
 for hemoperitoneum 118
 management of continued
   hypoperfusion 91
resuscitation fluids
 edema promotion effects
   143–144
 effect of normal saline on plasma
   volume 144
 normal saline and Plasma-Lyte
   compared 142
resuscitative thoracotomy, indications
   for 304–305
retained hemothorax
 diagnosis and management 446
 treatment following blunt chest
   trauma 306
retinol-binding protein, function as a
   negative acute phase protein
   178–179

retroperitoneal hematomas,
   indications for surgical
   exploration 311–312, *311*
retroperitoneal rectal injury,
   management 337, *338*
rhabdomyolysis, treatment 162
rib fractures
 incidence and consequences in
   elderly patients 465–466
 management in a patient with
   COPD 80–81
 management of flail chest
   450–451
Richmond Agitation and Sedation
   Scale (RASS) 127, **127**
 evaluation of delirium tremens
   **133**, 133
right atrial tracing, analysis
   8, *9*, *10*
right internal jugular dual lumen VV
   ECMO catheter,
   complications 28–29
right-sided heart failure associated
   with severe hypotension,
   therapeutic intervention
   8, 9
right-sided ventricular infarction
   45–48, 46, 47
risk ratio 487–488
rivaroxaban, rapid reversal in trauma
   patients 118–119, **118**
rocuronium
 mechanism of action 122, 123
 metabolism and elimination 72,
   97, **98**
 reversal drugs 107–108, *107*
Roux-en-Y gastric bypass
 anastomotic leak detection and
   treatment 368–369
 complications 417
 diagnosis of a perforated marginal
   ulcer 417
 diagnosis of acute postoperative
   obstruction 421
 diagnosis of postoperative enteric
   leaks 421–422
 internal hernia reduction 421
 internal herniation complication
   420–421
 intraoperative chlolecystectomy
   417–418
 intraoperative treatment of
   gallstones 417–418
 postoperative nutritional
   deficiencies 419, 420

 postoperative pulmonary
   embolus 420
 treatment of a perforated marginal
   ulcer 417

**S**
salicylate poisoning
 toxidrome 241–242
 treatment 241–242
sample size for randomized placebo-
   controlled blind trials
   483–484
scaphoid bone, management of
   occult fracture 323
scopolamine, antiemetic
   action 99
seat belt mark
 association with abdominal
   mesenteric injury
   379–380, *379*
 injuries associated with abdominal
   seat belt sign 310
second degree heart block (Mobitz
   type II) 36–37, *37*
sedation
 causes and treatment of
   hypotension 127
 optimum level during mechanical
   ventilation 127, **127**
 propofol infusion syndrome 125
 Richmond Agitation and Sedation
   Scale (RASS) 127, **127**
 weaning from 121–122
seizures, following traumatic brain
   injury 194
Selective Relaxant Binding Agents
   (SRBAs) 107
self-determination principle 491
sepsis 51–58
 diagnostic criteria 51
 following cystoprostatectomy
   339, *339*
 initial management 51
 major cause of vasodilation
   57–58
 pediatric patient protocolized
   emergency department sepsis
   guideline 227
 resuscitation of pediatric
   patients 459
 steroid treatment 146
 Surviving Sepsis Campaign
   recommendations 146
 therapeutics which effectively
   improve outcomes 56

sepsis-induced inflammatory cascade, role of the coagulation system 57

septic pelvic thrombophlebitis, diagnosis and management 223–224

septic shock
combination antibiotic therapy 92–93
comparison of epinephrine and dopamine treatment in children 231
definition 51
early clinical manifestations 74
indications for the use of corticosteroids 52
Surviving Sepsis Campaign guidelines 231
treatment of "cold" shock indicative of cardiovascular dysfunction 55
treatment of pediatric fluid-refractory septic shock 231
treatment of "warm" or vasodilatory shock 55
use of vasoactive agents 91–92
use of vasopressin 56–57

*Serratia* species
association with CRBSI 63
association with VAP 96
beta-lactamase production 105

severe pancreatitis, nutritional therapy 187–188

severe sepsis
combination antibiotic therapy 92–93
diagnostic criteria 51
early clinical manifestations 74
initial management 51

sevoflurane, potential side effects 124

Sheehan's syndrome 148

shock 15–21
early clinical manifestations 74
physiologic changes in various types of shock 59

shock state, relationship between oxygen delivery and oxygen uptake 13–14

shotgun wounds, type of vascular injuries associated with 334–335

sigmoid colon volvulus, recurrent 371–372

silver nitrate antimicrobial, side effects 428

silver sulfadiazine antimicrobial, side effects 428

skin and soft tissue infections (SSTIs)
most common identifiable cause 411
predictor of treatment failure and hospital mortality in MRSA SSTIs 410
severe SSTIs caused by diabetic foot infections 413
types of 409

small bowel, mesenteric injury from blunt trauma 379–380, *379*

small intestine 371–383

smoking, and cardiac risk 49

snakebite
Crotalinae (pit viper) antivenom administration 245–246
resolution of compartment syndrome caused by 245–246

sodium bicarbonate, indications for use 167

soft tissue infections 409–414

solid organ injuries
management in pediatric patients 463
use of anticoagulation 199

Specific Activity Scale 75

spinal anesthesia, postdural puncture headache 125–126

spinal cord injury (SCI)
complications of complete spinal cord injury 291–292
effects on the reproductive system 291–292
function spared with C7 transection 279
Jefferson fracture 295, *295*
pulmonary function testing 288
use of high-dose steroids 279–280

spinal cord injury without radiographic abnormality (SCIWORA), features in children 454–455

spinal shock
distinction from neural shock 21
presentation 21

spleen 398–402
anatomy 398

spleen injury

angioembolization 400–401

APSA guidelines for pediatric blunt trauma 234–235, *234*

contraindication to non-operative management 401

criteria for nonoperative management 308–309

indication for surgical intervention 399–400, *400*

Jehovah's Witness patient 401

management of 199

nonoperative management 263–264

pediatric patients 455, 457–458

presence of a blush on CT scan 399–400, *400*

splenic preservation in children 457–458

use of angiography in blunt trauma 263–264

use of anticoagulation 199

splenectomy
following gunshot wound to the spleen 338–339, *339*
indications for 401
locations for an accessory spleen 398
overwhelming postsplenectomy infection (OPSI) risk 401–402
predictors of a favorable response 398
vaccinations for splenectomy patients 313

splenic artery aneurysm, diagnosis and management 399

splenic artery embolization, following blunt trauma 263–264

splenic blush on CT, pediatric blunt abdominal trauma patients 231

splenic cyst, classification and management 399

spontaneous bacterial peritonitis, diagnosis and treatment 172

ST-elevation myocardial infarction (STEMI), acute stent thrombosis complication 440

standard deviation (SD) 484

*Staphylococcus aureus*
association with CRBSI 63
association with NSTIs 94–95
*see also* MRSA

*Staphylococcus epidermidis*
   association with CRBSI   63
   treatment of catheter-related
      bloodstream infection   53
Stark Laws   497
Starling equation   14
statin therapy, use in the
      perioperative period
      73–74
statistics   483–489
stent, patient with
   effect on subsequent non-cardiac
      surgery   75
   perioperative management of
      antiplatelet medications
      116–117
steroid therapy
   use in blunt traumatic brain
      injury   189
   use in sepsis   146
steroid-treated patients
   interventions to improve wound
      healing   149–150
   symptoms of bowel injury   149
stomach   359–369
stratified randomization   488
streptococcal toxic shock
      syndrome, choice of
      antibiotic   107
*Streptococcus pneumoniae*,
      association with VAP   96
*Streptococcus pyogenes*, association
      with NSTIs   94–95
stress and injury, phases of response
      to   177
stress ulcers in high-risk ICU
      patients, factors associated
      with increased incidence
      74–75
stroke volume, factors
      determining   4, *4*
stroke volume variability (SVV)
   factors affecting   60
   normal range of variation   60
Student's t-test   485
subarachnoid hemorrhage (SAH),
      symptoms and management
      282–283
subclavian artery injury
   commonly associated injuries
      301–302
   concomitant venous injury
      301–302
   management   302

subdural hematoma
   causes and management   282
   incidence and risk factors   282
subarachnoid hemorrhage, secondary
      to ruptured cerebral artery
      aneurysm   192
substituted judgment   491
   in end-of-life care   493–494
succinylcholine
   action as NMBA   107
   contraindication for burn
      victims   122
   mechanism of action   122, 123
   method of elimination   97, **98**
   risk of hyperkalemia and cardiac
      arrest   137
sugammadex, mechanism of
      action   107–108, *107*
suicidal hanging (non-lethal), common
      presenting injuries   291
suicide, rates among the elderly   471
sulfamylon acetate antimicrobial, side
      effects   427–428
sulfonylurea overdose, symptoms and
      treatment   244–245
superior mesenteric artery (SMA)
   treatment of penetrating trauma
      injury   373–374
   zones of the SMA   374
superior vena cava (SVC) syndrome,
      diagnosis and management
      446–447
supra-glottal airway devices (SADs),
      role in tracheal intubation
      293–294
surgeon autonomy   495–496
surgery
   anticoagulation management
      33–34, **34**
   prognostic models   169, **170**
surgery (non-cardiac)
   assessment for cardiovascular
      perioperative risk   75
   in patients that have received
      PCI   75
surrogate decision-making for
      patients   469–470
Surviving Sepsis Campaign
      guidelines   91, 92, 146
   for pediatric patients   459
syncope
   history of   36–37, *37*
   prevalence and etiologies in elderly
      people   473

syndrome of inappropriate
      antidiuretic hormone
      (SIADH), diagnosis and
      treatment   148–149
synthetic marijuana (Spice/K2),
      mechanism of action   250–251
systemic inflammatory response
      syndrome (SIRS)
   causes and treatment   20
   diagnostic criteria   20, 51
systemic vascular resistance (SVR)
   calculation   67
   definition   67
t-test   484

*t*
tachycardia, diagnosis   34–35, *34*
tacrolimus
   drug-drug interactions
      209–210, **210**
   immunosuppression in transplant
      patients   210
   mechanism of action   214–215
   side effects   215
Takotsubo's syndrome   36
tazobactam, antimicrobial activity
      105–106
telemedicine and telepresence for
      surgery and trauma   477–481
   applications for surgical
      telementoring   477–478
   benefits of implementation in
      critical care units   481
   electronic data communications
      networks   477
   real-time trauma
      resuscitation   480–481
   teletrauma support   479–480
   virtual intensive care   478–479
temperature management,
      intravascular versus surface
      cooling   157
temporary abdominal closure (TAC),
      methods and considerations
      312–313
temporary intravascular shunt (TIVS)
   duration of placement   329–330
   in combined skeletal and arterial
      injuries   333–334, *334*
   purpose of   329–330
tension pneumothorax
   diagnosis and management   447
   effect on central venous pressure
      (CVP)   66

tetanus, treatment for patients at risk   54

therapeutic hypothermia, indications and contraindications   155

thermodilution principle, use in pulmonary artery catheter   62–63

thiopental, mechanism of action   128

thoracic surgery   439–451

thoracic vascular injury   299–306

thoracotomy, indications for urgent/emergent thoracotomy   303

thrombocytopenia, heparin-induced (HIT)   100–101, 115–116

thromboelastography (TEG), use of rapid TEG in trauma patients   112, *112*

thromboembolism   199–208

thrombolytics, use in acute coronary syndromes   48

thrombosed external pile, diagnosis and management   381–382

thrombotic thrombocytopenic purpura (TTP), pregnant patient   222–223

thumb, replantation of traumatic amputations   323–324

thymoglobulin, side effects when used as induction agent   216–217

thyroid storm, etiologies, symptoms and management   148

tibia and fibula fracture

   indication for below-knee amputation   320

   indications of compartment syndrome   321

   limb salvage versus amputation   320

   pain following splinting   321

tibia fracture

   fasciotomy incision to decompress the leg compartments   322, *322*

   infection risk in open fractures   319–320, *319*

   timing of debridement of open fractures   320

tigecycline

   black box warning   108

   risk of death   108

   use in refractory *C. difficile* infection   100

time-to-event analysis   488–489, *489*

Tobin index   86

tocolytic associated pulmonary edema   226

torsade de pointes   41–42, *41–42*

total parenteral nutrition (TPN)

   constituents of   185

   efficacy in critically-ill and injured patients   181–182

   formulas   180

   guidelines on lipid use   182

   hypophosphatemia risk   141–142

   indications for the use of   180–181

   prophylactic antibiotics   93

   refeeding syndrome   141–142

tourniquet, use to control active bleeding   328–329

toxic shock syndrome, choice of antibiotic   107

toxicology   239–251

toxidromes

   management strategies   240–241

   salicilate poisoning   241–242

   signs for specific drug classes   240–241

tracheal injury

   airway management   297

   "clothesline" injury management   297

   penetrating injury   289–290

   tracheal laceration repair   292

tracheal intubation, actions following several failed attempts   293–294

tracheoesophageal fistula (TEF)

   diagnosis and management   448–449

   in intubated patients   448–449

tracheo-innominate fistula (TIF)

   diagnosis and treatment   445–446

   risk factors in tracheostomy   294–295

tracheostomy

   bleeding after the first 48 hours   445

   choice of technique   256–257

   complication rates in obese patients   416

   management of a dislodged tracheostomy tube   84

   ongoing hemorrhage from   445–446

potential early and late complications   257

   risk factors for tracheo-innominate fistula   294–295

tranexamic acid (TXA), use in trauma patients   110–111

transferrin, function as a negative acute phase protein   178–179

transfusion   109–119

   activation of massive transfusion protocol (MTP)   111–112

   blood component therapy   109

   definition of massive transfusion   111–112

   effects of liberal transfusion with PRBCs   111

   plasma for patient of unknown blood type   112–113

   PRBC transfusion in pediatric critically-ill patients   228–229

   prophylactic transfusion in trauma patients   109–110

   ratio and type of platelets   113

   respiratory distress during or after   110

   restrictive transfusion strategy   109–110

   stable trauma patient without active bleeding   109–110

   use of rapid thromboelastography (TEG) in trauma patients   112, *112*

   use of uncrossmatched type O blood in trauma patients   118

   *see also* massive transfusion

transfusion-associated acute lung injury (TRALI)   110

transfusion-associated circulatory overload (TACO)   110

transjugular intrahepatic portosystemic shunt (TIPS)

   stent stenosis risk   171

   use in intractable ascites   173

transplantation   209–217

   hyperacute rejection   213–214

   treatment of cytomegalovirus (CMV) infection   215–216

transthoracic echocardiography (TTE), assessment of pericardial effusion   261

trans-tracheal jet ventilation (TTJV)   293–294

trauma patients
  risk factors for developing
      pneumonia  94
  use of tranexamic acid (TXA)
      110–111
traumatic brain injury (TBI)
  avoiding secondary brain
      injury  191
  Brain Injury Guidelines (BIG)
      284–285, **285**
  brain oxygenation monitoring
      techniques  195
  Brain Trauma Foundation
      management guidelines  198
  criteria for brain death declaration
      494–495
  decompressive craniectomy
      283–284
  decreasing ICP without lowering
      BP  284
  disruption of cerebral
      autoregulation  196
  effects of fever in neurological
      injury  156
  identification in pediatric patients
      463–464
  initial management of acute head
      injury  277–279
  initial treatment of severe TBI  280
  intracranial pressure (ICP)
      monitoring  279
  management guidelines  191
  management of anticoagulated
      patients  285–286
  management of cerebral perfusion
      pressure  196
  management of elevated ICP in
      pediatric patients  196–197
  management of small
      injuries  284–285, **285**
  management using Brain Injury
      Guidelines (BIG)
      284–285, **285**
  objective of ICP monitoring
      189–190
  optimizing ICP and cerebral
      perfusion pressure (CPP)
      283–284
  predictor of poor outcome in
      gunshot wound to the brain
      191–192
  pregnant trauma patient  348
  recommended target cerebral
      perfusion pressure  280

  role of steroid therapy  189
  seizures following  194
  therapy for increased intracranial
      pressure (ICP)  280–281
  use of barbiturate therapy  194–195
  use of hypertonic saline  284
  use of progesterone therapy  196
  VTE risk and prophylaxis  283
traumatic diaphragmatic hernia
    (TDH), causes and
    presentation  299
traumatic head injury, drugs for
    rapid-sequence intubation
    72–73
traumatic venous injury, options for
    repair  332
tricuspid regurgitation, right atrial
    tracing  8, 9, *10*
tricyclic antidepressants (TCA)
  clinical presentation of TCA
      toxicity in overdose  239–240
  management of TCA
      overdose  471
  suicide risk in elderly people  471
triple contrast CT scan, indications
    and contraindications
    267–268
Trousseau sign  145
tubocurarine, metabolism and
    elimination  72
Type I error  485
Type II error  485
typhlitis, complication of
    chemotherapy  374–375

**u**
ultrasound  261–272
  guidance for central venous
      catheter (CVC) placement
      270–271
  use in initial assessment of trauma
      patients  262
umbilical hernia
  fluid leakage in patient with
      cirrhosis  404–405
  incarcerated/strangulated  381
  reduction of incarceration and
      repair  403
unfractionated heparin (UFH)
    anticoagulation  99–100
United States Uniform Anatomic Gift
    Act  496
unrecognised misplaced intubation
    (UMI), identifying  64–65

uremic bleeding, coagulopathy in
    uremic patients  116
ureteral injury from gunshot wound,
    treatment options
    341–342, **342**
urethral injury
  diagnosis in trauma patients  308
  indications and investigation
      337–338, *339*
  management of anterior and
      posterior urethral
      injuries  340
urinary tract infection (UTI), risk
    factors in catheterized
    patients  93–94
urologic trauma and disorders
    337–343

**v**
valproic acid overdose, symptoms
    and management  246
vancomycin
  antimicrobial action  104
  use in refractory *C. difficile*
      infection  100
  use in VAP  104–105
vancomycin-resistant *Enterococcus*
    (VRE), association with
    VAP  96
vascular injury
  abdominal  307–315
  evaluation and management  327
  hard and soft signs  327
  thoracic  299–306
vascular resistance, definition  67
vasoconstriction, role of endothelin-1
    in cardiogenic shock  58
vasodilation
  cause in sepsis  57–58
  effects of nitric oxide (NO)  57–58
  effects of vasodilators on cardiac
      function  3
  mechanism of action of
      dobutamine  62
vasopressin  15
  role in septic shock management
      56–57, 91–92
vasopressor-dependent septic shock,
    use of corticosteroids  52
vecuronium
  mechanism of action  122, 123
  metabolism and elimination
      72, **98**
  reversal drugs  107–108

venous access catheters, factors influencing optimal rate of volume resuscitation   3, *4*

venous thromboembolism (VTE)
ACCP prevention and treatment guidelines   205, 206
characteristics of VTE in pregnancy   223
incidence in the SICU   207
risk factors in pediatric patients   463
risk factors in pediatric trauma patients   232–233
risk in pregnancy and post-partum   201–202

venous thromboembolism (VTE) prophylaxis
criteria in pediatric patients   463
enoxaparin dosing and monitoring   207
in traumatic brain injury patients   283

ventilated patient, oxygen uptake/consumption (VO₂) calculation 18

ventilator-associated pneumonia (VAP)
choice and dose of antimicrobial agent   104
common causative organisms 55, 96
diagnosis   81
diagnostic criteria for quantitative microbiology   52
diagnostic use of bronchoscopy   258
duration of antibiotic therapy   90
empiric therapy   96
Infectious Disease Society of America (IDSA) guidelines for management   104–105, **104**
pathogens associated with early-onset VAP   52
prevention bundles   91
risk factors for MDR pneumonia   96
risk factors in the pediatric ICU   232
risk of multidrug resistant (MDR) pathogens   104–105, **104**
sources of causative bacteria   53
use of hospital antibiograms   104

ventilator support   79–88
addressing "bird's beak" pressure-volume curve   88, *88*
cardiopulmonary interactions 12–13
findings before postoperative spontaneous breathing begins   83
indicators for successful liberation from support   64
intraoperative ventilatory settings   83
management of respiratory acidosis   84
managing elderly patients   466
optimal level of sedation   127, **127**
parenchymal-pleural fistula (PPF) management   82
rapid shallow breathing index (RSBI)   64
waveform analysis   87, *87*
ventilator tidal volume setting for obese patients   416
ventral hernia, principles for repair   405
ventricular fibrillation
Brugada syndrome   35–36, *35*
following myocardial infarction 49–50, *49*
ventriculoseptal defect (VSD), post-myocardial infarction 44–45, *45*
ventriculostomy, management of elevated intracranial pressure   190
ventriculostomy catheters, incidence of infection from   192–193
vertebral artery, management of traumatic injury   295–296, *295*
*Vibrio* species, diagnosis of NSTI caused by   412
*Vibrio vulnificus*
association with NSTIs   94–95
symptoms and treatment of infection from seafood 211–212
video laryngoscopy, effect on first-chance intubation success rate   70
violence towards pregnant women, risk factors and consequences   435

virtue ethics   492–493, 495
vitamin B12 deficiency, risks related to nitrous oxide anesthesia   124
volume-cycled ventilation (VCV), prolonging the inspiratory time   81–82
volume resuscitation, management of continued hypoperfusion   91
volume status
indicators   60
management in trauma patients   340
vomiting, acid-base and electrolyte abnormalities caused by   136
VTE *see* venous thromboembolism

**w**

warfarin anticoagulation
rapid reversal in trauma patients   114
use in elderly trauma patients 466–467
weaning from sedation   121–122
Wells score for PE diagnosis   204
West lung zones   12
Westermark sign   80
whole bowel irrigation (WBI), prevention of absorption of drugs   239
Wilcoxon Rank Sum test   484, 485
Wolff–Parkinson–White syndrome 34–35, *34*
wound healing, impairment in steroid-treated patients   149–150
wrist injury, factors leading to poor outcomes   325
wrist pain
occult scaphoid fracture   323
without acute radiographic findings   323
wrong-site surgical procedures
protocol to prevent   73
risk factors for   73

**x**

Xarelto   *see* rivaroxaban
X-ray, use in pelvic fracture diagnosis   271

Made in the USA
Middletown, DE
01 October 2020